Surgery of the Elbow
– practical and scientific aspects

Edited by

DAVID STANLEY MBBS, BSc(Hons), FRCS

Upper Limb Surgeon in the Department of Orthopaedic Surgery,
Northern General Hospital, Sheffield and Honorary Lecturer
at the University of Sheffield, Sheffield, United Kingdom

NEVILLE R M KAY TD, FRCS

Formerly Consultant Orthopaedic Surgeon at the Royal Hallamshire Hospital,
Sheffield and Lecturer in Orthopaedic Surgery
at the University of Sheffield, Sheffield, United Kingdom

A member of the Hodder Headline Group
LONDON • SYDNEY • AUCKLAND
Co-published in the USA by Oxford University Press, Inc., New York

First published in Great Britain 1998
Arnold, a member of the Hodder Headline group,
338 Euston Road, London NW1 3BH
http://www.arnoldpublishers.com

Co-published in the United States of America by
Oxford University Press, Inc.,
198 Madison Avenue, New York, NY10016
Oxford is a registered trademark of Oxford University Press

British Library Cataloguing in Publication Data
A catalogue record for this book is available from the British Library

Library of Congress Cataloging-in-Publication Data
A catalog record for this book is available from the Library of Congress

ISBN 0 340 59805 0

1 2 3 4 5 6 7 8 9 10

Commissioning Editor: Annalisa Page
Project Editor: Catherine Barnes
Production Editor: Julie Delf
Production Controller: Helen Whitehorn
Project Manager: Jane Duncan

Composition by Scribe Design, Gillingham, Kent
Printed and bound in Great Britain by the Bath Press, Bath

This volume is gratefully and humbly dedicated to our teachers and our patients

Contents

Contributors

Andrew A Amis PhD, FIMechE
Reader in Orthopaedic Biomechanics, Biomechanics Section, Mechanical Engineering Department, Imperial College of Science, Technology and Medicine, London, UK

Champ L Baker MD
Orthopaedic Surgeon, The Hughston Clinic PC, Columbus, Georgia, USA

Piet de Boer MA, FRCS
Consultant Orthopaedic Surgeon, Head of Service, Department of Orthopaedic Surgery, Purey Cust, Nuffield Hospital, York, UK

Andrew A Brookes MD
The Hughston Clinic PC, Columbus, Georgia, USA

Frank D Burke MBBS, FRCS
Director of Hand Surgery, Pulvertaft Hand Centre, Derby and Visiting Professor in Hand Surgery, University of Derby, UK

S R Cannon FRCS, MCh(Orth)
Consultant Orthopaedic Surgeon and Chairman, The London Bone and Soft Tumor Service, Royal National Orthopaedic Hospital Trust, London, UK

Andy Carr ChM, FRCS
Consultant Orthopaedic Surgeon, Upper Limb Unit, Nuffield Orthopaedic Centre, Headington, Oxford, UK

Victor N Cassar-Pullicino LRCP, MRCS, MD, DMRD, FRCR
Consultant Skeletal Radiologist and Clinical Director, The Robert Jones & Agnes Hunt Orthopaedic Hospital, Oswestry, Shropshire, UK

Andrew H Crenshaw Jr MD
The Campbell Clinic, Department of Orthopaedic Surgery, Suite 101, Southhaven MS, USA

James R M Elliott MD, FRCS
Consultant Orthopaedic Surgeon, Musgrave Park Hospital, Belfast, Northern Ireland

Matthew Evans MBBS
Research Fellow, Department of Orthopaedic Surgery, Royal Children's Hospital, Flemington Road, Parkville, Victoria, Australia

Gary S Fanton MD
Orthopaedic Surgeon and Clinical Assistant Professor, Stanford University Hospital, Suite 110, Menlo Park, California 94025, USA

Mark P Figgie
Associate Attending, The Hospital for Special Surgery, New York, NY, USA

Bruce L Gillingham CDR, MC, USN
Director, Pediatric Orthopaedics, Naval Medical Center, San Diego, California, USA

Frank W Hagena MD, PhD
Director and Chairman Orthopaedic Hospital, Auguste-Viktoria Klinik, Bad-Oeynhausen, Germany

Douglas M Hedden MD, FRCS
Staff Surgeon, Division of Orthopaedic Surgery, The Hospital for Sick Children, 555 University Avenue, Toronto, Ontario, Canada

J S Hughes MBBS, FRACS(Orth), FA(Orth)A
Orthopaedic Shoulder & Elbow Surgery, Suite 12, McIntosh Street, Chatsworth, Sydney, Australia

Per Olof Josefsson MD, PhD
Consultant in Orthopaedic Surgery, Department of Orthopaedics, Malmo University Hospital, Malmo, Sweden

Jesse B Jupiter MD
Director, Orthopaedic Hand Service, Massachusetts General Hospital; Associate Professor of Orthopaedic Surgery, Harvard Medical School, Boston, Massachusetts, USA

Neville R M Kay TD, FRCS
Formerly Consultant Orthopaedic Surgeon at the Royal Hallamshire Hospital, Sheffield and Lecturer in Orthopaedic Surgery at the University of Sheffield, Sheffield, UK

H Kerr Graham MD, FRCS(Ed), FRACS
Professor of Orthopaedic Surgery, University of Melbourne; Director of Orthopaedics, Royal Children's Hospital, Parkville, Victoria, Australia

Hiroshi Kudo MD
Vice-President, Chief of of Orthopaedic Section, Sagamihara National Hospital, Sagamihara City, Kanagawa, Japan

A Lettin BSc(Hons), MS, FRCS
Consultant Orthopaedic Surgeon, Moat Farm, Cretingham, Woodbridge, Suffolk, UK

Ian W McCall MB ChB, FRCR
Professor of Radiological Sciences, University of Keele; Consultant Radiologist, Robert Jones & Agnes Hunt Orthopaedic Hospital, Owestry, Shropshire, UK

Allan Mishra MD
Clinical Instructor, Orthopaedic Surgery, Stanford University School of Medicine, Menlo Park, California, USA

David Propper MCRP, MD
ICRF Medical Oncology Unit Churchill, Oxford, Radcliffe Hospital, Headington, Oxford, UK

Wolfgang Ruther MD
Professor of Orthopaedics and Head of the Department of Orthopaedics, Rheumaklinik, Bad Bramstedt, Hamburg, Germany

Lech Rymaszewski FRS
Consultant Orthopaedic Surgeon, Stobhill NHS Trust, Glasgow, UK

WJW Sharrard MD, Chm, FRCS
Emeritus Professor of Orthopaedics, University of Sheffield, Sheffield, UK

Stephen R Soffer MD
Orthopaedic Surgeon and Director of Eastern Sports Medicine and Institute, Wyomising, Pennsylvania, USA

David H Sonnabend MBBS, BSc(Med), FRACS, FA(Orth)A
Chairman, Department of Traumatic and Orthopaedic Surgery, The Prince of Wales Hospital, Raundwick, New South Wales, Australia

David Stanley MBBS, BSc(Hons), FRCS
Upper Limb Surgeon, Department of Orthopaedic Surgery, Northern General Hospital, Sheffield; and Honorary Lecturer at the University of Sheffield, Sheffield, UK

Karl Tillmann MD
Orthopaedic Surgeon, Rheumaklinik, Bad Bramstedt, Germany

Amit R Tolat MS, FRCS, MCh(Orth), FCPS(Orth), Eur Dip Hand Surg
Senior Research Associate and Clinical Lecturer, BYL Nair Hospital, University of Bombay; Attending Orthopaedic Surgeon, St Elizabeth Hospital, Bombay, India

Verna Wright MD, FRCP
Emeritus Professor of Rheumatology, University of Leeds, Leeds, UK

Foreword

The elbow is one of man's most unique yet poorly understood articulations. The functional requirements of our ancestral hominid primates for stability throughout the arc of both forearm rotation and elbow flexion-extension led to a highly specialized anatomic unit. In fact, the elbow represents three distinct articulations enclosed in a single synovial-lined cavity which plays an integral role in the versatile manner in which we use our upper limb today.

The complexity of the anatomy of the elbow, coupled with its frequent adverse response to traumatic and inflammatory conditions, led to an air of pessimism regarding operative intervention. Even today, many standard orthopaedic texts suggest caution when considering surgical management of both traumatic or reconstructive problems of the elbow. Anecdotal information put forth as dogma abounds in discussions of conditions such as the stiff elbow, heterotopic bone, joint arthroplasty, or tendinopathies about the elbow.

Yet the advances in technology over the past two decades has led to substantial advances in our knowledge regarding the functional anatomy, kinesiology, and operative management of disorders of the elbow. Improvements in diagnostic modalities, such as three-dimensional imaging techniques as well as arthroscopic evaluations have led to much more accurate preoperative evaluations of a truly three-dimensional structure, heretofore often represented by two-dimensional conventional radiology.

Advances in extensile exposures, coupled with dramatic improvements in the small implants for internal fixation, have permitted a more predictable surgical treatment of traumatic injuries involving small articular fragments supported by a meagre amount of subchondral bone. Traditional expectations of outcome following traumatic injuries continue to be challenged by these advances in the surgical management of fractures as well as fracture-dislocations. A more extensive study of the structural and functional anatomy of the elbow, along with technological advances in joint arthroplasty, has seen major improvements in design features of total elbow arthroplasty – long thought to be among the most difficult and unpredictable of all joint arthroplasties.

Drs David Stanley and Neville RM Kay have assembled a comprehensive text on the elbow. With a truly international group of contributing authors, many of whom are well recognized for their expertise and contributions to various aspects of elbow pathology, the text presents an expansive view of both diagnostic as well as surgical management of the breadth of problems involving both the paediatric as well as adult elbow. The chapters dealing with the clinical problems present carefully indications, techniques and pitfalls of treatment. The Editors have clearly maintained a consistency of text emphasizing the appropriate use of technology which has evolved towards the end of this decade. This text, highlighted by its list of internationally renowned contributors, will provide great insight into the full expanse of problems of the elbow and will be the source of information that will provide direct benefits to patients for a long time to come.

Jesse B Jupiter MD
Director, Orthopaedic Hand Service,
Massachusetts General Hospital; Associate
Professor of Orthopaedic Surgery, Harvard Medical
School, Boston, MA, USA

Preface

Relative to the other major joints of the body, the elbow receives little attention in the medical literature. This book aims, at least in part, to redress the balance.

The authors who have contributed to the text come from many parts of the world and were chosen because of their expertise in particular fields of elbow surgery. They give a breadth to the book which we feel is unrivalled in other publications.

The topics covered provide practical guidance for surgeons faced with elbow abnormalities and specific clinical problems and with the help of the comprehensive references, guide the interested reader to a detailed study of most aspects of elbow surgery.

Thus, we hope to have produced a book that will not only enable the surgeon faced with a difficult elbow problem to obtain specific guidance allowing a confident treatment plan to be constructed, but will also provide assistance in evaluating the surgical options for the more commonly encountered elbow disorders.

Finally, for those with perhaps less experience of elbow surgery, each contributor has noted, wherever possible, their preferred treatment option.

David Stanley MBBS, BSc(Hons), FRCS
Neville R M Kay TD, FRCS

Acknowledgements

Few authors or editors of text books, who are actively engaged in a busy clinical practice, fully appreciate the significant effort which will be demanded of their colleagues, co-authors and families when they embark on a project such as this.

Whilst we could happily accept our own hopelessly optimistic estimate of the time scales involved, it is a tribute to all of those who have supported us in the preparation of this book that no hint of criticism has surfaced.

Particularly, we would like to thank our co-authors, all of whom have had to sacrifice family and professional commitments to produce their individual contributions.

Specifically we would like to thank Mr Stephen Hepple, who has been most helpful in acting as reference sub-editor and it is largely due to his efforts that the reference sections of this volume are accurate and comprehensive.

We are greatly indebted to Arnold, particularly Annalisa Page and Catherine Barnes who have helped us and guided us in the production.

Our special thanks must go to Mrs Denise Burton who typed and re-typed the manuscripts so willingly and carefully.

Finally, we bear a special debt of gratitude to our respective families who, for longer than we dare think, have allowed an editorial meeting most Sunday evenings.

We only hope that we have done justice to our publishers and contributors, but if there are any faults, these must be ours.

David Stanley MBBS, BSc(Hons), FRCS
Neville R M Kay TD, FRCS

CHAPTER 1

Embryology, growth, development and maturation of the elbow

WJW SHARRARD

Introduction

The skeletal elements of the limbs are derived from mesenchyme which first appears as a continuous mass in the limb bud on the 26th day after ovulation (Fig. 1.1). At this stage the developing embryo is approximately 3 mm from crown to rump.

Initially there is no differentiation into the primordia of individual bones, but during the following 30 days the limb buds elongate and the mesenchyme develops into muscle and centres of chondrification. The individual skeletal elements delineate rapidly with formation of the upper limb[1,2] (Fig. 1.2).

Prenatal development

The prenatal development of the elbow has been studied in considerable detail by Gray and

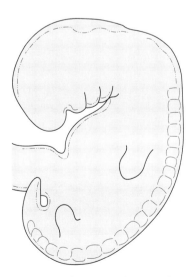

Fig. 1.1 A 30-day embryo. The limb buds are initially flipperlike, and consist of a core of mesenchyme and a covering layer of ectoderm.

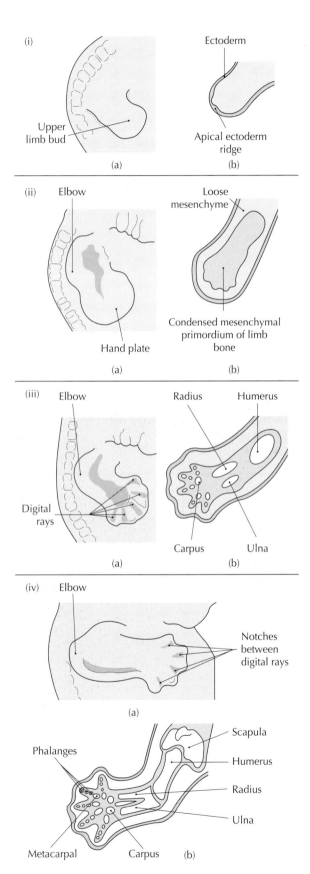

Fig. 1.2 The formation of the upper limbs with special reference to the elbow. The external appearance is shown in (ai) to (aiv) (right arm) whilst the internal development is shown in (bi) to (biv) (left arm) (i): 32 days, (ii): 36 days; (iii): 42 days; (iv): 48 days.

Gardner.[3] More recently Andersen,[4] and O'Rahilly and Gardner[5] have also made helpful contributions.

Chondrification is present in the shafts of the humerus, radius and ulna by the 6th intrauterine week in embryos of 12 mm but the site of the elbow joint still consists of an area of relatively undifferentiated interzonal mesenchyme. At this time, the lower end of the humerus shows enlargement in the region of the future condyles and, at 13 mm the shape of the coronoid and olecranon processes of the ulna can be recognised.

At 7.5 weeks, when the embryo measures 20 mm, the epiphyses are identifiable in precartilage and, by the 8th week, at 22 mm, the interzone between the radius and the humerus, and between the ulna and the humerus can be identified as the future site of the elbow joint. Cavitation starts to appear during the 9th week at 27 mm and is complete at the end of the 9th week at 30 mm length. The radiohumeral and ulnohumeral cavities are present at 33 mm but do not communicate with each other until about 1 week later. By the 10th week at 39 mm, the various cavities have united and are complete.

At the 30th week, the shafts of the humerus, radius and ulna are all well ossified and the cartilaginous form of the lower end of the humerus and the upper end of the radius and ulna is well established.

Muscles and tendons are well developed by the 9th week at the 28-mm stage. The motor and sensory nerve supply to the upper limb appears in association with the developing limb bud (Fig. 1.3).

The elbow develops in a position of 90 degrees of flexion but it is evident that all the elements required for elbow movement are probably present and can produce elbow movement by the 30th intrauterine week.

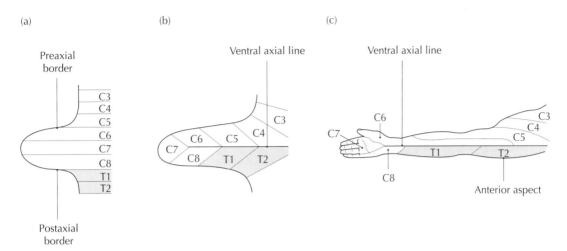

(a)

Preaxial
border

C3
C4
C5
C6
C7
C8
T1
T2

Postaxial
border

(b)

Ventral axial line

C3
C4
C5
C6
C7
C8
T1
T2

(c)

Ventral axial line

C6
C7
C3
C4
C5
C8
T1
T2

Anterior aspect

Fig. 1.3 The development of the upper limb dermatomes. The axial line indicates where there is no sensory overlap (a): 35 days; (b): 41 days; (c): adult dermatomal pattern.

Congenital and development abnormalities

Although the elbow joint and the superior radioulnar joint are relatively complex, severe developmental or congenital abnormalities of these joints are relatively rare.

Congenital humeroradial synostosis (congenital ankylosis of the elbow) in which the lower end of the humerus is fused to the ulna or the radius or both is very rare[6] (Fig. 1.4). It may be bilateral and is often associated with congenital ankylosis of other joints.[7] Fortunately the elbow is usually fused in some flexion and function is often acceptable.

Congenital radioulnar synostosis (Fig. 1.5) is uncommon and may take various forms between complete bony fusion of the upper end of the radius and ulna and a form of syndesmosis with a thick interosseous ligament resulting in loss of rotation of the forearm. The condition results from failure of separation of the upper ends of the cartilaginous rods destined to form the radius and ulna during the 7th intrauterine week of development.[8]

The only relatively more common congenital abnormality of the elbow is congenital dislocation or subluxation of the head of the radius. This may be anterior, posterior or lateral (Fig. 1.6). Anterior dislocation is the most common and although it has been suggested that this abnormality when unilateral does not exist without an associated general

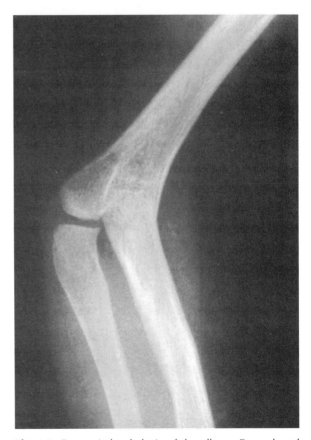

Fig. 1.4 Congenital ankylosis of the elbow. Reproduced from Ref. 14 with permission from Blackwell Scientific Publications, Oxford.

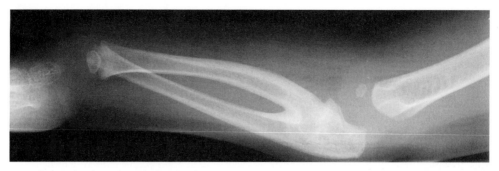

Fig. 1.5 Radiograph of a congenital radioulnar synostosis.

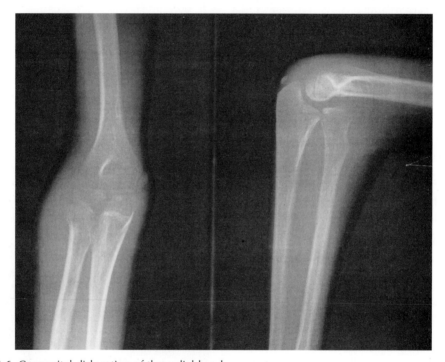

Fig. 1.6 Congenital dislocation of the radial head.

Table 1.1 Conditions associated with congenital dislocation of the radial head

Nail–patella syndrome	Chondroectodermal dysplasia
Nelson's syndrome	Congenital webbing of the elbow
Diaphyseal aclasis	Apert's syndrome
Klinefelter's syndrome	Silver's syndrome
Arthrogryposis	Cornelia de Lange's syndrome
Orofacial digital syndrome	Tibiofibula syndrome
Fetal face syndrome	König's syndrome
Acromesomelic dwarfism	Ehlers–Danlos syndrome
Kneist syndrome	Hemimelia

syndrome or other anomaly[9,10] the condition has been reported in apparent isolation.[11–13] More frequently, however, it occurs in association with other developmental anomalies of the upper extremity (Table 1.1). The varied aetiology suggests a germplasm defect.

Postnatal development

After birth, the most important anatomical changes concern the development and ossification of the lower humeral and the upper radial and ulnar epiphyses.

The lower end of the humerus is ossified by four ossific centres; the capitellum and lateral part of the trochlea, the medial epicondyle, the medial two-thirds of the trochlea and the lateral epicondyle (Fig. 1.7).

At birth all of the lower end of the humerus is cartilaginous. This is important since trauma during the first 6 months of life may result in displacement of the whole of the distal humerus which can be difficult to recognise radiologically.

The first ossific centre to appear is that for the capitellum and the lateral one-third of the trochlea. This appears in females at any time between the 1st and 11th month and in males at any time between the 1st and 28th month. The narrower medial portion of the lozenge-shaped epiphysis forms the lateral part of the trochlea whilst the lateral portion is closely associated with the lateral epicondyle. If, therefore, the capitellar epiphysis suffers displacement it almost invariably does so in one piece with the lateral epicondyle irrespective of whether the lateral epicondylar epiphysis is ossified. This anatomical arrangement may be referred to as the lateral condylar epiphysis. At its medial end, it more commonly separates from the medial two-thirds of the trochlea regardless of whether the trochlear epiphysis is ossified. Less commonly, the fracture–separation takes place through the middle or medial third of the capitellar epiphysis leaving the whole of the trochlear epiphyses intact. It blends with the trochlear and lateral epicondylar epiphyses at puberty and with the shaft of the humerus at 14 to 16 years.

The second ossific centre to appear at the lower end of the humerus is that for the medial epicondyle which appears between the 5th and 8th year in females and between the 6th and 9th year in males. It is completely extracapsular and is always completely separate from the remainder of the lower humeral epiphysis. The common flexor origin is attached to it and the ulnar nerve runs immediately behind it. It can be completely detached from the humerus without disturbing the remainder of the epiphysis and is liable to be incarcerated into the elbow joint when the joint is laterally dislocated. When the remainder of the components of the lower humeral epiphysis blend together and subsequently fuse with the humeral shaft, a tongue of bone extends distally between the lower humeral epiphysis and the medial epicondylar epiphysis which does not fuse with the shaft until the 20th year of life.

The third ossific centre to develop is that for the medial two-thirds of the trochlea. This appears between the 7th and 11th years in females and the 8th and 13th year in males. It almost always first forms in two parts, each of which has its own blood supply – the lateral part from vessels derived from the metaphysis and the medial part from structures attached to the medial epicondyle, a feature that may affect the pattern of avascular necrosis of the trochlea. It blends with the capitellar epiphysis at puberty and with the humeral shaft at 14 to 16 years.

The fourth ossific centre to develop is that for the lateral epicondyle which develops between the 8th and 11th year in females and between the 9th and 13th year in males. It is extracapsular and gives origin to the attachment of the common extensors and the middle portion of the lateral ligament.

Within 6 months it blends with the capitellar epiphysis and then with the humeral shaft at puberty. Its very brief separate existence means that fracture–separation of the lateral epicondylar epiphysis is rare.

The centres of ossification of the lower end of the humerus always appear in the same time sequence – first the capitellum, then the medial (internal) epicondyle, then the trochlea and finally the lateral (external) epicondyle.

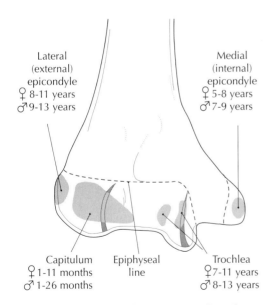

Lateral (external) epicondyle
♀ 8-11 years
♂ 9-13 years

Medial (internal) epicondyle
♀ 5-8 years
♂ 7-9 years

Capitulum
♀ 1-11 months
♂ 1-26 months

Epiphyseal line

Trochlea
♀ 7-11 years
♂ 8-13 years

Fig. 1.7 The mean time of appearance of ossific centres at the lower end of the humerus. Note the mnemonic CITE together with the average figures: 1 (Capitellum); 7 (Internal epicondyle); 10 (Trochlea) and 11 (External epicondyle).

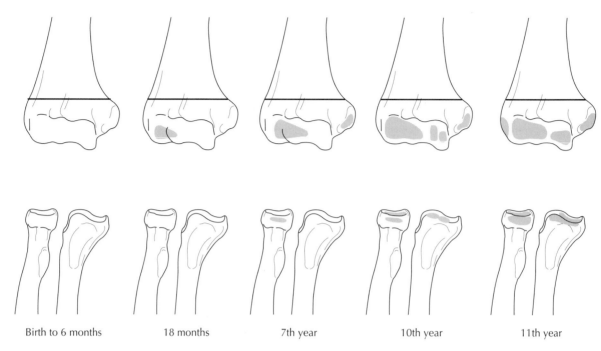

Birth to 6 months   18 months   7th year   10th year   11th year

Fig. 1.8 Stages in the ossification of the epiphyses at the elbow joint.

The centre of ossification for the upper end of the radius appears at the 4th year of life in females and at the 5th or 6th year in males (Fig. 1.8). A particular feature of the epiphysis is that it is entirely intracapsular and, like the upper end of the femur, it is very liable to develop avascular necrosis because of damage to its intracapsular supplying vessels. It joins the shaft between the 14th and 17th year of life.

The centre of ossification of the tip of the olecranon appears, usually in two parts, at the 9th year of life in females and the 11th year in males (Fig. 1.8). It fuses with the shaft at the 14th and 16th years respectively.

Knowledge of the normal times of ossification of the epiphyses in the region of the elbow joint is essential in the diagnosis of traumatic lesions of the elbow in childhood.[14] When doubt exists it is wise to x-ray the opposite normal elbow, for comparison with the injured side.

References

1. Lewis WH. The development of the arm in Man. *Am J Anat* 1901; **1:** 145–84.
2. O'Rahilly R, Gardner E The timing and sequence of events in the development of the limbs in the human embryo. *Anat Embryol* 1975; **147:** 1–23.
3. Gray DJ. Gardner E Prenatal development of the human elbow joint. *Am J Anat* 1951; **88:** 429–69.
4. Andersen H Histochemical studies of the histiogenesis of the human elbow joint. *Acta Anat* 1962; **51:** 50–68.
5. O'Rahilly R, Gardner E The initial appearance of ossification in staged human embryos. *Am J Anat* 1972; **134:** 291–301.
6. Mnaymneh WA Congenital radiohumeral synostosis. A case report. *Clin Orthop* 1978; **131:** 183–4.
7. Jacobsen St, Crawford A.H Humeroradial synostosis. *J Pediatr Orthop* 1983; **3:** 96–8.
8. Mital MA Congenital radioulnar synostosis and congenital dislocation of the radial head. *Orthop Clin North Am* 1976; **7:** 375–83.
9. Lloyd-Roberts GC, Bucknill TM Anterior dislocation of the radial head in children. Aetiology, natural history and management. *J Bone Joint Surg (Br)* 1977; **59B:** 402–7.
10. Mardam-Bey T, Ger E Congenital radial head dislocation. *J Hand Surg* 1979; **4:** 316–20.
11. Almquist EE, Gordon LH Blue AI Congenital dislocation of the head of the radius. *J Bone Joint Surg (Am)* 1969; **51A:** 1118–27.
12. Kelly DW Congenital dislocation of the radial head. Spectrum and natural history. *J Pediatr Orthop* 1981; **1:** 295–8.
13. Gattey PH, Wedge JH Unilateral posterior dislocation of the radial head in identical twins. *J Pediatr Orthop* 1986; **6:** 220–1.
14. Sharrard WJW Fractures and joint injuries – Part 1: General principles and upper limb injuries. In: *Paediatric orthopaedics and fractures.* Oxford: Blackwell Scientific Publications, 1993: 1365–467.

Anatomy of the elbow

PIET DE BOER

Introduction

The elbow is a complex synovial joint formed by the articular surfaces of the distal humerus, and proximal ulna and radius. It comprises the humeroulnar, humeroradial and proximal radioulnar joints. Flexion and extension movements occur predominantly at the humeroulnar joint whilst pronation and supination are features of the humeroradial and proximal radioulnar joints.

The primary function of the elbow is the positioning of the hand in space such that it can be used both as a grasping and tactile organ. To this end elbow movements are dependent upon the muscle groups that cross the joint whilst the neurovascular structures that lie in close proximity provide innervation to the more distal segment of the upper limb.

In this chapter the surgically relevant anatomy is described.

Skin

The skin covering the elbow is different on the flexor and extensor surfaces. The skin is thickened on the extensor aspect of the elbow especially in those occupations which apply pressure to the skin of the posterior aspect of the elbow. The Langer's lines on the two aspects of the elbow are also fundamentally different. On the anterior aspect of the elbow the Langer's lines run longitudinally, whilst posteriorly they run transversally. Although the skin incisions made parallel to Langer's lines heal with much less scar formation than those which are at 90 degrees to these lines the siting of skin incisions around the elbow is determined by the required surgical exposure rather than healing and cosmesis.

Subcutaneous tissues

The subcutaneous tissues of the elbow are also fundamentally different on the flexor and extensor aspects. On the flexor surface of the elbow there is a complex system of veins (Fig. 2.1). Superiorly these veins are organised into the basilic and cephalic veins. The basilic vein passes up the arm deep to the superficial fascia and the cephalic vein runs up the arm on the lateral side of the biceps superficial to the superficial fasica. It eventually ends up in the groove between the deltoid and

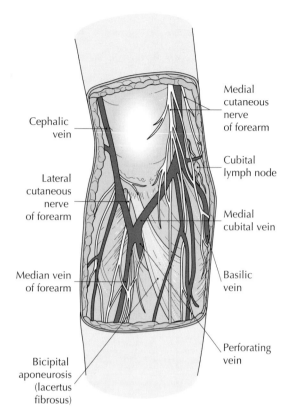

Cephalic vein

Lateral cutaneous nerve of forearm

Median vein of forearm

Bicipital aponeurosis (lacertus fibrosus)

Medial cutaneous nerve of forearm

Cubital lymph node

Medial cubital vein

Basilic vein

Perforating vein

Fig. 2.1 The anterior aspect of the right elbow showing the subcutaneous structures. The superficial complex of veins and the cutaneous nerves should be noted.

pectoralis major. Superficial dissection on the flexor aspect of the elbow will inevitably involve mobilisation and ligation of these structures. Posteriorly no significant superficial veins occur.

There are numerous cutaneous nerves crossing the elbow, some of which will need to be protected during superficial dissection. The lateral cutaneous nerve of the forearm which is the terminal branch to the musculocutaneous nerve emerges from the lateral side of the biceps muscle about a hand's breadth above the elbow. It is at risk during anterior and anterolateral approaches to the elbow. The medial antibrachial cutaneous nerves run across the anterior aspect of the elbow accompanying branches of the basilic vein. Although if possible these should be preserved, damage to them will not cause significant distal sensory impairment. Posteriorly there are no significant superficial nerves although it should be noted that the ulnar nerve whilst deep to the deep fascia is still extremely near the skin of the posterior aspect of the elbow.

Bursae

Bursae at the elbow occur in association with both superficial and deep structures. Posteriorly the most commonly recognised bursa, the olecranon bursa, lies between the olecranon process and the subcutaneous tissues. It is not present at birth and first appears at the age of 7 years.[1] Clinically it may become inflamed giving rise to olecranon bursitis. Other subcutaneous bursae that have been described are the medial epicondylar and lateral epicondylar bursae.

Of the deep bursae the most constant separates the tuberosity of the radius from the biceps tendon. This is the bicipitoradial bursa. Another, the radio-humeral bursa, lies between the capsule of the radiohumeral joint and the deep surface of extensor carpi radialis brevis. This has been implicated in the aetiology of tennis elbow.[2,3]

Other smaller and less constant bursae have been described but rarely cause clinical problems.

Muscles

Four groups of muscles cross the elbow joint.

1. The main flexors of the elbow cross the anterior aspect of the joint. They are supplied by the musculocutaneous nerve.
2. The extensor of the elbow crosses the posterior aspect of the joint. It is supplied by the radial nerve.
3. The flexor/pronator group of muscles cover the anteromedial aspect of the joint. They are supplied by the median and ulnar nerves.
4. The extensor of the wrist and fingers together with supinator are found laterally. They are supplied by the radial and posterior interosseous nerves.

ANTERIOR MUSCLE GROUP (Fig. 2.2)

Brachialis

The brachialis arises from the front of the lower two-thirds of the humerus between the medial and lateral intermuscular septa. It inserts into the coronoid process and tuberosity of the ulna. Although its principle nerve supply is from the musculocutaneous nerve the lateral fibres usually receive innervation from the radial nerve.[4]

Clinically the muscle is of interest since it is often damaged following elbow dislocation and may subsequently be the site of myositis ossificans.[5]

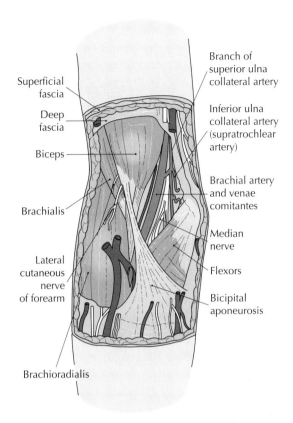

Fig. 2.2 The anterior muscle group and the associated neurovascular structures of the right elbow. The relationship of the biceps tendon, brachial artery and median nerve is clearly seen.

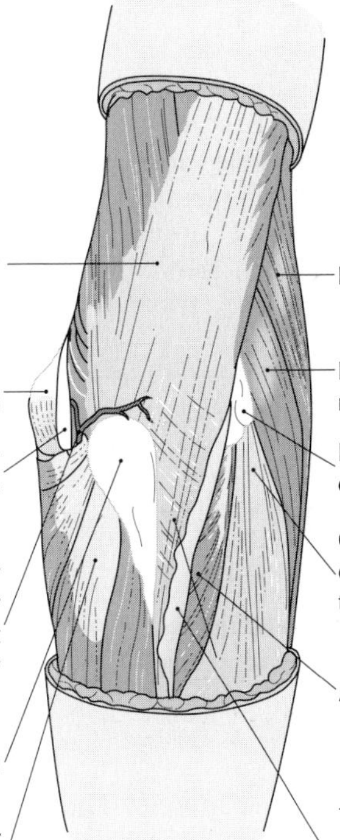

Fig. 2.3 The posterior aspect of the right elbow. The triceps muscle is the principle extensor of the elbow. The ulna nerve passes behind the medial epicondyle.

Biceps brachii

The biceps brachii arises from two heads. The long head has its origin at the supraglenoid tubercle within the shoulder whilst the short head arises from the apex of the coracoid process of the scapula. The muscle inserts via an easily palpable tendon into the bicipital tuberosity of the radius. The bicipitoradial bursa is adjacent to the insertion and is an important surgical landmark in anterior approaches to the proximal third of the radius. Arising from the medial border of the tendon is a sheet of extremely tough fascia known as the bicipital aponeurosis (lacertus fibrosus). This inserts into the deep fascia over the medial side of the forearm and the subcutaneous border of the upper end of the ulna. The bicipital aponeurosis separates the superficial veins of the antecubital fossa from the underlying brachial artery.

In addition to functioning as a flexor of the elbow the biceps brachii is also a powerful supinator.

POSTERIOR MUSCLE GROUP (Fig. 2.3)

Triceps

The triceps muscle has an extensive origin which consists of three separate heads. The long head arises from the infraglenoid tubercle of the scapula, the lateral head has a linear attachment from the upper border of the radial groove of the humerus whilst the medial head takes origin from the whole of the posterior surface of the humerus below the radial groove together with the adjacent medial and lateral intermuscular septa. The medial head lies deep to the lateral and long heads. The muscle inserts via a tendon onto the olecranon and subcutaneous surface of the ulna, extending for a considerable distance below the elbow joint.

The long and lateral heads are innervated by the radial nerve before it enters the radial groove whilst the medial head is supplied by the radial nerve distal to the groove.

The function of the muscle is active extension of the elbow joint.

Anconeus

The anconeus muscle arises from the posterior aspect of the lateral epicondyle and inserts into the lateral dorsal surface of the proximal ulna. The branch of the radial nerve which innervates the medial head of the triceps also supplies the anconeus.

Although the anconeus has been considered to be an extensor of the elbow[6] it is more likely to function as a joint stabiliser.[7]

MEDIAL MUSCLE GROUP (Fig. 2.4)

The medial group of muscles arise from the medial epicondyle of the humerus.

Pronator teres

This is a two headed muscle. The superficial belly arises from the medial epicondyle of the humerus and from the lower part of the medial supracondylar ridge. The deep belly arises from the medial border of the coronoid process of the ulna. It inserts into the middle of the lateral convexity of the radius.

The muscle is innervated usually by two branches from the median nerve. Of interest clinically is the fact that the median nerve enters the forearm by passing between the two heads of pronator teres, and it is at this site that the median nerve can be compressed. This gives rise to one of the causes of median nerve entrapment.

In addition to being a pronator of the arm the muscle has also been shown to be a weak flexor of the elbow.[8,9]

Flexor carpi radialis

The flexor carpi radialis arises from the common flexor origin distal to pronator teres. It inserts into the bases of the second and third metacarpals. It is innervated by the median nerve and is a flexor of the wrist.

Palmaris longus

The palmaris longus arises from the medial epicondyle and inserts into the apex of the palmar aponeurosis and flexor retinaculum. It is supplied by the median nerve. It is a flexor of the wrist and also tightens the palmar aponeurosis. In 10% of cases seen the muscle is absent.[10]

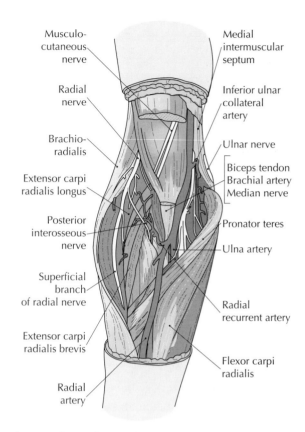

Fig. 2.4 The medial and lateral muscle groups of the right elbow. It is important to note the relationship of the radial, posterior interosseous and median nerves to the muscles.

Flexor carpi ulnaris

The flexor carpi ulnaris lies on the medial border of the forearm. It arises as two heads from the common flexor origin and from the upper two-thirds of the posterior subcutaneous border of the ulna. Distally it inserts into the pisiform and thence into the hamate and medial aspect of the fifth metacarpal base. It is supplied by the ulnar nerve which it overlies in the forearm. Its action is flexion and ulnar deviation of the wrist.

Flexor digitorum superficialis

This large muscle lies deeper than the other muscles of this group. It has a humeroulnar head which arises from the common flexor origin, the ulnar collateral ligament of the elbow joint and the medial aspect of the coronoid process. In addition there is a radial head which arises from the anterior oblique line on the radius. Distally the muscle divides into four tendons which insert into the base of the middle phalanges of the second to fifth fingers. It is supplied by the median nerve. The action of flexor digitorum superficialis is to produce flexion of the middle and then the proximal phalanx. In addition it also flexes the wrist.

LATERAL MUSCLE GROUP (Fig. 2.4)

Brachioradialis

The brachioradialis arises from the upper two-thirds of the lateral supracondylar ridge of the humerus. It crosses the elbow joint forming the lateral border of the cubital fossa and inserts into the radial styloid process. It is supplied by the radial nerve. It is a powerful flexor of the elbow and is strongest with the arm in the midprone position.

Extensor carpi radialis longus

The origin of extensor carpi radialis longus is from the lower third of the lateral supracondylar ridge of the humerus. It runs down the forearm under the brachioradialis and is inserted into the base of the second metacarpal. It is supplied by the radial nerve and is an extensor of the wrist. Clinically this muscle is of interest since in combination with the extensor carpi radialis brevis it has been implicated in the pathology of tennis elbow.[11]

Extensor carpi radialis brevis

The extensor carpi radialis brevis arises from the common extensor origin and passes down the forearm to insert into the base of the third metacarpal. It is supplied by the posterior interosseous nerve and is a wrist extensor. Clinically the origin of the muscle is considered to be the primary site of pathology in tennis elbow.[12]

Extensor digitorum communis

The extensor digitorum communis arises from the common extensor origin and inserts into the extensor expansion of the fingers. It is supplied by the posterior interosseous nerve and is an extensor of the digits and wrist.

Extensor carpi ulnaris

The extensor carpi ulnaris arises as two heads from the common extensor origin and also by an aponeurotic attachment to the posterior subcutaneous border of the ulna. The tendon inserts into the ulna side of the base of the fifth metacarpal bone. It is supplied by the posterior interosseous nerve and is a powerful extensor of the wrist and ulna deviator.

Supinator

The supinator muscle passes around the upper end of the radius to form part of the floor of the cubital fossa. It arises as two heads from the common extensor origin and from the supinator crest on the ulna. The fibres pass laterally and then anteriorly around the lateral aspect of the upper third of the radius to be attached to its anterior surface as far medially as the anterior oblique line. The muscle is supplied by the posterior interosseous nerve and as its name suggests the muscle is a supinator of the forearm.

In order to gain access to the extensor surface of the forearm the posterior interosseous nerve passes between the two heads of supinator. This is of importance clinically since surgical exposure of the proximal radius can put the nerve at risk.[13] In addition, as the nerve passes between the two heads of the supinator it is covered by a fibrous arch known as the arcade of Frohse. This can be responsible for compressive lesions of the posterior interosseous nerve.[14] The nerve may also be compressed in this region secondary to adjacent synovial proliferation[15] or bursal swelling.[16]

Internervous planes

Surgical approaches to the elbow can utilise the intermuscular planes between these four groups of muscles. Between the anterior and lateral muscle groups there exists an internervous plane since the anterior group is supplied by the musculocutaneous nerve and the lateral group is supplied by the radial nerve. This intermuscular and internervous plane is used in the anterolateral approach when the interval between the brachialis and the brachioradialis muscle is used. Between the anterior and the medial muscle groups an internervous plane also exists. The medial approach to the elbow utilises this plane between the brachialis supplied by the musculocutaneous nerve and the pronator teres muscle supplied by the median nerve. There is also a potential internervous plane between the extensor carpi ulnaris supplied by the posterior interosseous nerve and the anconeus muscle supplied by the radial nerve. This plane is utilised in the posterolateral approach to the head of the radius.

Neurovascular structures

Three major nerves cross the elbow joint. The median nerve runs down the anterior aspect of the elbow joint (Fig. 2.2). It enters the cubital fossa on the medial side of the brachial artery lying underneath the brachialis muscle. It is crossed by the bicipital aponeuroses and leaves the region of the elbow joint between the two heads of the pronator teres.

The radial nerve crosses the front of the elbow between the brachialis and brachioradialis (Fig. 2.4). It divides into its terminal branches in the cubital fossa. The major muscular branch (the posterior interosseous nerve) enters the forearm between the two heads of the supinator muscle. The superficial radial nerve, which is nearly all sensory, descends down the lateral side of the forearm under cover of the brachioradialis muscle.

The ulnar nerve is the only major neurovascular structure to traverse the elbow on its posterior aspect (Fig. 2.3). It runs in a groove on the back of the medial epicondyle. It enters the forearm by passing between the two heads of flexor carpi ulnaris and may become entrapped at this site. The nerve may also be vulnerable to direct compression due to its superficial position as it passes behind the medial epicondyle. A valgus deformity of the elbow will stretch the nerve producing a partial or complete palsy.

The brachial artery enters the cubital fossa medial to the biceps tendon and lateral to the median nerve (Fig. 2.4) It lies on the brachialis muscle. The artery divides into its two terminal branches the radial and ulnar arteries, half way down the cubital fossa. The radial artery runs down the medial aspect of the biceps tendon lying on the supinator to disappear down the forearm under the cover of the brachioradialis. It is closely tethered to the brachioradialis muscle by a series of small transversally running vessels which may need to be ligated during surgical approaches to the proximal radius. The ulnar artery exits the cubital fossa by passing deep to the deep head of the pronator teres.

The elbow joint

OSTEOLOGY

It is the shape and orientation of the articular surfaces of the distal humerus and proximal radius and ulna that allows flexion, extension, pronation and supination movements to occur at the elbow joint.

The distal humerus has two articular facets. Laterally the capitellum is almost spheroidal in shape and is separated from the medial trochlea by a groove. It articulates with the radial head. The trochlea is pulley shaped and is larger medially than

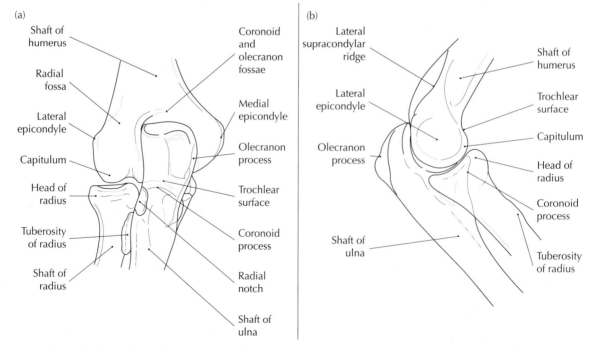

Fig. 2.5 The articular surface of the distal humerus. The humeral facets do not lie at right angles to the humeral shaft but are orientated 30 degrees anteriorly with approximately 6 degrees of valgus and 5 degrees internal rotation.

laterally. It articulates with the proximal ulna. These humeral facets do not lie at right angles to the humeral shaft but are oriented 30 degrees anteriorly with approximately 6 degrees of valgus and 5 degrees of internal rotation (Fig. 2.5).

The proximal radius is a cylindrical head which is concave to fit with the convexity of the capitellum. The proximal ulna has two projections the olecranon and the coronoid process. Between these is a saddle-shaped articular surface which is usually deficient of hyaline cartilage in its mid-portion where it is covered by fatty tissue. On the lateral surface of the coronoid process is a concave cylindrical facet for the head of the radius.

The angle formed by the long axis of the humerus and ulna when the elbow is extended is referred to as the carrying angle. This is a valgus angulation of between 11 degrees and 16 degrees. It is usually slightly greater for females than males. On full flexion the angulation reverses such that the forearm becomes on average 6 degrees varus to the upper arm. This shift from a valgus angle in extension to a varus angle in flexion occurs at 60 degrees flexion.[17]

JOINT CAPSULE

The joint capsule is attached to the proximal edges of the coronoid and radial fossae anteriorly and to the edges of the olecranon fossa posteriorly. The distal attachments are to the anterior margin of the coronoid process, the annular ligament and the margins of the trochlear notch. The capsule is lined by a synovial membrane but is separated from it by fatty tissue in the coronoid and olecranon fossae.

LIGAMENTS

Ulnar collateral ligament

The ulnar collateral ligament is triangular in shape and consists of three bands. By far the strongest is the anterior band which runs from the medial epicondyle of the humerus to the medial border of the coronoid process. The posterior band joins the medial epicondyle to the medial border of the olecranon whilst the middle band connects the two (Fig. 2.6).

Radial collateral ligament

The radial collateral ligament originates from the lateral epicondyle and inserts into the annular ligament (Fig. 2.7).

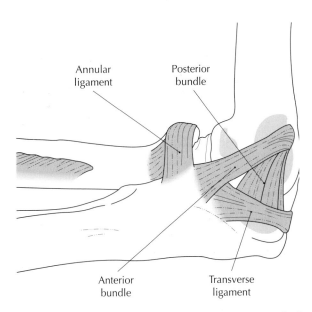

Fig. 2.6 The ulna collateral ligament. It is composed of an anterior, posterior and middle band.

Annular ligament

The annular ligament is a strong band which encircles the head and neck of the radius holding it in the superior radioulnar joint. The ligament is attached to the anterior and posterior margins of the radial notch of the ulna (Fig. 2.7).

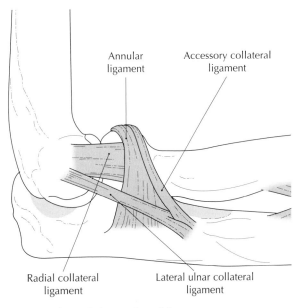

Fig. 2.7 The radial complex of ligaments.

Lateral ulnar collateral ligament

The lateral ulnar collateral ligament was first described by Morrey and An in 1985.[18] It arises from the lateral epicondyle, blends with fibres of the annular ligament and then arches superficial and distal to the annular ligament to be inserted into the tubercle of the crest of the supinator on the ulna. It provides stability to the humeroulnar joint (Fig. 2.7).

Minor ligaments

The accessory lateral collateral ligament, quadrate ligament, and oblique cord have all been described but appear to be of minor importance when compared with the other more substantial ligamentous structures.

References

1. Chen J, Alk D, Eventov I, Weintroub S Development of the olecranon bursa: An anatomic cadaver study. *Acta Orthop Scand* 1987; **58:** 408–9.
2. Osgood RB Radiohumeral bursitis epicondylitis epicondylalgia (tennis elbow): A personal experience. *Arch Surg* 1922; **4:** 420–33.
3. Carp L Tennis elbow (epicondylitis) caused by radio humeral bursitis. *Arch Surg* 1932; **24:** 905–22.
4. Gray H *Anatomy descriptive and applied* (35th edn). Warwick R, Williams PL (eds) Philadelphia: WB Saunders Co, 1980.
5. Thompson HC 111, Garcia A Myositis ossificans: Aftermath of elbow Injuries. *Clin Orthop* 1967; **50:** 129–34.
6. Travill A An electromyographic study of the extensor apparatus of the forearm. *Anat Rec* 1962; **144:** 373–6.
7. Basmajian JV, Griffin WR Function of anconeus muscle. *J Bone Joint Surg* 1972; **54A:** 1712–4.
8. An KN, Hui FC, Morrey BF, Linscheid RL, Chao EY Muscles across the elbow joint: A biomechanical analysis. *J. Biomechs* 1981; **14**(10): 659–69.
9. Basmajian JV, Travill A Electromyography of the pronator muscles in the forearm. *Anat Rec* 1961; **139:** 45–9.
10. Reimann AF, Daseler EH, Anson BJ, Beaton LE The palmaris longus muscle and tendon: A study of 1600 extremities. *Anat Rec* 1944; **89:** 495–505.
11. Nirschl RP, Pettrone F Tennis elbow: The surgical treatment of lateral epicondylitis. *J Bone Joint Surg* 1979; **61A:** 832–9.
12. Nirschl RP Tennis elbow. *Orthop Clin North Am* 1973; **4:** 787–800.
13. Strachan JH, Ellis BW Vulnerability of the posterior interosseous nerve during radial head resection. *J Bone Joint Surg* 1971; **53B:** 320–3.
14. Capener N The vulnerability of the posterior interosseous nerve in the forearm – A case report and anatomic study. *J Bone Joint Surg* 1966; **48B:** 770–3.
15. Field JH Posterior interosseous nerve palsy secondary to synovial chondromatosis of the elbow joint. *J Hand Surg* 1981; **6**(A): 336–8.
16. El-Hadidi S, Burke FD Posterior interosseous nerve syndrome cause by a bursa in the vicinity of the elbow. *J Hand Surg* 1987; **12B:** 23–4.
17. Poll RG Souther-Strathclyde total elbow arthroplasty. Thesis, Leiden, 1994.
18. Morrey BF, An KN Functional anatomy of the elbow ligaments. *Clin Orthop* 1985; **201:** 84–90.

CHAPTER 3

Biomechanics of the elbow

ANDREW A AMIS

Introduction

An appreciation of elbow biomechanics is important in the clinical assessment of patients who present with elbow pain and disability. In particular, biomechanical principles must be considered in the primary treatment of elbow fractures and when late reconstruction is planned. The decision to excise a comminuted radial head following trauma whilst clinically appropriate will have a significant effect on force transmission across the elbow joint. Distal humeral reconstruction without appreciation of the normal orientation of the humeral articulation alters the biomechanics of the elbow by affecting the muscle moment arm geometry.

In addition these principles must also be applied in the treatment of chronic inflammatory elbow disease. In the same way that force transmission requires consideration when excision of the radial head is undertaken for trauma the same principle applies when the procedure is performed in association with synovectomy of the elbow. Biomechanical assessments are also vital when prosthetic replacement becomes necessary for these patients.

In this chapter the biomechanics of the normal elbow are discussed with reference to trauma management and the use of elbow arthroplasties.

Functional anatomy – the form of the articulation related to elbow motion

FLEXION–EXTENSION

The overall shape of the elbow articulation is such that the resulting motion is akin to a hinge during flexion–extension, with both the radius and ulna sliding over approximately circular-sectioned surfaces, the axis of motion being positioned near to the centre of the circular section. The distal humerus is hollowed-out anteriorly and posteriorly to allow an increase in the range of flexion–extension motion before it is limited by impingement. The coronoid process and the rim of the radial head fit into the anterior humeral fossae in extreme flexion, and the olecranon process into a posterior fossa in extension. This allows a normal range of motion of 0 to 142 degrees (the mean of published measurements)[1] with active flexion limited by apposition of the tensed flexor muscles. Glanville and Kreezer[2] have noted that this range is increased by a mean of 5 degrees with passive flexion of the elbow.

Hyperextension is more common in females and a mean difference of 8 degrees has been noted between the sexes.[3] This tendency has also been associated with the presence of a supratrochlear foramen, that links the coronoid and olecranon fossae.[4] Children have an average of 6 degrees hyperextension[5] and advancing age leads eventually to a loss of 5 degrees flexion motion in middle age.[6]

In the past there has been much debate as to whether the different parts of the humeral articular surfaces are positioned along a single axis, or whether they are actually circular in section. These concerns are now resolved and a detailed study of the articular geometry[7,8] has shown that sagittal sections of the distal humerus are circular within a close tolerance (typically within 0.2 mm on diameter). Examination of the positions of the centres of these circles across the width of the distal humerus has shown them all to be located within 1.2 mm of a straight line. The radius and ulna must therefore be moving around a common flexion–extension axis, and thus are unable to move relative to each other.

One deviation from circular geometry has been described by Yamaguchi[9] He noted the progressive erosion of the central part of the articular cartilage of the trochlear notch, leading with advancing age to two separate cartilage areas. Although the olecranon and coronoid articular facets are not then on a circle, they still allow the humeral trochlea to rotate about a single axis of flexion, within 0.3 mm. Thus, for all practical purposes, the articular surfaces of the distal humerus are uniaxial. The reason for the confusion in the past is that parts of the circular geometry are obscured by the sweeping-in of the condylar butresses, and by the medial face of the trochlea not being perpendicular to the axis. These factors lead to an asymmetrical or even spiral appearance.

THE CARRYING ANGLE

Observations on the anatomy of the articulation led to many different hypotheses for the variation in carrying angle, normally defined as the lateral deviation of the forearm from the sagittal plane of the humerus. This deviation is largest at full extension, being an average of 11 degrees in adult males and 14 degrees in adult females.[1] In both sexes it increases from the childhood value of approximately 6 degrees.[10] Confusion regarding carrying angle variation has arisen in the past because of lack of geometrical rigour, particularly lack of control of humeral rotation, which affects measurements with the elbow flexed (a factor which makes it impossible for example to measure elbow valgus in a rheumatoid patient with a flexion deformity).

Amis *et al.*[11] linked their three-dimensional measurements to the articular geometry of cadaver limbs by use of templates fitted to the joint surfaces and to the axis of the goniometer, thus allowing correction of rotational inaccuracies. This work showed that the forearm follows a single plane in space, that is tilted from the humerus by a half of the carrying angle; i.e. the humeral articulation is tilted into valgus by half of the carrying angle, thus bisecting the angle between arm and forearm. This simple geometry leads to the carrying angle decreasing as the elbow flexes (Fig. 3.1).

Experimentation with a piece of folded card will show that this arrangement leads to the forearm overlying the arm in full flexion. Interestingly, this geometry had been recorded a century ago.[12] The practical consequence of this is that an elbow prosthesis can be made with simple uniaxial geometry, and it will accurately recreate the carrying angle variation if its axis is inclined by approximately 6 degrees from being perpendicular to the humerus. Tuke *et al.*[13] used templates to tilt the axis by 7 degrees in both humerus and ulna, in order to obtain a 14 degree carrying angle. This permitted the hand to reach the shoulder in full elbow flexion.

Work *in vitro* has also shown that the collateral ligaments allow some varus–valgus freedom at the elbow, which corresponds to approximately 9 degrees of carrying angle variation. This is difficult to elucidate *in vivo*, but is an integral part of forearm rotation movements.

FOREARM ROTATION

Forearm rotation is normally defined in terms of arcs of pronation and supination with the hand in the sagittal plane and the elbow flexed 90 degrees. The mean ranges of pronation/supination at the wrist are 76/80 degrees and at the hand 77/106

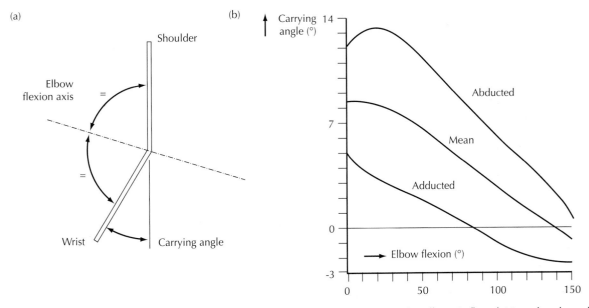

(a)

Shoulder

Elbow
flexion axis

=

=

Wrist

Carrying angle

(b)

↑ Carrying
angle (°)

Abducted

Mean

Adducted

→ Elbow flexion (°)

Fig. 3.1 The carrying angle is maximal at full elbow extension and decreases as the elbow is flexed. Note that the collateral ligaments allow some 9 degrees varus–valgus freedom. Redrawn after Ref. 11 with permission.

degrees.[1] The hand can rotate further if the elbow is extended, but this then includes glenohumeral rotation, and the rotation within the elbow is reduced.[14]

It is normally taken that forearm rotation is the result of the radius swinging around a stationary ulna. However, if this were the case, then the little finger would remain on the anatomical axis of rotation, that passes from the centre of the capitellum to the centre of the distal ulna, close to the ulnar styloid. This would lead to a transposition of the hand in space. Observation of actual motion shows that the hand rotates in one place, with the longitudinal rotation axis effectively being through the centre of the wrist. In order for this to be true, it seems that the ulna must move, into abduction during pronation and adduction during supination (Fig. 3.2). Some observers have felt that, since the humeroulnar joint is close-fitting, this ulnar motion must originate from small humeral rotations. That

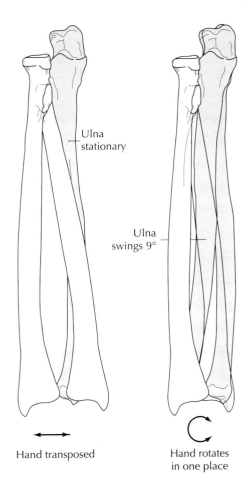

Ulna
stationary

Ulna
swings 9°

Hand transposed

Hand rotates
in one place

Fig. 3.2 Forearm rotation: if there were no movement in the humeroulnar joint, then the hand would move around an axis passing through the little finger. The rotation effectively occurs at the centre of the wrist, keeping the hand in one place, which entails humeroulnar circumduction movements.

this is not true was demonstrated by Ray *et al.*,[15] who pinned the humeral epicondyles to an x-ray jig and then did double-exposures as the subject rotated the forearm. They found humeroulnar abduction–adduction motion of 9 degrees. This lateral freedom corresponded exactly to the varus–valgus laxity measured by Amis *et al.*[11] during their carrying angle studies, and represents collateral ligament slackness allied to a sloppy fit of the trochlear notch onto the trochlea. Heiberg[16] disarticulated the wrists of cadavers, and showed that the ulna and radius effectively circle around each other during forearm rotation, while Dwight[17] proved that the ulnar motion was circumduction. He showed that the circular path of the ulna in space was composed of varying contributions of flexion–extension and abduction–adduction.

The shapes and sizes of the bones

HUMERUS

Street and Stevens[18] recognised that the distal humeral articulation had a constant shape, that was geometrically similar in all sizes of elbow, and this was the basis of their humeral hemiarthroplasty. Unfortunately, the dimensions which they published were not those of the natural articulation, but of their implant, and this had been altered to help ensure adequate function. The dimensions given were a smaller trochlear diameter and larger capitellum, in order to fit into the natural trochlear groove and to articulate against an eroded or resected radius. A survey of the humeral articular geometry on radiographs and cadavers yielded the shape shown in Fig. 3.3.[11] This indicates that any dimension follows in fixed proportion to the width of the humeral articulation.

An attempt was made to extend this analysis proximally, and thus provide data on the cavity for the intramedullary fixation of prosthetic stems. Unfortunately it was found that the shape and size of the bone was very variable away from the articular surfaces. For example, heavily built males had humeral bone stock of greater diameter and cortical thickness than females. There was also much variation in the shape of the condyles. This combined with carrying-angle variations that involved different valgus orientations of the articulation relative to the diaphysis, meant that there was only a small tapered volume proximal to the centre of the articulation that was common to all elbows.

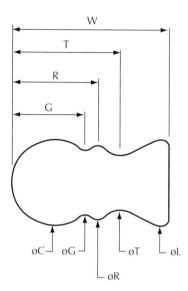

Dimension	Mean	Standard deviation	Correlation coefficient	Cadaver survey
T	66.2	2.7	0.92	66.5
R	48.1	2.4	0.90	46.5
G	38.4	2.6	0.82	-
øC	53.9	4.4	0.70	51.1
øG	45.1	4.3	0.59	-
øR	50.7	3.8	0.73	48.9
øT	40.5	4.1	0.56	39.4
øL	63.2	6.3	0.59	62.2

Results of survey of 100 radiographs

All dimensions expressed as % of 'W'

Fig. 3.3 The shape of the articular surfaces of the distal humerus is constant, and any dimension can be predicted from the overall size of the articulation. Redrawn after Ref. 11 with permission.

It is well known that the humeral articulation is not in line with the medullary cavity when seen in a lateral projection, this offset allowing some space that delays impingement of the flexor muscles as the forearm approaches full elbow flexion. The axis passing through the centre of the articulation is approximately in line with the extended line of the anterior humeral cortex. Some elbow joint replacements have neglected to keep this flexion–extension axis in the correct place. Usually, they tend to bring the axis posteriorly, so that the hinge point in the prosthetic trochlea is located more within the condyles. Although this design feature may help to create a stable fixation, it upsets the normal muscle moment arm geometry. This could explain why

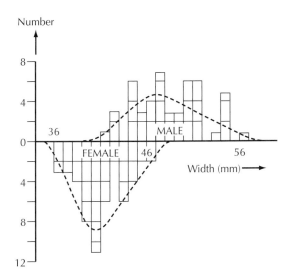

Fig. 3.4 The size distribution of the elbow. Male joints are significantly larger than female. Redrawn after Ref. 11 with permission.

some implants can suffer posterior dislocation, due to slackening of the anterior capsule, which is normally tensed by passing over the anterior bulk of the joint. Abnormal axis placement has also been found to lead to decreased strength after elbow replacement.[19]

As well as the data on the shape of the articulation, Amis *et al.*[11] measured the sizes of 100 elbows from anteroposterior radiographs. The size was defined as the medial–lateral width between the points where the articular cartilage surfaces contacted, i.e. between the capitellum and the rim of the radial head laterally, and between the medial lip of the ulnar trochlear notch and the trochlea. The radiographs were all taken with the elbow resting on the film cassette, and with a source to film distance of 1 metre. Analysis showed that the radiographic dimensions had to be multiplied by 0.95 ± 0.01 (0.96 for large elbows, 0.94 for small), leading to the size distribution shown in Fig. 3.4. It is seen that male elbows are significantly larger than females, with mean sizes of 48.1 mm and 40.6 mm, respectively.

ULNA

The dimensions of the proximal ulna are shown in Fig. 3.5. As expected, the width of the articular surface is related to that of the humeral articulation, as is the position of the intercept between the axis along the medullary cavity and the flexion axis. Note, however, that the lateral deviation of the ulna is quite variable, ranging from 6 to 23 degrees away

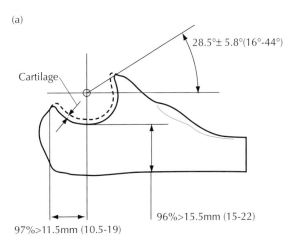

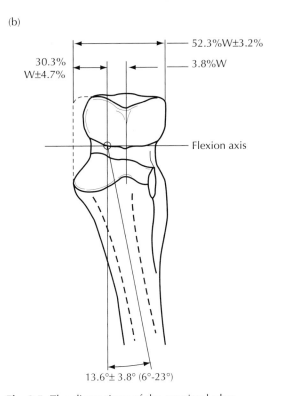

Fig. 3.5 The dimensions of the proximal ulna.

from the sagittal plane. This leads to there being only a very small area common to all joints.

The dimensions shown are for normal joints, and it should be appreciated that the rheumatoid elbow when being considered for joint replacement will have suffered bone loss. Thus, although the olecranon is shown with a depth greater than 15 mm, this refers to the central ridge which is the area that is lost by erosion. There is less bone depth to either side.

The height of the coronoid process is also important, since this controls any tendency for the elbow to dislocate posteriorly – a complication seen following joint replacement,[20] particularly if the axis is displaced into the humerus, thereby slackening the anterior capsule.

RADIUS

Since the radial head fits onto the humeral articulation, its diameter is related to the width of the elbow. From radiographic measurements, after allowing 1.5 mm for cartilage thickness, the radial head diameter is noted to be 53 ± 3% of the width of the elbow joint when viewed in an anteroposterior direction with the forearm supinated. The head is slightly oval when viewed end-on, due to the facet of the radioulnar joint, which adds material outside of the concave end-face area. Other dimensions, such as the thickness of the head and the diameter and length of the neck, can also be correlated to the head diameter. The thickness of the head is approximately 48% of the diameter, but there is a wide variation of neck size for a given head. Some radial necks can be fitted into the medulla of others that have the same size head. For an average head size of 24 mm diameter, the medullary cavity is 9 ± 3 mm diameter, and the outer diameter of the neck is 14 ± 2 mm. In general the impression gained was that females tend to have more delicate bones supporting the radial head, while some large males have a column-like configuration, with the neck continuing distally almost at the diameter of the head. The morphology also suggests that the rim of the radial head is more vulnerable to fracture in females, since because of its size it overhangs the radial neck to a greater extent than occurs in males.

Elbow joint forces during various activities

REVIEW OF ELBOW FORCE ANALYSES

Initial work on elbow joint forces suggested that the capsule would take much of the load, rather than the joint surfaces.[18] However, even a simple engineering analysis shows that the muscles are acting at a great mechanical leverage disadvantage, which leads to large muscle forces compressing the joint during normal activities.

In 1973, Groh[21] obtained maximal flexion–extension strength curves and used the data in a two-dimensional force analysis of the elbow. He used previously published muscle moment arm data, which he combined into a single 'flexor muscle action', leading to a maximum flexor force prediction of 2.55 kN at 30 degrees flexion, and a maximum triceps tension of 2.1 kN. Although he did not calculate the joint forces, the data can be used to find a maximum elbow force of 2.3 kN. Groh noted that use of the single 'flexor muscle' led to inaccurate directions being predicted for the forces, leading to high loads on the tip of the coronoid. He suggested that more accurate work should include the forearm muscles, that would centre the forces, for example, into the radial head. Groh predicted larger forces on the radial head than on the ulna, and that the resultant force on the humerus would act onto the distal aspect when the elbow was extended, swinging onto the anterior aspect as the elbow flexed.

Although he did not show any details of how the forces were calculated, Schlein[22] said that 40% of the elbow force passed through the humeroradial joint, and 60% through the humeroulnar joint. Of greater concern, though, were the torsional forces, that he felt would break the bond between bone and the fixation cement of elbow arthroplasties.

Elbow forces during flexion were examined by Walker,[23] who allowed for biceps and brachialis actions when supporting 10 N in the hand. He predicted joint forces of 428 N at 45 degrees flexion and 215 N at 90 degrees. Since this analysis did not include any muscles passing along the forearm, the forces were predicted to act onto the distal aspect of the humerus. Walker also noted that the compressive load during a pushing action would be transmitted directly to the capitellum, with no muscle actions needed, if the force were in line with the forearm. However, if the push force were angled 10 degrees into flexion, a triceps action of 1.6 times the external force would be needed to resist the flexion effect, adding to the force on the elbow.

Nicol *et al.*[24] examined forces and motion during daily activities such as reaching and pulling, and obtained data on the loads imposed on the limb. When the elbow joint forces were calculated, allowance was made for brachialis, biceps and brachioradialis in flexion, and triceps in extension. Forces were predicted to act mainly on the humeroulnar joint, thus potentially underestimating the radial head forces.

Following from the work of Paul[25] on the hip there was much activity in biomechanics. It became appreciated that one of the crucial aspects of force analysis results from there being more muscles crossing most joints than are strictly necessary. It could be argued, for example, that brachialis action makes biceps redundant in elbow flexion, assuming that a maximal force is not needed. The consequence of this redundancy is that there will be more forces acting on and around the joint than can be analysed by normal engineering equations of equilibrium. Thus some scheme must be used, that allows the redundancy to be overcome. This has led to optimisation criteria being hypothesised, which could explain how the body chooses the relative contributions of co-operating muscles. Ideas such as minimising the joint force or minimising the energy expenditure have been tried, particularly in relation to the hip. This has sometimes been in conjunction with attempts to relate electromyographic findings to muscle forces,[26,27] but this unfortunately is not an exact procedure. In contrast to the lower limb, where the activity being analysed is usually walking, and does not require maximal muscle actions, it is often the case in the upper limb that maximal strength is exerted, particularly for elderly patients, who may struggle to grip or move objects. In this circumstance, the redundancy problem is eased if it is hypothesised that muscle forces are in proportion to their sizes; specifically, to the 'physiological cross-sectional area'. This takes account of the fibre pennations in muscles when estimating how many muscle fibres are present. This approach was used by Alexander and Vernon[28] in the leg. In the upper limb it led to an analysis of the relative sizes (and hence strengths) of the muscles crossing the elbow.[29,30] These data thus allowed the relative forces of co-operating muscles to be calculated, and this allowed the force–equilibrium equations to be solved while including all of the muscles crossing the elbow joint.

ELBOW FORCES IN FLEXION

In order to predict the elbow joint forces during flexion, data is needed on the magnitude of the external forces acting on the hand, knowledge of which muscles are active, and on the geometry of the anatomical structures that are relevant. In particular the moment arms of the muscles as they pass across the joint need to be determined.

Maximal force actions of the upper limb have been studied in depth, usually as part of the ergonomic design of controls in vehicles. The work of Hunsicker[31] was comprehensive, finding a mean maximum elbow flexion strength of 270 N force on a handle at 60 degrees elbow flexion, which dropped to approximately 200 N at the extremes of the range of flexion–extension. These were 'isometric' forces, that were obtained by acting on a fixed handle. Muscle has a velocity–tension relationship, that drops as the speed of muscle shortening increases, and is raised by a forced muscle

extension against a contraction.[32,33] Hill[32] found that the strength when resisting a forced muscle elongation could be twice the isometric strength, and this may explain avulsion fractures of the olecranon insertion of the triceps.

The strength data of Hunsicker[31] was for fit young men. Elkins et al.[34] found that females had 55% of male elbow flexion strength. Since most elbow joint replacements are for rheumatoid patients, who will also be older than the population tested by most researchers, Amis et al.[35] reported on the elbow flexion strength of 102 rheumatoid patients. They were split between in- and outpatients, and thus were representative of the rheumatoid population as a whole. Some had little problem with the elbow, while others were in severe pain. They applied force to a fixed wide soft strap, that was placed over the wrist in 30 degrees supination with the elbow at 90 degrees flexion. Male inpatients had strength of 98 ± 46 N and outpatients 146 ± 76 N, while the females had strengths of 57 ± 41 N in both groups. These results suggested that rheumatoid patients had approximately 45% of normal strength.

In order to flex the elbow, there must be contraction of a number of muscles, of which the brachialis, brachioradialis, biceps and pronator teres, are the most important. The biceps and pronator teres also have antagonistic forearm rotation actions in addition to elbow flexion effects. It is also normally the case that forcible elbow flexion entails lifting or pulling an object in the hand, and this, in turn, requires actions from the digital flexor muscles and the carpal muscles, to stabilise the wrist against the transverse shearing forces imposed by the external load. Many of the tendons which cross the wrist to act on bones of the hand have origins proximal to the elbow, and so these actions, which are integral to elbow flexion, impose forces on the elbow along the direction of the forearm. Electromyographic studies, as reviewed by Basmajian,[36] have shown that elbow movements do not always invoke actions from all of the possible muscles. This appears to occur when the hand is unloaded. As the load increases, so all the muscles contract forcibly, both to flex the elbow and to grasp the object in the hand.[37] The many tendons crossing the wrist were investigated electromyographically by Dempster and Finerty.[38] They found that the muscles contracted maximally in the direction from which a transverse force was applied, with activation reducing progressively to approximately 50% on either side of this. In addition the antagonistic muscles on the opposite aspect of the wrist were activated 30%, thus providing stability with a net action opposing the load.

The moment arms of the muscles crossing both wrist and elbow were estimated on dissected limbs by Amis *et al.*,[29] who digitised cross-sections at elbow and wrist, and assumed the muscles acted in straight lines. The moment arm data produced was compared with that already published, and found to be in reasonable agreement.[21,39] Muscle paths around the elbow are shown in Fig. 3.6.

The equilibrium analysis for elbow efforts has also been studied.[40] Since the wrist is effectively a ball joint, the many tendon tensions must produce equilibrium against the load imposed while also maintaining the hand position against lateral displacement. This is achieved primarily by a combination of the finger flexors and the carpal extensors. The wrist and hand muscles attach

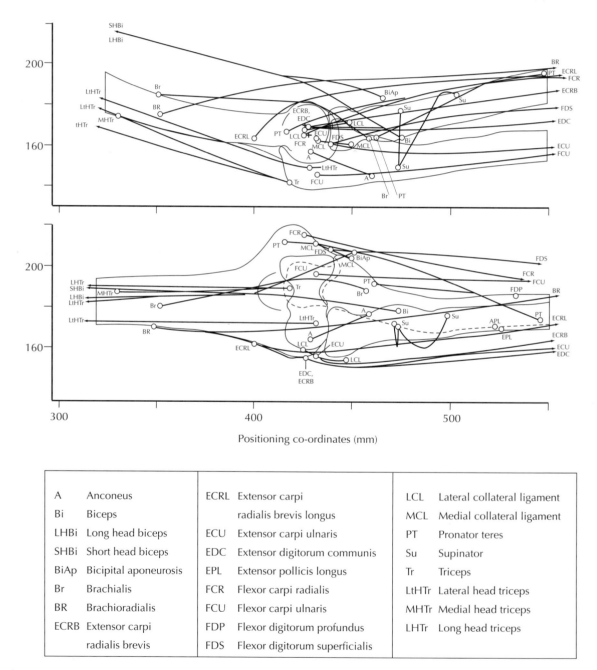

Positioning co-ordinates (mm)

A	Anconeus	ECRL	Extensor carpi	LCL	Lateral collateral ligament
Bi	Biceps		radialis brevis longus	MCL	Medial collateral ligament
LHBi	Long head biceps	ECU	Extensor carpi ulnaris	PT	Pronator teres
SHBi	Short head biceps	EDC	Extensor digitorum communis	Su	Supinator
BiAp	Bicipital aponeurosis	EPL	Extensor pollicis longus	Tr	Triceps
Br	Brachialis	FCR	Flexor carpi radialis	LtHTr	Lateral head triceps
BR	Brachioradialis	FCU	Flexor carpi ulnaris	MHTr	Medial head triceps
ECRB	Extensor carpi	FDP	Flexor digitorum profundus	LHTr	Long head triceps
	radialis brevis	FDS	Flexor digitorum superficialis		

Fig. 3.6 Muscle paths around the elbow: each line represents the centroid of the muscle's cross-section. Redrawn after Ref. 29 with permission.

close to the elbow flexion–extension axis, so have little effect on flexion–extension equilibrium, although they do compress the joints. The radius is also akin to a mast with stabilising guylines around it. It tends to impose a medial force onto the head of the ulna, since both pronator teres and biceps pass medially to the capitellum. This is reflected in the large medial facet of the coronoid process, that resists this load. The elbow flexor muscle forces were scaled-up, in proportion to their physiological cross-sections, until equilibrium was attained against the hand forces measured by Hunsicker.[31] Allowance was also made for some triceps antagonism, which Messier *et al.*[26] suggested would act to stabilise the elbow.

It is not surprising that when the muscle paths were considered, the joint forces were predicted to act primarily in the sagittal plane. Almost equal forces were noted to act on the coronoid process and head of radius (Fig. 3.7). It can be seen that large forces act axially onto the distal aspect of the humerus when the elbow is near extension, and that the forces diminish as the elbow is flexed, and then act onto the anterior aspect. Both the radial head and coronoid forces were predicted to act at approximately 20 degrees posterior to a distal direction, at the base of the coronoid and at the posterior rim of the radial head. This balance of forces results from the humeroulnar joint being compressed by the brachialis and common flexor muscles, while the radius has biceps, pronator teres and brachioradialis inserting into it. This force

analysis was based on a neutral position of forearm rotation, and it is likely that the humeroulnar joint will be exposed to a greater proportion of the forces if flexion is analysed with the forearm supinated. This arises primarily because the wrist flexors are loaded more directly. Conversely, flexion with the forearm pronated involves the hand pulling via the fingers, and the combined actions of the external force and the finger flexors will create a large wrist flexion action, that must be resisted by the extensor carpi muscles, that act to compress the humeroradial joint.

ELBOW FORCES IN EXTENSION

The triceps is the strongest muscle in the upper limb, and provides almost the entire elbow extension action. Most of the resulting tension acts onto the olecranon process, and thus the main elbow joint force, which can exceed 3 kN, acts into the trochlear notch, peaking when the elbow is being extended through 120 degrees flexion.[40] There are also forces arising from the forearm muscles, that act to stabilise the hand, plus the lateral head of the triceps, which passes along the lateral aspect of the olecranon and dissipates into the fascia overlying the supinator muscle. These actions contribute to a humeroradial force which peaks at approximately 1 kN. The triceps has a relatively small moment arm about the elbow extension axis, approximately 20 mm, and thus the muscle forces must be high.

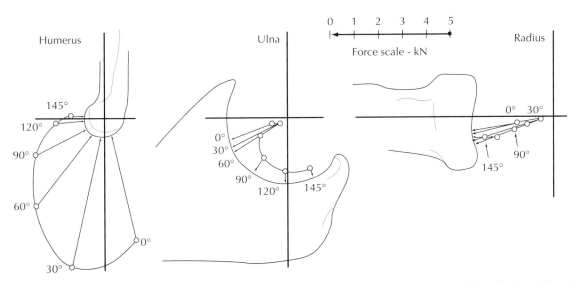

Fig. 3.7 Forces acting on the humerus, radial head and coronoid during maximal isometric elbow flexion efforts in adult male subjects. Redrawn after Ref. 49 with permission.

With biceps stabilising antagonism equal to 7% of triceps tension,[26] the humeroulnar force exceeds 20 times the load at the hand, with the force on the humerus reaching 24 times the external load. This great ratio occurs when extension is from a flexed posture, since the triceps tendon will then have been wrapped around the waist of the trochlea, and have the smallest moment arm.[29]

ROTATION ACTIONS OF THE HUMERUS, WITH THE ELBOW FLEXED

This is the situation which has been implicated in causing loosening of the humeral intramedullary fixation stems of hinge prostheses. If the pectoral muscles contract maximally, to squash a box held between the hands with the elbows flexed 90 degrees, a force of 218 ± 100 N can be exerted.[31] The opposite action, pulling the hands apart, can exert a force of 156 ± 81 N.

Inward rotation causes a force to be applied to the palm of the hand, and this leads to wrist flexor muscle actions. These, in turn, help to stabilise the humeroulnar joint. However, the rotation torque on the humerus is sufficient to cause the coronoid to be lifted from the trochlea, causing a medial collateral ligament tension of approximately six times the external load, 1.3 kN. This action must be counteracted by the humero-radial joint being compressed, and a force of 1.8 kN can act.[40] This shows the advantage of the width of the distal humerus, since the torque exerted by the muscles must be resisted by a force couple acting between the medial collateral ligament tension and the radial head compression.

Radial head excision reduces the effective width of the articulation, and so greater forces will be concentrated onto the lateral edge of the coronoid process.[41] This can lead to an increase in valgus angulation at the elbow after trauma[42] and in rheumatoid patients.[43] The valgus collapse is resisted by tension in the anterior band of the medial collateral ligament (Fig. 3.8). This effect will also raise the forces acting on the fixation of any narrowly based prosthesis, resulting in a greater risk of loosening.

If forearm abduction is analysed, as though the subject is attempting to tear an object apart, it is apparent that the hands must act strongly to grasp the object with the fingers. This action flexes the wrist, and so the wrist and forearm extensor muscles are tensed by this activity as they counteract this tendency.

The geometry of the hand is such that the finger tendons work at a mechanical disadvantage, leading to relatively high muscle forces for a small external

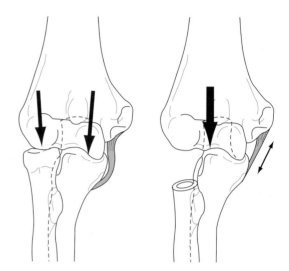

Fig. 3.8 During normal flexion efforts, the elbow acts as a balanced bicondylar joint. With radial head excision, medial collateral ligament tension increases to resist valgus collapse. Redrawn after Ref. 41 with permission.

load. The result of this is that this action does not pull the radial head away from the capitellum. The extensor carpii muscles maintain it in position, and so no lateral collateral ligament action is required. This finding, which contrasts markedly with the situation at the medial collateral ligament, reflects the relative morphology of the ligamentous structures, which are, at best, insubstantial on the lateral aspect.

LIFTING A SUITCASE

Prior to force analyses, it was usually thought that the 'suitcase lift' would tend to pull an elbow prosthesis out of its fixation. This is not the case, however, since the forearm is actually under compression during a pulling action. This surprising result arises from the mechanical disadvantage of the flexor tendons as they pass close to the axes of the joints of the fingers. To resist a pulling load of 530 N, the tendons exert a tension of approximately 920 N, or 390 N compressing the wrist. When actions to stabilise the wrist are also included, the wrist compression increases, and the net result is a small compressive load on the elbow. This arises from the wrist and finger muscles which originate from the humerus.[40] It would be a different story if the load were to hang on a wrist strap, since little muscle action would then be required.

Forces acting along the forearm

The structure of the forearm is adapted to transmitting compressive loads from the hand to the elbow, such as when pushing – or in a fall onto the outstretched hand. This situation was analysed by Halls and Travill,[44] who found that the radius transmitted 50–70% of the force applied to the hand. One drawback of this experiment was that the load was aligned with the axis of the forearm and any deviation from that alignment would cause the force distribution to change. This effect is likely to be caused by the valgus angulation of the carrying angle, and in a fall forwards onto the hand the normal posture is one of inward rotation of the humerus with a semi-pronated forearm. This posture causes the lateral aspect of the elbow to be uppermost at the moment of impact, and this leads to medial collateral ligament tension and compression force on the radial head – hence the frequency of radial head fractures in this situation.[45]

An experiment in which forces were applied at a range of directions found that 73% of the load passed to the radial head when the load was aligned with the forearm, but that deviations of the line of force could cause the load to pass entirely to the radial head or to the coronoid, depending on the direction.[46] If the force vector passed beyond the medial or lateral extent of the elbow, then stability demanded collateral ligament tension, which was more effective at resisting valgus loading, and this tension increased the load on the elbow.

The role of the interosseous membrane has been debated, with regard to its efficiency at transmitting axial forces from radius to ulna after radial head excision, and thereby resisting proximal migration of the radius, that might disrupt the distal radioulnar joint. This has been hypothesised in view of the slanting orientation of the fibres of the membrane. Axial loading of cadaver forearms has shown that the humeroradial joint had a stiffness of 1400 N/mm. Following radial head excision, the stiffness of the forearm was reduced to 200 N/mm, which would thus allow significant proximal excursions of the radius to result from muscle actions.[47] It was then shown that a metallic radial head replacement restored the normal axial forearm stiffness, preventing proximal radial migration after trauma. Silicone rubber implants have also been used to replace the radial head, but these are too soft to transmit much force without deforming and result in the interosseous membrane continuing to take most of the axial loads.[47]

Radial head excision is often used as part of synovectomy in rheumatoid surgery, and examination of the literature shows that this does not cause problems in these patients with low mechanical demands. There is some evidence, however, that the elbow can drift into valgus as the coronoid process erodes under the elevated loads imposed on it,[43] and that proximal radial migration is more likely in the post-trauma patient, leading to wrist symptoms.[42,48]

Practical applications

An understanding of the biomechanics of the elbow is essential for the acute management of fractures and also in late reconstruction. This is perhaps best exemplified in the management of radial head fractures where excision of the radial head will result in increased force transmission across the ulnohumeral articulation. In reconstruction of complex fractures it is important to appreciate that the distal humeral articulation does not lie at right angles to the humeral shaft but is orientated 30 degrees anteriorly with approximately 6 degrees of valgus and 5 degrees of internal rotation. Failure to achieve an anatomical reconstruction will affect elbow movement and prevent restoration of the normal carrying angle.

The direction of normal muscle pull has been detailed and is of practical importance in the treatment of neuromuscular disorders. These often require tendon transfers and when such surgery is contemplated it is important not only to choose an innervated muscle but also one whose direction of pull can be appropriately re-routed to provide effective joint movement.

Finally the development and design of elbow prostheses for the treatment primarily of inflammatory elbow disease is also dependant on a thorough and detailed appreciation of normal elbow biomechanics.

References

1. Amis AA, Miller JH The elbow. Measurement of joint movement. *Clin Rheum Dis* 1982; **8:** 571–93.
2. Glanville AD, Kreezer G The maximum amplitude and velocity of joint movements in normal male human adults. *Hum Biol* 1937; **9:** 197–211.
3. Hertzberg HTE Engineering anthropology. In: *Human engineering guide to equipment design.* Cott HP, Kinkade RG (eds) Washington: US Govt Printing Office, 1972.
4. Zimmer EA *Borderlands of the normal and early pathologic in skeletal roentgenology.* New York, London: Grune and Stratton, 1968.

5. Silverman S, Constine L, Harvey W, Grahame R Survey of joint mobility and *in vivo* skin elasticity in London schoolchildren. *Ann Rheum Dis* 1975; **34:** 177–80.

6. Boone DC, Azen SP Normal range of motion of joints in male subjects. *J Bone Joint Surg* 1979; **61A:** 756–9.

7. Amis AA Biomechanics of the upper limb and design of an elbow prosthesis. PhD Thesis Leeds 1978.

8. Amis AA Biomechanics of the elbow. In: *Joint replacement in the shoulder and elbow*. Wallace WA (ed) Oxford: Butterworth-Heineman, 1996: 105–26.

9. Yamaguchi B The bipartite tendency of the articular surface of the trochlear notch in the human ulna. *Okajimas Folia Anat Jap* 1972; **49:** 23–35.

10. Smith L Deformity following supracondylar fractures of the humerus. *J Bone Joint Surg* 1960; **42A:** 235–52.

11. Amis AA, Dowson D, Wright V, Miller JH, Unsworth A An examination of the elbow articulation with particular reference to the variation of the carrying angle. *Engng Med* 1977; **6:** 76–80.

12. Potter HP The obliquity of the arm of the female in extension. The relation of the forearm with the upper arm in flexion. *J Anat Physiol* 1895; **29:** 488–91.

13. Tuke MA, Roper BA, Swanson SAV, O'Riordan S The ICLH elbow. *Engng Med* 1981; **10:** 75–8.

14. Salter N, Darcus HD The amplitude of forearm and of humeral rotation. *J Anat* 1953; **87:** 407–18.

15. Ray RD, Johnson RJ, Jameson RM Rotation of the forearm: an experimental study of pronation and supination. *J Bone Joint Surg* 1951; **33A:** 993–6.

16. Heiberg J The movements of the ulna in rotation of the forearm. *J Anat Physiol* 1884; **19:** 237–86.

17. Dwight T The movement of the ulna in rotation of the forearm. *J Anat Physiol* 1884; **19:** 186–9.

18. Street DM, Stevens PS A humeral replacement prosthesis for the elbow. *J Bone Joint Surg* 1974; **56A:** 1147–58.

19. Morrey BF, Askew RPT, An K-N Strength function after elbow arthroplasty. *Clin Orthop* 1988; **234:** 43–50.

20. Ewald FC, Jacobs MA Total elbow arthroplasty. *Clin Orthop* 1984; **182:** 137–42.

21. Groh H Proceedings 1. Elbow fractures in the adult. (a) Anatomy biomechanics of the elbow joint. *Hefte zu Unfallheilkund* 1993; **114:** 13–20.

22. Schlein AP Semiconstrained total elbow arthroplasty. *Clin Orthop* 1976; **121:** 222–9.

23. Walker PS *Human joints and their artificial replacements*. Springfield, Illinois: CC Thomas, 1977.

24. Nicol AC, Berme N, Paul JP A biomechanical analysis of elbow joint function. In: *Joint replacement in the upper limb*. Bury St Edmunds: I Mech E Press, 1977: 45–51.

25. Paul JP Bioengineering studies of the forces transmitted by joints. Part 2 Engineering analysis. In: *Biomechanics and related engineering topics*. Kenedi RM (ed) Oxford: Pergamon Press, 1965: 369–80.

26. Messier RH, Duffy J, Litchman HM, Pasley PR, Soechting JF, Stewart PA The electromyogram as a measure of tension in the human biceps and triceps muscles. *Int J Mech Sci* 1971; **13:** 585–98.

27. Hof AL, van den Berg JW Linearity between the weighted sums of the EMGs of the human triceps surae and the total torque. *J Biomechs* 1977; **10:** 529–39.

28. Alexander R McN, Vernon A The dimensions of knee and ankle muscles and the forces they exert. *J Hum Mov Studies* 1975; **1:** 115–123.

29. Amis AA, Dowson D, Wright V Muscle strengths and musculoskeletal geometry of the upper limb. *Engng Med* 1979; **8:** 41–8.

30. An KN, Hui FC, Morrey BF, Linscheid RL, Chao EY Muscles across the elbow joint: a biomechanical analysis. *J Biomechs* 1981; **14:** 659–69.

31. Hunsicker P Arm strength at selected degrees of elbow flexion. *Tech Rep* 54–548, Ohio: Wright Air Development Center, Wright-Patterson Air Force Base, 1955.

32. Hill AV The mechanics of voluntary muscle. *Lancet* 1951; **261:** 947–51.

33. Elftman H Biomechanics of muscle. *J Bone Joint Surg* 1966; **48A:** 363–77.

34. Elkins EC, Ledan UM, Wakim KG Objective recording of the strength of normal muscles. *Arch Phys Med* 1951; **32:** 639–47.

35. Amis AA, Hughes S, Miller JH, Wright V, Dowson D Elbow joint forces in patients with rheumatoid arthritis. *Rheumatol Rehab* 1979; **18:** 230–4.

36. Basmajian JV *Muscles alive* (2nd edn). Baltimore: Williams and Wilkins, 1967.

37. Long C, Conrad PW, Hall EA, Furler SL Intrinsic-extrinsic muscle control of the hand in power grip and precision handling. An electromyographic study. *J Bone Joint Surg* 1970; **52A:** 853–67.

38. Dempster WT, Finerty JC Relative activity of wrist moving muscles in static support of the wrist joint: an electromyographic study. *Am J Physiol* 1947; **150:** 595–606.

39. Wilkie DR The relation between force and velocity in human muscle. *J Physiol* 1949; **110:** 249–80.

40. Amis AA, Dowson D, Wright V Elbow joint force predictions for some strenuous isometric actions. *J Biomechs* 1980; **13:** 765–75.

41. Amis AA, Dowson D, Wright V, Miller JH The derivation of elbow joint forces and their relation to prosthesis design. *J Med Engng Technol* 1977; **3:** 229–34.

42. Taylor TKF, O'Connor BT The effect on inferior radio-ulnar joint of excision of head of radius in adults. *J Bone Joint Surg* 1964; **46B:** 83–8.

43. Rymaszewski LA, Mackay I, Amis AA, Miller JH Long term effects of radial head excision in rheumatoid arthritis. *J Bone Joint Surg* 1984; **66B:** 109–13.

44. Halls AA, Travill A Transmission of pressures across the elbow joint. *Anat Rec* 1964; **150:** 243–7.

45. Amis AA, Miller JH The mechanisms of elbow fractures: an investigation using impact tests *in vitro*. *Injury* 1995; **26:** 163–8.

46. Amis AA, Miller JH, Dowson D, Wright V Axial forces in the forearm: their relationship to excision of

the head of the radius. In: *Mechanical factors and the skeleton*. Stokes IAF (ed) London: J Libbey, 1981: 29–37.

47. Knight DJ, Rymaszewski LA, Miller JH, Amis AA Primary replacement of the fractured radial head with a metal prosthesis. *J Bone Joint Surg* 1993; **75B:** 572–6.

48. McDougall A, White J Subluxation of inferior radio-ulnar joint complicating fracture of radial head. *J Bone Joint Surg* 1957; **39B:** 278–87.

49. Amis AA, Miller JH Design, development and clinical trial of a modular elbow replacement incorporating cement-free fixation. *Engng Med* 1984: **13** 175–9.

CHAPTER 4

Clinical assessment of the elbow

DH SONNABEND, JS HUGHES

Introduction

In the assessment of elbow abnormalities a detailed history of both current and previous elbow problems is essential. This should be followed by a methodical examination together with specific provocation manoeuvres in order that an accurate diagnosis of the elbow disorder might be reached. The process is enhanced by the clinician's 'mind's eye' picturing the anatomy, thereby enabling meaningful palpation of the soft tissues and bony landmarks. This chapter outlines a systematic approach to clinical assessment of the elbow. The technique of examination and commonly elicited clinical signs are discussed.

History

HISTORY OF PRESENTING ILLNESS

The majority of patients with elbow disorders present with either pain, local tenderness or an inability to perform a certain task or manoeuvre. These symptoms may occur in isolation or be part of a combined disability.

When taking a history, the patient's age, hand dominance and duration of symptoms should be determined. In addition, comment should be sought as to whether the symptoms are the result of a single injury or cumulative minor trauma. This is important since pathology associated with a single injury usually differs from that following repetitive trauma.

The clinician should also determine whether the patient is able to perform activities of daily living and whether work practices or sport and leisure pursuits have affected the situation. This is of relevance since certain of these may result in particular elbow problems and thus provide a clue to the likely diagnosis[1] (Table 4.1).

The nature of any pain should be noted with attention paid to its quality, location, radiation and where it occurs in the arc of movement. The effect of previous non-operative measures including analgesia, non-steroidal anti-inflammatory drugs and steroid injections should also be recorded.

Table 4.1 Sports and activities associated with injuries to the elbow

Tennis/racquet sports
  Lateral epicondylitis (improper backhand or serving with a pronated forearm), lateral overload/radiocapitellar degenerative changes.
  Medical collateral ligament laxity (repeated forehand strokes).
  Pronator syndrome (dominant arm sports).

Throwing/baseball
  Lateral compartment compression overload (osteochondritis dissecans, usually involving the capitellum, but also radial head or both – 'little leaguer's elbow').
  Valgus overload (medical collateral ligament tears and laxity).
  Hyperextension (postero-medial impingement and apophysitis of the olecranan ossific centre).
  Ulna neuritis.
  Posterior interosseous nerve entrapment.
  Pronator syndrome (dominant arm sports).

Javelin
  Valgus overload (medical collateral ligament rupture)

Weight lifting.
  Fast concentric contractions with hand weights or eccentric hyperextension, both can produce ruptures of the biceps tendon.
  Pronator syndrome (dominant arm sports) esp with curls.

Rock climbing
  Brachialis tendonitis.

Gymnastics
  Lateral compartment compression (osteochondritis dissecans), especially with vaulting.
  Acute dislocations.
  Medial tension overload.
  Posterior interooseous nerve entrapment.

Contact sports
  Hyperextension and valgus injuries (elbow dislocation, coronoid shear fractures).

Golf
  Lateral epicondylitis (overplaying/poor swing mechanics).
  Medial epicondylitis.
  Pronator syndrome (dominant arm sports).

Swimming backstroke (hyperextension).

Wrestling
  MCL ruptures.

Musicians
  Lateral epicondylitis (esp violinists and wind instruments).

Modified from Ref. 1.

The patient should be asked to demonstrate manoeuvres which reproduce the symptoms and also asked about methods employed to bring relief.

Whilst spontaneous descriptions of symptoms are ideal, certain symptoms are of such critical relevance that if necessary they should be sought by specific questioning. Crepitus and locking or recurrent swelling may be indications of mechanical derangement or intra-articular inflammation. Some elbow instabilities are obvious by the patient's description. Others may be described as giving way, or result in the sensation of a 'dead arm' when loading the elbow. Loss of grip strength in particular is significant but not specific. For example, an overly extensive lateral epicondyle release might relieve lateral epicondylitis but precipitate postero-lateral instability. This may be suggested by a change of symptoms after surgery.

Finally, the patient should be asked about legal proceedings or worker's compensation since both of these may have a significant effect on the likely outcome.

PAST HISTORY

A review of past medical history should note other joint injuries or the presence of chronic inflammatory disease. Specific questions concerning other joint swellings, rashes and ocular problems may also be relevant. Where inflammatory disease is suspected, a systems review should be undertaken.

Some elbow conditions are associated with a generalised 'mesenchymal syndrome', particularly in women in the fourth decade of life. In this condition, however, multiple upper limb problems, including lateral and medial epicondylitis, ulnar nerve compression at the elbow, rotator cuff pathology, carpal tunnel syndrome and stenosing tenosynovitis of the fingers and thumbs frequently co-exist. The presence of any one of these conditions should direct questioning to the remaining sites.

FAMILY HISTORY

A family history of inherited disorders such as osteochondromatosis or haemophilia should be noted.

GENERAL HEALTH

A brief review of the patient's general health is important. Systemic ligamentous laxity (hypermobility) pre-disposes to generalised joint instability.[2]

Any obvious musculoskeletal asymmetry, including limb atrophy (due to disuse or neurological disease) or hypertrophy (which may reflect dominant limb sport) should be noted. Dysmorphic features may suggest a syndromal diagnosis. Other joint abnormalities should be sought. Shoulder and cervical spine problems frequently produce pain in the region of the elbow and therefore these regions should always be carefully assessed.

Clinical examination of the elbow

LOCAL INSPECTION

The posture in which the patient holds the elbow should be noted. Skin overlying the elbow may provide some clues. The scaly lesions of psoriasis and the paper-like scars of Ehlers–Danlos syndrome may be obvious. Dilated veins may overlie underlying mitotic lesions. Adjacent swellings, including rheumatoid nodules or supratrochlear lymph nodes (lying along the course of the basilic vein) may direct attention to associated inflammatory disease.

POSITIONING

Elbow anatomy is generally best appreciated with the joint flexed to 90 degrees. Since it is necessary to move the shoulder and elbow during the examination, it is preferable to have the patient sitting or lying, rather than standing (Fig. 4.1). This effectively fixes the patient's torso, and prevents the patient from 'following his arm around the room'.

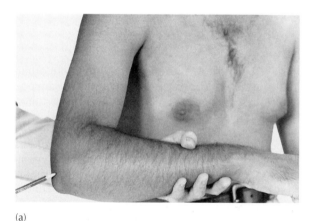

(a)

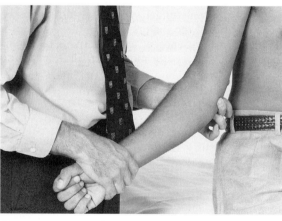

(b)

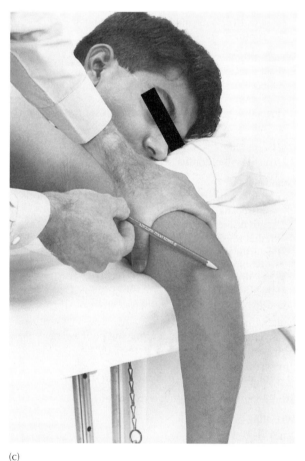

(c)

Fig. 4.1 Examination of the elbow should be performed with stabilisation of the arm: (a) examination of the lateral aspect; (b) medial and anterior structures; (c) the posterior structures are examined by positioning the patient prone, abducting the shoulder 90 degrees and stabilising the upper arm and with the elbow flexed.

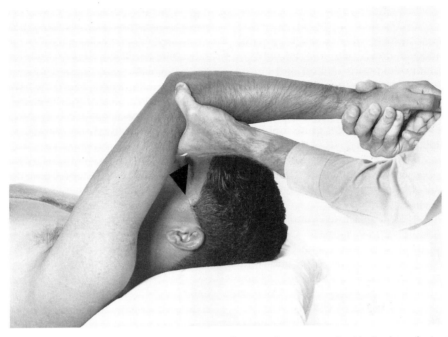

Fig. 4.2 Posterolateral rotatory instability of the elbow is demonstrated with the lateral pivot shift test. The patient lies supine with the arm overhead. A combination of axial compression, as well as valgus and supination movements are applied to rotate and subluxate the humeroulnar joint. The manouvre should be repeated with the forearm pronated and the symptoms compared.

With the examiner standing in front of the patient, the anterior and lateral aspects can be palpated. This should be performed methodically, identifying bony and soft tissue landmarks.

The posterior and medial aspects can be examined in a number of ways. Standing behind the patient with the shoulder abducted and extended, the elbow joint can be inspected and palpated. Alternatively, with the patient lying supine and the arm fully elevated overhead, the posterior, posterolateral and posteromedial aspects of the flexed elbow can be palpated. In addition, instability manoeuvres can be performed (Fig. 4.2). Assessment of posterior elbow pathology may be enhanced by examination with the patient prone, the shoulder abducted to 90 degrees, and the upper arm held fixed to the bed (Fig. 4.1). With the elbow flexed over the edge of the bed, the forearm can then be moved on a fixed upper arm. The patient's face should be observed for signs of pain or apprehension.

PALPATION

With the patient appropriately positioned, the elbow can be carefully palpated. This process is enhanced by the fact that much of the elbow is subcutaneous.

While the anterior, posterior and medial aspects of the elbow deserve careful attention, it is the lateral aspect of the elbow which yields most information to palpation. The examiner should develop a systematic approach to palpation of the elbow, and it is suggested that this begins at the top of the lateral supracondylar ridge. Walking one's fingers down the ridge, the lateral epicondyle is reached. The common extensor tendon and the lateral collateral ligament can be palpated and signs of lateral epicondylitis sought. The contour of the lateral condyle is noted. The adjacent muscle bellies of the forearm extensors can be examined as one progresses to the lateral aspect of the radiohumeral joint.

The infracondylar recess and adjacent radial head warrants careful attention. Next, the olecranon is palpated, and its relationship to the epicondyles assessed. Further, medially between the olecranon and the medial epicondyle the ulnar nerve and medial collateral ligaments are palpated. From the medial epicondyle, the examination extends both proximally and anteriorly, to review the many structures of the anticubital fossa, completing the circumnavigation of the elbow. For descriptive purposes this 'continuum' is subdivided into lateral and medial, anterior and posterior.

LATERAL

The lateral supracondylar ridge is easily palpable and can be followed down onto the lateral epicondyle, the common extensor tendon and lateral collateral ligament. If a non-union of a lateral condyle fracture is present the elbow may appear to have only mild restriction of movement. The bulbous lateral condyle fragment is quite mobile. If the condyle is held fixed to the shaft of the humerus, the range of movement is often dramatically reduced. The degree of mobility of the lateral segment is better appreciated with flexion, extension, supination and pronation.

The extensor carpi radialis brevis and extensor carpi radialis longus can be assessed by resisted wrist extension in neutral and radial deviation respectively. Tenderness over the 'mobile wad' (brachioradialis, extensor carpi radialis longus and brevis) must be interpreted carefully as it is normally a sensitive region. The course of the posterior interosseous nerve can be palpated. The infracondylar recess is palpated for an effusion or synovitis, and occasionally bony debris can also be palpated at this site.

The radial head is best appreciated while supinating and pronating the forearm.

The most frequent congenital abnormality of the elbow is a radial head dislocation,[3,4] of which 50% are bilateral.[5] The condition is often associated with overall shortening of the forearm. When this is present other abnormalities and dysmorphic features that frequently occur with it should be looked for as part of the examination.

Radial head dislocation acquired in childhood may closely resemble congenital radial head dislocation.[6]

The distinction between the congenital condition and a longstanding missed Monteggia fracture dislocation is not always easily made. Volar angulation (posterior bow) deformity of the ulna is usually associated with posterior subluxation or dislocation of the radial head. Midshaft ulnar bowing is usually apparent but deformity close to the elbow joint may be difficult to discern. If suspected, the patient should be examined prone. Patients with cerebral palsy often have a flexed pronated forearm, with an associated posterior dislocation of the radial head.

The most common fracture about the elbow is that of the radial head. It is associated with point tenderness, a haemarthrosis and pain on movements. Malunion of a radial head fracture may result in loss of full elbow extension and often restriction of forearm rotation. A palpable prominence over the radial head, or apparent enlargement of the radial head may suggest a 'stellate' or comminuted fracture. If the malunion has resulted

Table 4.2 Causes of an enlarged radial head

Post-surgical in a growing child
Post-traumatic (radial head fracture, lateral condyle fracture, heterotopic ossiffication)
Synovitis producing epiphyseal overgrowth (e.g. haemophilia)
Synovitis of chronic inflammatory disease (e.g. rheumatoid arthritis)
Osteoarthritis (hypertrophic)
Osteochondroma (sessile or pedunculated)
Developmental (type 1 chronic posterior subluxation of the radial head)
Tumours (giant cell tumours, aneurysmal bone cyst, fibrous dysplasia)

in an eccentrically increased diameter of the radial head, camming of the radial head may occur at the radioulnar articulation with restriction of forearm rotation. Gross radiocapitellar crepitus suggests a significant step in the articular surface or an occult osteochondral lesion of the capitellum. Such lesions often lodge in the coronoid fossa and may produce a mechanical block to full flexion. The causes of an enlarged radial head are shown in Table 4.2. Clinically the enlargement is usually readily apparent on palpation and rotation of the forearm.

MEDIAL

The medial epicondyle, ulnar nerve and medial collateral ligament are the next structures to be palpated. Enlargement of the medial epicondyle may result from a childhood fracture, and as on the lateral side an ununited fracture may result in a mobile bony fragment which lies anteromedial to the distal humerus.

The ulnar nerve is best identified proximal to the cubital tunnel, and then followed distally through the groove and between the two heads of flexor carpi ulnaris. Compression may occur at multiple sites. Ulnar neuritis is often seen in association with other conditions (osteoarthritis, rheumatoid arthritis, medial epicondylitis, elbow instability and fracture dislocations), and these should be sought. In addition any adjacent surgical scars should be reviewed to exclude iatrogenic causes. Common compression sites include the cubital tunnel and between the two heads of the flexor carpi ulnaris. Ulnar nerve irritation is demonstrated by a Tinel's sign, which is usually best elicited at the point of maximal nerve tenderness.

An enlarged ulnar nerve suggests a peripheral neuropathy and a general neurological examination should be undertaken.

In certain situations, gross displacement of the ulnar nerve needs to be considered. If the ulnar nerve has been mobilised as part of a previous surgical procedure, such as in attempted salvage of gross valgus deformity, the nerve may spontaneously displace lateral to the olecranon and lie over the posterior aspect of the elbow well away from its anatomical position. Similarly, the possibility of the nerve having been transposed anteriorly should be entertained whenever a surgical scar is evident on the medial or posterior aspect of the elbow.

The common flexor muscles should then be palpated. Tenderness over the belly of pronator teres may suggest a diagnosis of the pronator syndrome (Chapter 21).

ANTERIOR

When examining the anterior aspect of the elbow it is important to appreciate that the skin flexion crease is approximately 1cm distal to the joint axis.

Structures that can be palpated anteriorly include: the brachioradialis, the lateral cutaneous nerve of the forearm, the biceps tendon and the lacertus fibrosus, the brachial artery (medial to the biceps tendon), the median nerve (medial to the artery) and the anterior surface of the brachialis (deep to biceps).

POSTERIOR

Viewed from behind with the elbow extended, the tip of the olecranon process and the medial and lateral epicondyles form a straight line (Fig. 4.3A). With the elbow flexed to 90 degrees these landmarks form an isosceles triangle, with the base perpendicular to the long axis of the limb (Fig. 4.3B). Palpation of these three points allows assessment of malunions and non-unions of the supracondylar and intercondylar region. A grossly prominent olecranon process suggests a posterior dislocation of the elbow.

The olecranon fossa is palpated with the elbow flexed to 30 degrees. This unlocks the olecranon from the fossa. Further flexion produces overtensioning of the triceps tendon and interferes with palpation. The triceps insertion is readily palpable on the olecranon. Partial rupture of the tendon may be difficult to detect, except for localised tenderness or a mobile flake of bone. An inability to extend the elbow, in the presence of a contracting

(a)

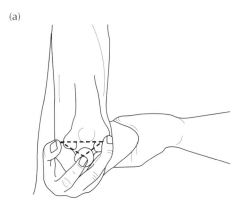

(b)

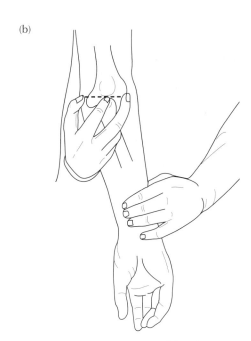

Fig. 4.3 The normal orientation of the olecranon process and medial and lateral epicondyles. (a) With the elbow extended a straight line is formed. (b) With the elbow flexed an isosceles triangle is produced.

triceps muscle belly and a palpable defect indicates complete rupture (Chapter 16).

The olecranon bursa overlies the olecranon process and proximal ulna and is the largest of the bursae described around the elbow (Chapter 2). It is a frequent site of pathology.

Painless swelling of the bursa may be associated with a bony spur at the triceps insertion. The bursa may fill with debris, in which case palpation produces crepitus. Sepsis of the bursa is not uncommon, particularly following trauma or surgery. If sepsis is suspected, aspiration and laboratory examination may be indicated. Even in the presence of septic bursitis, the elbow joint may have a good range of movement, distinguishing the condition from septic arthritis (Chapter 29). Solid gouty tophi may also be present in the olecranon bursa, with the diagnosis usually being apparent in the context of systemic disease.

PALPATION – SWELLING OF THE ELBOW

The position of maximal joint volume is 80 degrees of flexion.[7] If a tense effusion or haemarthrosis is present, such as following an intra-articular fracture, the elbow will assume this position, to minimise discomfort. If the capsule has been breached, however, the intra-articular pressure is released. Extensive haematoma and swelling occur and the range of comfortable movement is paradoxically increased.

Subtle effusions are best detected by looking for the sulcus of the infracondylar recess. The recess is sited distal to the lateral condyle, adjacent to the lateral aspect of the olecranon and the radial head. It is obliterated by intra-articular distension, regardless of whether this is fluid or synovium.

Mild synovitis may be palpated in the infracondylar recess laterally. If the synovitis is extensive (e.g. inflammatory arthropathies), the proliferative synovium may track beneath the annular ligament and extend along the radial neck and interosseous membrane. It may occasionally produce a posterior interosseous nerve lesion and a soft-tissue forearm mass. If there is synovial crepitus distal to the radial head the extensive nature of the synovitis should be assessed further with ultrasound or computed tomography (CT). The same process can produce a large antecubital cyst. Proliferative synovitis can occasionally become intraosseous and produce a pathological fracture of the olecranon or one of the condyles (usually capitellum). For this reason tenderness over the proximal olecranon should be assessed radiologically.

Synovitis may occasionally produce elbow instability secondary to ligament attrition, but instability in inflammatory disease results more commonly from loss of bony architecture. Instability signs in patients with inflammatory arthropathies are usually associated with joint crepitus.

RANGE OF MOVEMENT

The humeroulnar joint is a modified hinge allowing flexion and extension together with a small amount of internal and external rotation. Clinically the range of movement can be measured in a highly reproducible manner, with a goniometer. With both forearms supinated the extremes of active and passive flexion and extension can be demonstrated. The normal elbow extends to 0 degrees and flexes to 140 degrees (± 10 degrees). Hyperextension is recorded as a negative integer. If hyperextension is greater than 10 degrees, it suggests hypermobility or periarticular deformity. A loss of full extension is often the earliest sign of an intra-articular elbow problem.

Both elbows should always be compared since even subtle unilateral loss of range of movement is significant. The post-traumatic stiff elbow usually has an extra-articular aetiology with a restricted, but pain-free range of movement. The presence of pain should suggest an additional intra-articular component.

A discrepancy between the passive and active range of movement suggests a loss of strength due to a neurological lesion or musculotendinous complex rupture. Gross differences in range of movement obtained in the examination room and under anaesthetic suggest a reflex pain inhibition or a conversion reaction.

FOREARM ROTATION

Forearm rotation is demonstrated by flexing both elbows to 90 degrees, whilst adducting the arms to the body to block any compensatory shoulder movements. Passive and active rotation of the distal radius and ulna is then assessed and any associated crepitus noted. Supination is generally greater than pronation; 85 degrees of supination and slightly less pronation is normal, but considerable variation occurs. Where pronation or supination is abnormal, the other joints of both upper limbs should be assessed. The functional significance of any reduction of range is dependent upon the normality or otherwise of these adjacent joints. For example, a partially recovered Erb's palsy may leave an internal rotation deformity of the shoulder in association with a flexion contracture of the elbow, exacerbating the functional deficit of restricted supination.

AXIAL ALIGNMENT

The normal carrying angle varies with gender, averaging 10 degrees valgus for males and 13 degrees valgus for females.[8,9] The angle can only be adequately assessed with the elbow in full extension. A flexion deformity may hide angulatory pathology, and hyperextension may give the impression of deformity. Valgus angulation beyond the normal carrying angle may be the result of an epiphyseal plate injury or abnormality, lateral condyle non-union, local impaction associated with a childhood supracondylar fracture, or valgus overload and local growth retardation in the developing skeleton. Varus deformity detected in full elbow extension is always abnormal and may result from malunion of a supracondylar fracture, or growth arrest on the medial side of the distal humerus.

Morrey and Chow[10] have shown that flexion of the normal elbow is accompanied by a change from valgus to a few degrees of varus. Any shortening of the lateral or medial supracondylar column of the humerus produces not only a change in the carrying angle in full extension but also a change in the axis of rotation of elbow flexion. Consequently shortening of the lateral column (such as following a lateral condyle non-union) results not only in increased valgus with the arm extended but also increased varus with elbow flexion. Shortening of the medial supracondylar column produces the opposite effect. Bowing of the long bones of the upper limb, such as may occur in Paget's disease, also alters the alignment of the elbow joint.

ROTATIONAL DEFORMITY

Rotational deformity is often overlooked. Rotation may occur either at the shoulder joint or 'in the humerus'. If both shoulders are normal, asymmetrical ranges of rotation indicate humeral rotational deformity. This deformity is elegantly demonstrated by the technique described by Yamamoto *et al.*[11] (Fig. 4.4).

The examiner stands behind the patient with the elbow at 90 degrees and the forearm behind their back. The patient bends forward whilst the shoulder is held in full extension. Each shoulder is maximally internally rotated. Increased internal rotation is measured as the angle between the forearm and the horizon of the back. It is frequently increased in malunited supracondylar fractures. A supracondylar fracture with internal rotation greater than 45 degrees, may demonstrate bony impingement of the medial supracondylar ridge on the coronoid, blocking elbow flexion at approximately 90 degrees.

FOREARM LENGTH AND RADIOULNAR DISSOCIATION

Radial head pathology, including resection, subluxation and dislocation, may be associated with radioulnar dissociation. In the acute episode, with failure of the radial head, the line of injury may pass through the radiocapitellar joint, along the interosseous membrane to the distal radioulnar joint. As well as the obvious elbow injury (e.g. radial head fracture or dislocation), the distal radioulnar joint and interosseous membrane may also be damaged. Thus, a distal radioulnar joint disruption is highly significant. With the normal wrist in neutral rotation, a significant amount of anteroposterior translocation of the distal ulna relative to the radius is possible because of the diametral mismatch of the sigmoid notch of the radius and the head of the ulna. This translocation is significantly reduced by full

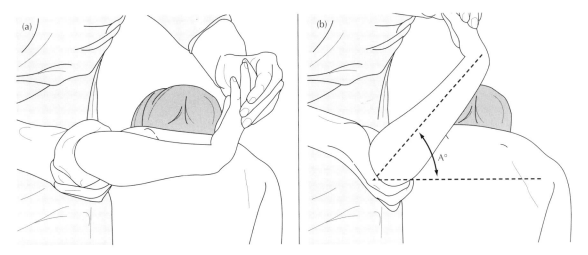

Fig. 4.4 The assessment of rotational deformity. The patient is bent forward whilst fully extending the shoulder. With the elbow flexed to 90 degrees the forearm is normally parallel to the ground (a). If there is increased internal rotation in the humerus then the acute angle between the axis of the forearm and the horizontal is a measure of the internal rotation deformity (b).

pronation or supination, which wind up the ligament complexes. Loss of this mechanism may indicate a distal radioulnar joint disruption. Other signs of distal radioulnar joint pathology include an 'ulna plus' deformity at the wrist and dorsal subluxation of the distal ulna. Carpal impingement is associated with pain on ulnar deviation or wrist pronation (which produces ulnar lengthening) and restriction of forearm rotation.

If signs of a distal radioulnar joint derangement occur in the presence of a radial head fracture or dislocation, acute radioulnar dissociation should be suspected. Early diagnosis of this condition allows early treatment which improves the prognosis. If, however, the injury occurs prior to skeletal maturity and is unrecognised, secondary changes occur in the forearm bones which can be very difficult to treat when eventually the problem is appreciated.

STENGTH

Four basic tests can be used to assess strength about the elbow. They provide only a gross estimate but this is usually sufficient for clinical needs. For research purposes more accurate and quantitative assessment can be undertaken.

Flexion is tested with the elbow flexed to 90 degrees and the forearm in neutral rotation. Flexion is then resisted. At the same time the biceps tendon should be observed for any loss of continuity. Extension is tested in a similar position but in the reverse direction. If extension is very weak then gravity should be excluded or the arm placed overhead and extension tested against gravity. Flexion is usually stronger than extension in the normal limb.

Testing forearm rotation is performed with the elbow flexed to 90 degrees and in neutral rotation. Pronation and supination are resisted by fixing the forearm at the wrist. Normally supination is slightly stronger than pronation.

Provocation manoeuvres and tests for common conditions

Provocation tests are applied to support or exclude specific diagnoses.

LATERAL EPICONDYLITIS

The lateral musculotendinous unit is highly susceptible to overuse and tension overload injuries, especially in middle-aged athletes. Lateral epicondylitis

may present as an acute, chronic or acute-on-chronic condition. If acute it may be associated with localised swelling and heat. Range of movement is often normal, although there may be pain at extremes of extension.[12]

- Tenderness is localised to a point a few millimetres anterior and superior to the lateral epicondyle, in the region of the attachment of the extensor carpi radialis brevis. Although some discomfort can be felt posterior to the epicondyle, tenderness is never elicited here unless the triceps tendon is involved.
- Passive volar flexion of the wrist with elbow extension and pronation causes pain localised to the lateral epicondyle.
- Resisted extensor carpi radialis brevis (wrist extension in neutral) and extensor digitorum communis (middle finger extension), and to a lesser extent extensor carpi radialis longus (wrist extension in radial deviation) cause pain localised to the lateral aspect of the elbow (Fig. 4.5).
- Pinch grip, especially between thumb and middle finger, is often painfully weak.
- Injection of 2 ml of 1% lignocaine to the attachment of extensor carpi radialis brevis (i.e. an extra-articular injection) produces significant reduction in signs for the duration of the local anaesthetic.

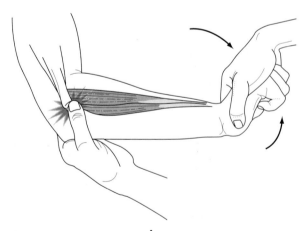

Fig. 4.5 The lateral epicondylitis provocation sign. Resisted wrist extension results in localised pain over the lateral epicondyle.

MEDIAL EPICONDYLITIS

The medial musculotendinous unit is susceptible to injury. Medial and lateral symptoms often co-exist and either may predominate.

- Tenderness is localised to the tendinous attachment of the common flexor origin to the medial epicondyle, usually within the pronator teres or flexor carpi radialis.
- Resisted wrist flexion or a tightly clenched fist causes pain.
- Passive extension of the wrist and elbow causes pain at the medial epicondyle.

There may be secondary limitation of movement.

- Ulnar neuritis may be present.
- It should be noted that the valgus stress test does not cause pain.

BICEPS PATHOLOGY AT THE ELBOW (DISTAL BICEPS TENDINITIS, PARTIAL AND COMPLETE TEAR)

Biceps rupture at the elbow is not uncommon (Chapter 16). The disruption usually occurs at the attachment of the tendon to the radial tuberosity, although it can occur in the mid-substance of the tendon or at the musculotendinous junction. Both complete and partial ruptures occur.[13] Most occur acutely, although occasionally the rupture can be preceded by weeks or months of elbow discomfort. It is usually produced by a sudden eccentric flexion contraction. At the time of injury, acute pain is experienced in the middle of the cubital fossa, and if treatment is delayed, a chronic ache develops. The muscle belly retracts proximally, leaving a palpable defect. The biceps tendon is normally palpable during elbow flexion. If it is ruptured, the tendon cannot be felt, although medially, the lacertus fibrosus may still be intact and palpable. This can be differentiated from the biceps tendon by its diffuse and superficial insertion into the forearm fascia.

A complete tear of the biceps is associated with weakness of supination. With the elbow at 90 degrees, however, the patient may still have more than 50% of normal supination strength. Elbow flexion is also weakened, but to a lesser extent. In cases of partial rupture, which may precede total disruption, the tenderness is localised to the radial tuberosity. This is best palpated by flexing the elbow, maximally pronating the arm, and palpating the tuberosity from the dorsal aspect of the forearm. This area is normally moderately tender and comparison should be made with the asymptomatic side before pathology is diagnosed. Not surprisingly, resisted supination and passive stretch of the tendon by elbow extension and pronation, also cause pain. Occasionally, a sensation of crepitus can be detected with repeated pronation and supination of the elbow in 90 degrees of flexion.

If a partial tear is suspected, selective local anaesthetic injection to the region of the radial tuberosity, may aid diagnosis. This is performed by passing the needle from the volar aspect, along the radial border of the tendon on to the radial tuberosity under x-ray or CT control. Although the injection relieves pain, it does not restore strength, enabling differentiation between tendon pathology and radial tuberosity bursitis. In the latter condition, when the local anaesthetic eliminates pain, strength is temporarily restored.

BRACHIALIS FASCIITIS

Certain athletic and recreational pursuits, such as mountain climbing or gymnastics, involve repetitive eccentric brachialis contraction. Brachialis tension is maintained, while allowing the elbow to extend in weight-bearing situations. Anteromedial elbow pain may occur, associated with resisted elbow flexion. Tenderness is present over the brachialis fascia on the anterior aspect of the muscle belly. This is felt behind the biceps tendon from the medial side. This site is well proximal to that of biceps rupture, and the fasciitis may be distinguished from a partial disruption of the biceps by selective local anaesthetic injection to the site of tenderness. The local anaesthetic at this site relieves the pain of the fasciitis, but not that of biceps disruption. Entrapment of the lateral cutaneous nerve of the forearm is differentiated by its tenderness at the lateral border of the biceps tendon which is quite localised and occasionally associated with distal paraesthesia or numbness.

ELBOW INSTABILITY

The understanding of elbow instability is evolving. Various patterns occur, possibly representing variations of a basic injury mechanism. O'Driscoll and co-workers[14] have presented a concept of elbow instability as a circle of soft tissue injury from lateral to medial, occurring in three stages. Although this may be an oversimplification, this concept allows an appreciation of the different instabilities produced by various combinations of ligament injuries (Chapter 15).

Stage 1   The ulnar part of the lateral collateral ligament is disrupted resulting in posterolateral subluxation which self reduces.

Stage 2   The disruption extends medially, both posteriorly and anteriorly but not involving the medial collateral ligament. This permits incomplete dislocation, with the coronoid process perched in the trochlea groove. This can be easily reduced by the patient.

Stage 3A   All structures around to and including the posterior bundle of the medial collateral ligament are disrupted. This permits posterolateral rotatory dislocation. The intact anterior bundle of the medial collateral ligament provides valgus stability, and the elbow is stable as long as the forearm is pronated.

Stage 3B   The entire medial collateral ligament complex is disrupted. The elbow is unstable in extension.

Instability can also be classified in terms of directional failure with valgus, posterolateral rotatory and varus instability being the most common.

VALGUS INSTABILITY

The anterior bundle of the medial collateral ligament is the primary valgus stabiliser of the elbow with the radial head acting as a secondary stabiliser.[15] Failure of the ligament either acutely or via attenuation gives rise to instability. Throwing athletes (especially those with ligamentous laxity) are at high risk of valgus or medial overload injuries.

Valgus stability is assessed with the trunk of the patient fixed and the shoulder maximally externally rotated. The elbow is flexed to 30 degrees to unlock the olecranon from the olecranon fossa and minimise the contribution of bony congruity to stability. As a valgus force is applied, the medial collateral ligament is palpated and local tenderness and laxity noted (Fig. 4.6).

Tenderness is usually felt over the medial collateral ligament especially at its distal insertion. Infrequently the tenderness is proximal, and in this situation an unfused medial apophysis should be suspected. Laxity is usually graded according to severity. Grade I 0–5 mm, Grade II 5–10 mm and Grade III more than 10 mm. Occasionally crepitus may be felt at the medial collateral ligament as the elbow is flexed and extended. This may indicate calcific deposits within the medial collateral ligament complex. There may be a localised Tinel's sign.

Posterior impingement secondary to valgus instability should also be evaluated. This can be determined during testing for valgus instability since, if present, pain and crepitus will be produced as the elbow is extended. This same manoeuvre is much more sensitive under x-ray control. Subtle forms of valgus instability may be best appreciated at arthroscopy during this manoeuvre.

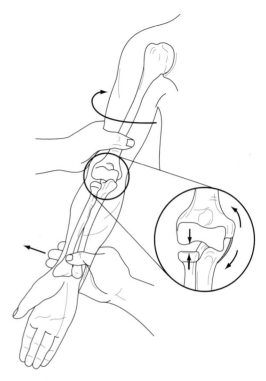

Fig. 4.6 Valgus instability is demonstrated with the valgus stress test. With the elbow flexed 30 degrees, and the shoulder fully externally rotated a valgus force is applied to the elbow. Redrawn after Ref. 18 with permission from WB Saunders Company, Philadelphia.

Increasing laxity of the anterior bundle of the medial collateral ligament results in progressive valgus deformity. A flexion contracture of the elbow may develop together with secondary degenerative changes which primarily affect the radiocapitellar joint.

Sometimes it can be difficult to distinguish between valgus instability and posterolateral instability. Such a situation can be clarified by performing the valgus stress test with the forearm in pronation. This manoeuvre obliterates any posterolateral instability allowing the distinction to be made.

POSTEROLATERAL ROTATORY INSTABILITY

This instability should be considered if there has been a history of trauma (sprain or full dislocation), recurrent locking or clunking, or if it has occurred following lateral release or radial head excision. There is also a subgroup of people with ligamentous laxity who also develop this form of instability following a

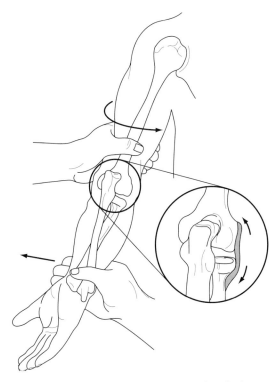

Fig. 4.7 Varus instability is demonstrated with the varus stress test. With the elbow flexed 30 degrees the shoulder is fully internally rotated to fix the humerus and a varus force is applied. Redrawn after Ref. 18 with permission from WB Saunders Company, Philadelphia.

traumatic dislocation. The lateral humeroulnar ligament, part of the lateral collateral ligament complex is the primary posterolateral stabiliser.[14]

Posterolateral rotatory instability of the elbow is demonstrated with the lateral pivot shift test. The patient lies supine with the arm overhead. A combination of axial compression, as well as valgus and supination moments are applied to rotate and subluxate the humeroulnar joint. These forces are maintained from a fully extended position and when the elbow flexes past a certain point (usually 30 to 60 degrees) it reduces with a palpable clunk (Fig. 4.2). Most people, however, demonstrate marked apprehension before allowing this degree of subluxation. The execution of this manoeuvre is virtually identical to the pivot shift of the knee if performed with the patient lying and the arm elevated overhead.[14] This test is more dramatic and sensitive if performed as part of an examination under anaesthetic with x-ray control. The sign is obliterated if the arm is pronated. In the more severe form of this instability, flexion extension is not required and pure forearm supination in 90 degrees of flexion is all that is required to demon-

strate the ulna rotating off the humerus (this is best seen in the lateral projection using an image intensifier). Dislocation with transient locking of the radial head behind the capitellum may produce a wedge-shaped defect in the posterior aspect of the capitellum, analogous to the Hills–Sachs lesion of the humeral head. (This lesion is visible radiographically, and may occasionally be palpable.)

Sometimes the lateral pivot shift test produces pain or apprehension without an obvious 'clunk'. In this situation the symptoms may be due to pathology at or adjacent to the inferior or posteroinferior aspect of the capitellum, rather than instability. If there is a bony abnormality at that site, it may impinge on the rim of the radial head, producing pain during the pivot shift manoeuvre. Similarly, following dislocation, osteochondral debris can collect at that site, with the same effect. These problems can be excluded by radiology (plain film, tomogram or CT scan) and a careful examination under anaesthetic.

VARUS INSTABILITY

The radial collateral ligament part of the lateral collateral ligament complex is the main varus stabiliser of the elbow. It is demonstrated by fully internally rotating the glenohumeral joint and flexing the elbow joint to unlock the olecranon. A varus stress is applied to the elbow, and any opening of the lateral joint space noted (Fig. 4.7). The degree of laxity is best quantitated with x-ray control.

Impingement

Impingement of the olecranon process occurs in a variety of settings, including instability, osteoarthritis and following hyperextension injury. In valgus instability, the impingement is generally posteromedial. Hyperextension, particularly with repetitive extension overload activities (as in tennis and throwing) produces a similar effect. Osteophytic encroachment of the olecranon fossa produces impingement wherever the osteophytes meet. Loose bodies may produce a similar result.

To elicit impingement, the end point of elbow extension should be noted. A gentle push beyond that end point reproduces the patients symptoms. To demonstrate posteromedial impingement a slight valgus load should be added to the extension force. Tenderness may be present along the posteromedial joint line or, with the elbow flexed, in the olecranon fossa. Occasionally loose bodies may be palpated, anteriorly or posteriorly, with associated palpable synovial hypertrophy. A history of occasional locking caused by the loose bodies, aids this diagnosis, and ulnar nerve symptoms and signs are not uncommon.

Anterior osteophyte formation can produce impingement in front of the elbow, between the enlarged coronoid process and the obliterated coronoid fossa. Occasionally the small radial fossa superior to the anterior aspect of the capitellum may fill with osteophytes, and impingement may occur with the radial head, in full flexion. The differentiation between anterior coronoid impingement and anterior radial head impingement is clinically very difficult and is best made radiologically. Either type of anterior impingement is associated with some loss of elbow flexion, and anterior pain on gentle pushing beyond the comfortable extreme of flexion.

Diffuse anterior or posterior compartment osteophytosis produces progressive loss of movement. Initially there is loss of full extension, due to both bony block and also secondary capsular fibrosis. Pain in the mid-range of elbow movement is a late sign of osteoarthritis and is usually of an aching character. Multiple loose bodies suggest a diagnosis of synovial osteochondromatosis or, if the elbow is grossly deranged, a neuropathic joint.

Articular abnormalities involving the humeroulnar and radiocapitellar joints

Assessment of the articular surfaces is enhanced by considering the medial and lateral compartments separately. It is usually possible to clinically distinguish between radiocapitellar and humeroulnar symptoms. When radiology shows diffuse pathology, it is important to determine which compartment, lateral or medial, is responsible for symptoms. If the symptoms are localised, significant benefit may be achieved by minor surgical intervention, which can avoid or postpone a major reconstruction. Where osteochondral pathology exists, clinical assessment aids both the diagnosis and selection of treatment.

Valgus stress testing can provoke radiocapitellar symptoms. The site and extent of pathology can be assessed by the arc of crepitus on flexion and extension. If the patient 'makes a fist', this increases the compressive force across the radiocapitellar joint. If this manoeuvre increases pain or crepitus it is of further localising value. There may be tenderness along the joint line, and the anterior and posterior

aspects of the capitellum may be palpated with the elbow extended and flexed, respectively. Some radiocapitellar lesions can be palpated.

Medial compartment (humeroulnar) articular lesions may be assessed by noting pain and crepitus throughout flexion and extension, particularly when performed against resistance in the plane of the arm. This may be achieved by asking the patient to hold a weight in the hand while flexing and extending the elbow. The increased load increases the forces across the joint, compressing the surfaces. Gross loss of bony architecture can produce 'pseudo instability' in the presence of intact collateral ligaments (e.g. rheumatoid disease).

Selective injections to differentiate or confirm diagnoses

Diagnostic selective injections of local anaesthetic to special sites about the elbow may be helpful if doubt exists as to the clinical diagnosis.

Generally the first step is to identify whether the problem is intra- or extra-articular. This can be acertained by intra-articular injection of local anaesthetic at the infracondylar recess. With this clarified the most common use of injection techniques is in the assessment of lateral elbow pain.[16] Less frequently, selective injections may be valuable in the investigation of pain at other sites (Table 4.3).

Small volumes (approx 1–3 ml) of lignocaine are necessary to avoid diffusion and more distant anaesthetic effects. Accurate injection is essential and this can be best achieved by the use of x-ray or CT control.

Table 4.3 Selective local anaesthetic injections in the assessment of elbow pain

The differentiation of extra or intra-articular problems:
Lateral epicondylitis
Revision lateral release
Posterior interosseous nerve entrapment
Lateral cutaneous nerve of the forearm entrapment
Radial tuberosity bursitis/partial biceps tendon tear
Brachialis fasciitis
Partial triceps avulsion
Wound neuromas

Neurological assessment

Examination of the elbow should always include a neurological assessment of the upper limb. This is important since elbow pain may at times be referred from more proximal structures – classically the neck. In addition, entrapment neuropathies are not uncommon and should always be considered whenever the elbow is examined (Chapter 21). Primary neurological disorders may also affect the elbow and although uncommon must not be forgotten as a cause of elbow dysfunction (Chapter 22).

Clinical assessment of the patient with a total elbow arthroplasty

The clinical assessment of patients following total elbow arthroplasty may be undertaken at routine follow-up, for the assessment of instability, or after the sudden or gradual development of pain or loss of strength.

Assessment of the painful total elbow arthroplasty is difficult. In this particular situation it is advisable to obtain new radiographs before any provocative manoeuvres are undertaken. The examiner must be absolutely certain whether the arthroplasty is constrained, semi-constrained or unconstrained before physical examination. While documentation of range of movement, including flexion–extension and pronation–supination is important, it should be remembered that a successful elbow arthroplasty is not necessarily associated with a 'full range of movement'. Recent change in range is more significant than the absolute range.

The stability of the prosthesis should be assessed. With unconstrained prostheses, instability is usually self-evident, and provocation manoeuvres should be undertaken only with extreme caution, ideally under x-ray control. If a translocation (subluxation or dislocation) of the articulation has occurred there is often surprisingly little pain. Flexion may be near normal but extension is both weak and restricted.

If a patient presents with a dislocated elbow arthroplasty which is reducible under anaesthetic, the opportunity should be taken to assess under x-ray control whether the instability is due to primary ligamentous pathology (medial, lateral or combined insufficiency), component placement, or loosening.

Triceps function following total elbow arthroplasty is variable and important. Different surgical approaches produce different end-results, and many patients undergoing total elbow arthroplasty do not regain normal or even near normal triceps strength. It is important to ask the patient whether there has been a recent loss of strength. Patients with constrained and semi-constrained prostheses may achieve reasonable function with almost no elbow extensors, by using gravity to extend the elbow. In these situations, however, progressive flexion contractures often occur. With unconstrained and some semi-constrained prostheses, loss of triceps integrity may precipitate instability.

If prosthetic loosening is suspected, the joint should be put through gentle anterior and posterior draw tests, and repeated resisted elbow flexion. These manoeuvres can produce toggling of the components and reproduce pain, suggesting prosthetic loosening. Pain or tenderness at a site corresponding to the proximal end of the humeral component or the distal end of the ulnar stem suggests impending periprosthetic fracture and requires a check radiograph.

If sepsis is suspected the usual laboratory tests should be undertaken with urgency. Redness or swelling overlying any part of the elbow should be viewed with suspicion. An inflamed or swollen olecranon bursa in particular, even without discharge, should be regarded as evidence of an infected underlying total elbow arthroplasty until proven otherwise.

Whenever examining a total elbow arthroplasty, the position and function of the ulnar nerve should be reviewed and recorded. In addition it is important to know whether or not the nerve was transposed at the time of surgery.

Assessment of disability

Traditionally, scoring systems have been used to measure the results of elbow surgery, particularly arthroplasty. More recently, there has been a trend towards the use of outcome criteria rather than scores in the assessment of surgical results. The reasons behind this are several. The criteria sought depend upon the condition being treated. Outcome studies also assess the benefit or otherwise of surgery in restoring or enabling basic functions, such as combing the hair, using a knife and fork normally or dressing independently. Potential patients concerns are more meaningfully addressed if patients can be told the likelihood of regaining certain functions than if they are told what an average increase in elbow score might be for a proposed procedure. Outcome studies will provide patients with hard data on which to base their choice of treatment. With funding for medical services becoming increasingly scarce in many societies, it is important to be able to quantitate and present the potential benefits of surgery in a comprehensible and palatable form. Outcome studies are particularly appropriate for this purpose.

The daily activities which we assess depend on the function of the upper limb as a unit. Positioning the hand in space depends on both the shoulder and elbow. To some extent, a normal shoulder can accommodate some loss of elbow function, and vice versa. Whilst the loss of a few degrees of elbow extension might not dramatically alter a patient's 'sphere of reach', the loss of 45 degrees of elbow flexion has a significant effect. In particular, the shoulder and elbow combine to place the hand on the head, to the mouth, or to the perineum. It is because of this association between shoulder and elbow function, that we have found the 'simple shoulder test' popularised by Matsen and co-workers to be valuable in the assessment of altered upper limb function.[17] The Mayo elbow evaluation[18] is a simple means of assessing basic functions of the upper limb, as it incorporates this simple test and also range of movement, strength, stability and pain. Questions may be asked of the patient directly, or may be presented in the form of a short questionnaire to be filled out prior to consultation.

Questions used to assess elbow function should address multiple parameters, including pain, range of motion, stability, strength and function, as well as patient satisfaction. It is often useful to employ linear analogue scales (0–10) to help patients quantitate symptoms, especially pain. While it is scientifically desirable to quantitate the strength (and changes in strength) of various movements, including flexion, extension, pronation and supination, this is often not practicable in a clinical setting. If available, spring tensiometers and grip-strength measurements can provide a more objective assessment.

Clinicians are frequently asked to assess impairment or disability for medico-legal purposes. Some jurisdictions rely on predetermined guidelines, which vary in the USA for example, from State to State. Impairment is 'the alteration of an individual's health status, as assessed by medical means' while disability is 'assessed by non-medical means, and is an alteration of an individual's capacity to meet personal, social or occupational demands or statutory or regulatory requirements'.[19] The American Medical Association has provided guidelines to help estimate percentage disability of elbow function. These take into account range of movement, neurovascular abnormalities, bone and joint deformities, joint instability and weakness. Whilst discussion of medico-legal assessment is beyond the brief of this publication, interested readers are referred to *Guides to the evaluation of permanent impairment* (American Medical Association).[19]

References

1. Andrews JR, Whiteside JA Common elbow problems in the athlete. *J Orthop Sports Phys Ther* 1993; **6:** 289–95.
2. Beighton P, Graham R, Bird H *Hypermobility of joints.* Berlin: Springer-Verlag 1983.
3. Fox KW, Griffin LL Congenital dislocation of the radial head. *Clin Orthop* 1960; **18:** 234–43.
4. Mardam-Bey T, Ger E Congenital radial head dislocation. *J Hand Surg* 1979; **4:** 316–20.
5. Almquist EE, Gordon LH, Blue AL Congenital dislocation of the head of the radius. *J Bone Joint Surg (Am)* 1969; **51A:** 1118–27.
6. Good CJ, Wicks MH Developmental posterior dislocation of the radial head. *J Bone Joint Surg (Br)* 1983; **65B:** 64–5.
7. O'Driscoll SW, Morrey BF, An Kn Intra-articular pressure and capacity of the elbow. *Arthroscopy* 1990; **6:** 100–3.
8. Beals RK The normal carrying angle of the elbow. *Clin Orthop* 1976; **119:** 194–6.
9. Keats TE, Teeslink R, Diamond AE, Williams JH Normal axial relationships of the major joints. *Radiology* 1966; **87:** 904–7.
10. Morrey BF, Chow EY Passive motion of the elbow joint. *J Bone Joint Surg (Am)* 1976; **58A:** 501–8.
11. Yamamoto I, Ishii S, Usui M, Ogino T, Kaneda K Cubitus varus deformity following supracondylar fracture of the humerus: a method for measuring rotational deformity. *Clin Orthop* 1985; **201:** 179–85.
12. Nirschl RP Elbow tendinosis/tennis elbow. *Clin Sports Med* 1992; **4:** 851–70.
13. Bourne MH, Morrey BF Partial rupture of the distal biceps tendon. *Clin Orthop* 1991; **271:** 143–8.
14. O'Driscoll SW, Morrey BF, Korinek S, An KN Elbow subluxation and dislocation: A spectrum of instability. *Clin Orthop* 1992; **280:** 186–97.
15. Morrey BF, An KN, Tanaka S Valgus stability of the elbow. A definition of primary and secondary constraints. *Clin Orthop* 1991; **265:** 187–95.
16. Morrey BF Reoperation for failed surgical treatment of refractory lateral epicondylitis. *J Shoulder Elbow Surg* 1992; **1:** 47.
17. Matsen FA, Foo FH, Hawkins RJ The shoulder: A balance of mobility and stability. *Am Acad Orthop Surg* 1993; 501–18.
18. Morrey BF, An KN, Chao EYS Functional evaluation of the elbow. In: *The Elbow and its Disorders.* Morrey BF (ed) Philadelphia: WB Saunders Co, 1993: 86–97.
19. American Medical Association: *Guides to the evaluation of permanent impairment* (3rd edn). Washington: AMA, 1990.

CHAPTER 5

Imaging of the elbow

VN CASSAR-PULLICINO, IW MCCALL

Introduction

Despite the expansion of various imaging techniques, evaluation of the elbow joint still relies heavily on routine radiographic procedures. Plain radiographs are the most cost effective initial approach to diagnostic imaging. They provide information on the bone and joint components, and their respective relationships in the static state. Ectopic calcification, loose bodies and soft tissue swelling may also be clearly identified.

For further investigation, fluoroscopy, tomography, computed tomography (CT), arthrography, and ultrasound, have been shown to be of value. These techniques, however, should only be undertaken to answer specific diagnostic questions. In addition it is essential that the investigator is well aware of the complex anatomy of the elbow in order to allow accurate interpretation of abnormal findings.

Radiographic anatomy

The elbow joint is a complex synovial joint comprising the humeroulnar, humeroradial, and the proximal radioulnar joints. The articular surfaces of the distal humerus (capitellum and trochlea) are convex, while those of the radius and ulna are concave. The subchondral bone is covered by hyaline cartilage. It is important to recognize that the apex of the coronoid process is also covered by cartilage and is not the site of attachment of the capsule or brachialis muscle both of which attach slightly more distally. A fracture of the coronoid process ('beak') indicates intra-articular trauma due to dislocation and not avulsive injury (Fig. 5.1).

The coronoid and radial fossae are indentations on the anterior aspect of the distal humerus which receive the coronoid process of the ulna and radial head respectively when the elbow is flexed, while the posterior olecranon fossa receives the olecranon process of the ulna when the elbow is fully extended. The elbow fat pads are lodged in these fossae (Fig. 5.2) and are dynamically involved and affected by joint motion. It is this structural design which allows the elbow a flexion range of about 140 degrees to be achieved from the completely extended position. The complex anatomical arrangement inevitably gives rise to the superimposition of bony outlines on plain films and therefore sophisticated methods of imaging are often required to fully assess the bony anatomy and

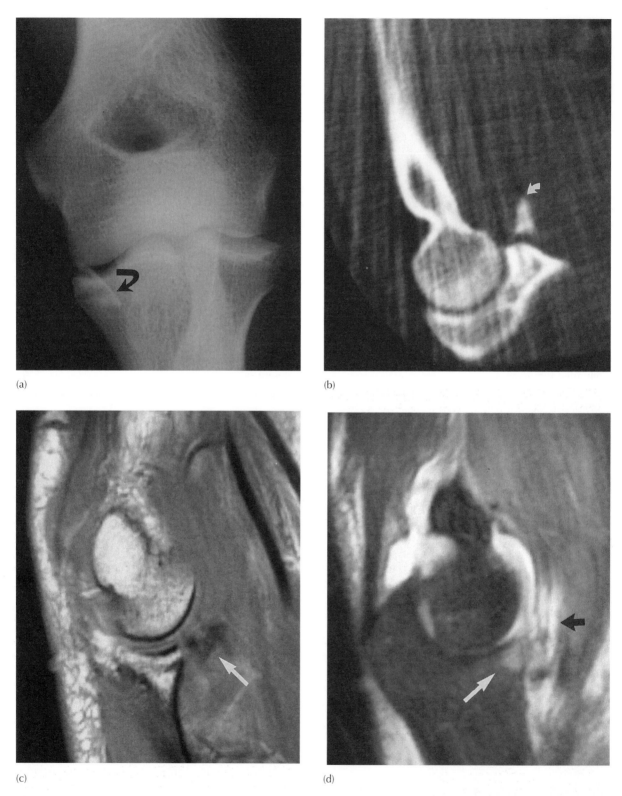

(a)

(b)

(c)

(d)

Fig. 5.1 Coronoid process fracture separation indicating a relocated elbow dislocation. (a) Anteroposterior view of the elbow; (b) direct sagittal CT image; (c) T1 sagittal MRI; (d) short T1 inversion recovery (STIR) sagittal MRI showing the fracture fragment, capsular disruption, effusion, and marrow oedema at the base of the coronoid process. The 'beak' is shown to be intra-articular (black arrow).

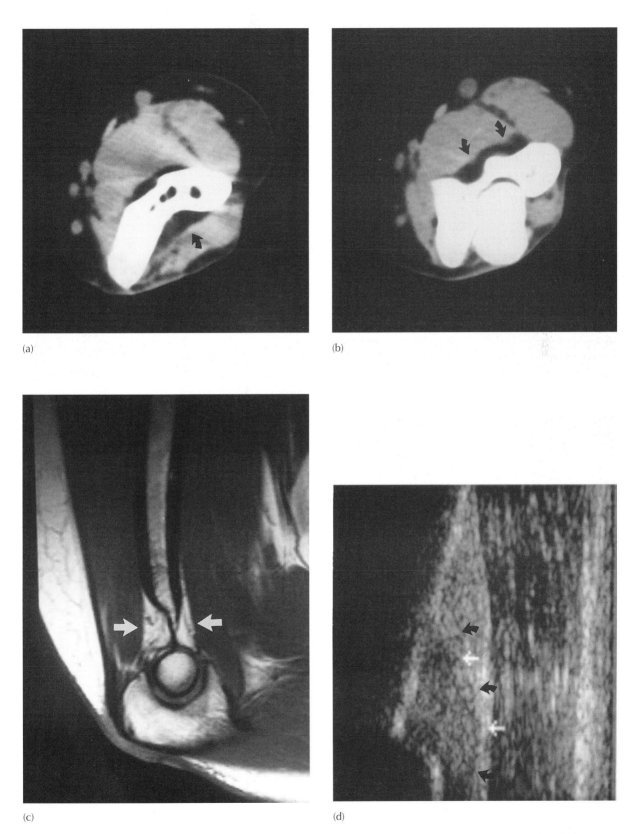

Fig. 5.2 CT (a), (b), MRI (c), and ultrasound (d), appearances of normal fat pads in the coronoid, radial and olecranon fossae.

Table 5.1

Plain radiography
    Routine
        Anteroposterior and lateral
    Additional views
        radial head-capitellum
        external and internal obliques
        ulnar sulcus
Fluoroscopy
    Stress views
Tomography
    Conventional linear or complex motion
Computed tomography
    (CT) + Arthrography
Arthrography
    Single or double contrast (contrast medium or air) +
    tomography
Ultrasound
Scintigraphy
Magnetic resonance imaging (MRI)

exclude intra-articular disease. The imaging techniques available in evaluating elbow disorders are outlined in Table 5.1.

Plain films

To fully assess the elbow joint at least two tangential radiographic views should be obtained. The anteroposterior view with the arm fully extended and the forearm supinated is supplemented by a lateral view with the arm in 90 degrees of flexion. In cases of trauma these views may need to be complimented by internal and external obliques. If the patient is unable to fully extend the elbow anteroposterior views of the humerus and then the forearm should be obtained.

The anteroposterior radiograph in supination demonstrates the medial and lateral epicondyles, the radiocapitellar articular surface, the trochlear articular surface and at least a portion of the olecranon fossa. In addition the valgus carrying angle between the ulna and humerus is also shown. Normally, the long axis of the forearm forms a valgus angle of between 11 and 16 degrees with the long axis of the arm. The anteroposterior radiograph also demonstrates that the humeral articular surface is not quite perpendicular to the humeral shaft making a valgus angle of between 5 and 7 degrees to the long axis of the humerus (Fig. 5.3). It is for this reason that a true lateral view of the joint requires the beam to be directed distally by about 7 degrees.

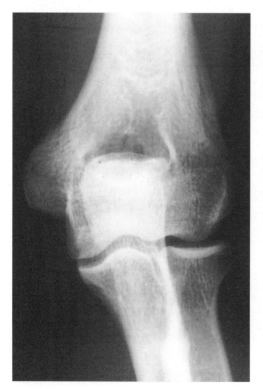

(a)

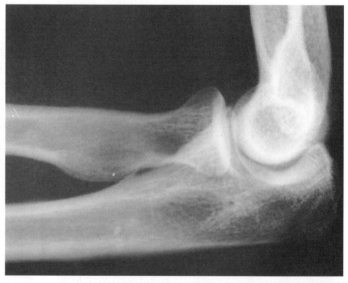

(b)

Fig. 5.3 Normal adult elbow. On the anteroposterior view (a) the humeral articular surface makes a valgus angle (5–7 degrees) with the long axis. If the lateral view is obtained without correcting for this, (b) the joint space is not optimally visualised.

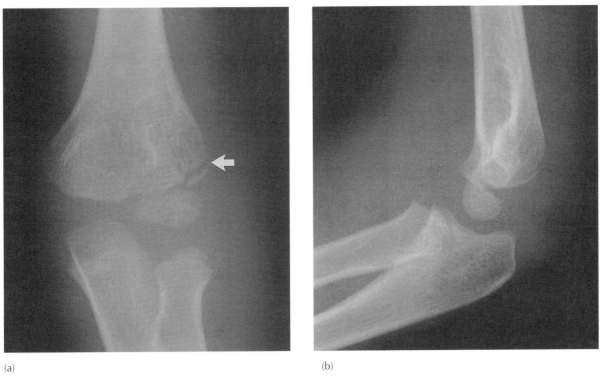

(a)   (b)

Fig. 5.4 Salter-Harris type II fracture of the distal humeral epiphysis. Note the metaphyseal fracture on the anteroposterior view (a), and the posteroinferior location of the capitellar ossification centre on the lateral view (b).

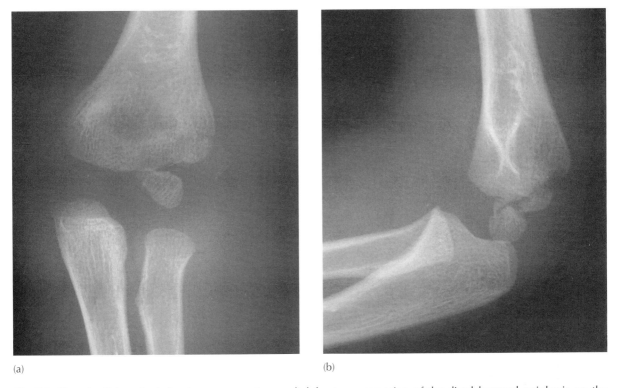

(a)   (b)

Fig. 5.5 'Pseudo dislocation' due to severe posteromedial fracture separation of the distal humeral epiphysis on the anteroposterior (a), and lateral (b) views.

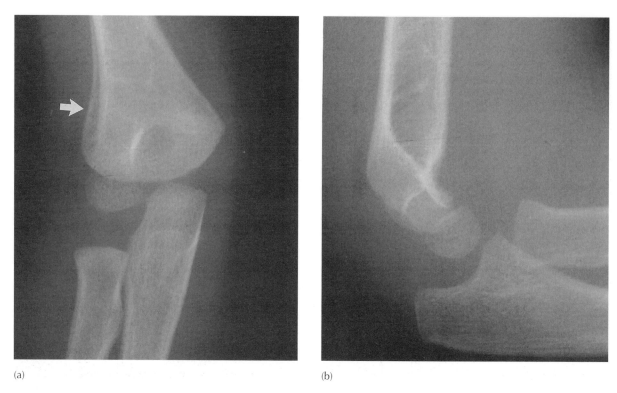

(a)   (b)

Fig. 5.6 A 3-year-old infant with periosteal reaction and increased valgus on the anteroposterior view (a), and anterior migration of the capitellum (b) on the lateral view.

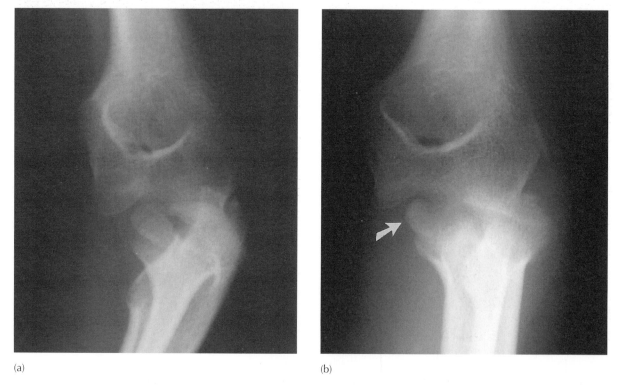

(a)   (b)

Fig. 5.7 Dislocation of the elbow (a) with unsatisfactory reduction appearances (b). The avulsed medial epicondyle is located intra-articularly preventing adequate reduction.

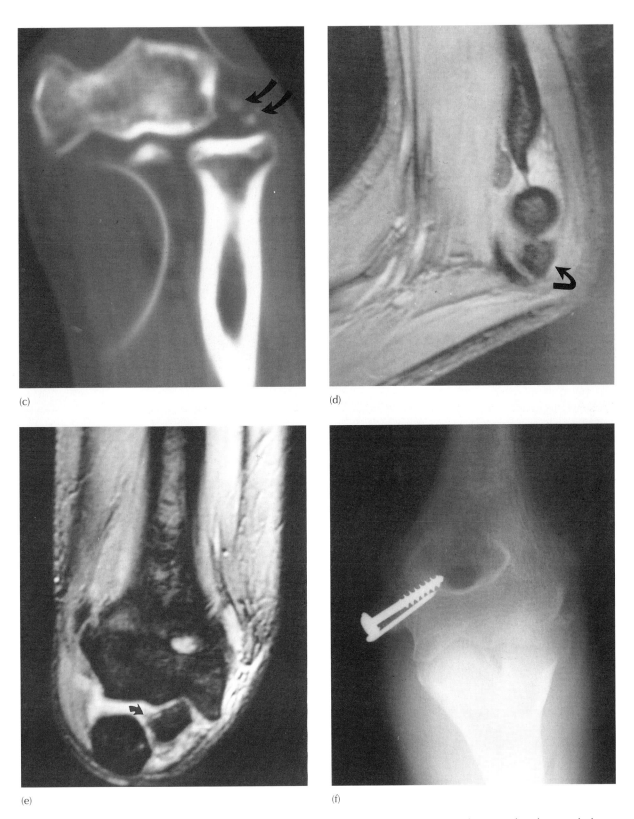

(c)

(d)

(e)

(f)

Fig. 5.7 continued CT reveals further intra-articular fragments laterally (c), while MRI in the sagittal and coronal planes (d) (e), confirms the location and the status of the ossification centre of the medial epicondyle. Open reduction and fixation of the medial epicondyle was required (f).

During development of the elbow joint there are three epiphyseal centres (trochlea, capitellum and radial head) and three apophyseal centres (medial and lateral epicondyles and olecranon). In children it is essential to recognise the four secondary ossification centres of the distal humerus on the anteroposterior view, namely the capitellum, the medial and lateral epicondyles, and the trochlea. The usual order in which these centres appear and the age in which they become radiographically visible are important factors in the evaluation of injuries to the elbow[1] (Chapter 1). Displacement of these secondary centres of ossification is important in the diagnosis of trauma to the paediatric elbow[2] (Figs 5.4, 5.5, 5.6, 5.7). The epicondyle always ossifies before the trochlea. In a child between 4 and 8 years

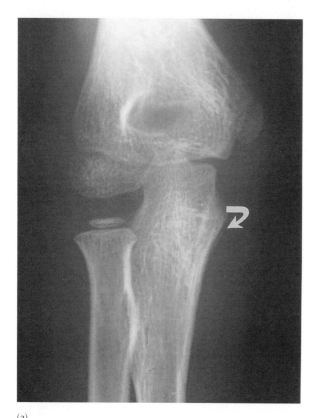

(a)

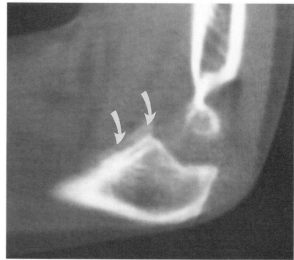

(b)

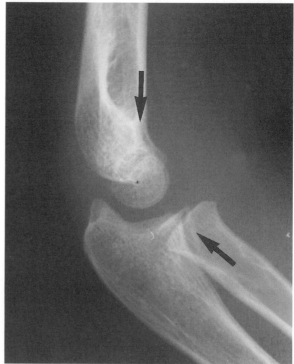

(c)

Fig. 5.8 Periosteal reaction 1 week after trauma seen on the anteroposterior view (a) and direct sagittal CT image (b) in a 6-year-old child. Note the normal relationship of the anterior humeral cortical line and long axis of the radius, in relation to the capitellum on the lateral view (c).

of age, an ossicle in the region of the trochlea (before this centre should appear) without any evidence of the ossification centre of the medial epicondyle, must indicate that the ossification centre of the medial epicondyle has been avulsed and displaced into the joint to lie in the trochlear position. Comparative assessment with radiographs of the contralateral asymptomatic elbow can be crucial in identifying trauma to the elbow joint.

The lateral view demonstrates the distal humerus, the elbow joint and the proximal forearm. It also allows good views of the coronoid process of the ulna as well as the olecranon. However, due to the overlap of bony structures it is limited in the information it provides with particular respect to the posterior half of the radial head and the coronoid process. Following trauma a lateral radiograph with the horizontal beam technique may demonstrate a lipohaemarthrosis indicating the presence of an intra-articular fracture.[3] In acquiring plain films, the central x-ray beam needs to be centred over the joint. Inclusion of the elbow and wrist joint at the time of acquiring views of the traumatised forearm bones is proper and safe practice, as long as the joints are examined by separate radiographic views.

In the evaluation of plain radiographs, several important lines, relationships and contours are routinely assessed. The articular surface of the humerus as shown on the lateral view projects anteriorly forming an angle of 140 degrees with the mid shaft of the humerus. Thus when the anterior humeral line is drawn along the anterior surface of the humeral cortex it passes through the middle third of the capitellum (Fig. 5.8). This configuration is lost in a supracondylar fracture which is commonly associated with posterior displacement of the capitellum and therefore the anterior humeral cortical line falls on the anterior one-third of the capitellum or anterior to it (Fig. 5.4). Configuration is usually lost in distal humeral fractures due to displacement of the fracture components. In addition, the radiocapitellar line bisecting the radial head and neck should always pass through the middle third of the capitellum irrespective of elbow position or radiographic views. Absence of this relationship indicates subluxation or dislocation of the radial head.

FAT PADS

The anterior and posterior fat pads are intracapsular but extrasynovial. Elevation or displacement of the fat pads as judged on the lateral projection allows evaluation of joint distension[4,5] (Fig. 5.9). There are two fat pads anteriorly over the coronoid and radial fossae respectively which are superimposed on the lateral radiograph producing a single

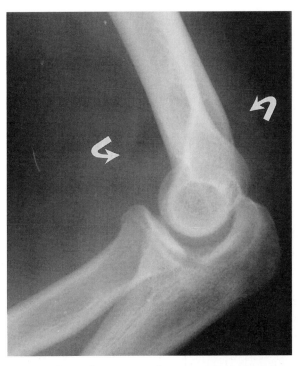

Fig. 5.9 Elevated anterior and posterior fat pads indicative of intra-articular fluid.

triangular lucent configuration (Fig. 5.2). The anterior fat pad is routinely visualised on the lateral view of the elbow immediately anterior and parallel to the humeral cortex. The single posterior fat pad overlying the olecranon fossa is not seen in the lateral projection with the elbow in flexion, but is routinely seen if the elbow is examined in extension. A visible posterior fat pad on the lateral view in the flexed elbow is always abnormal. Regardless of the patient's age, displacement of the normal position of these fat pads around the elbow provides a useful diagnostic clue to the presence of an intra-articular fracture.[6] Fluid within the elbow joint elevates the inferior aspect of the posterior fat pads and this is often also associated with elevation of the anterior fat pad (Fig. 5.10).

The supinator fat stripe is seen on the normal lateral radiograph with the elbow in flexion as a thin lucent line parallel to the ventral aspect of the proximal third of the radius. It is elevated, widened or blurred in virtually all cases of radial head fracture.[7]

ADDITIONAL VIEWS

Oblique views are performed by internal and external rotation of the forearm with the patient positioned in the anteroposterior plane. These allow

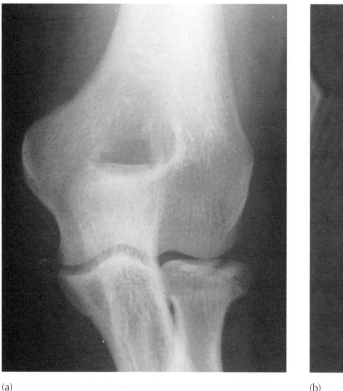

(a)

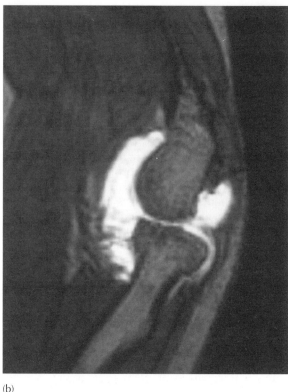

(b)

Fig. 5.10 Radial head fracture seen on the anteroposterior view (a), and by follow-up MRI sagittal image (b). Note residual deformity and intra-articular fluid.

improved visualisation of the trochlea, olecranon and coronoid process on the internal oblique film whilst the radiocapitellar and radioulnar joints, as well as the coronoid tubercle and medial epicondyle are better seen on the external oblique view.

The radial head–capitellum view overcomes the major limitation of the standard lateral view by projecting the radial head in a cranial direction, free of overlap by the coronoid process.[8] This allows complete visualisation of the radial head, easier identification of fractures and better visualisation of bony and soft tissue anatomy. After positioning the patient for a routine lateral view the tube is angled 45 degrees towards the shoulder joint with the elbow flexed and the thumb pointing vertically. It is helpful in demonstrating trauma to the posterior half of the radial head, capitellum, and coronoid process. It is particularly indicated when displaced fat pads are seen on the lateral view without an identifiable fracture.[9,10]

The ulnar sulcus view is an axial view which is obtained by flexing the patient's elbow to 110 degrees, and placing the forearm on the cassette. The x-ray beam is directed perpendicular to the cas-

sette. It enables visualisation of the epicondyles, ulnar sulcus and radiocapitellar and ulnatrochlear articulations.

Fluoroscopy/stress views

In patients with suspected instability secondary to ligament disruption with or without intra-articular bony injury, varus and valgus stress views under fluoroscopic control can provide very helpful diagnostic information (Fig. 5.11). However, 33% of patients with symptomatic medial elbow instability due to ulnar collateral ligament injuries do not demonstrate any valgus instability on preoperative stress radiographs.[11] In avulsive injury to the epicondyles and olecranon process, fluoroscopy can be of value in the assessment of intra-articular loose bodies. After proper positioning of the elbow, changes in the articular space and displacement of fractures can be assessed during stress testing, with spot films taken in the neutral position and following valgus and varus stress. Normally the joint space

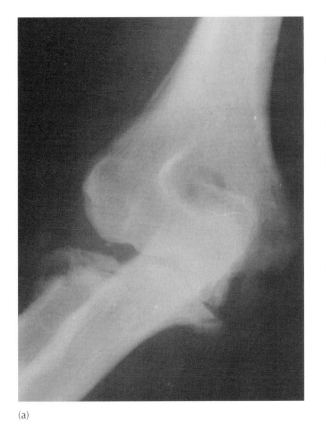

(a)

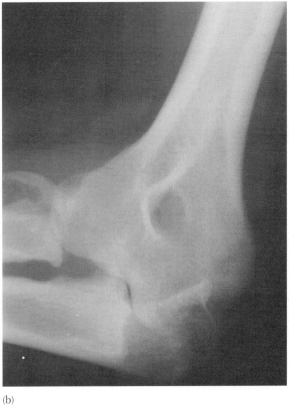

(b)

Fig. 5.11 Instability following a radial head fracture treated by excision. Neutral anteroposterior view (a), shows new bone formation and osteoarthritis at the humeroulnar joint. On valgus stress views the ulna and radius virtually dislocate, indicating ulnar collateral ligament disruption (b), treated by titanium head replacement and ligament reconstruction (c).

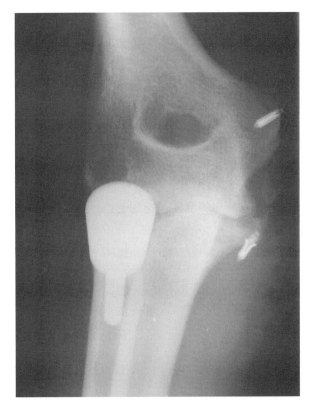

(c)

does not open. If significant pain is present adequate stress views may only be obtained after local anaesthetic has been injected into the painful area, or by performing the assessment under general anaesthesia.

Tomography

Conventional tomographic techniques employing linear, elliptical, spiral, or even more complex pluridirectional methods can provide thin sections in both the anteroposterior and lateral projection to aid in the study of the subchondral and articular contours of the elbow joint. They allow the delineation of complex fractures extending into the elbow joint, assess the exact position of fragments, and the degree of comminution. Even in the presence of internal fixation, conventional tomography is useful in assessing the healing process and in identifying complications such as non-union and/or secondary infection. Prior to CT this technique played a significant role in the detection of calcified loose bodies and in the accurate definition of osteochondritic abnormalities. It can also be employed following arthrography to define more clearly the articular and capsular anatomy.

Conventional tomography does, however, have two disadvantages compared with CT. The intricate curvilinear anatomy confined in a small volume still leads to superimposition and difficulty in interpreting and detecting subtle abnormalities with or without the presence of intra-articular contrast medium. When combined with arthrography, linear tomography still requires projections in two planes with a long examination time and increased radiation dose. The prolonged examination time results in a degradation of image quality due to resorption of injected contrast medium. Furthermore, difficulties arise in keeping a painful elbow still as tomography in multiple planes is required.

Computed tomography

Computed tomography provides exquisite bony detail in the axial plane and also provides useful data on the adjacent soft tissues. Depending on the clinical state of the patient and the range of joint movement, the axial CT can be done with the elbow in extension or in flexion. The olecranon fossa and the radiocapitellar and humeroulnar articulations are well assessed. In flexion the humerus is examined in the axial plane while at the same time coronal slices of the proximal radius and ulna are produced along their longitudinal axis. Injured elbows are normally held in flexion, but when possible, additional scans of the extended joint should also be obtained in order to assess the olecranon–trochlear articulation and the superior radioulnar joints in the axial plane. The CT protocol can be varied to tailor the clinical requirements. In the examination of a palpable para-articular mass non-contiguous 4–8 mm sections are usually sufficient (Figs 5.12, 5.13), while thin (2 mm) continuous section slices are employed in the exclusion of small lesions such as osteoid osteomas (Fig. 5.14). In adult elbow trauma, CT has been shown to provide additional important information not available on plain radiography in 45% of cases altering the diagnosis and management in 31% of patients.[12] It determines the intra or extra-articular nature of the fractured fragments before and after reduction, and can do so through plaster casts. Although not usually undertaken, CT should ideally routinely be done after reduction of an elbow dislocation to exclude intra-articular fragments of bone (Figs 5.15, 5.16). When plain films reveal an effusion but no visible fracture, CT will often identify an occult radial head fracture. In the non-traumatised adult painful elbow, plain CT after normal plain film radiography is rarely productive.

In the further evaluation of trauma to the paediatric elbow CT infrequently changes the therapy regime based on clinical findings and conventional radiography.[13] It only helps in confirming the suspicions raised by clinical examination and plain film. However, computed arthrotomography as an adjunct to paediatric arthrography provides additional information in the evaluation of 67% of chronic conditions of the elbow.[14]

Although CT is optimal in demonstrating the intra-articular contour, intra-articular contrast medium is normally required to help define articular, subchondral and capsular abnormalities.[15] The routine use of CT immediately after standard elbow arthrography provides thin, detailed sections of the contrast-enhanced intra-articular anatomy, which are rapidly generated and recorded on a compact easy-to-visualise format. Variation of the window settings optimises bone and soft tissue detail while multiplanar analysis can be done at a later date, eliminating the need to reposition the elbow. This reduces the time span and improves the image quality when compared with conventional arthro-tomography.[16] Following the acquisition of single orientation axial CT images, 2-D and 3-D re-formatting can be employed (Fig. 5.16). The acquisition of continuous thin (2 mm or less) slices optimises the quality of the reconstructed images in the other planes, but is not as good as the resolution and sharpness provided by direct CT imaging. In selected patients, direct sagittal assessment can provide very useful information, particularly in the assessment of osteochondritis dissecans, and in helping differentiate loose bodies from osteophytic spurs (Fig. 5.17).

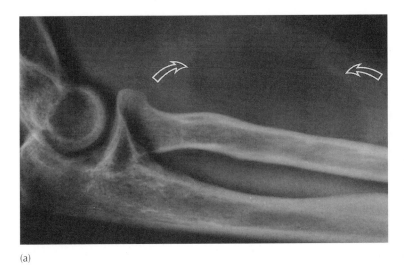

(a)

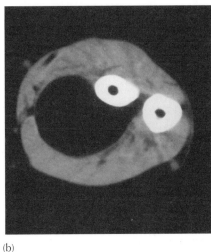

(b)

Fig. 5.12 Benign lipoma appearing as a radiolucent soft tissue mass on plain film (a) and confirmed by low CT attenuation of fat consistency (b).

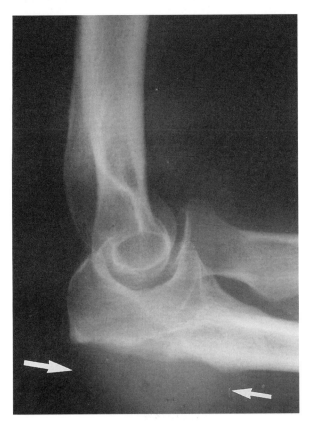

(a)

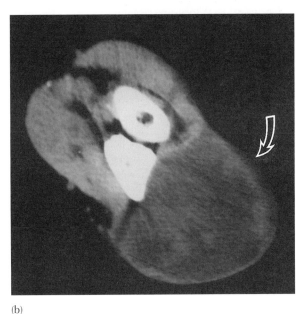

(b)

Fig. 5.13 Pleomorphic liposarcoma appearing as a large soft tissue mass with adjacent bone destruction on the lateral view (a). The mass lacks the low CT attenuation features of fat (b).

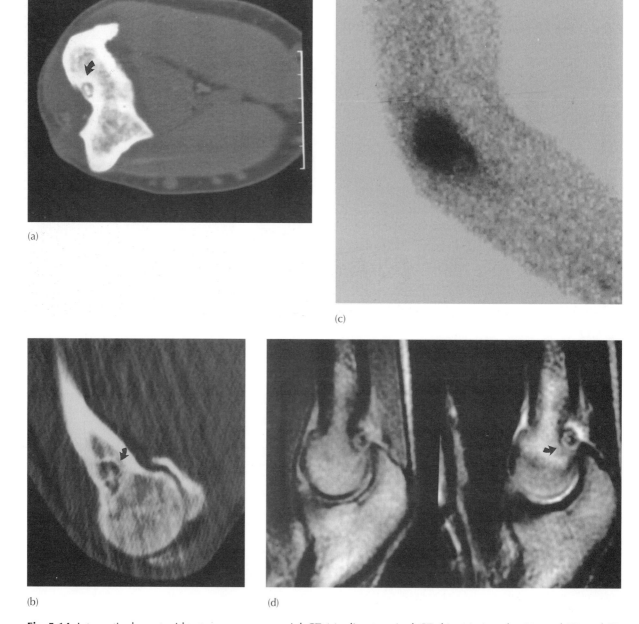

(a)

(c)

(b)   (d)

Fig. 5.14 Intra-articular osteoid osteoma seen on axial CT (a), direct sagittal CT (b), scintigraphy (c), and T1 and T2 sagittal MRI images (d). The CT shows the mineralised centre of the osteoid osteoma.

Arthrography

Elbow arthrography was first described by Lindblom in 1952.[17] In 1962, Del Buono and Solarino[18] reported the use of double contrast arthrography in the assessment of intra-articular lesions of the elbow.

Elbow arthrography can provide useful information about the capsule, its capacity, the synovium, and the articular contour and thickness (Fig. 5.18). If performed within 24–48 hours after

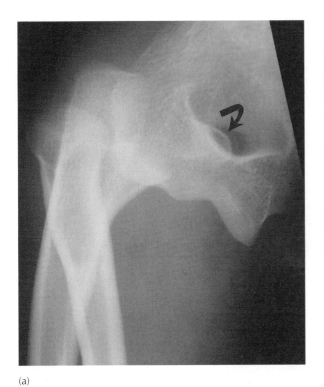

(a)

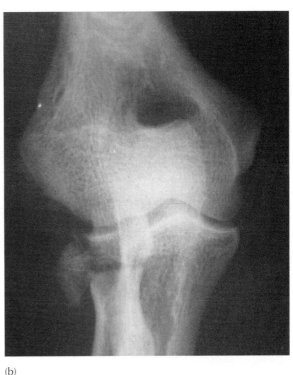

(b)

Fig. 5.15 Anteroposterior view of dislocated elbow (a). The intra-articular fractures are often best visualised on the post-reduction film (b) which clearly demonstrates the medial condylar fragment and radial neck fractures in this case. The curvilinear opacity (curved arrow) overlying the olecranon fossa suggests an intra-articular fragment.

injury, ligamentous and capsular tears may be demonstrated.[19,20] Although conventional arthrography is difficult to interpret because of the superimposition of structures, variations in technique and imaging adjuncts have improved its diagnostic yield. Single or preferably double contrast arthrography combined with tomography (arthrotomography)[21] or CT (computed arthrotomography) have proved very useful in demonstrating chondral abnormalities, osteochondritis dissecans, radiolucent and radiopaque osteochondral bodies, extra-articular sites of calcification, as well as synovial and capsular abnormalities including the evaluation of juxta-articular lesions (Table 5.2). There is no doubt that CT if available is better than pluridirectional tomography as an adjunct to elbow arthrography. Indeed a study which reassessed conventional tomography before and after arthrography, concluded that arthrotomography rarely improved the diagnostic accuracy of non-contrast methods.[22]

The choice of contrast material employed is highly dependent on the clinical setting. Negative contrast agents (air) or positive contrast agents (contrast medium) can be used in isolation or in combination to produce single or double contrast

Table 5.2 Indications for arthrography

Loose bodies: Detection, size, site and number
Location of juxta-articular calcification: intra-articular or extra-articular
Articular cartilage assessment
Delineate communication with para-articular soft tissue lesions
Assess joint capacity
Exclude synovial abnormalities

arthrography. Air alone will suffice if the indication for arthrography is to localise the presence, size and number of intra-articular osseous loose bodies, and differentiate them from extra-articular sites of ossification (Fig. 5.19). Air alone is also used in patients who are allergic to contrast medium. Tomography or CT is routinely employed after air arthrography. In single contrast techniques employing contrast medium, 5–8 cc are required in the demonstration of capsular tears, ligamentous disruption, the communication with para-articular cysts, as well as chondral loose bodies and synovial abnormalities. Double con-

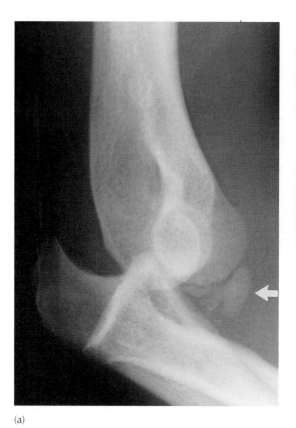

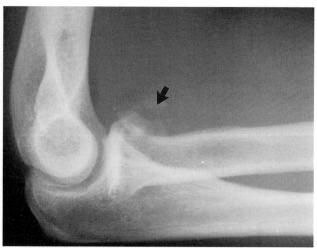

(b)

(a)

Fig. 5.16 Elbow dislocation with fracture fragmentation of the coronoid process as seen on the immediate lateral (a). Following reduction the coronoid fracture remains separate (b) which is confirmed on the three-dimensional reconstruction (c).

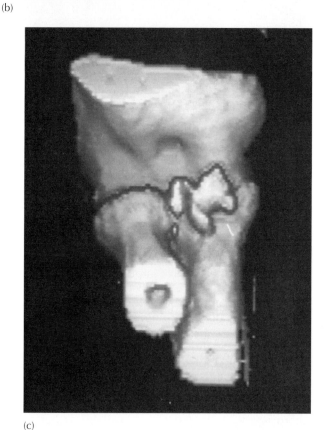

(c)

trast arthrography, however, provides more detailed assessment of the articular surface and synovial lining and detects smaller osteochondral abnormalities. In this double contrast technique, 0.5–1 cc of contrast medium are injected followed by 8–10 cc of air. The instillation of air is monitored fluoroscopically so that maximum distension is ensured with complete filling of the olecranon recess and radioulnar joint. In the presence of discomfort a lesser amount of contrast medium is injected as this often indicates the presence of diminished joint capacity due to post-traumatic capsulitis. The addition of 0.3 ml of 1 in 1000 concentration of adrenaline with the contrast medium delays absorption and optimises the quality of the examination. This is especially helpful if

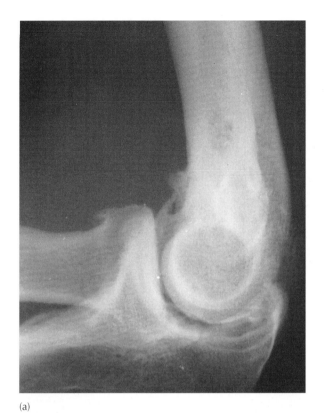

(a)

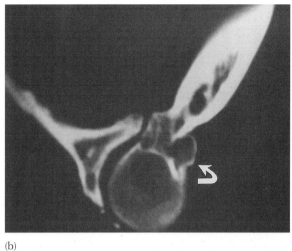

(b)

Fig. 5.17 Primary osteoarthritis of the elbow shown on the lateral view (a). Direct sagittal CT (b) clearly reveals the extent and critical location of the osteophytes in the coronoid and olecranon fossae.

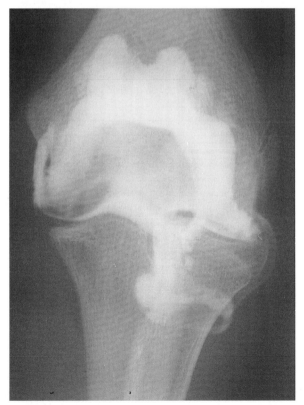

(a)

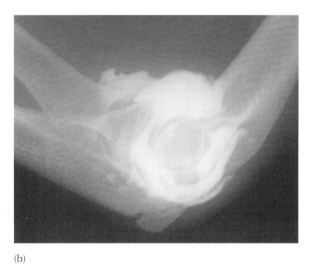

(b)

Fig. 5.18 Elbow arthrogram. Normal appearance of a single contrast study in the anteroposterior view (a), and lateral projections (b), depicting the humeroulnar, radio-capitellar, and superior radioulnar articulations. Note the synovial recess in the supinator fossa which is contiguous with the joint.

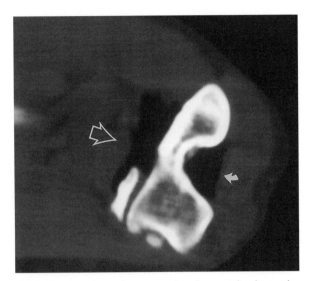

Fig. 5.19 CT air arthrogram. In the axial plane the injected air is seen as low CT attenuation distending the capsule anteriorly and posteriorly. There is a large intra-articular loose body while the separate ossicle lying medially is outside the joint.

tomography or CT are routinely performed after the conventional arthrogram.[23] Following the instillation of contrast medium the elbow is initially studied fluoroscopically to exclude instability of the joint and loose bodies. Routine films including anteroposterior, lateral, and oblique views are obtained. Varying the position of the humerus by elevating it above the head or employing a more dependent position maximises the value of the double contrast technique. The complex anatomy results in the superimposition of normal and abnormal structures and requires conventional or computed tomography to accurately delineate the arthrographic anatomy.

NORMAL FINDINGS

The normal joint capacity is between 15 and 25 cc. This is increased in patients with chronic instability, neuropathic arthropathy, and rheumatoid disease, and is conversely decreased in patients with post-traumatic fibrosis, flexion contractures and para-articular myositis ossificans. The distended joint capsule shows two anterior projections over the radial and coronoid fossae of the humerus while the posterior recess of the capsule is particularly deep behind the olecranon fossa and the radial head. The borders of the recesses are smooth with two exceptions; the anterior border of the coronoid process is crenated in appearance during flexion, while the border adjacent to the medial collateral ligament is also normally irregular in outline.[24] The joint space communicates with the superior radioulnar joint through the annular recess formed by the extrinsic compressive effect of the annular ligament (Fig. 5.18). The radioulnar recess extends between the proximal portions of the radius and ulna. Articular cartilage of uniform thickness covers the subchrondral surfaces of the humerus, radius and ulna, except for a normal defect in the articular cartilage of the mid portion of the trochlear notch of the ulna where the subchondral bone appears irregular. The latter is of variable size, can involve most of the trochlear notch, and should not be misinterpreted as pathological in nature. The articular surfaces are best delineated when thinly coated by contrast and outlined by air. The articular cartilage of the capitellum is limited to its anterior and inferior surfaces, whereas cartilage is present on the anterior, inferior and posterior contours of the trochlea. Optimal visualisation of the radial articular surface is provided when the arm is elevated while conversely the humeral articular outline is best seen with the arm dependent.

ARTHROGRAPHIC ABNORMALITIES

In chondral disease, arthrography, especially with CT establishes the diagnosis, and determines the exact site and extent of damage.[25] In cases with plain film evidence of osteochondritis dissecans, the CT arthrogram reliably identifies if the cartilage overlying the damaged bone is intact, fissured, fractured, separated, or detached. Furthermore, the exact number, size and sites of loose body location are readily documented by CT arthrography. Loose bodies are easily detectable whether they are chondral or osteochondral in nature. Osteochondral loose bodies may have a small, bony component, and the actual size of the entire fragment is usually much larger than first suggested on the plain films.[26] The superior contrast resolution of computed arthrotomography allows more accurate differentiation between intra-articular cartilaginous loose bodies and osseous loose bodies from osteophytes. The state of the subchondral bone and the presence of cystic change is optimally assessed. Although axial CT is routinely employed, direct sagittal images optimally demonstrate the osteochondral abnormality as they are better at assessing the convexity of the humeral condyles. The demonstration of an unossified distal humeral epiphysis is silhouetted against the contrast medium allowing assessment of fractures and separation of the distal humerus in early childhood.[27–29]

Ultrasound

High resolution real time sonography of the musculoskeletal system is of particular value in detecting effusions and depicting unossified cartilage. Real time systems equipped with 7.5 MHz transducers are best suited for this purpose. Although limited in application, sonography can in selected clinical settings produce invaluable help in the management of elbow problems. The elbow can be studied in multiple sagittal, coronal and transverse planes from the anterior, posterior, medial and lateral aspects. Depending on the limitations imposed by the clinical setting, dynamic assessment is possible, as is comparison with the contralateral side. In the presence of para-articular and articular swellings, ultrasound clearly differentiates echo free fluid from echogenic solid tumours, and also differentiates intra-articular from extra-articular fluid accumulations. Intra-articular calcification (loose bodies and synovial osteochondromatosis) and extra-articular calcification (myositis ossificans) are detected by virtue of their reflectivity. In instances of trauma, apart from depicting intra-articular fluid, ultrasound also demonstrates the relationship of the fluid to the fat pads.[30-33] The fat pads appear as echogenic triangular structures lying within the radial, coronoid, and olecranon fossae. The articular cartilage is normally seen as a thin echo poor line between the lower end of the fat pad and subchondral bone and should not be mistaken for an effusion (Fig. 5.20). The normal morphological alterations which occur in elbow movement can be assessed dynamically by real time ultrasound. The anterior fat pads are contained within their fossae by the brachioradialis tendon with the elbow extended making them accessible to the ultrasound transducer. In elbow flexion, the triceps tendon presses the posterior fat pad into the olecranon fossa, while on extension the olecranon process of the ulna compresses, deforms and elevates the fat pad. It is for this reason that the reliability of a displaced posterior fat pad as an indicator of an intra-articular disease only applies when the elbow is in the flexed position. Although the presence of intra-articular fluid is commonly associated with radiographic evidence of elevated fat pads, this is not the case in 13% of conditions associated with an intra-capsular effusion.[10] Confirming the absence of a joint effusion can spare children unnecessary attempts at needle aspiration.

Sonography allows adequate visualisation of the bone–soft tissue interface due to the large differences in acoustic impedance. The bony contour is easily visualised and any cortical disruption is indicative of an underlying fracture. Moreover, in the traumatised paediatric elbow, ultrasound allows the demonstration of bony contour, disruption of the physis, and maintenance of articular relationships. This is particularly useful in the infant since plain film assessment of the injured distal humeral epiphysis is difficult prior to the appearance of the ossification centres.[34] Furthermore, before the appearance of the ossification centre of the capitellum, its alignment with the radius cannot be ascertained (Fig. 5.20). Consequently fracture separation involving the distal humeral epiphysis (usually posteromedial) may be misdiagnosed as a 'posterior' dislocation of the elbow in the infant age group[35] (Fig. 5.5). The differentiation of dislocation from fracture and a complete detachment of the cartilaginous components of the epiphysis previously required arthrography.[36] The ability to visualise the cartilaginous radiolucent component in its unossified state make ultrasonography a useful tool in the evaluation of suspected fractures and dislocations in young children (Figs 5.5, 5.20). In addition it allows monitoring after reduction and during the healing phase. Ultrasonography also has a limited role in the assessment of the overlying cartilage in instances of osteochondritis dissecans.[37] It has also been used in the assessment of ulnar nerve entrapment within the ulnar sulcus. The technique allows visualisation of the posterior aspect of the medial condyle, measurement of the tunnel dimensions and identification of the ulnar nerve.

Nuclear medicine

The standard technique for isotope examination of the elbow as with the remainder of the skeleton, utilises ^{99}Tc-labelled methylene diphosphonate. The elbow is scanned within 3 minutes of the intravenous injection which must obviously be performed in a vein away from the symptomatic joint to avoid misdiagnosis of any extravasted isotope as a 'hot lesion'. This early phase provides an assessment of the vascularity of the elbow and the activity is increased in any condition which increases vascular flow such as trauma, synovitis, infection, vascular tumours which include arteriovenous malformation, haemangioma or osteoid osteoma and neurogenic alteration of blood flow (Fig. 5.14). The bone phase is assessed at 3 hours after clearance of the isotope from the soft tissue. Increased bone production with or without increased vascularity will produce increased uptake and therefore activity of the ^{99}Tc MDP. This phase is particularly useful for identifying occult bone trauma which is always active after 72 hours, and bone producing tumours such as osteoid osteoma. More chronic infections will produce increased bone phase activity but if destruction predominates the scan may not be significantly active.

The use of single photon emission computed tomography (SPECT) may increase the sensitivity of the examination in demonstrating mild increases in activity compared with planar scanning but the superficial nature of the elbow and its relatively small size does not benefit from the axial spatial differentiation of sites of activity.

In cases of suspected infection or inflammation cell labelling techniques may be used. These include indium III or ^{99}Tc HMPAO-labelled leucocytes or granulocytes.

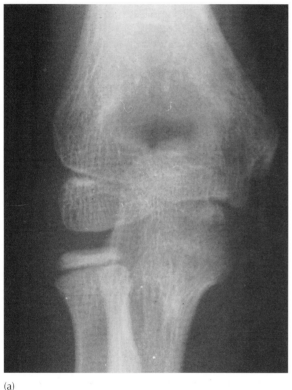

(a)

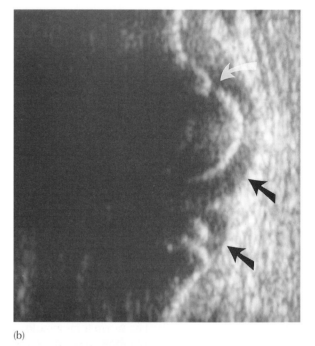

(b)

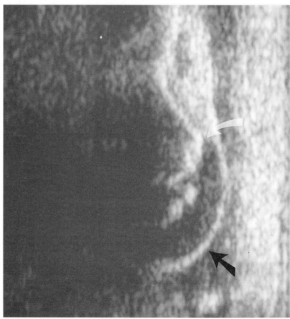

(c)

Fig. 5.20 Normal 10-year-old child's elbow (a). On the anteroposterior view the ossification centres of the capitellum, radius, medial epicondyle and trochlea are clearly visualised. Direct sagittal ultrasound assessment through the humeroradial and humeroulnar joints, showing ossified and unossified components of the capitellum and radial head (b) and trochlea (c). Note optimal visualisation of the physis (curved white arrow).

Imaging at 3 hours and 24 hours will demonstrate accumulation of isotope with an active infection but will not differentiate from active non-infective synovitis in all cases. Chronic tuberculous arthritis may produce either no increase or even a negative uptake in some cases.

Magnetic resonance imaging

Magnetic resonance imaging (MRI) of the elbow can clearly depict the intra-articular and extra-articular anatomy.[38,39] The improved soft tissue contrast resolution and the possibility of imaging the elbow directly in all three planes provides significant advantages over other techniques including CT.[40] Dedicated surface coils and pulse sequences designed to demonstrate contrast differences between normal and abnormal tissues help to identify abnormalities, and stage the pathology within the articular and osseous structure. Evaluation of soft tissues including muscle, ligament, tendon, and neurovascular structures is best achieved by MRI. It is also the modality of choice for the detection and assessment of soft tissue and bone neoplasms around the elbow joint. The injection of intra-articular gadolinium mixed with saline can also produce an MR arthrogram to help identify loose bodies and defects in the articular surface (Fig. 5.21). Extra-articular soft tissue inflammation and/or bursitis can be demonstrated. Capsular and ligamentous integrity are well shown and enhanced by the presence of an associated joint effusion. Furthermore, in the paediatric elbow, MRI has great potential in helping to identify the extent of damage to the physis in the growing skeleton. It also has the advantage of not being reliant on ionising radiation although relatively long imaging times frequently necessitate sedation of the young child.[41]

IMAGING TECHNIQUE

The patient is best scanned in a supine or posterior oblique position with the arm at the side. However, this is only possible when software allows the use of off-centre placement of surface coils. The prone position with the arm extended overhead produces patient discomfort and the resultant images are degraded by motion artefact. A circular surface coil is ideal for localised evaluation of the joint. Depending on the clinical problem the elbow may be positioned in flexion, pronation, or supination to enhance the value of the MR examination. In the assessment of the biceps tendon insertion for example, the flexed elbow displays the anatomy optimally in the sagittal plane, while axial imaging provides further information in pronation and supination. Comparative assessment with the asymptomatic elbow can be obtained by using dual coils which allow simultaneous examination of the joints without loss of image quality or increase in acquisition time.

The pulse sequences and image planes depend on the generation of the MR scanner and degree of sophistication of its software, as well as the clinical problem and condition of the patient's elbow. The T2 weighted images are usually obtained in the axial and sagittal planes using spin echo techniques (SE 2000/20–30, 60–80). Some authors recommend the use of dual echo with the long TR producing proton density images. If used this may obviate the need for TI weighted sequences. Soft tissue contrast is superior with this pulse sequence so the likelihood of overlooking an abnormality is remote. The T1 weighted sequences (SE 500, 20) in either the axial, coronal or sagittal plane are then obtained depending on the clinical symptomatology and findings of the T2 sequences. Additional sequences may be added depending on the clinical problem. Short T1 inversion recovery (STIR) sequences, are usually useful in the coronal plane. They cause suppression of the fat signal enhancing the depiction of subtle pathological processes due to the additive effects of T1 and T2 contrast which increase the contrast resolution. Furthermore, chemical shift fat suppression techniques may be added to various pulse sequences to improve visualisation of the hyaline articular cartilage. Optimal visualisation of loose bodies are provided by T2 weighted gradient echo sagittal sequences. Gradient echo 3-D volume acquisition allows the acquisition of thin axial images which can be re-formatted in the other two planes on a computer satellite work station. These sequences tend to have poor soft tissue contrast and produce magnetic susceptibility artefacts in the postoperative state.

Imaging abnormalities

OSTEOCHONDRITIS DISSECANS

This lesion is reliably detected and staged by MRI (Figs 5.22, 5.23). Unstable lesions are characterised by fluid encircling the osteochondral fragment on T2 weighted images, while loose *in situ* lesions always have a subchondral cyst beneath the osteochondral fragment.[42] Unstable osteochondral lesions may fragment and migrate throughout the joint as loose bodies (Fig. 5.24). These are easily identified if they are large in the presence of an effusion. Conversely, MRI may miss the presence of small loose bodies in the absence of an effusion. Theoretically, intra-articular loose bodies should be diagnosed by virtue of their mobility. Definitive mobility after patient re-positioning and re-scan- ning can be shown in osteochondral lesions which are truly free within the joint. However, after a variable period most osteochondral fragments fail to persist as loose bodies, attaching themselves to synovium by fibrosis or embedding in neighbouring hyaline cartilage or bone.[29]

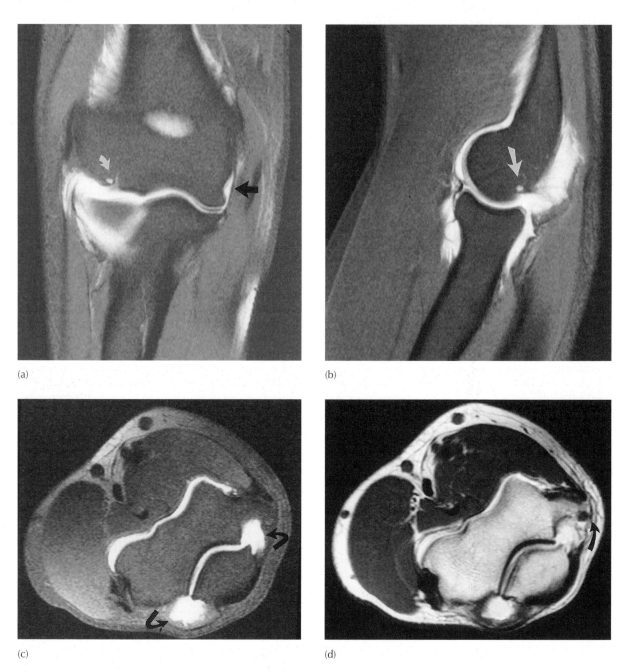

(a)

(b)

(c)

(d)

Fig. 5.21 Magnetic resonance arthrogram utilising dilute gadolinium solution. There is a small subchondral cyst at the posterior limit of the articular cartilage on the capitellum (a), coronal, and (b) sagittal T1 fat suppressed images. The close relationship of the ulnar nerve as it lies behind the medial epicondyle to the distended joint capsule is also well seen in the axial plane (c) (d).

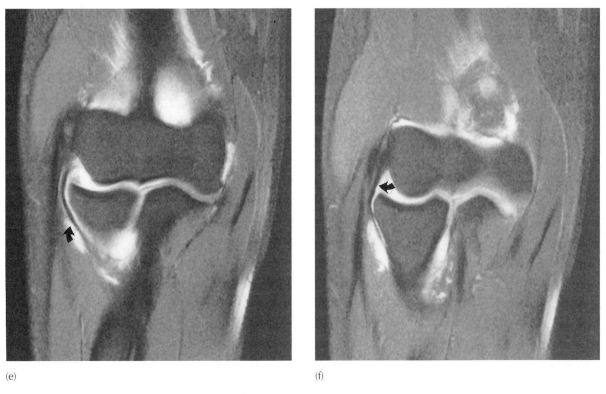

(e) (f)

Fig. 5.21 continued Optimum detail of capsular and ligamentous structures is afforded. Note accurate delineation of radial and ulna collateral ligaments (e), (f).

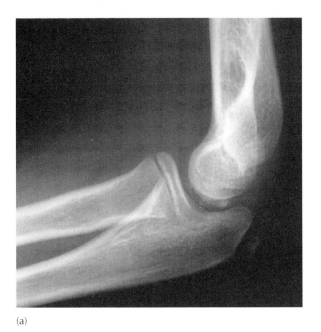

(a)

Fig. 5.22 Oseochondritis dissecans of the capitellum seen on the lateral view (a) and sagittal MR images (b) with small loose body formation (arrow).

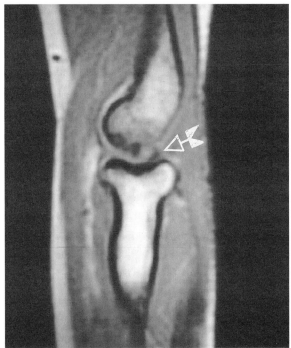

(b)

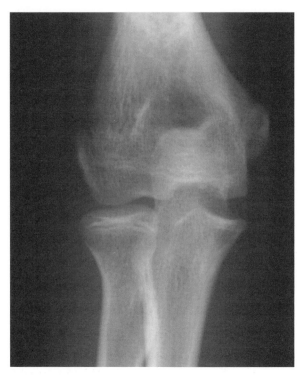

Fig. 5.23 Osteochondritis dissecans of the elbow occasionally involves the trochlea.

BONE INJURY

Plain radiography with conventional or computed tomography is usually sufficient in the detection and classification of osseous injury. Radiographically occult or overlooked fractures are easily identified by ^{99}Tc MDP isotope scanning and may also be demonstrated by MRI. Occult fractures in the marrow (bone bruise)[43] and stress fractures can also be detected by MRI.[44] Cortical changes are most obvious on T2 images having high signal intensity compared with the dark cortical intact bone. As marrow fat is suppressed on these sequences, marrow oedema, fluid or blood, will produce a stellate area of high signal intensity on T2 sequences and low signal on T1 sequences. Compression fractures of the trabeculae, however, have a low signal on both T1 and T2 sequences. By virtue of the superior contrast resolution STIR sequences detect marrow injury optimally compared with proton density and gradient echo studies which can mask the presence of signal alterations due to trauma (Fig. 5.1). In the healing process, MRI can monitor new bone formation and differentiate between fibrous union and non-union. In fibrous union the signal intensity is decreased on both T1 and T2 sequences, but in a non-union the

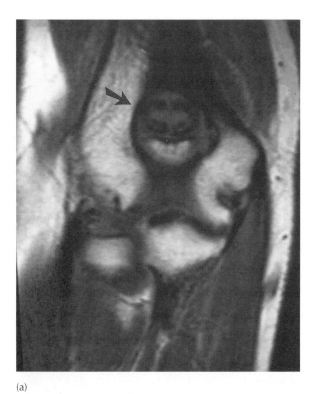

(a)

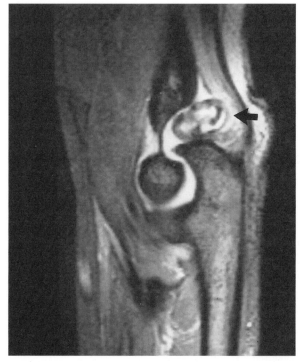

(b)

Fig. 5.24 Large osteochondral loose body in the olecranon fossa not appreciated on plain films, but elegantly seen on coronal T1 (a), and sagittal T2 (b) MRI images.

T2 study shows increased signal due to fluid along the fracture. In paediatric trauma, MR can exclude the presence of supracondylar fractures and help define combined injury to the growth plate and unossified epiphysis.

AVASCULAR NECROSIS

Osteochondrosis of the capitellum (Panner's disease) is seen in young males (age 5–10 years) affecting focally the anterior central portion at the point of maximal contact with the radial head. It is characterised by fragmentation and decreased signal of the ossifying capitellum on T1 weighted images (Fig. 5.25). Follow-up MR scans reveal a return to normal marrow signal with little or no residual deformity of the capitellar articular surface. In the adult type of avascular necrosis, the T1 sequence initially shows the necrotic area as isointense with normal marrow but surrounded by a low intensity rim due to hyperaemia. This appears high in signal on the T2 study. In the established chronic state mixed resorption and new bone formation will give rise to variable MR appearances. The overlying articular cartilage is well delineated, but subtle fissuring and defects are better visualised on the T2 weighted sequence. Alternatively T1

sequences with intra-articular gadolinium especially with fat suppression, will show these features.

TENDONS AND LIGAMENTS

Tendon injuries are more common in the upper extremity. Trauma to the biceps and triceps tendons at their insertions are easily detected by MRI. The technique is particularly useful when the clinical diagnosis is equivocal: MRI differentiates partial from complete ruptures, determines the size of the gap, and the location of the tear. Axial and sagittal imaging utilising T2 weighted or STIR sequences are best for this assessment.

Inflammation or partial tears of the common extensor and flexor tendons produce the common syndromes of lateral (tennis elbow) and medial (golfer's elbow) epicondylitis (Fig. 5.26). The underlying pathology is a combination of repetitive tendon degenerative tears with repair by scar tissue rather than a true 'tendinitis'. In tendon degeneration, there is normal or increased thickness with increased T1 signal intensity, which does not increase or alter on the T2 sequences. Partial tears are characterised by tendon thinning with surrounding fluid best seen on the T2 images. A fluid filled gap between the tendon and its bony attachment indicates a complete detachment.

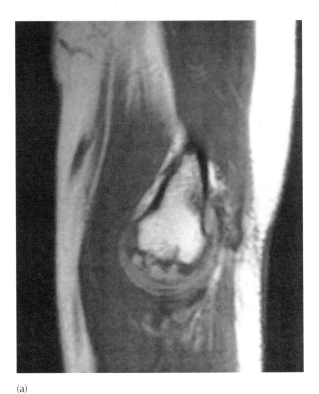

(a)

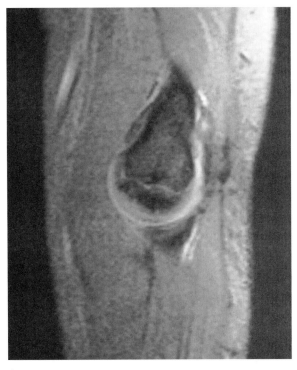

(b)

Fig. 5.25 Panner's disease of the capitellum. MRI utilising T1 (a), and T2 (b) sequences in the sagittal T2 (b) MRI images.

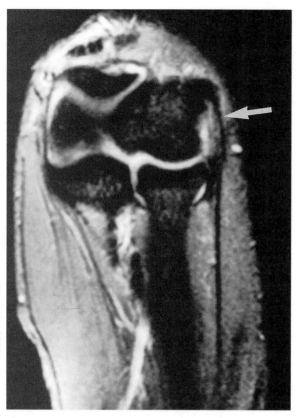

Fig. 5.26 Lateral 'epicondylitis'. Coronal MRI employing a STIR sequence showing oedema in the tendinous common extensor origin.

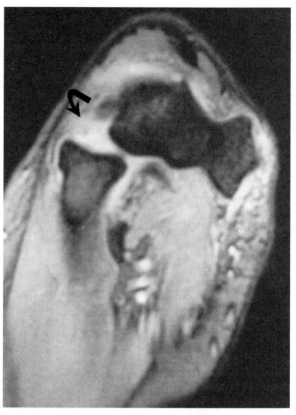

Fig. 5.27 Magnetic resonance appearance of dislocated radial head with associated rupture of the radiocollateral ligament utilising coronal sequences.

Acute injury to the medial collateral ligament not uncommonly accompanies lateral compartment bone contusions.[45] The status of the anterior bundle of the medial collateral ligament (the primary stabiliser to valgus stress) can be determined by axial and coronal images. The majority of the tears are intrasubstance in nature while a small proportion are true distal avulsion. In chronic medial collateral ligament degeneration the ligament is thickened with foci of calcification, and osteophytes are seen at the insertion in the coronoid process.[46]

Ruptures of the lateral collateral ligament may occur particularly in association with radial head dislocation (Fig. 5.27).

NERVE ENTRAPMENT SYNDROME

The presentation of nerve entrapment syndromes is one of chronic pain with or without neurologic signs. The radial, median and ulnar nerves can be compressed in their course at the elbow joint by a variety of processes ranging from fibrous adhesions, bursal enlargement, ganglia, trauma, inflammation, osteophytes and neoplasms (Fig. 5.28). The ulnar nerve can often be well assessed on axial MR as it crosses the cubital tunnel. The floor of the tunnel is composed of the capsule and posterior fibres of the medial collateral ligament. Thickening of these soft tissues together with medial epicondylar osteophytes can cause entrapment of the ulnar nerve. The roof of the tunnel is formed by the cubital tunnel retinaculum which if absent allows anterior dislocation of the nerve over the medial epicondyle during flexion with secondary friction neuritis. If the retinaculum itself is thickened the nerve is also compressed during flexion. Lastly, the anomalous muscle, anconeus epitrochlearis can replace the retinaculum resulting in a further cause of compression of the ulnar nerve.

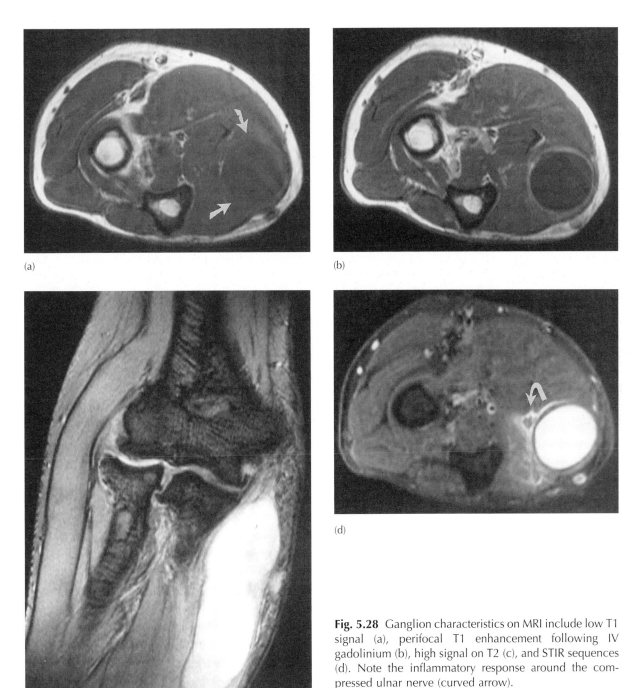

(a)

(b)

(c)

(d)

Fig. 5.28 Ganglion characteristics on MRI include low T1 signal (a), perifocal T1 enhancement following IV gadolinium (b), high signal on T2 (c), and STIR sequences (d). Note the inflammatory response around the compressed ulnar nerve (curved arrow).

References

1. McCarthy SM, Ogden JA Radiology of post-natal skeletal development V1: Elbow joint, proximal radius and ulna. *Skeletal Radiol* 1982; **9:** 17–26.
2. Peterson CA, Peterson HA Analysis of the incidence of injuries to the epiphyseal growth plate. *J Trauma* 1972; **12:** 275–81.
3. Yousefzadeh DK, Jackson JH Jr Lipohaemarthrosis of the elbow joint. *Radiology* 1978; **128:** 643–5.
4. Norrell HG Roentgenologic visualisation of the extra-capsular fat. Its importance in the diagnosis of traumatic injuries to the elbow. *Acta Radiol* 1954; **42:** 205–10.
5. Murphy WA, Siegel MJ Elbow fat pads with new signs and extended differential diagnosis. *Radiology* 1977; **124:** 659–65.

6. Bohrer SP The fat pad sign following elbow trauma: Its usefulness and reliability in suspecting 'invisible' fractures. *Clin Radiol* 1970; **21:** 90–4.

7. Rogers SL, Macewan DW Changes due to trauma in the fat plane overlying the supinator muscle: a radiographic sign. *Radiology* 1969; **92:** 954–8.

8. Greenspan A, Norman A The radial head-capitellum view: Useful technique in elbow trauma. *Am J Radiol* 1982; **138:** 1186–8.

9. Pitt MJ, Speer DP Imaging of the elbow with an emphasis on trauma. *Radiol Clin North Am* 1990; **28:** 293–305.

10. Khon AM Soft tissue alterations in elbow trauma. *Am J Radiol* 1959; **82:** 867–74.

11. Conway JE, Jobe FW, Glousman RE, Pink M Medial instability of the elbow in throwing athletes. *J Bone Joint Surg* 1992; **74A:** 67–83.

12. Franklin PD, Dunlop RW, Whitelaw G, Jacques E Jr, Blickman JG, Shapiro JH CT of the normal and traumatised elbow. *J Comput Ass Tomogr* 1988; **12:** 817–23.

13. Blickman JG, Dunlop RW, Sanzone CF, Franklin PD Is CT useful in the traumatised paediatric elbow? *Paediatr Radiol* 1990; **20:** 184–5.

14. Brody AS, Ball WS, Towlin RB Computed arthrotomography as an adjunct to paediatric arthrography. *Radiology* 1989; **170:** 99–102.

15. Holland P, Davies AM, Cassar-Pullicino VN Computed tomographic arthrography in the assessment of osteochondritis dissecans of the elbow. *Clin Radiol* 1994; **49:** 231–5.

16. Singson RD, Feldman F, Rosenberg ZS Elbow joint: Assessment with double contrast CT arthrography. *Radiology* 1986; **160:** 167–73.

17. Lindblom K Arthrography. *J Foc Radiol* 1952; **3:** 151–63.

18. Del Buono MS, Solarino GB Arthrography of the elbow with double contrast media. *Ital Clin Ortop* 1962; **14:** 223–32.

19. Pavlov H, Ghelman B, Warren R Double contrast arthrography of the elbow. *Radiology* 1979; **130:** 87–95.

20. Johansson O Capsular and ligamentous injuries of the elbow joint: A clinical and arthrographic study. *Acta Chirug Scand* 1962; **287**(Suppl): 17–20.

21. Eto RT, Anderson PW, Harley JD Elbow arthrography with the application of tomography. *Radiology* 1975; **115:** 283–8.

22. Teng MM, Murphy WA, Gilula LA, Destouet JM, Edelstein G, Monsees B, Totty WG Elbow arthrography: A reassessment of the technique. *Radiology* 1984; **153:** 611–3.

23. Hudson TM Elbow arthrography. *Radiol Clin North Am* 1981; **19:** 227–41.

24. Arvidson H, Johansson O Arthrography of the elbow joint. *Acta Radiol* 1955; **43:** 445–52.

25. Blane CE, Ling TF Jr, Andrews JC, Dipietro MA, Hensinger RN Arthrography in the post-traumatic elbow in children. *Am J Radiol* 1984; **143:** 17–21.

26. Milgram J, Rodgers L, Miller J Osteochondral fractures: mechanisms of injury and fate of fragments. *Am J Radiol* 1978; **130:** 651–8.

27. Akbarnia BA, Silberstein MJ, Rende RJ, Graviss ER, Luisir A Arthrography in the diagnosis of fractures of the distal end of the humerus in infants. *J Bone Joint Surg* 1986; **68:** 599–602.

28. Hansen PE, Barnes DA, Tullos HS Arthrographic diagnosis of an injury pattern in the distal humerus of an infant. *J Paediatr Orthop* 1982; **2:** 569–72.

29. Rogers LF, Rockwood CA Jr Separation of the entire distal humeral epiphysis. *Radiology* 1973; **106:** 393–400.

30. Thomas EA, Cassar-Pullicino VN, McCall IW The role of ultrasound in the early diagnosis and management of heterotopic bone formation. *Clin Radiol* 1991; **43:** 190–6.

31. Cassar-Pullicino VN McClelland M, Badwan DAH, McCall IW, Pringle RG, El Masry W Sonographic diagnosis of heterotopic bone formation in spinal injury patients. *Paraplegia* 1993; **31:** 40–50.

32. Miles KA, Lamont AC Ultrasound demonstration of the elbow fat pads. *Clin Radiol* 1989; **40:** 602–4.

33. Barr LL, Babcock DS Sonography of the normal elbow. *Am J Radiol* 1991; **157:** 793–8.

34. Markowitz R, Davidson RS, Harty MP, Bellah RD, Hubbard AM, Rosenberg HK Sonography of the elbow in infants and children. *Am J Radiol* 1992; **159:** 829–33.

35. Welk LA, Adler RS Case report 725. *Skeletal Radiol* 1992; **21:** 198–200.

36. Dias JJ, Lamont AC, Jones JM Ultrasonic diagnosis of neonatal separation of the distal humeral epiphysis. *J Bone Joint Surg* 1988; **70B:** 825–8.

37. Bruns J, Lussenhop S Sonographische darstellung AM, Ellbogenelenk Freie gelenkkorper und osteochondrosis dissecans. *Ultraschall in Med* 1993; **14:** 58–62.

38. Bunnell DH, Fisher DA, Bassett LW, Gold RH, Ellman H Elbow joint: Normal anatomy of MR images. *Radiology* 1987; **165:** 527–31.

39. Middleton WD, Macrander S, Kneeland JB, Froncisz W, Jesmanowicz A, Hyde JS MR imaging of the normal elbow: Anatomic correlation (1987). *Am J Radiol* 1987; **149:** 543–7.

40. Murphy BJ MR imaging of the elbow. *Radiology* 1992; **185:** 525–9.

41. Jaramillo D, Hoffer FA, Shapiro F, Rand F MR imaging of the fractures of the growth plate. *Am J Radiol* 1990; **155:** 1261–5.

42. De-Smet AA, Fisher DR, Burnstein MI, Graf BK, Lange RH Value of MR imaging in staging osteochondral lesions of the talus (osteochondritis dissecans). *Am J Radiol* 1990; **154:** 555–8.

43. Yao L, Lee JK Occult intra-osseous fracture: detection with MR imaging. *Radiology* 1988; **167:** 749–51.

44. Lee JK, Yao L Stress fractures: MR imaging. *Radiology* 1988; **169:** 217–20.

45. Mirowitz SA, London SI Ulnar collateral ligament injury in baseball pitchers: MR imaging evaluation. *Radiology* 1992; **185:** 573–6.

46. Timmerman LA, Schwartz ML, Andrews JR Preoperative evaluation of the ulnar collateral ligament by magnetic resonance imaging and computed tomography arthrography. *Am J Sports Med* 1994; **22:** 26–31.

CHAPTER 6

Arthroscopy of the elbow

ANDREW A BROOKS, CHAMP L BAKER

Introduction

Arthroscopy of the elbow was first described by Burman[1] in 1931. He initially believe that arthroscopically this joint was 'unsuitable for examination,' but later revised his opinion after he successfully visualized the anterior compartment of the elbow in cadavers. In 1971, Watanabe[2] developed the 1.7 mm needle scope for use in small joints and later, Ito[3] and Maeda[4] described various arthroscopic surgical approaches to the elbow. In the USA, Andrews and Carson,[5] Johnson,[6] Guhl,[7] and Poehling et al.,[8] helped further refine the technique and increased the number of applications such that now, diagnostic and therapeutic arthroscopy of the elbow are well-accepted techniques for an ever-increasing number of elbow disorders.

Indications and contraindications

Elbow arthroscopy may at times be helpful in the assessment of the painful elbow. More commonly it is used therapeutically for 1) the removal of loose bodies; 2) the evaluation and treatment of osteochondral lesions; 3) the management of valgus extension overload syndrome; 4) partial synovectomy in inflammatory arthritis; 5) arthrolysis; 6) management of selected fractures; and 7) lavage of septic arthritis.

The major contraindication to elbow arthroscopy is any significant distortion of normal bony or soft tissue anatomy such that the local neurovascular structures cannot be safely avoided (e.g. previous ulnar nerve transposition) or the joint space cannot be adequately distended. Joint distension is essential to displace the nerves away from the portal sites. Severe ankylosis that prevents entry into or manipulation of the joint and the presence of local skin infection are also contraindications to elbow arthroscopy.

Preoperative planning

The key elements of preoperative planning for elbow arthroscopy are similar to any other type of surgical procedure. A thorough history and physical examination should always be undertaken with special care being taken in the assessment of the ulnar nerve for anterior subluxation. This occurs in approximately 15–20% of the population and this altered position puts the nerve at risk when establishing an anteromedial portal. Appropriate radiographs should also be performed. Standard radiographs taken at The Hughston Clinic include anterioposterior, lateral, and axillary views. We have not found more sophisticated imaging studies such as arthrography, magnetic resonance imaging (MRI), or computed tomography (CT) scan to be of value in the majority of cases.

Operative planning, positioning and instrumentation

Although elbow arthroscopy can be performed as an outpatient procedure under a regional block, a general anaesthetic is preferred. General anaesthesia allows complete muscle relaxation about the elbow during the procedure neurologic examination to be performed immediately after surgery.

We prefer to position the patient prone with the shoulder abducted 90 degrees and the arm supported in a foam bolster[9] (Fig. 6.1). A pneumatic tourniquet is placed on the involved arm at the mid-humerus level and the elbow is flexed 90 degrees. This allows maximal distension of the intra-articular space. Alternatively, the patient can be positioned supine with the shoulder abducted 90 degrees and in neutral rotation with the elbow in 90 degrees of flexion. The hand and forearm are placed in a prefabricated plastic wrist gauntlet that is connected to an overhead suspension device with 5lb (2 kg) of traction (Fig. 6.2).

The prone position offers several significant advantages. The arm is held in a more stable position, avoiding the unstable pendulum effect inherent in a suspended setup. Access to the posterior

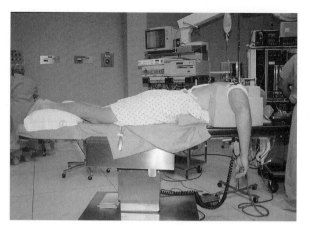

Fig. 6.1 A patient in the prone position for elbow arthroscopy.

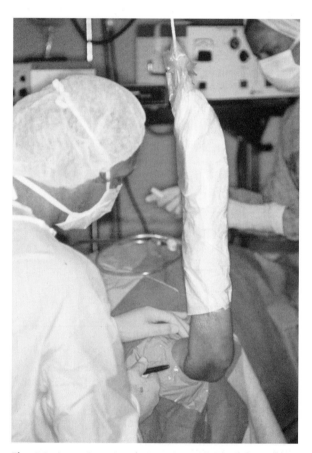

Fig. 6.2 A patient in the supine position for elbow arthroscopy.

chamber is facilitated by avoiding the need to operate in an uphill direction and, with the olecranon facing the surgeon, the prone position allows a more intuitive approach to manipulating

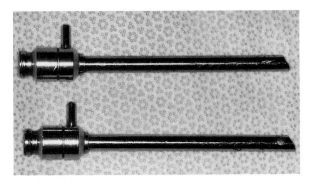

Fig. 6.3 Non-vented cannulas (top), rather than vented cannulas (bottom), should be used in the elbow to prevent fluid extravasation into soft tissue.

instruments within the joint. With the patient in the prone position, the proximal medial portal can be used as the initial viewing portal. This allows the instruments to enter the joint more parallel to the neurovascular structures, which may protect these structures during establishment of the portal. Finally, if arthrotomy is indicated the elbow is simply moved to a 90 degrees–90 degrees position and stabilised on an arm board. A standard Kocher approach can then be used. If a posterior approach is indicated the patient does not require repositioning.

The equipment required for elbow arthroscopy is similar to that used in other joints. A standard 4.0 mm, 30 degrees videoscope allows excellent visualization of the elbow joint. It is also helpful to have a 2.7 mm arthroscope available for viewing in smaller spaces, such as the lateral compartment as seen through the direct lateral portal. Interchangeable cannula systems for both the 4.0 and 2.7 mm arthroscopes should be used. These cannulas should be non-vented to avoid fluid extravasation into the soft tissues (Fig. 6.3). A cannula system eliminates the need for repeated entries into the joint when switching viewing and working portals. This minimizes risk of injury to the local anatomy and decreases fluid extravasation and swelling. The trocars used with the cannulas should be conical and blunt tipped, the sharp-tipped trocars pose an unnecessary risk to local nerves and vessels and are not needed for joint entry.

Hand-held instruments, such as probes, grasping forceps, osteotomes and punches are commonly used and in addition motorized synovial resectors and bone burrs may sometimes be required. Where possible, instruments should be inserted through cannulas to avoid multiple capsular punctures and reduce the risk of neurovascular injury.

Anatomy

GROSS ANATOMY

The topographical anatomy of the elbow is fully described in Chapter 2. However, for surgeons undertaking arthroscopy of the elbow it is essential to be aware of the important landmarks around the elbow in order that the arthroscopic portals can be safely established. For this reason the gross anatomy relevant to arthroscopy of the elbow is reviewed in this chapter.

The antecubital fossa is formed by three muscular borders. The lateral border is formed by the 'mobile wad of three': the brachioradialis, the extensor carpi radialis longus, and the extensor carpi radialis brevis. The medial border of the fossa is formed by the pronator teres, which originates from the medial epicondyle. The superior border of the fossa is defined by the biceps brachii.

The lateral and medial humeral epicondyles as well as the olecranon process of the proximal ulna are easily palpable. By pronating and supinating the forearm, the radial head can be palpated 3–4 cm distal to the lateral epicondyle. On the lateral aspect of the elbow, a triangle is formed by the lateral epicondyle, olecranon, and radial head. At the centre of this triangle is a 'soft spot', through which initial joint distension is performed.

The posterior aspect of the elbow comprises the triceps brachii and its tendon along with the tip of the olecranon. The anconeus muscle sits posterolaterally and – originates on the lateral epicondyle and posterior elbow capsule; it inserts on the proximal ulna.

The sensory nerves around the elbow originate from various levels of the brachial plexus. The medial brachial cutaneous nerve pierces the deep fascia midway down the arm on the medial side and supplies sensation to the posteromedial aspect of the arm to the level of the olecranon. The medial antebrachial cutaneous nerve separates into anterior and posterior branches and supplies skin sensation on the medial side of the elbow and forearm. The lateral antebrachial cutaneous nerve exists between the biceps and brachialis muscles and divides into anterior and posterior branches to supply the elbow and lateral half of the forearm. The posterior antebrachial cutaneous nerve originates from the radial nerve and courses down the lateral side of the arm to supply the posterolateral aspect of the elbow and posterior surface of the forearm.

The median nerve courses into the antecubital region on the medial aspect of the brachial artery and biceps tendon. As it exits the antecubital fossa, it disappears between the two heads of the pronator teres and distally beneath the flexor digitorum superficialis.

The radial nerve spirals around the posterior humeral shaft, penetrates the lateral intermuscular septum, and descends anterior to the lateral epicondyle between the brachioradialis and brachialis. In the antecubital region it divides into two branches. A superficial sensory branch supplies the dorsoradial wrist and posterior surface of the thumb, index, and middle fingers and sometimes the radial side of the ring finger. The deep motor branch descends deeply to wind around the posterolateral radial neck, enters the supinator and emerges as the posterior interosseus nerve.

The ulnar nerve penetrates the medial intermuscular septum in the distal third of the arm; it then courses behind the medial epicondyle, resting on the superficial aspect of the ulnar collateral ligament, and travels distally between the flexor carpi ulnaris and flexor digitorum superficialis.

The brachial artery descends into the elbow region on the anterior aspect of the brachialis muscle, just medial to the biceps tendon. At the level of the radial head, the artery bifurcates into the radial and ulnar arteries.

PORTAL ANATOMY

The most commonly used portals in elbow arthroscopy include the direct lateral, supermedial, anterolateral, superolateral, anteromedial, posterolateral, and straight posterior.

DIRECT LATERAL

The direct lateral portal is the standard initial site for distention of the joint before entry with the arthroscope. The portal site is located in the middle of the triangle formed by the lateral humeral epicondyle, the olecranon process, and the radiohumeral joint (Fig. 6.4). The direct lateral portal passes through the anconeus muscle when used to view the radiocapitellar joint, but it passes between the anconeus and tricep muscles when it is being used to visualize the posterior chamber (unpublished data, Brooks *et al.*, 1993). The only neurovascular structure at risk with this portal is the posterior antebrachial cutaneous nerve, which passes within an average of 7 mm.[10]

This portal is useful in viewing the radiocapitellar joint, particularly when using a 2.7 mm arthroscope, but we have found it most helpful as a viewing portal for working in the posterior chamber, particularly with the patient in the prone position.

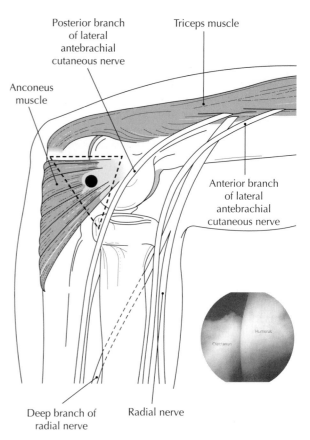

Fig. 6.4 The direct lateral portal is established in the middle of a triangle formed by the lateral epicondyle, the olecranon, and the radial head. Visible structures include the olecranon and humerus in the posterior compartment. This figure is reproduced in colour in the colour plate section.

Superomedial

The superomedial, or proximal medial, portal is located 2 cm proximal to the medial humeral epicondyle (Fig. 6.5). The arthroscopic cannula with its trocar is inserted anterior to the intermuscular septum. The surgeon keeps the cannula in contact with the anterior humerus and directs the trocar toward the radial head during insertion. A recent cadaver study[10] showed that the median nerve lies within 19 mm of the cannula in a distended joint; without distention the average distance is approximately 12 mm. The ulnar nerve was an average of 21 mm from the cannula when the joint is distended. The medial antebrachial cutaneous nerve was an average of 6 mm from this portal with the elbow distended and in 90 degrees of flexion.[10]

The superomedial portal provides superb visualization of the anterior compartment of the elbow.

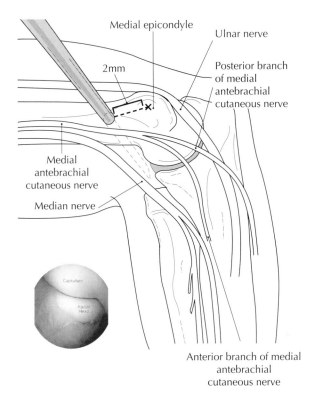

Fig. 6.5 The superomedial portal is established approximately 2 cm proximal to the medial humeral epicondyle. Visible structures include the capitellum and radial head. This figure is reproduced in colour in the colour plate section.

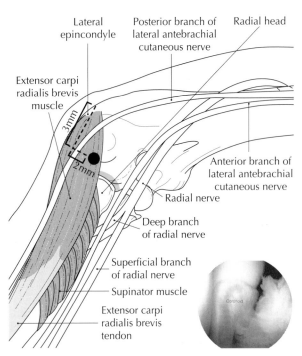

Fig. 6.6 The anterolateral portal is established approximately 3 cm distal and 2 cm anterior to the lateral humeral epicondyle. Visible structures include the coronoid process of the ulna. This figure is reproduced in colour in the colour plate section.

Visualisation of the radial head is facilitated with pronation and supination of the forearm. It is also useful as a working portal when viewing through the anterolateral portal and can be used as a high-flow irrigation portal when viewing through the posterolateral portal.

Anterolateral

The anterolateral portal is established in the sulcus between the radial head and capitellum anteriorly, approximately 3 cm distal and 2 cm anterior to the lateral humeral epicondyle.[11] The cannula passes through the extensor carpi radialis brevis and the supinator as it courses posterolateral to the radial nerve. The radial nerve can be as close as 3 mm to this portal even in distended specimens.[12] The posterior antebrachial cutaneous nerve is normally an average of 2 mm from the arthroscopic sheath.[13]

The anterolateral portal provides an excellent view of the medial capsule, medial pilca; coronoid process, trochlea, and coronoid fossa (Fig. 6.6).

Posterolateral

The posterolateral portal is located approximately 3 cm proximal to the tip of the olecranon, just superior and posterior to the lateral humeral epicondyle at the lateral border of the triceps. The cannula is directed towards the olecranon fossa. Neurovascular structures at risk with this portal include the medial brachial cutaneous and posterior antebrachial cutaneous nerves, which are an average of 25 mm from this portal.[13] The ulnar nerve is approximately 25 mm from this portal and as long as the cannula stays lateral to the posterior midline this nerve is not at risk.

The posterolateral portal allows viewing of the olecranon tip, olecranon fossa, and posterior trochlea.

Straight posterior

If necessary a straight posterior portal can be established 2 cm medial to where the posterolateral portal traverses the centre of the triceps tendon. This portal passes within 23 mm of the posterior antebrachial cutaneous nerve and within 25 mm of the ulnar nerve.[14] This portal can be helpful for removing impinging osteophytes and loose bodies from the posterior elbow joint.[15]

Diagnostic elbow arthroscopy

TECHNIQUE

After administration of general anaesthesia, the patient is positioned prone and chest rolls are used for stabilization. The patient's head and neck are stabilized with pillows to keep the airway open. A tourniquet is placed on the arm and the arm is supported in a foam holder with the elbow flexed 90 degrees. The elbow is carefully examined for any evidence of instability, and the range of motion is documented. After sterile preparation and draping is completed, landmarks including the medial and lateral humeral epicondyles, ulnar nerve, and radial head are outlined with a surgical marking pen. It is helpful to map out the various portals with the aid of a centimeter ruler. A rubber elastic bandage is used to exsanguinate the arm, and the tourniquet is inflated to 250 mm Hg. The joint is distended through the direct lateral or 'soft spot' portal using an 18-gauge spinal needle and instilling 30–40 ml of saline. Confirmation of intra-articular joint placement is made by either observing backflow from the needle or, alternatively, the elbow can be observed to extend and supinate as fluid is injected.

There are several precautions that, if followed, facilitate safer creation of arthroscopic portals about the elbow. First, always establish new portals in a fully distended joint; this provides maximal clearance from adjacent neurovascular structures (Fig. 6.7). Second, when creating portals, only incise the skin with the scalpel blade and use haemostats to spread the subcutaneous tissue in a longitudinal direction to move sensory nerves out of the way; a blunt trocar is used to penetrate the subcutaneous fat and muscles and enter the joint. Finally, when possible, establish portals only once and use cannulas to maintain the portal tract for passage or instruments.

In order to reduce the risk of missing intra-articular pathology it is wise when arthroscopically examining the elbow to do so systematically. We begin our arthroscopic examination of the elbow from the superomedial portal. This we believe has several advantages over starting laterally. In particular there is less risk to the local neurovascular structures (the radial nerve is only 4 mm from the arthroscope in the anterolateral portal but the median nerve is 23 mm from the anteromedial portal).[11] Also, there is less fluid extravasation because the superomedial portal traverses predominantly tendinous tissue and a fibrous portion of the forearm flexor muscles. This thicker tissue minimizes fluid extravasation more effectively than the softer, thinner radial capsule. Finally, the majority

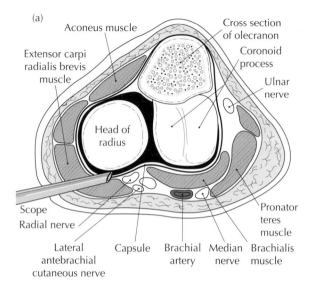

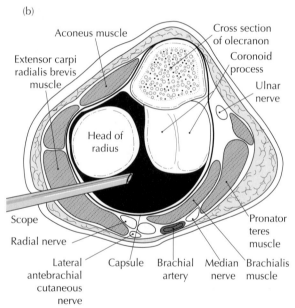

Fig. 6.7 (a) Non-distended and (b) distended joint illustrating the importance of obtaining full joint distension. With the arthroscope in the anterolateral portal, the cannula passes very close to neurovascular structures in the non-distended joint.

of elbow lesions tend to be located in the lateral compartment, which is visualized better from the medial side of the joint.

After establishment of this initial portal, the anterior compartment of the elbow is carefully examined. The lateral capsule, radial head, capitellum, and radial fossa are initially visualized. As the arthroscope is withdrawn medially, the coronoid and its humeral articulation can be seen. The anterior capsule is then inspected by rotating the lens of the camera. Next, the anterolateral portal is established using an outside-in technique; proper portal location is initially determined with an 18–gauge spinal needle. Alternatively, this portal can be established in an inside-out manner by advancing a Wissinger rod through the lateral capsule. After the skin is incised a cannula is retrograded into the joint. This second portal can be used as a working or viewing portal. It is important to visualize the anterior compartment through both medial and lateral portals to obtain a complete examination. If the radiocapitellar joint needs closer visualisation, this is easily done by changing to a 2.7 mm arthroscope and establishing a direct lateral portal while maintaining high inflow through the already created superomedial portal.

After the anterior compartment has been evaluated, the posterior compartment is entered through the posterolateral or, alternatively, the direct lateral portal. If a second working portal is needed posteriorly, we use the straight posterior approach, which is placed through the centre of the triceps, 3 cm proximal to the olecranon tip. The posterior chamber is sometimes difficult to visualize initially and may require debridement with a motorized shaver before an adequate examination can be performed.

After completion of the procedure, the tourniquet is deflated and the wounds are dressed with adhesive bandages or skin tape. We do not instill the joint with local anaesthetic because local extravasation can affect the postoperative nerve examination. A soft dressing and sling are routinely applied, and the patient is discharged on the day of surgery. The patient is permitted to remove the dressing after 48 hours and can shower if there is no active wound drainage.

REHABILITATION

Physical therapy exercises are usually initiated on the day of surgery. The programme is modified according to the extent of the procedure that was performed, but the basic goal of all therapy is to return the patient or athlete to activity quickly and safely. The physical therapy programme must be tailored to the individual patient, but it should follow a certain progression of phases.

Initially, during the first 2 weeks, the goal of rehabilitation should be to restore range of motion (especially extension), minimize pain and inflammation, and avoid atrophy of the surrounding muscles. Patients are instructed on hand, wrist, and elbow exercises to be performed three times a day.

These include grip strengthening with putty, wrist flexor and extensor stretching, wrist curls with a 1lb (500 g) weight in flexion and extension, and radial wrist curls with the ulnar border of the forearm resting on the table. Inflammation can be minimized early with judicious use of local ice-packs for several days.

The second phase of therapy usually occurs between 2 and 4 weeks after surgery. During this time the therapist continues to emphasize progressive elbow mobility and improved strength. Stretching exercises are continued to maintain flexion and extension, along with pronation and supination. Strengthening exercises with use of isotonic muscle contractions are emphasized at this phase, and shoulder rotator cuff strengthening is begun.

The final phase usually begins 4–6 weeks after surgery and is directed at progressively increasing activities to prepare the patient for unrestricted functional participation. The final phase of therapy is only initiated when the patient has achieved full range of motion and has minimal pain and tenderness. The goals of this phase are to increase the patient's total arm strength, power and endurance. If the patient is a throwing athlete, a throwing programme is initiated.

COMPLICATIONS

Complications from elbow arthroscopy can and do ccur, but they are usually associated with surgeon inexperience, poor technique, or lack of understanding of local anatomy. The list of complications that can occur is similar to other arthroscopic procedures, but the majority of reported complications are neurovascular in nature. Lynch et al.[13] reported a series of 21 elbow arthroscopies in which there was one transient low radial nerve plasy believed to be a result of overdistension of the joint, one transient low median nerve palsy believed to be secondary to use of local anesthetic, and one neuroma of the medial antebrachial cutaneous nerve that ultimately required resection. Cascells[16] described a case in which the use of motorised instruments posteromedially led to irreparable ulnar nerve damage. Thomas et al.[17] described a radial nerve injury, and Papilion et al.[18] have reported a case of compression neuropathy of the radial nerve during elbow arthroscopy. Small[19] reported only one neurovascular complication, a radial nerve injury, in a survey of 569 elbow arthroscopies performed by members of the Arthroscopy Association of North America.

In our series of more than 200 elbow arthroscopies, we have not had a single neurovascular complication. We did have one patient develop massive heterotopic bone anteriorly following an arthroscopic arthrolysis whilst a second patient developed a postoperative olecranon bursitis.

Most of the complications associated with elbow arthroscopy can be avoided by strictly adhering to proper surgical technique. Attention to detail is paramount. Successful elbow arthroscopy requires a thorough understanding of local anatomy, meticulous mapping of local landmarks on the skin, maintaining joint distention during establishment of portals and passage of instruments, and keeping the elbow flexed to 90 degrees during the majority of the procedure in order to keep the neurovascular structures in the antecubital fossa relaxed. If these procedures are followed, the surgical morbidity of elbow arthroscopy should be low.

Therapeutic elbow arthroscopy

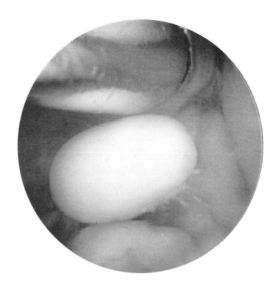

Fig. 6.8 A loose body in the elbow as seen through the arthroscope. This figure is reproduced in colour in the colour plate section.

REMOVAL OF LOOSE BODIES

Removal of loose bodies is the most common indication for elbow arthroscopy (Fig. 6.8). The loose bodies occur as a result of joint surface fragmentation[20] and cause pain, loss of motion (typically extension), swelling, catching and occasional locking if the fragment is free within the joint. Most loose bodies are visible radiographically, but the radiographs will be negative if the loose bodies are non-calcified cartilaginous lesions. Patients should be informed preoperatively that occasionally the loose body may not be found at surgery or there may be additional loose bodies that may produce symptoms in the future. Finally, there is the possibility of recurrence of loose bodies, especially if the underlying primary disease is an ongoing process (i.e. degenerative joint disease or synovial chondromatosis).

There are several technical points that may be helpful in finding loose bodies in the elbow. The location of loose bodies is often dictated by the underlying disease. For example, loose bodies seen with osteochondritis dissecans are often located laterally near the capitellum or radial head. Loose bodies caused by fractures are usually located near the site of fracture, such as the coronoid, radial head, or tip of the olecranon. Loose bodies associated with synovial chondromatosis will usually be found in the anterior portion of the joint.

If a loose body is suspected to be within a certain compartment but is not seen, it is helpful to place a shaver with full suction in the compartment, this may help evacuate the loose body. It is critical to thoroughly examine every compartment and gutter of the joint in search of loose bodies. Occasionally, loose bodies can migrate from one compartment to another during the procedure. Larger fragments sometimes have to be sectioned with an osteotome before removal.

EVALUATION AND TREATMENT OF OSTEOCHONDRAL LESIONS

Osteochondritis dissecans of the elbow, or Panner's disease, typically involves the young throwing athlete or gymnast. There has been much confusion about the terminology for discussing these lesions. We believe this stems from some authors separating osteochondritis dissecans and Panner's disease into two separate entities. Most likely, these terms refer to two different stages of the same disease, which affects the endochondral ossification of the epiphyseal growth centre.[21]

The cause of this pathologic process is probably repetitive microtrauma to a vulnerable epiphysis with a precarious blood supply. These lesions usually involve the capitellum, but occasionally osteochondral lesions can involve the radial head as well. Whether the original osteochondral lesion advances to a frank osteochondritis dissecans with joint incongruity and associated loose body formation depends on several factors, including age of patient at disease onset and the nature of the trauma associated with the lesion.[21]

The typical patient is aged 12–16 years and complains of dull pain on the lateral aspect of the elbow with loss of motion (typically extension). The patient may also complain of catching or locking of the elbow. Examination reveals occasional swelling, limited motion, and tenderness over the radiocapitellar joint. Radiographs often show irregularity of the capitellar surface and occasional radiolucencies can be seen. Some cases may warrant more sophisticated imaging such as MRI.

Indications for surgery in osteochondritis dissecans are failure of conservative treatment, the presence of loose bodies, and a locked elbow. The entire procedure is performed arthroscopically and involves simple excision of loose or detached cartilage along with chondroplasty of the crater with a motorised burr and drilling with a K-wire. If no evidence of disease is identified anteriorly, it is important to visualise the posterior capitellum through a posterolateral portal.[22]

MANAGEMENT OF VALGUS EXTENSION OVERLOAD

The repetitive forces of pitching can lead to unnatural stresses across the elbow joint that can result in osteochondral changes of both the olecranon and distal humerus. These changes can result in a chronic extension overload with a mechanical block between the tip of the olecranon and olecranon fossa causing loss of full extension. Andrews coined the term valgus extension overload to describe this combination of bony hypertrophy and soft tissue contractures.[23] Specifically, an osteophyte on the posteromedial aspect of the tip of the olecranon with concomitent impingement on the olecranon fossa creates a 'kissing lesion', which is an osteochondral defect on the trochlea of the humerus.[23] This is a direct result of the tremendous repetitive valgus forces generated during the acceleration phase of pitching as the elbow goes into extension.

The typical patient is a baseball pitcher in his mid-twenties who complains of posterior elbow pain during the acceleration and follow through phases of pitching. Physical examination reveals a flexion contracture, pain over the tip of the olecranon posteriorly, and pain with valgus stress and extension. Lateral radiographs usually reveal a posterior osteophyte on the olecranon tip. A posteromedial osteophyte may be seen on the axial view.

The ulnar nerve lies within the posteromedial gutter and is only separated from the bone by a thin capsule and ligamentous tissue. Therefore, great care must be taken when using motorised instruments in this area.

SYNOVECTOMY

Approximately 20–50% of patients with rheumatoid arthritis have involvement of the elbow.[24] About half of these patients will have pain and associated loss of motion. The majority of patients can be treated conservatively with non-steroidal anti-inflammatory drugs (NSAIDs), physical therapy, and judicious use of intra-articular corticosteroid injections. However, in patients where pain relief is not obtained with the usual conservative therapies, operative intervention can be beneficial, particularly if the destruction of the articular cartilage is minimal. There have been reports of no recurrence of pain for at least 6 years after open synovectomy of the elbow,[24] thus it is reasonable to expect comparable results with an arthroscopic approach.

Care must be taken when performing arthroscopic synovectomy with motorised instruments since the capsule is often quite thin in rheumatoid patients and the neurovascular structures in close proximity can be at risk.

ARTHROLYSIS

Flexion contractures of the elbow can be a serious problem both functionally and cosmetically. The cause is often related to trauma, but it may also be the result of degenerative and inflammatory arthritis.

The clinical presentation varies, but all patients will usually complain of decreased motion in flexion or extension or occasionally both. It is important to delineate the cause of the contracture as this may affect treatment. To this end radiographs can be helpful.

Treatment initially is conservative using NSAIDs, stretching and splinting. In cases where this conservative approach fails, arthroscopic release and thorough joint debridgement can be helpful in properly selected cases.[25–27] This procedure is technically demanding and does require considerable experience in order that it can be performed safely. The elbow capsule is released from its anterior humeral attachment along with adhesions from the radial head and coronoid. In most cases there is extensive scarring posteriorly in the olecranon fossa with osteophyte formation within the fossa and at the tip of the olecranon. This remaining scar tissue is debrided and osteophytes are resected with a motorised burr. Postoperatively, the patient is splinted in full extension and supination for 24 hours. After 24–48 hours, passive and active motion is initiated.

MANAGEMENT OF SELECTED FRACTURES

Certain fractures around the elbow can be successfully treated with arthroscopy.[28] Radial head fractures are now commonly treated with an arthroscopic procedure. Excision of osteochondral fracture fragments and evaluation of the degree of fracture displacement are also indications for arthroscopy. Some minimally displaced fractures can be reduced and stabilised arthroscopically with percutaneous pinning or other forms of internal fixation. However, the most common indication for elbow arthroscopy in this setting is removal of fracture debris blocking elbow motion.

LAVAGE OF SEPTIC ARTHRITIS

Acute sepsis of the elbow requires urgent and effective treatment if destruction of the joint is to be prevented. Although this can be undertaken by an open procedure arthroscopy enables the efficient collection of pus samples for microscopy culture and sensitivity, and allows the thorough irrigation and debridgement of the joint. In addition suction drains and irrigation cannulae can be inserted through the arthroscopic portals.

Future developments

As our understanding of the elbow continues to grow and technology continues to advance, our capacity to correct problems of the elbow with arthroscopic techniques will naturally expand. We are at the brink of some major advancements in the evaluation and treatment of elbow disorders. Many surgical procedures currently being performed in an open manner will undoubtedly be adapted for an arthroscopic approach. We are already seeing this with treatment of radiocapitellar arthrosis, arthrolysis and arthroscopic ulnohumeral arthroplasty.[29] It is conceivable in the near future that liagmentous tightening procedures, fracture treatment with arthroscopic bioabsorbable devices, and biological joint replacement will be common procedures performed in the elbow with the aid of the arthroscope.

References

1. Burman MS Arthroscopy or the direct visualization of joints. *J Bone Joint Surg* 1931; **13**: 669–95.
2. Watanabe M Arthroscopy of small joints. *J Jpn Orthop Assoc* 1971; **44**: 908.
3. Ito K The arthroscopic anatomy of the elbow joint. *Arthroscopy* 1979; **4**: 2–9.
4. Maeda Y Arthroscopy of the elbow joint. *Arthroscopy* 1980; **5**: 5–8.
5. Andrews JR, Carson WG Arthroscopy of the elbow. *Arthroscopy* 1985; **1**: 97–107.
6. Johnson LL Elbow arthroscopy. In: *Arthroscopic surgery: Principles and practice.* St Louis: Mosby, 1986, 1446–77.
7. Guhl JF Arthroscopy and arthroscopic surgery of the elbow. *Orthopedics* 1985; **8**: 290–6.
8. Poehling GG, Whipple TL, Sisco L, Goldman B Elbow arthroscopy: A new technique. *Arthroscopy* 1989; **5**: 222–4.
9. Baker CL, Shalvoy RM The prone position for elbow arthrocopy. *Clin Sports Med* 1991; **10**: 623–8.
10. Adolfsson L Arthroscopy of the elbow joint: A cadaveric study of portal placement. *J Shoulder Elbow Surg* 1994; **3**: 53–61.
11. Boe S Arthroscopy of the elbow. Diagnosis and extraction of loose bodies. *Acta Orthop Scand* 1986; **57**: 52–3.
12. Lindenfeld TN Medial approach in elbow arthroscopy. *Am J Sports Med* 1990; **18**: 413–7.
13. Lynch GJ, Meyers JF, Whipple TL, Caspari RB Neurovascular anatomy and elbow arthroscopy: Inherent risks. *Arthroscopy* 1986; **2**: 190–7.
14. Cohen B, Constant CR Extension-supination sign in prearthroscopic elbow distention. *Arthroscopy* 1992; **8**: 189–90.
15. Andrews JR, St Pierre Rk, Carson WG Arthroscopy of the elbow. *Clin Sports Med* 1986; **5**: 653–62.
16. Cascells SW Neurovascular anatomy and elbow arthroscopy: Inherent risks, editors comments. *Arthroscopy* 1987; **2**: 190.
17. Thomas MA, Fast A, Shapiro D Radial nerve damage as a complication of elbow arthroscopy. *Clin Orthop* 1987; **215**: 130–1.
18. Papilion JD, Neff DS, Shall LM Compression neuropathy of the radial nerve as a complication of elbow arthroscopy: A case report and review of the literature. *Arthroscopy* 1988; **4**: 284–6.
19. Small NC Complications in arthroscopy. On knee and other joints. *Arthroscopy* 1986; **2**: 253–8.
20. Milgram JW The development of loose bodies in human joints. *Clin Orthop* 1977; **124**: 292–303.
21. Singer KM, Roy SP Osteochondrosis of the humeral capitellum. *Am J Sports Med* 1984; **12**: 351–60.
22. Ruch DS, Poehling GG Arthroscopic treatment of Panner's disease. *Clin Sports Med* 1991; **10**: 629–36.
23. Wilson FD, Andrews JR, Blackburn TA, McClusky G Valgus extension overload in the pitching elbow. *Am J Sports Med* 1983; **11**: 83–8.
24. Porter BB, Richardson C, Vaino K Rheumatoid arthritis of the elbow: The results of synovectomy. *J Bone Joint Surg* 1974; **56B**: 427–37.
25. Nowicki KD, Shall L Arthroscopic release of post traumatic flexion contracture in the elbow: A case report and review of the literature. *Arthroscopy* 1992; **8**: 544–7.

26. Jones GS, Savoie FH Arthroscopic release of flexion contractures (arthrofibrosis) of the elbow. *Arthroscopy* 1993; **9:** 277–83.

27. Timmerman LA, Andrews JR Arthroscopic treatment of post traumatic elbow pain and stiffness. *Am J Sports Med* 1994; **22:** 230–5.

28. O'Driscoll SW, Morrey BF Arthroscopy of the elbow: Diagnostic and therapeutic benefits and hazards. *J Bone Joint Surg* 1992; **74A:** 84–94.

29. Redden JF, Stanley D Arthroscopic fenestration of the olecranon fossa in the treatment of osteoarthritis of the elbow. *Arthroscopy* 1993; **9:** 14–16.

CHAPTER 7

Surgical approaches to the elbow

PIET DE BOER, DAVID STANLEY

Introduction

All surgical approaches are based on the anatomy of the structures to be exposed and their soft tissue coverings. Thus a detailed knowledge of the surgical anatomy of the elbow is critical if operative procedures are to be performed successfully.

The best surgical approaches exploit internervous planes. These planes were first described by Henry[1] and lie between muscles supplied by different nerves. Their significance in operative surgery, lies in the fact that the planes can be used along their entire length without risk of denervation of the adjacent muscles. Henry[1] characterised approaches using these planes as being extensile and although his concepts are best applied in the forearm and upper arm his principles nevertheless apply at the elbow.

In this chapter each surgical approach will be structured in an identical way:

Indication for surgery
As with all operations the surgical approach should be determined by the indication for operative treatment. It is therefore important to have a clear appreciation of the pathological process occurring at the elbow in order that the most appropriate surgical approach is undertaken.

Position of the patient
This is critical for successful exposure and should be achieved before the patient is prepared for surgery.

Surgical landmarks and incision
The skin incision is based on the surgical landmarks. It should be long to avoid unnecessary tension when the soft tissues are retracted and unless they cross the flexor crease should be straight or gently curved.

Dissection
A layered approach to dissection is strongly recommended. Each layer of the dissection must be fully exposed before going on to the deeper structures, ensuring that the exposure does not get progressively smaller as it becomes deeper. For this reason the description of the surgical dissection has been divided into superficial and deep dissections.

Dangers
The dangers of each surgical approach are described in order to reduce the risk of operative complications.

Enlargement of the approach
This can be achieved by local measures such as repositioning retractors or extensile measures in which the approach is extended to include adjacent structures.

Tourniquets

The majority of elbow operations are performed with a tourniquet which should be well padded to prevent blistering of the underlying skin. Exanguination of the limb can be achieved either by elevation for 5 minutes or by the use of a soft rubber exsanguinator. The inflated pressure of the tourniquet should be approximately 275 mm Hg. The tourniquet should not be left in place for more than 1 hour, and should not be used at all for patients with peripheral vascular or sickle cell disease.

Posterior approach

Indications for surgery
The posterior approach to the elbow provides the best exposure of the bony structures of the elbow joint. It is the most appropriate approach for many traumatic conditions and is used for the fixation of distal humeral fractures, the treatment of non-unions, the operative reduction of unreduced elbow dislocations and the treatment of post-traumatic ankylosis. In addition it is the most commonly used approach for elbow arthroplasty and the debridement of the osteoarthritic elbow.

Variations in surgical technique either involve splitting or reflecting the triceps mechanism[2–6] or necessitate an osteotomy of the olecranon.[7,8] For traumatic conditions an olecranon osteotomy provides excellent exposure. This technique, however, is inappropriate for the insertion of a total elbow arthroplasty where integrity of the ulna is essential. In this situation the triceps will require reflection or splitting in order to provide adequate joint exposure. A more limited posterior approach is used for the treatment of osteoarthritis of the elbow[9–11] (Chapter 28).

Position of the patient
The posterior approach to the elbow can be undertaken with the patient supine and the arm draped free across the chest (Fig. 7.1a). Alternatively the patient can be positioned prone on the operating table with the arm abducted 90 degrees and the elbow flexed to 90 degrees allowing the forearm to hang vertically (Fig. 7.1b). The preferred position,

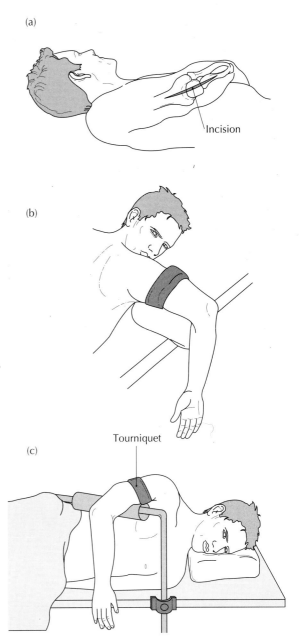

Fig. 7.1 The patient can be positioned in several ways for the posterior approach to the elbow. (a) Supine with the arm draped free across the chest. (b) Prone with the arm abducted 90 degrees, the elbow flexed 90 degrees and the forearm hanging vertically. (c) Lateral with the arm supported on a bolster the elbow flexed 90 degrees and the forearm hanging vertically.

however, is with the patient lateral, the upper arm supported on a bolster and with the elbow flexed to 90 degrees and the forearm hanging free (Fig. 7.1c). This provides the same excellent exposure that is obtainable with the prone position but avoids the anaesthetic hazards.

Surgical landmarks and incision
Before the incision is made the surgical landmarks of the posterior aspect of the elbow should be palpated. In particular the olecranon and its relationship to the medial and lateral epicondyles should be identified and the position of the ulnar nerve noted (Fig. 7.2).

The skin incision should be centred at the level of the olecranon and should begin approximately 10cm proximally. It should avoid passing directly over the tip of the olecranon since scars in this region can be troublesome. As such, therefore, the incision should either begin in the midline and curve gently around the olecranon finishing over the subcutaneous surface of the ulna or it should be a straight incision centred just lateral or medial to the tip of the olecranon (Fig. 7.3). The authors preferred incision is just medial to the tip of the olecranon. This does not place the ulnar nerve at risk providing it has been previously palpated and providing the incision is carefully performed. The advantage of this approach is that it avoids raising large skin flaps over the tip of the olecranon.

Superficial dissection
The fascia overlying the triceps is incised and the ulnar nerve identified by palpation. The nerve is then carefully dissected so that it is clearly seen

throughout its course as it passes behind the medial epicondyle.

The further management of the ulnar nerve varies depending on whether it is to be fully mobilised and transposed anteriorly[12,13] or whether as is the authors' preference it is to be allowed to remain in its normal anatomical position.[6,14] If anterior transposition is to be undertaken soft rubber slings are carefully passed around the nerve to facilitate the mobilisation and transposition procedure. If the nerve is to be left in its anatomical position then frequent reference to the nerve should be made during the deep dissection in order to prevent it being inadvertently damaged.

Deep dissection
The deep dissection depends on which surgical approach is being undertaken.

TRICEPS SPLITTING

This approach often referred to as the Campbell posterior approach involves splitting the triceps muscle and tendon down to the tip of the olecranon. The dissection is then continued subperiosteally with lateral reflection of anconeus and medial reflection of flexor carpi ulnaris (Fig. 7.4). Steiger and Gschwend[5] modified this technique by raising osteoperiosteal flaps from the olecranon (Fig. 7.5).

Van Gorder[3] advised dissecting an inverted V shaped flap of the triceps aponeurosis and reflecting this distally (Fig. 7.6). The remaining fibres of the triceps are then split in the midline and reflected from the humerus.

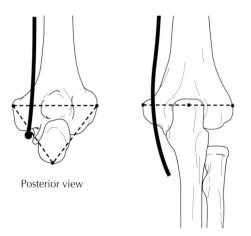

Fig. 7.2 The sugical landmarks of the posterior aspect of the elbow.

Posterior view

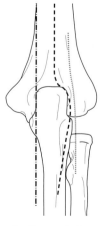

Fig. 7.3 Incisions for the posterior approach to the elbow.

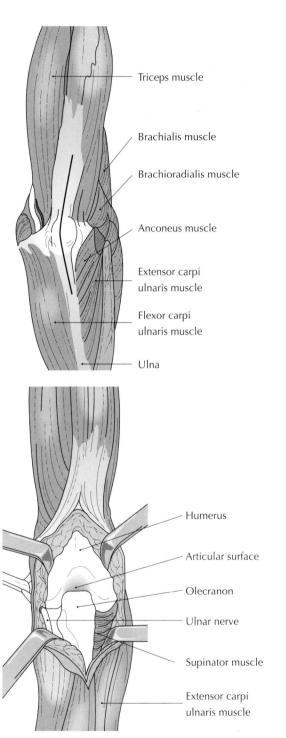

Fig. 7.4 The Campbell triceps splitting posterior approach to the elbow.

- Triceps muscle
- Brachialis muscle
- Brachioradialis muscle
- Anconeus muscle
- Extensor carpi ulnaris muscle
- Flexor carpi ulnaris muscle
- Ulna

- Humerus
- Articular surface
- Olecranon
- Ulnar nerve
- Supinator muscle
- Extensor carpi ulnaris muscle

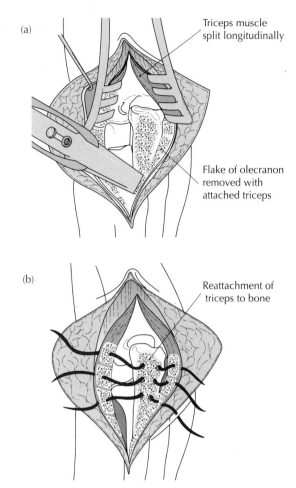

(a)
- Triceps muscle split longitudinally
- Flake of olecranon removed with attached triceps

(b)
- Reattachment of triceps to bone

Fig. 7.5 The Gschwend posterior approach to the elbow.

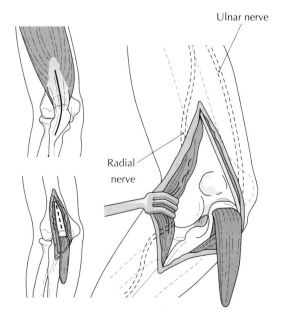

- Ulnar nerve
- Radial nerve

Fig. 7.6 The Van Gorder posterior approach to the elbow.

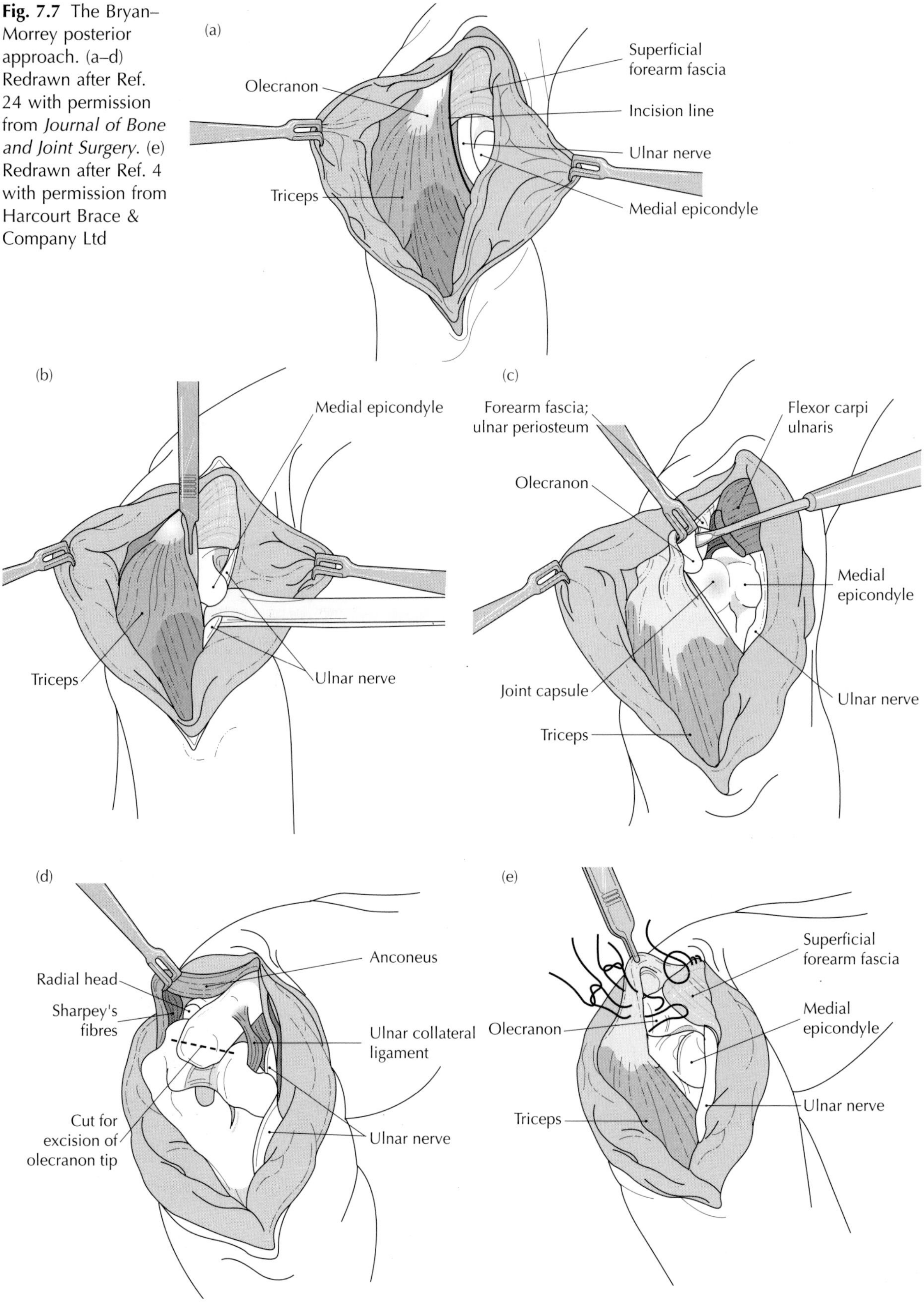

Fig. 7.7 The Bryan–Morrey posterior approach. (a–d) Redrawn after Ref. 24 with permission from *Journal of Bone and Joint Surgery*. (e) Redrawn after Ref. 4 with permission from Harcourt Brace & Company Ltd

(a)
Olecranon
Superficial forearm fascia
Incision line
Ulnar nerve
Medial epicondyle
Triceps

(b)
Medial epicondyle
Triceps
Ulnar nerve

(c)
Forearm fascia; ulnar periosteum
Olecranon
Flexor carpi ulnaris
Medial epicondyle
Joint capsule
Triceps
Ulnar nerve

(d)
Radial head
Sharpey's fibres
Anconeus
Ulnar collateral ligament
Ulnar nerve
Cut for excision of olecranon tip

(e)
Superficial forearm fascia
Medial epicondyle
Olecranon
Triceps
Ulnar nerve

TRICEPS REFLECTING

Bryan and Morrey[4] described a triceps reflecting posterior approach to the elbow. This involves identifying the medial aspect of the triceps which is then elevated. The dissection is continued through the superficial fascia of the forearm down onto the periosteum of the medial aspect of the proximal ulna. The periosteum is then carefully reflected laterally (Fig. 7.7). Wolfe and Ranawat[6] described a similar approach but raised an osteoanconeus flap. The dissection involved a longitudinal incision along the subcutaneous border of the ulna dividing the anconeus fascia at its origin. The incision was then carried medially across the olecranon and a wafer of bone with the attachment of the triceps tendon was reflected from the olecranon using a sharp osteotome or oscillating saw (Fig. 7.8).

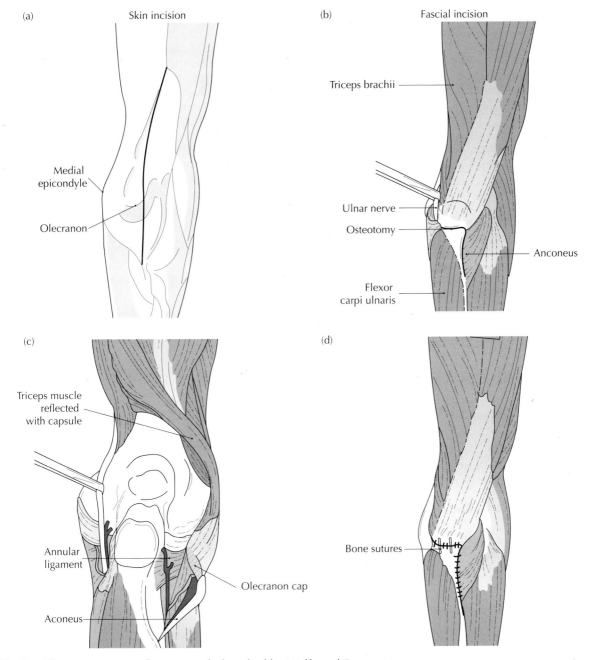

Fig. 7.8 The osteoanconeus flap approach described by Wolfe and Ranawat.

OLECRANON OSTEOTOMY

The transolecranon approach to the elbow was originally described by MacAusland.[7] It provides excellent exposure for the operative treatment of distal humeral fractures.

Having identified and protected the ulnar nerve, a 3.2 mm drill hole is made from proximal to distal in the ulna medullary canal. The olecranon is then osteotomised with a saw in the mid portion of the sigmoid notch, and the olecranon and triceps reflected proximally. The olecranon is reattached to the ulna at the end of the procedure using a cancellous screw inserted through the previously prepared drill hole (Fig. 7.9).

A variation in the method of osteotomising the ulna involves making a V shaped incision in the olecranon periosteum with the apex of the V facing distally. The olecranon is then divided creating a V-shaped osteotomy. This is achieved with an oscillating saw until the articular surface of the olecranon has almost been breached. At this point the osteotomy is completed using an osteotome. This technique provides better keying of the bone when the olecranon is reattached at the end of the procedure and prevents reduction of the diameter of the sigmoid notch which will occur if the saw blade is taken completely through the olecranon.

An extra-articular osteotomy of the olecranon has been recommended by the A-O group.[8] This, as with the other osteotomy approaches, involves initial pre-drilling of the ulna in order to facilitate reattachment of the olecranon at the end of the procedure. The triceps insertion onto the ulna is then identified and an extra-articular oblique osteotomy performed. The olecranon fragment and attached triceps muscle is then reflected proximally (Fig. 7.10).

Dangers

The ulnar nerve is the structure most at risk. Careful initial dissection with either anterior transposition or protection if the nerve is not transposed should ensure its safety. It is at greatest danger during the insertion of K wires or screws if local soft tissues snag around the drill. In addition it is

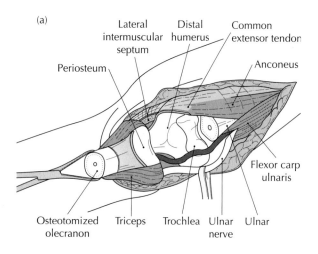
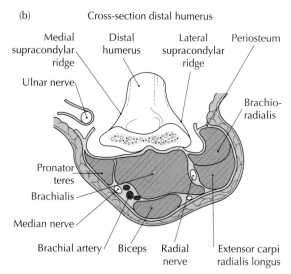

Fig. 7.9 The transolecranon approach described by MacAusland.

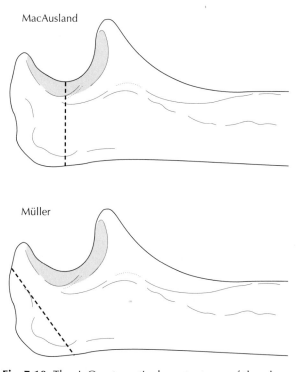

Fig. 7.10 The A-O extra-articular osteotomy of the ulna.

also at risk if its blood supply is compromised during mobilisation or if slings placed around the nerve are forcibly retracted. The median nerve and brachial artery lie anterior to the distal humerus. They should not be at risk providing any anterior dissection of the distal humerus is performed in a periosteal plane. The radial nerve is only at risk if the stripping of the triceps is carried proximally into the middle third of the humerus. At this level the radial nerve traverses the posterior aspect of the bone running from proximomedially to distolaterally.

Enlargement of the approach

The posterior approach can be extended proximally to allow exposure of the distal third of the humerus. Above this level the radial nerve traverses the operative field. The approach can be extended distally along the subcutaneous border of the ulna to explore the entire length of this bone. Although rarely indicated, enlargement of the approach may be required for a patient with a distal humeral and proximal ulna fracture.

Posterolateral approach

Indications for surgery

The posterolateral approach to the elbow is indicated for the treatment of Monteggia fracture dislocations, the fixation of radial head fractures, lateral ligament reconstructions and open elbow synovectomies.

The technique most commonly used, and the one that will be described here is the Boyd approach.[15] Modifications of this have been reported.[16–18] In addition Wadsworth[19] has described an extensive posterolateral approach.

Position of the patient

With the patient in the supine position the arm is abducted and placed on an arm board. The Wadsworth extensive posterolateral approach, however, requires the patient to be prone with the arm abducted and elbow flexed 90 degrees.

Surgical landmarks and incisions

The lateral epicondyle of the humerus should first be palpated and below this at a distance of approximately 2.5 cm the radial head will be found. To facilitate identification of the radial head the forearm can be pronated and supinated and the radial head will be noted to rotate beneath the palpating thumb.

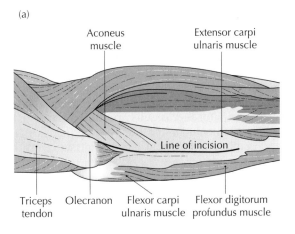
(a)

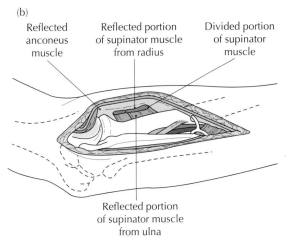
(b)

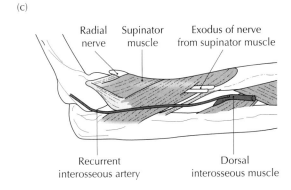
(c)

Fig. 7.11 The Boyd posterolateral approach.

The incision commences approximately 1 cm posterior to the lateral epicondyle and continues distally curving beside the lateral tip of the olecranon down onto the subcutaneous border of the ulna.

Superficial dissection

The skin flaps are raised to expose the superficial muscle mass and the anconeus and extensor carpi ularis muscles are identified. These are stripped subperiosteally from the ulna and reflected volarward. The forearm is fully pronated.

Deep dissection

The supinator is released subperiosteally from its ulnar insertion and also reflected in a volar direction. This protects the posterior interosseous nerve. As the supinator is released care should be taken to avoid detachment of the ulnar component of the lateral collateral ligament which is attached to the ulna in this region (Fig. 7.11).

The surgical technique for the Wadsworth extensive posterolateral approach is shown in Fig. 7.12.

Dangers

The only significant danger of this approach lies in damaging the posterior interosseous nerve. The risk of this is reduced by pronation of the forearm which keeps the nerve as far away from the dissection as possible. If the arm is supinated the nerve is brought closer to the plane of dissection.

(a)

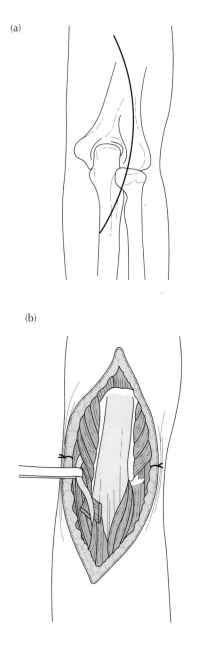

(c)

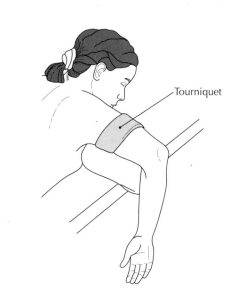

Tourniquet

(b)

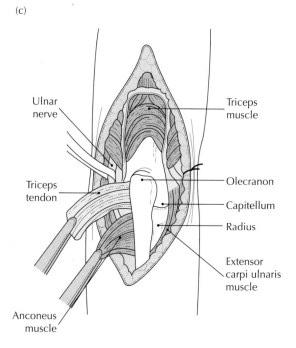

Ulnar nerve

Triceps muscle

Triceps tendon

Olecranon

Capitellum

Radius

Extensor carpi ulnaris muscle

Anconeus muscle

Fig. 7.12 Wadsworth's extensive posterolateral approach.

Enlargement of the approach

The approach can be enlarged proximally and distally. Proximal extension is achieved by increasing the incision and dissecting down directly onto the lateral supracondylar ridge. The muscles can then be reflected anteriorly and posteriorly to give exposure of the distal humerus. If greater exposure of the radius is required the recurrent interosseous artery is ligated and the muscle mass is reflected volarly. This technique provides continued protection of the posterior interosseous nerve.

Lateral approach

Indication for surgery

The lateral approach to the elbow provides excellent exposure for the fixation of lateral condylar and radial head fractures and Monteggia fracture dislocations. It can also be used for excision of the radial head, open synovectomy and repair of the lateral collateral ligament.

Several approaches have been described[20,21] but the safest and most commonly used is that described by Kocher.[22]

Position of the patient

The patient is positioned supine with the arm abducted and placed on an arm board. The elbow is comfortably flexed and forearm pronated in order to display the lateral aspect of the elbow.

Surgical landmarks and incision

The lateral supracondylar ridge of the humerus, lateral epicondyle and radial head should be palpated before surgery is commenced.

The incision should begin 5 cm proximal to the elbow joint over the lateral supracondylar ridge. It should extend distally along the ridge, over the radial head and approximately 5 cm distal to the radial head it should curve posteriorly to end at the posterior border of the ulna.

Superficial dissection

The superficial dissection is taken between the triceps muscle posteriorly and the brachioradialis and extensor carpi radialis longus muscles anteriorly. This enables exposure of the lateral condyle and the capsule over the lateral aspect of the joint. Distally the extensor carpi ulnaris is separated from the anconeus.

Deep dissection

The periosteum is reflected from the anterior and posterior surfaces of the distal humerus together with anterior reflection of the common extensor

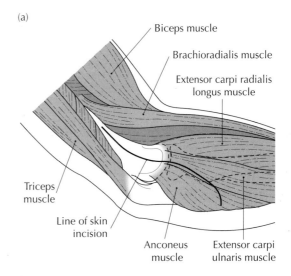

(a)

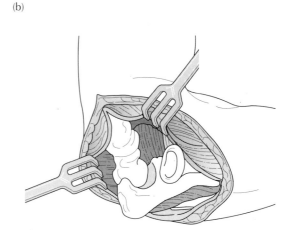

(b)

Fig. 7.13 The Kocher lateral approach.

muscles from the lateral epicondyle. The joint capsule can now be incised enabling visualisation of the joint and appropriate exposure of the radial head and neck. If further exposure of the joint is required the anconeus muscle can be reflected subperiosteally from the proximal ulna and the joint can then be dislocated (Fig. 7.13).

The Campbell modification of this approach involves reflecting the common extensor origin distally by osteotomizing the lateral epicondyle (Fig. 7.14).

Dangers

The posteror interosseous nerve is at risk during dissection of the proximal radius, and the ulnar nerve may be damaged during dislocation or reduction of the elbow joint.

(a)

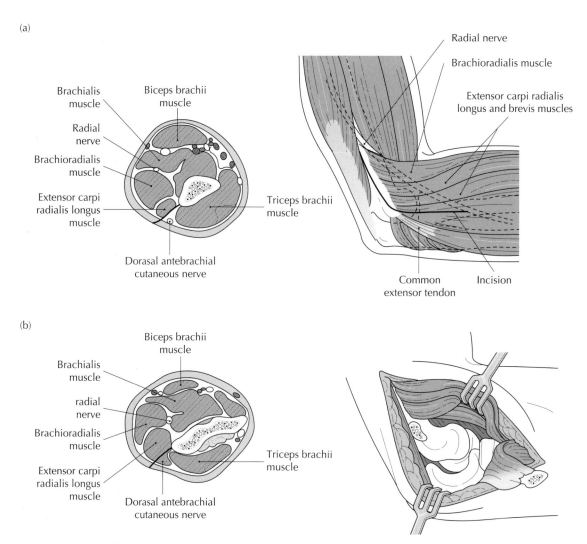

Brachialis muscle

Biceps brachii muscle

Radial nerve

Brachioradialis muscle

Extensor carpi radialis longus muscle

Dorasal antebrachial cutaneous nerve

Triceps brachii muscle

Radial nerve

Brachioradialis muscle

Extensor carpi radialis longus and brevis muscles

Common extensor tendon

Incision

(b)

Biceps brachii muscle

Brachialis muscle

radial nerve

Brachioradialis muscle

Extensor carpi radialis longus muscle

Dorasal antebrachial cutaneous nerve

Triceps brachii muscle

Fig. 7.14 The Campbell lateral approach. The lateral epicondyle is osteotomized.

Enlargement of the approach

The Kocher lateral approach can be converted to an extensile posterolateral approach to the entire distal humerus. This is achieved by extending the incision proximally and dissecting down onto the proximal lateral supracondylar ridge. Anterior and posterior reflection of the attached muscles allows exposure of the distal humerus.

Anterior approach

Indications for surgery

The anterior approach to the elbow that is commonly used is that described by Henry.[1] It is a variant of the exposure originally described by Fiolle and Delmas (cited by Henry[1]). The approach permits the fixation of anteriorly displaced fractures, the release of post-traumatic anterior capsular contractures, the excision of tumours and exploration for entrapment syndromes.

Position of the patient

The patient is positioned supine with the arm abducted and resting on an arm board. The forearm is supinated.

Surgical landmarks and incisions

The structures that must be palpated prior to commencing the operation are the brachioradialis muscle and the biceps tendon. The position of the flexor skin crease should also be noted.

The skin incision begins approximately 5 cm proximal to the flexor skin crease at the anterior margin of the brachioradialis muscle. The incision

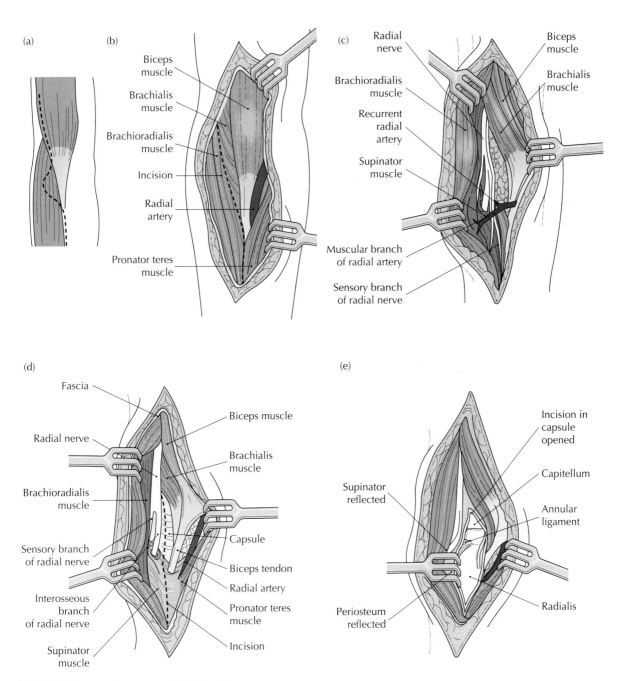

Fig. 7.15 The anterior approach to the elbow.

extends distally in an 'S' shape turning medially at the level of the flexor skin crease and then distally once more at the level of the biceps tendon. The incision ends approximately 5 cm distal to the flexor crease.

Superficial dissection
The superficial fascia is divided and the interval between brachioradialis laterally and biceps and

brachialis medially is developed. More distally the interval between brachioradialis and pronator teres is identified.

Deep dissection
Blunt dissection between the muscle groups enables identification of the radial nerve on the inner aspect of the brachioradialis muscle. The pronator teres is retracted medially revealing the

radial artery together with its muscular and recurrent branches. These should be ligated to prevent haematoma formation. The biceps tendon and brachialis muscle are retracted medially allowing visualisation of the supinator muscle. With the forearm fully supinated supinator is released from the anterior aspect of the radius by subperiosteal disection. The capsule is incised and the entire anterior aspect of the elbow joint is visualised (Fig. 7.15).

Dangers
The radial nerve is at risk during this approach. The nerve must be identified proximally in the interval between brachioradialis and brachialis before any deep dissection is performed. The posterior interosseous nerve is at risk during dissection of the proximal third of the radius. As such it is important that all dissection should be carried out with the forearm fully supinated in order to take the nerve away from the site of dissection. It is critical to identify the origin of the supinator muscle from the anterior aspect of the radius before beginning subperiosteal stripping. Cutting blindly into the muscle will result in damage to the nerve. Forcible retraction of the supinator muscle should also be avoided

as this may produce a traction injury to the posterior interosseous nerve.

The muscular and recurrent radial branches of the radial artery are also at risk with this approach. The branches should be ligated to allow mobilisation of the artery. Avulsion of any of these branches may result in postoperative haematoma formation with in extreme cases, the development of compartment syndrome.

Enlargement of the approach
This is the most extensile approach in the elbow joint. The approach actually forms a link between the anterior approach to the forearm and the anterolateral approach to the humerus. To extend the approach proximally the incision is extended and the biceps muscle is retracted medially. The brachialis muscle is split in its midline (medial half supplied by the musculocutaneous nerve and the lateral half by the radial nerve) allowing exposure of the anterior aspect of the humerus. Distally the approach can be extended by increasing the incision and then developing the plane between the brachioradialis muscle and the pronator teres muscle. This enables exposure of the anterior aspect of the radius.

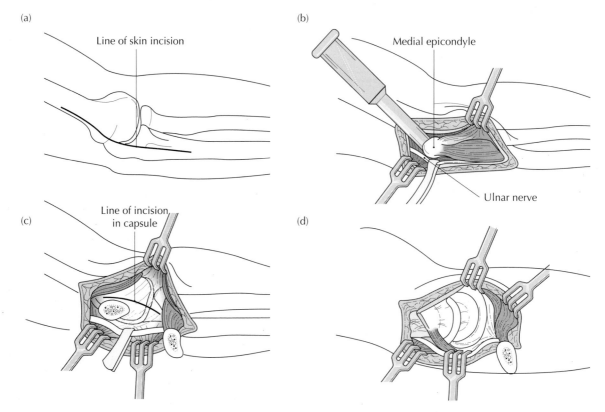

Fig. 7.16 The medial approach to the elbow. This was described independantly by Molesworth and Campbell.

Medial approach

Indications for surgery

The indications for the medial approach to the elbow are limited. It is used most frequently for the fixation of medial epicondylar fractures but has also been used for the removal of medial joint loose bodies (now more commonly removed arthroscopically) and the occasional exploration of the medial joint compartment when this is symptomatic.

The approach was described independently by Molesworth[23] and Campbell.[2]

Position of the patient

The operation is performed with the patient in the supine position. The arm is abducted and the shoulder externally rotated such that the medial epicondyle faces anteriorly. Finally the elbow is flexed to 90 degrees and the forearm supported on a Mayo table. Landmarks which must be identified are the ulnar nerve and medial epicondyle. Having done this a 10 cm gently curved incision centred on the medial epicondyle can be performed. The surgical approach utilises an internervous plane proximally between the brachialis muscle (musculocutaneous nerve) and the triceps muscle (radial nerve) and distally between the brachialis muscle (musculo cutaneous nerve) and the pronator teres muscle (median nerve).

Superficial dissection

The ulnar nerve is palpated as it passes behind the medial epicondyle, and is mobilised. The anterior skin flap is dissected to expose the superficial flexor muscles and the interval between the pronator teres muscle and the brachialis muscle is identified. A periosteal elevator is placed beneath the medial collateral ligament in order to be certain that when the medial epicondyle is osteotomized the ligament remains attached to the medial epicondyle. Thus at the end of the procedure when the medial epicondyle is reattached to the humerus stability of the elbow is restored.

Deep dissection

With the ulnar nerve protected the medial epicondyle is osteotomized and turned distally with its attached muscles. This should be undertaken with care to avoid damage to the median nerve or its branches. Finally the dissection is completed by developing the plane between the brachialis muscle anteriorly and the triceps posteriorly. The capsule is incised and the joint examined. By applying a valgus stress to the elbow almost the entire joint can be visualised (Fig. 7.16).

At the end of the procedure the medial epicondyle is screwed back to its anatomical position on the humerus.

Dangers

The ulnar nerve is at risk when performing the osteotomy of the medial epicondyle. The nerve must be carefully dissected out and gently retracted before the osteotomy is performed. At greater risk, however, is the median nerve. This sends branches into the superficial flexor muscles particularly pronator teres, and forceful retraction of the muscle mass may produce a traction injury to the nerve. It is also important when undertaking the medial epicondylar osteotomy to avoid dividing the medial collateral ligament. This is the most important stabilising structure of the elbow and damage will result in instability.

Enlargement of the approach

The approach can be enlarged in two ways. Local exposure can be improved by releasing the joint capsule from the humerus. This will enable more extensive visualisation of the joint.

The approach can be extended proximally by developing the plane between triceps and the brachialis muscle. Distal extension, however, cannot really be achieved. This is due to the innervation of the superficial flexor muscles by branches from the median nerve. The approach allows exposure of the insertion of brachialis into the coronoid process of the ulna but cannot be used for more distal approaches to the ulnar shaft.

References

1. Henry AK *Extensile exposure* (2nd edn). Baltimore: Williams and Wilkins, 1957.
2. Campbell WC Incision for exposure of the elbow joint. *Am J Surg* 1932; **15:** 65-7.
3. Van Gorder GW Surgical approach in supracondylar 'T' fractures of the humerus requiring open reduction. *J Bone Joint Surg* 1940; **22:** 278-92.
4. Bryan RS, Morrey BF Extensive posterior exposure of the elbow: A triceps-sparing approach. *Clin Orthop* 1982; **166:** 188–92.
5. Steiger JU, Gschwend N, Bell S GSB elbow arthroplasty: A new concept, and six years experience. In: *Elbow joint.* Kashiwagi D (ed) Amsterdam: Elsevier Science Publishers BV (Biomedical Division), 1985: 285–94.
6. Wolfe SW, Ranawat CS The osteo-anconeus flap: An approach for total elbow arthroplasty. *J Bone Joint Surg* 1990; **72A:** 684-8.
7. MacAusland WR Ankylosis of the elbow, with report of four cases treated by arthroplasty. *J Am Med Assoc* 1915; **64:** 312-8.

8. Muller ME, Allgower M, Willenegger H *Manual of internal fixation: Technique recommended by the AO-Group*. New York: Springer-Verlag, 1970.

9. Kashiwagi D Osteoarthritis of the elbow joint – intra-articular changes and the special operative procedure, Outerbridge – Kashiwagi Method (0-K method). In: *Elbow joint*. Kashiwagi D (ed) Amsterdam: Elsevier Science Publishers BV (Biomedical Division), 1985: 177-88.

10. Stanley D, Winson IG A Surgical approach to the elbow. *J Bone Joint Surg (Br)* 1990; **72B:** 728-9.

11. Morrey BF Primary Arthritis of the elbow treated by ulno humeral arthroplasty. *J Bone Joint Surg* 1992; **74B:** 409-13.

12. Kudo H, Iwano K, Nishino J Cementless or hybrid total elbow arthroplasty with titanium-alloy implants. *J Arthroplasty* 1994; **9:** 269-78.

13. Morrey BF, Adams RA Semi constrained elbow replacement arthroplasty: Rationale, techniques and results. In: *The elbow and its disorders*. Morrey BF (ed) Philadelphia: WB Saunders Co, 1993: 648-64.

14. Jonsson B, Larsson S Elbow arthroplasty in rheumatoid arthritis. *Acta Orthop Scand* 1990; **61:** 344-7.

15. Boyd HB Surgical exposure of the ulna and proximal third of the radius through one incision. *Surg Gynecol Obstet* 1940; **71:** 86-8.

16. Gordon ML Monteggia fracture. A combined surgical approach employing a single lateral incision. *Clin Orthop* 1967; **50:** 87-93.

17. Pankovich AM Anconeus approach to the elbow joint and the proximal part of the radius and ulna. *J Bone Joint Surg* 1977; **59A:** 124-6.

18. Gschwend N Our operative approach to the elbow joint. *Arch Orthop Traumat Surg* 1981; **98:** 143-6.

19. Wadsworth TG A modified posterolateral approach to the elbow and proximal radio ulnar joints. *Clin Orthop* 1979; **144:** 151-3.

20. Kaplan EB Surgical approaches to the proximal end of the radius and its use in fractures of the head and neck of the radius. *J Bone Joint Surg* 1941; **23:** 86-92.

21. Campbell WC, Edmonson AS, Crenshaw AH (eds) *Campbells operative orthopaedics in surgical approaches* (6th edn), Vol 1. St Louis: CV Mosby Co, 1971: 117.

22. Kocher T *Text-book of operative surgery* (3rd edn). (Stiles HJ and Paul CB Transl) London: A and C Black, 1911.

23. Molesworth WHL An operation for the complete exposure of the elbow joint. *Brit J Surg* 1930; **18:** 303-7.

24. Morrey BF, Bryan RS, Dobbyns JH, Linscheid RL. Total elbow arthroplasty. A five-year experience at the Mayo Clinic. *J Bone Joint Surg* 1981; **63A:** 1050–63.

CHAPTER 8

Fractures of the distal humerus in children

BRUCE L GILLINGHAM, DOUGLAS M HEDDEN

Introduction

Elbow fractures are among the most common injuries sustained by children since they are always involved in activities that imperil this joint. The risk of injury has been further increased recently by the advent of roller blades.

Following injury, assessment is complicated by radiolucent chondroepiphyses which can make accurate diagnosis difficult. Thus a significant potential for morbidity exists. Knowledge of the complex anatomy of the developing elbow and the myriad ways in which it can be injured is essential for successful treatment. To a large degree, the patient's functional outcome depends on maintaining a high index of suspicion for occult injury and instituting timely and appropriate treatment.

In this chapter fractures of the distal humerus are discussed. Subsequent chapters will deal with paediatric elbow dislocations, fracture dislocations and proximal radius and ulna fractures.

Mechanism of injury

The anatomy of the elbow is much more complicated than most joints and it is this which can cause confusion for the treating clinician.

The elbow has more secondary centres of ossification than any other joint which also contributes to the confusion and misdiagnosis. Many fractures involve a large cartilaginous fragment which will not be visible on plain radiographs. As a result, identification of the fracture line can be very difficult.

Knowledge of when the secondary centres of ossification appear is very helpful (Chapter 1, Fig. 8.7) in understanding fracture patterns. In the case of the medial epicondyle fracture this can avoid a disastrous result. Knowing that the medial epicondyle should be present and not seeing it should make the clinician look carefully for an intra-articular fragment. It is helpful to x-ray the opposite side but this may often be avoided if the specific anatomy is understood.

The pattern of the fracture which occurs in cartilage is often difficult to ascertain on plain radiography and thus other forms of imaging become mandatory for some lesions. The radiograph only shows the osseous structure. Intra-articular contrast to outline the cartilage is very helpful. However, an arthrogram in the young child often requires an anaesthetic and we have found ultrasound a very useful alternative to further delineate the fracture anatomy. Magnetic resonance imaging (MRI) may also be used but it is expensive, and often less readily available.

Injuries of the elbow may be caused by direct or indirect trauma to the elbow. Most flexion supracondylar fractures are caused by a direct blow to the back of the elbow whereas most extension supracondylar fractures are caused by a fall on the outstretched hand which puts a hyperextension force on the elbow. In addition, the elbow may also be subjected to varus and valgus as well as supination and pronation stresses. Many injuries are caused by a combination of forces leading to complex fracture patterns.

Distal humeral epiphyseal separation

Although once thought to be a rare injury, fracture separation of the distal humeral epiphysis has probably been underreported due to misdiagnosis and failure of recognition.[1]

Macafee reported three cases of infantile supracondylar fracture in 1967.[2] These were later determined to be injuries of the distal humeral epiphysis rather than true supracondylar fractures.[3] This injury has been reported in the newborn and in children up to the age of 13 years.[4–10] The peak incidence, however, is from birth to 2½ years of age.[3]

The first description of fracture-separation of the distal humeral epiphysis was credited to Gurlt in 1818 by Stimson.[11] The first complete description of the injury differentiating it from elbow dislocation and supracondylar fracture was by R.W. Smith in 1850.[12] Since that time there have been case reports of small numbers of patients by many authors.[1–4,6–10,13–21] The largest series to date included 16 patients.[3]

The distal humeral growth plate has a smooth, transverse interface with the metaphysis.[22] Fracture-separation of the distal humeral epiphysis is thought to occur due to a shear stress across this interface. Siffert reproduced the injury in two stillborns with hyperextension in one specimen and a backward thrust of the forearm with the elbow flexed to 90 degrees in another. In both specimens the posterior periosteal attachment between the humeral metaphysis and epiphysis remained intact.[10]

Rogers and Rockwood implicated both a fall on the outstretched hand as well as lifting or pulling the forearm as the means by which shear stress is produced.[20] In infants and younger children forces applied to the elbow are more likely to be rotatory shear in nature. This type of force rather than pure bending forces most often causes physeal failure.[23] Rotary shear characteristically occurs in birth trauma and child abuse.[3] Both are reported causes of this injury.[1,3–7,9,10,14,15,20.]

Non-accidental trauma is a common cause of distal humeral physeal separation, particularly in younger children.[1,14,15,20] In DeLee's series, child abuse was documented or suspected as a cause in six of the 16 fractures.[3] Any suspicion of child abuse should be pursued with appropriate clinical evaluation and referred for investigation by the appropriate child protection agency.

CLINICAL PRESENTATION

The biggest challenge in treating this injury lies in correctly recognizing it. Delay in diagnosis and misdiagnosis are common.[1,3,5,8,14,16,18,20] Younger children usually sustain a Salter-Harris I physeal injury (Fig. 8.1) which is most commonly confused with an elbow dislocation. In older children a Salter–Harris type II injury occurs and is frequently misdiagnosed as a Salter–Harris type IV injury of the lateral condyle (Fig. 8. 2). A mistaken diagnosis can lead to unnecessary surgical intervention, exposing the child to otherwise avoidable risks. In one series, five of seven patients were initially misdiagnosed. Four of these patients were taken to the operating room for open reduction and internal fixation of presumed lateral condyle fractures.[16] DeLee *et al.* reported on 16 cases, eight of which were initially misdiagnosed.[3]

Maintenance of the normal triangular relationship between the olecranon and the medial and lateral condyles on palpation of the elbow through a range of motion has often been cited as a means of differentiating epiphyseal separation from an elbow dislocation.[10] Post-traumatic swelling superimposed on an already chubby elbow, however, often makes this determination difficult.

The increased warmth created by the inflammatory response to the fracture may lead to a presumptive diagnosis of a septic elbow, particularly in smaller children. Absence of fever, and a normal laboratory evaluation with only slight elevation of the erthrocyte sedimentation rate will help rule this out.

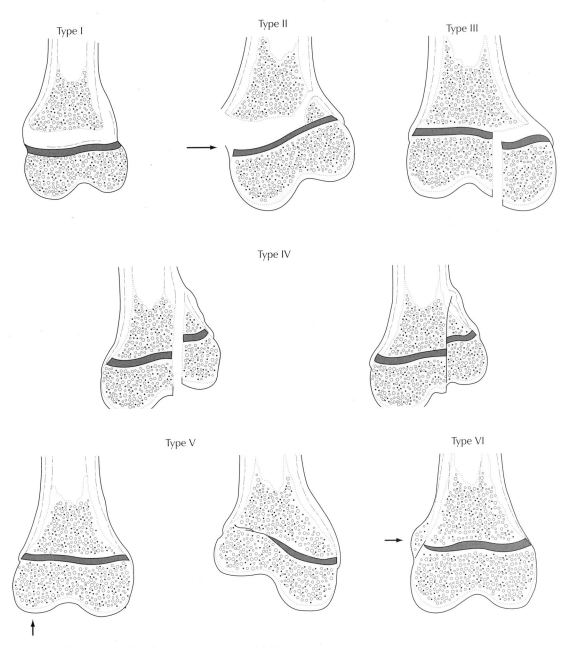

Fig. 8.1 The Salter–Harris classification of epiphyseal injuries.

The presence of 'muffled crepitus' is considered a classic finding in distal humeral separation. This is produced by the relatively smooth opposing surfaces of the cartilaginous separation moving on one another. To avoid increased trauma to the child and the physis, however, this examination should not be performed. In a baby who will not move the arm the presence of a grasp reflex or hand and wrist movement helps rule out an injury to the brachial plexus from birth trauma.

ASSESSMENT/INVESTIGATION

Until the appearance of the ossific nucleus of the capitellum appears (between 3 and 9 months of age) diagnosis by plain x-rays can be difficult.[24] On the anteroposterior radiograph the relationship between the radius and ulna will be preserved but they are displaced in relation to the distal humerus. Although all possible directions of displacement have been reported, the overwhelming majority are

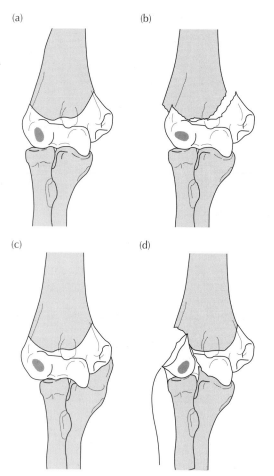

Fig. 8.2 Elbow injuries in children that can be clinically confused. (a) Normal elbow. (b) Sepation of entire distal humeral epiphysis (Salter–Harris type I). (c) Dislocation of the elbow. (d) Lateral condylar fracture. Redrawn after Ref. 19 with permission from *Journal of Bone and Joint Surgery*.

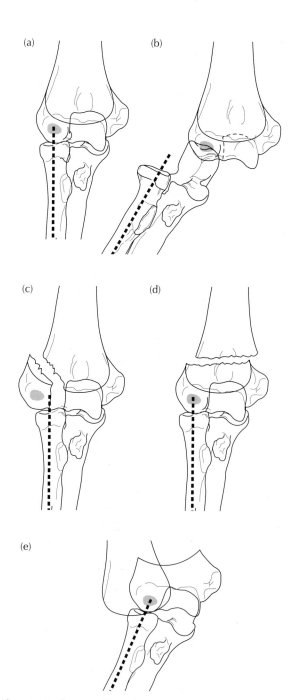

Fig. 8.3 Radiocapitellar relationship. (a) Normal. (b) Left elbow dislocation. (c) Displaced fracture of the lateral condyle. (d) Supracondylar fracture. (e) Right distal humeral epiphyseal separation. Redrawn after Ref. 121 with permission from *Journal of Bone and Joint Surgery*.

translated posteromedially.[3,10,18] By contrast, in a dislocation of the elbow the forearm will usually be displaced laterally. The alignment between the radial head and capitellum is the key radiographic relationship to bear in mind when distinguishing transphyseal separations from other elbow injuries, particularly dislocation and lateral condyle fractures. On a radiograph of a normal elbow a line drawn along the long axis of the radius intersects the capitellum regardless of the position of the elbow (Fig. 8.3). In distal humeral epiphyseal separations this relationship is maintained whereas in elbow dislocation and displaced lateral condyle fractures this relationship is disrupted. Prior to the radiographic appearance of the capitellum, however, no such diagnostic key exists. A less specific radiographic clue to this injury is foreshortening of the cartilage space between the distal end of the humerus and

forearm on an anteroposterior radiograph when compared with the uninjured side.[10]

An arthrogram can be an useful aid in correctly differentiating distal humeral epiphyseal separations from other elbow injuries when plain radiographs are not diagnostic.

Ultrasound has also been reported as a means of identifying distal humeral epiphyseal separations, particularly in neonates.[6,25] In addition to being non-invasive, the risks of anaesthesia and ionising radiation are avoided.

In identifying the position of the cartilaginous distal humeral epiphysis MRI may also prove useful. Children in the age group for whom this would be most beneficial, however, would require anaesthesia in order for an adequate study to be performed.[22]

MANAGEMENT OPTIONS

The goal of treatment is to realign the distal humeral epiphysis with the metaphysis. The majority of patients reported in the literature have had satisfactory outcomes after closed reduction and a short period of 3 weeks cast immobilization.[3–5,7–9,15,18,20] In fact, acceptable results have been obtained in patients who were diagnosed late with persistent displacement and who received no manipulation.[3,8,14]

When recognized early, closed reduction is recommended. In cases where significant elbow swelling precludes adequate elbow flexion a period of traction has been used prior to closed reduction.[3,14,19]

Percutaneous pinning is indicated if the elbow is judged to be unstable after reduction. This is less likely than with supracondylar humeral fractures as the separated surfaces are much broader.[3] DeJager and Hoffmann advocated routine percutaneous pinning after closed reduction for children under 2 years of age in order to allow immediate clinical assessment of the carrying angle.[5] This provides information not available radiographically in this age group. Their review of six series of patients disclosed residual cubitus varus in 12 of 48 patients, ten of whom were under 2 years of age.[5]

Open reduction is rarely indicated in a closed injury. McIntyre, however, advocates open reduction when diagnostic confusion exists or difficulty occurs in achieving reduction, particularly in older patients.[8] Interposed brachialis muscle has been reported to block reduction in at least one case.[4] Several patients in the literature were treated with open reduction due to misdiagnosis of the injury as an irreducible elbow dislocation or lateral condyle fracture. Owing to concern that a good reduction was difficult to obtain and document, Mizuno *et al.* advocate routine 'gentle open reduction' and pinning through a posterior osteocartilaginous approach. This method, however, is not widely practised.[19]

AUTHORS' PREFERRED MANAGEMENT/SURGICAL TECHNIQUE

In the younger child, in whom the diagnosis may remain in doubt, we perform an arthrogram under general anaesthesia. A small-gauge needle is used to introduce 0.5–1.0 cc of contrast medium into the joint from a lateral approach, using the 'soft-spot' present within the triangle formed by the radial head, olecranon and lateral condyle.[26] An image intensifier is then used to obtain anteroposterior, lateral and oblique radiographs. These will demonstrate a normal radiocapitellar relationship with evidence of posteromedial translation of the epiphysis in relation to the humeral shaft. No intra-articular step-off will be present as would be seen with most lateral condyle fractures.[1,15,19]

A closed reduction is then performed. Distal traction is applied to correct axial malalignment followed by flexion and pronation of the forearm to tighten the postero-medial hinge and 'lock in' the reduction.[3,10,18]

If persistent instability is present, percutaneous pinning is performed. Single lateral and medial pins are generally sufficient.

If the ulnar nerve and medial epicondyle are not palpable two lateral pins are inserted. The arm is then extended to assess the carrying angle and allow comparison with the contralateral arm. A posterior and stirrup-type splint are applied in approximately 70 degrees of flexion. The pins should be removed in the outpatient clinic after 3 weeks.

Open reduction is reserved for open fractures and the rare irreducible separation.

COMPLICATIONS

Cubitus varus is the most common complication of distal humeral epiphyseal separations.[1,3,5,8,10,14,16,18] This is believed to occur as a result of uncorrected medial tilt of the distal fragment as is also commonly seen in supracondylar fractures.[3,16] Hyperaemic overgrowth of the lateral aspect of the distal humerus has also been hypothesized. Growth plate injury is a less likely aetiology as the varus malalignment is non-progressive.[3,16]

Several authors report a functionally insignificant loss of motion, primarily at the extreme of extension but also occasionally of flexion. DeLee found that the largest measurable loss of elbow motion was in patients immobilized for more than 3 weeks, the period of time usually considered adequate for healing of an epiphyseal fracture.[3]

Growth arrest is uncommon. The entire epiphyseal growth plate usually remains with the epiphysis and thus physeal damage is rare.[22]

Few neurovascular complications have been observed, presumably because the relatively smooth surfaces of the separated cartilaginous surfaces are less likely to injure adjacent nerves and vessels than bony spikes. However, as with any paediatric elbow injury, vigilant monitoring for neurovascular compromise must be maintained.

Supracondylar fractures

Supracondylar fractures of the distal humerus are the most common elbow fracture in the paediatric age group and often they require operative management. The potential for serious complications also creates more anxiety than almost any other fracture.

They can be divided into extension- and flexion-type injuries. In the extension-type the distal fragment is posterior to the shaft. These occur approximately 95% of the time. In the flexion-type the distal fragment is anterior to the shaft.

The extension-type are thought to occur due to hyperextension of the elbow with the olecranon acting as a lever of the distal humerus as it locks into the olecranon fossa. The rarer flexion-type are most probably due to a fall on to the point of the elbow.

Extension type injuries are most commonly classified according to Gartland's classification system.[27] This is based on the degree of displacement of the distal fragment. Type 1 fractures are undisplaced and are often difficult to visualise (Fig. 8.4). In type 2 fractures there is anterior angulation such that the fracture line opens up on the anterior cortex but the posterior cortex remains intact. This is a greenstick-type fracture. In type 3 fractures there is no bony contact. The distal fragment is totally displaced from the shaft. In type 2 and 3 fractures there is usually also displacement medially or laterally. There may be varus or valgus angulation and there may be a rotatory malalignment as well. Extension type supracondylar fractures with posteromedial displacement and internal rotation of the distal fragment are the most common.

CLINICAL PRESENTATION

The child with an undisplaced fracture may present with an unwillingness to move the elbow and with tenderness in the supracondylar region. In contrast, a child with a type 3 fracture often presents in pain and is distressed. The elbow is often extremely swollen although much of the apparent swelling may be due to the proximal fragment being displaced into the subcutaneous tissue.

In the severely displaced fracture there will be bruising on the anterior aspect of the elbow, and the skin may appear about to be broken by the proximal spike of bone which has lacerated the brachialis muscle. Indeed it is important not to miss a small puncture wound which by definition makes the fracture compound.

ASSESSMENT/INVESTIGATION

The child must be examined carefully for both vascular and neurological complications. The pulses must be palpated and the vascular status of the hand should be assessed. The colour, warmth, sensation and movement of the hand should be documented. Capillary refill should be noted but it is important to be aware that venous back-flow may give a false sense of viability.

Pulse oximetry may give some additional information but only when used as an adjunct to careful clinical examination. The turgor and tenderness of the forearm compartments should be noted for later reassessment. The vascular complications of this fracture may be due to either acute ischaemia or the development of a compartment syndrome.

Careful neurologic examination of the radial, ulnar and median nerves should be performed. Special attention should be given to the anterior interosseous nerve since there is no sensory deficit with a complete nerve palsy. Examination of the child may be very difficult but every attempt should be made, since a nerve deficit noted postoperatively will have a significantly different impact on the child's parents if it was not recorded preoperatively.

Neural injury associated with these fractures is not uncommon and has been reported in the range 5–19%.[28] The radial nerve is the most commonly injured followed by the median and ulnar nerves.[29] Cramer *et al.* found anterior interosseous nerve palsies in 15% of displaced supracondylar fractures in their series.[30] This is a much higher incidence than previously noted and probably relates to the fact that this neuropraxia is easily overlooked.

Radiographic assessment should be performed, after the limb has been appropriately splinted.

In Type 1 injuries the thin hairline fracture may be difficult to identify and it is therefore important to look for evidence of blood in the joint. The presence on the lateral x-ray of anterior and posterior fat pads which are displaced is indicative of an intra-articular fracture.

In type 2 and 3 fractures determining the amount of displacement, angulation and rotation of the

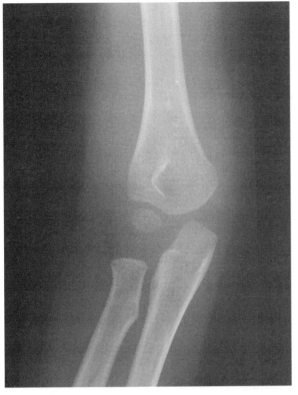

(a)

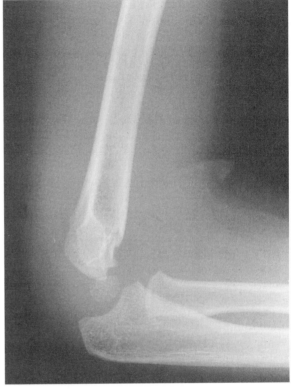

(b)

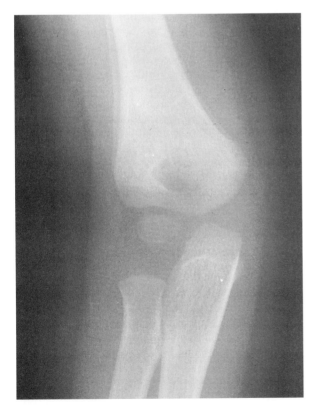

(c)

Fig. 8.4. (a) Type 1 supracondylar fracture. Nearly imperceptible fracture line present medially. (b) Lateral view. Note torus type fracture posteriorly. (c) Follow-up radiograph at 3 weeks. Note subperiosteal new bone formation medially and laterally.

fracture is important. In completely displaced fractures this is less of an issue but in the type 2 fractures a decision will have to be made as to whether the fracture is in an acceptable position.

Anteroposterior and lateral x-rays are mandatory with medial and lateral oblique views often contributing significantly to the understanding to the fracture. An intercondylar split fracture should always be considered and positively excluded.

The alignment on the anteroposterior x-ray will assess varus and valgus alignment as well as displacement and rotation. The lateral x-ray allows assessment of posterior displacement as well as rotation. Inequality of the widths of the proximal and distal segments is suggestive of malrotation. Comminution of the medial and lateral columns must be assessed since, even in a minimally displaced type 2 fracture, comminution of the medial pillar may be the clue to underlying varus angulation.

Assessment of varus and valgus may be difficult radiographically and it may be that clinical assessment of the carrying angle compared with the other side is the most valuable. Baumann's angle has been used to assess the varus and valgus angulation of the distal fragment but it can be inaccurate due to positioning.[31] On the lateral x-ray assessment of the anterior humeral line and the lateral humerocapitellar angle (normal 25–65 degrees) is possible.[32] The anterior humeral line should pass through the middle to posterior one-third of the capitellar ossification centre.

In the healed fracture assessment of varus and valgus can be performed with the child holding his elbows at his side and flexed to 90 degrees.[33] The maximum supination and pronation is measured and compared with the other side. The average between the loss of pronation and gain in supination equals the varus malunion. If there is a valgus malunion supination is lost and pronation is gained.

MANAGEMENT OPTIONS

The management of type 1 fractures is uncontroversial. These are stable injuries which will not displace. Application of a posterior splint with the elbow in 90 degrees flexion for 3 weeks will allow the child's arm to heal well without complication. Following this, the child should undergo supervised mobilisation of the elbow. During this phase a removable splint can be used for support and protection if the child is anxious or at risk of falling. The parents should be advised, however, that continuous splinting after 3 weeks is not recommended as it may lead to prolonged or even permanent stiffness in the elbow.

Type 2 fractures which demonstrate no varus or valgus malalignment and minimal extension such that the anterior humeral line still passes through the capitellar ossification centre may be treated in a similar manner as type 1 fractures. The elbow should be flexed beyond 90 degrees and the fracture reassessed at 1 week since some of these may displace.

Controversy exists over what should be done for displaced type 2 fractures which require a closed reduction. Reducing these is easily achieved as they are out to length and just need to be pushed forward. This is best accomplished by flexing the elbow to 90 degrees and gently pushing on the medial and lateral condyles of the distal humerus to bring them forward into their normal position. After reduction the anteroposterior x-ray must be checked to make sure there is no varus or valgus angulation due to comminution of the pillars. The further treatment is then either in a posterior splint in more than 90 degrees flexion or percutaneous pin fixation.[34,35]

The treatment of type 3 fractures has even more options. These are variously managed by closed reduction and splinting, traction and delayed splinting, traction and delayed closed reduction and splinting, traction and delayed closed reduction and pinning, closed reduction and percutaneous pinning and open reduction and pinning.[36,37]

Closed reduction and splinting of type 3 fractures is no longer recommended. The reduction may be obtained but it is difficult to maintain. The elbow must be flexed well beyond 90 degrees often up to 120 degrees. This may obliterate the radial pulse putting the child at risk for ischaemia. In addition, it impedes venous return increasing the likelihood of compartment syndrome. Kurer and Regan reported only 49% excellent results with this technique.[38]

Traction can be performed with the elbow abducted 90 degrees and the elbow either extended or flexed 90 degrees. Overhead traction can also be employed. It may be applied with skin tapes or with an olecranon pin or screw. Good results have been obtained with traction and it may be the safest form of treatment for the surgeon who only rarely treats these injuries.[39] The traction should be maintained until early union is established (usually 2 weeks) after which posterior splinting should be performed. Alternatively it can be maintained for 3-4 days until the swelling decreases making closed reduction easier and percutaneous pinning safer. Sutton *et al.* compared the results of traction and percutaneous pinning and found that the results were similar with over 90% satisfactory results.[39] They did show, however, that the cost to the health care system was much less if these fractures were pinned acutely.

In the percutaneous pinning technique the placement of the pins also varies. Some use two lateral pins while others use crossed pins, one in the medial and one in the lateral column. Zionts *et al.* have shown that two crossed K-wires provide the maximum stability.[40] These should cross above the fracture line and should be in the column and not passing through the olecranon fossa. If, because of inability to feel the medial epicondyle, two lateral pins are used they should be placed parallel and not crossed.[40]

There is interest in absorbable pins for the treatment of these fractures but Bostman *et al.* have shown that current devices have insufficient strength to maintain the reduction.[41]

The management options for flexion type supracondylar fractures are the same except that splintage in extension is necessary. These are difficult to treat as they are best reduced in extension making it difficult to obtain a lateral radiograph to assess the reduction in that plane.

AUTHORS' PREFERRED MANAGEMENT

Type 1 fractures are managed in a posterior splint with the elbow in 90 degrees of flexion for 3 weeks. The splint is then converted to a removable splint which is used for an additional 3 weeks while the child is up and about. The parents are encouraged to remove the splint at other times to allow the child to regain a range of motion.

Type 2 fractures which are minimally displaced with mild extension and no varus or valgus are treated in a similar fashion to type 1 fractures but are placed in more flexion (120 degrees). They are checked at 1 week with a radiograph in order to assess displacement. If this increases they are treated in the same way as displaced fractures.

Type 2 fractures which are more displaced such that the anterior humeral line does not pass through the ossification centre of the capitellum or if varus or valgus malalignment is present are treated in the operating room with closed reduction and percutaneous pinning. One pin is placed in the lateral column and one in the medial column such that the pins cross above the fracture line. While others engage the far cortex our preference is to penetrate it. This we believe gives better fixation. Care must be taken not to go too far beyond the medial cortex in order to prevent damage to the ulnar nerve.

Type 3 fractures are also treated with closed reduction and percutaneous pinning (Fig. 8.5). If reduction cannot be obtained then open reduction should be performed. This may be accomplished from either the medial or lateral side. Once reduc-

tion has been obtained it should be maintained by pin fixation of the fracture.

Injuries associated with a nerve palsy at the time of presentation are treated in a similar fashion. The nerve palsy is followed clinically as most are neuropraxias and will recover spontaneously. If after 3 months there is no recovery, nerve conduction studies are undertaken and the nerve is explored.

Children presenting with a pulseless white hand are immediately taken to the operating room for closed reduction. If after reduction the hand is well perfused the fracture is pinned and the child carefully observed. If however, the child's hand is still not adequately perfused the brachial artery is explored through an anterior approach. An on-table arteriogram may be necessary as part of this procedure and should therefore be anticipated in the operative preparation. All children should be carefully observed postoperatively for evidence of compartment syndrome and immediately decompressed should this develop.

SURGICAL TECHNIQUE

Under general anaesthesia the arm is placed on a radiolucent arm board and prepared as if for an open reduction. Any further radiographic views may then be obtained using the image intensifier. Correction of translation, rotation and tilt is obtained and longitudinal traction applied on the forearm with the elbow in extension. Countertraction is applied to the humerus. Once the fracture is out to length it can be brought forward and flexed to lock it into position. If there is any resistance to flexion the position of the fracture should be checked using the image intensifier. Resistance may imply that the fracture is still posteriorly displaced and any further attempts at flexion may trap the brachial artery or median nerve. Once the fracture is felt to be reduced the hand should be pronated if the original displacement was posteromedial. If it was posterolateral supination may make the reduction more stable. An anteroposterior image should then be taken with the elbow flexed. Although there is overlap on this view it is usually possible to see the reduction adequately. A lateral x-ray obtained by externally rotating the entire upper extremity at the shoulder is also undertaken. Assessment of the anterior humeral line and the lateral humerocapitellar angle may then be made. Internal and external oblique x-rays done in about 30 degrees of rotation will help assess the lateral and medial column respectively. Any small adjustments may be made by slightly unflexing the elbow and pushing posteriorly on the appropriate pillar. If a major adjustment needs to

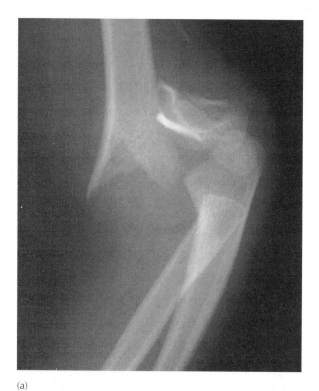

(a)

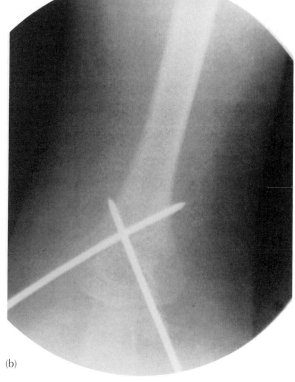

(b)

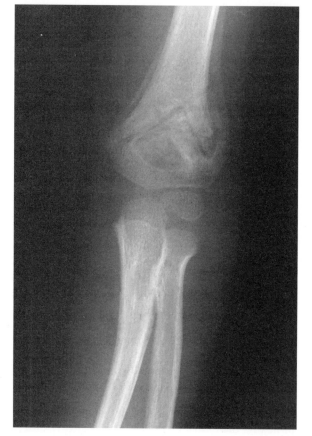

(c)

Fig. 8.5 (a) Type 3 supracondylar fracture. Note complete displacement and rotation of distal fragment. (b) Intraoperative view after closed reduction and percutaneous pinning. (c) Follow-up at 3 weeks. Pins have just been removed. Extensive subperiosteal new bone formation is present.

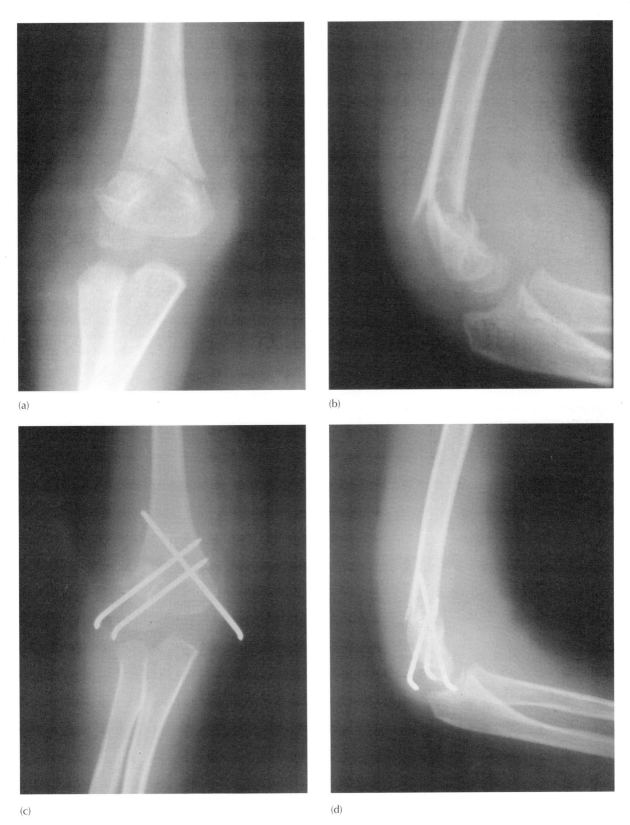

(a)

(b)

(c)

(d)

Fig. 8.6 Flexion type supracondylar humerus fracture. (a) Anteroposterior view. (b) Lateral view. (c, d) Immediately after closed reduction and percutaneous pinning.

be made it will be necessary to extend the elbow and repeat the manoeuvres.

Once the reduction is adequate the lateral pin is inserted. If the metaphyseal fragment is large enough the wire should enter above the growth plate and pass up the lateral column avoiding the olecranon fossa. The pin is advanced until the opposite cortex is encountered at which stage the position is checked using the image intensifier. If it is satisfactory the pin should be advanced further until the far cortex has just been penetrated. The medial pin is then inserted. The medial epicondyle is palpated and the ulnar nerve identified and protected. This can be achieved by extending the elbow which displaces the nerve away from the epicondyle. Using the thumb, the nerve can then be held posteriorly displaced as the pin is inserted into the epicondyle. Since the epicondyle is a posterior structure the pin should be directed slightly anteriorly. The pin on the lateral side is a good guide to the angulation required. The pin should pass up the medial column such that it crosses the lateral wire above the fracture site. It too should just perforate the opposite cortex.

Once both pins are in place the elbow may be completely extended and an anteroposterior image taken to assess varus and valgus angulation. The carrying angle may be assessed clinically.

The pins are then grasped with a needle holder and bent over using a metal suction tip. They are dressed with betadine-soaked gauze and removed in the clinic 3 weeks later. If the medial epicondyle is not palpable then a small incision should be made on the medial side of the elbow so that the medial pin can be safely and accurately inserted.

After pin fixation the elbow may be placed in a posterior splint in 45 degrees of flexion in order to allow good arterial inflow and venous outflow.

Flexion supracondylar fractures usually require reduction in extension (Fig. 8.6). Visualisation on the anteroposterior image is easy but obtaining a lateral image is much more difficult. If the anteroposterior image is satisfactory a lateral pin should be inserted and then gentle flexion of the elbow will allow a lateral image to be obtained. If adequate the medial pin should be inserted. Postoperatively these injuries are treated in the same way as the extension fractures.

COMPLICATIONS OF SURGERY

Malunion rather than non-union is a problem in supracondylar fractures. Failure to obtain and maintain an adequate reduction is the leading cause of late deformity with cubitus varus being the most common problem. This is almost always associated

with rotation of the distal fragment such that the medial portion is displaced posteriorly. Residual cubitus varus is primarily a cosmetic deformity and most do not worsen with time. If correction is requested several different techniques are available.[42]

As pointed out by Wilkins this procedure is exacting and results are sometimes less than expected.[42]

Stiffness is mentioned as a complication of this fracture but if immobilisation is kept to no more than 3 weeks this should not be a problem.

Myositis ossificans is an extremely uncommon complication which gradually improves with time. Nerve injuries following surgery should be treated promptly. Median nerve injuries which were not present preoperatively should be explored through an anterior approach (Chapter 7) since the nerve may have been trapped in the fracture site at reduction. The ulnar nerve may also become entrapped but is more usually damaged by the fixation pins. The nerve may either be transfixed by the pin or if the pin has been placed with the elbow extended subsequent flexion of the elbow may stretch the nerve around the pin. Prompt removal of the pin is necessary with replacement of either another medial pin or placement of a second and possibly a third lateral pin. Radial nerve damage secondary to pin fixation has also been recorded. There is no agreement on whether a nerve felt to be injured due to pin placement should be explored but Royce *et al.* have suggested that most will recover if treated conservatively.[43]

Medial epicondyle fractures

Injuries to the medial epicondylar apophysis are relatively common, comprising approximately 10% of all elbow injuries.[44] Only supracondylar fractures (58%) and lateral condylar injuries (13%) occur more frequently.[45] Fracture of the medial epicondyle is an injury of late childhood and adolescence, characteristically occurring between the ages of 9 and 14 years. The peak incidence is at 11–12 years of age.[46-53] Boys are affected four times more frequently than girls.[47,51,53]

The medial epicondyle is a secondary centre of ossification which appears between the ages of 5 and 9 years and fuses with the humeral shaft during the 20th year of life (Chapter 1). This early appearance and late closure over a very active period of growth in a child's life contributes to the high incidence of injury, particularly in adolescence. The medial epicondyle's importance stems from its role as the origin of the forearm flexor and pronator muscles as well as the ulnar collateral ligament. The ulnar nerve lies in a groove on its posterior aspect explaining the frequency of associated partial or complete ulnar nerve lesions.

Medial epicondylar injuries are generally the result of a fall onto an outstretched arm with the elbow in extension. Hyperextension of the wrist and fingers places an added tension force on the epicondyle through the forearm flexor muscles. These forces are accentuated by the normal valgus carrying angle of the elbow in extension (Fig. 8.7).[29,51] The weakest link, the physis, fails in tension and the apophysis is avulsed creating a Salter–Harris type I injury (Fig. 8.8). The associa-

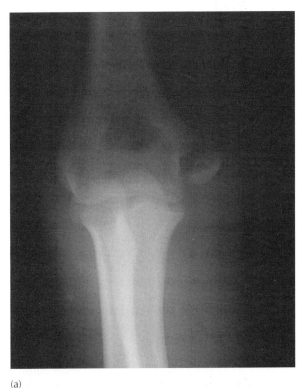

(a)

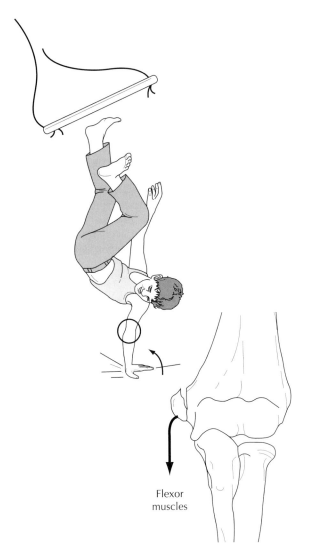

Flexor
muscles

Fig. 8.7 Medial epicondyle fracture mechanism of injury. Fall onto outstretched arm with fingers forced into hyperextension placing tension on forearm flexor musculature leading to avulsion of medial epicondyle. Redrawn after Ref. 104 with permission from JB Lippincott Co, Philadelphia.

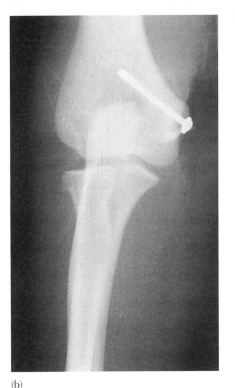

(b)

Fig. 8.8 (a) Medial epicondylar avulsion associated with valgus instability. (b) After treatment with open reduction, internal fixation with cancellous screw and washer.

tion of a valgus angulated radial neck and olecranon fractures with medial epicondyle injuries supports this mechanism.[49,50,54] If displaced, the fragment will be pulled inferiorly toward the joint by the flexor muscles. In those cases with sufficient valgus stress to cause medial opening of the joint the apophysis can be pulled laterally and downward into the joint where it will become trapped. This is very likely in the 50% of cases in which the avulsion occurs in association with an elbow dislocation. The epicondylar fragment has been found to be incarcerated in the joint in approximately 15–18% of all medial epicondyle fractures.[29] The elbow dislocation may reduce spontaneously or be reduced by a well-meaning bystander. As a result, the severity of the injury may not be appreciated by the examining physician who is unaware of the true nature of the injury. A high index of suspicion must be maintained given the likelihood of an incarcerated fragment.

A direct blow may also cause a fracture. This will most often result in comminution but little displacement of the apophysis.[55]

Chronic stresses on the medial epicondyle such as those generated by the flexor-pronator muscle group in teenage pitchers can cause a fatigue fracture with separation of the apophysis. This is radiographically demonstrated by widening and irregularity of the physis compared with the contralateral side.[56] If the injury is long-standing there may be hypertrophy of the distal humerus with acceleration of bone growth. The bone age of the elbow will exceed the patient's chronological age.[55] Treatment in this circumstance entails rest until symptomatic relief occurs. Attention to proper throwing mechanics on returning to pitching or changing to a non-pitching position is recommended.

Significant ligamentous instability can accompany medial epicondyle injuries. Ligament and soft tissue damage is often far more extensive than x-rays would suggest.[57,58] A gravity stress test x-ray can be a valuable diagnostic tool to rule out previously unappreciated medial ligamentous laxity.[58] It has been proposed that if not recognised and treated, functional lengthening of the ligament due to healing with a fibrous union in a displaced position will result in chronic valgus instability.[57,58]

CLINICAL PRESENTATION

In undisplaced fractures tenderness to direct palpation and local soft tissue swelling are usually present. In minimally to moderately displaced fractures increased soft tissue swelling reflecting the increased energy of the injury occurs.

Palpable crepitus caused by the movement of the fragment on its metaphyseal base may be elicited. The fragment in severely displaced fractures may be freely mobile, although significant soft tissue swelling may preclude palpation of the fragment. A block to full extension suggests an incarcerated fragment after spontaneous relocation of an elbow dislocation. Careful radiographic evaluation is necessary to correctly characterise the extent of the injury.

As with any elbow injury a complete neurological examination of the upper extremity is essential. Testing ulnar nerve function is particularly important prior to any intervention. Paresthesias and weakness of the ulnar innervated hand muscles is common and most likely reflects nerve contusion. In severe cases the ulnar nerve can become entrapped in the joint along with the apophyseal fragment.[59]

ASSESSMENT/INVESTIGATION

Standard anteroposterior and lateral radiographs are obtained. Oblique views are also helpful given the posterior attachment of the medial epicondyle on the medial column of the distal humerus.

A number of anatomic and developmental anomalies can complicate the accurate radiographic diagnosis of medial epicondyle injuries. Occasionally, ossification of the medial epicondyle may begin eccentrically mimicking an avulsion with slight displacement. Comparison x-rays will generally resolve this issue. Other clues are helpful. The presence of a posterior fat pad sign suggests a fracture. Its absence, however, may represent a false negative since the elbow capsule does not always extend to cover the entire medial epicondyle. This is particularly true in older children as the epicondyle migrates proximally.[60] In addition, an effusion will not be present if the injury is extra-articular. Loss of parallelism between the ossification centre and the metaphysis suggests true displacement associated with avulsion. Loss of a clearly defined physeal border of the apophysis implies avulsion accompanied by fragment rotation.[61] Inferior displacement on an anteroposterior radiograph also suggests a characteristic avulsion by the flexor-pronator muscles.

The presence of a metaphyseal flake strongly suggests a Salter–Harris type II avulsion fracture.[55,62] It is important to realise, however, that the medial epicondylar apophysis is one of the few that can avulse without an associated metaphyseal fragment. Indeed some authors feel that the presence of a metaphyseal flake heralds a Salter–Harris IV fracture of the medial condyle.[60,63]

Not infrequently, ossification of the medial epicondyle is multicentric giving a fragmented appearance to its centre. The rare fracture through the centre of the apophysis should be discernible by the sharpness of the fracture line, associated soft tissue swelling and if intracapsular, a positive fat pad sign.[61]

The most important determination to be made in evaluating medial epicondylar injuries is whether or not the fragment is incarcerated in the joint (Fig. 8.9). As discussed, the elbow may spontaneously reduce after a dislocation and entrap the apophysis. The associated pain and muscle spasm may prevent the patient co-operating with clinical evaluation and prevent good antero-posterior elbow x-rays from being obtained. The fragment may be obscured on the lateral view by the overlying olecranon. Smith proposed obtaining two anteroposterior views. One with the central beam centred on the distal humerus and the other on the proximal forearm.[59] Clues to the entrapment of the fragment are its complete absence from its usual metaphyseal location. If the fragment appears at the level of the joint it must be considered to be partially or totally within the joint until proven otherwise.[64] The displaced apophysis has been mistaken for the ossification centre of the trochlear epiphysis. This error can be avoided by realising that the trochlear centre should never ossify before the medial epicondylar centre.[62]

Another important consideration is to rule out the presence of a medial condyle fracture masquerading as an epicondylar injury. Medial condyle injuries are Salter–Harris IV type fractures extending from the capitellotrochlear groove to the medial supracondylar ridge. Distinguishing between these is usually of concern in younger children prior to the ossification of the trochlear epiphysis. The presence of a significant effusion, demonstrated by a positive fat pad sign suggests an intra-articular fracture. Isolated medial epicondylar fractures are extra-articular and rarely produce a significant effusion.[65] In addition, medial epicondyle fractures are unusual in children prior to 8 or 9 years of age. Significant epicondylar displacement in this age group must be assumed to represent a condylar fracture. An arthrogram can help to rule out intra-articular involvement and differentiate these fractures.

Clinically suspected valgus instability can be confirmed with a gravity stress x-ray.[57,58] With the patient supine on the x-ray table and the arm abducted 90 degrees the shoulder and arm are externally rotated 90 degrees. It is important to flex the elbow to 30 degrees to eliminate the stabilising force of the olecranon. Sedation may be required in the acutely injured patient.

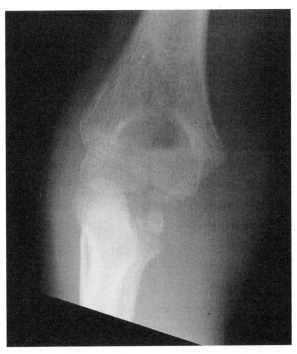

(a)

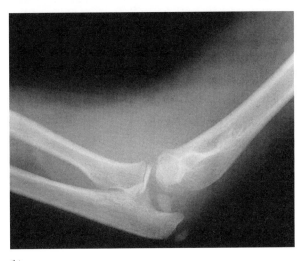

(b)

Fig. 8.9 (a, b) Fracture of medial epicondyle with entrapment in elbow joint.

MANAGEMENT OPTIONS

For undisplaced and minimally displaced fractures immobilisation for comfort in a removable posterior long arm splint for the first 7–10 days after the injury should be provided. The patient should be encouraged to come out of the splint to begin early elbow range of motion with progressive use of the elbow as tolerated. As Smith and Joyce demonstrated in 1950 a loss of 5–10 degrees of extension can occur in approximately 20% of patients.[51] Length of immobilisation was felt to be the primary factor in development of stiffness in these patients.[51] Clinical suspicion of instability should be evaluated with a gravity stress x-ray.

At the other end of the spectrum, patients who have completely avulsed the apophysis in association with an elbow dislocation with evidence of entrapment in the joint should have open reduction of the fragment. Successful closed reductions have been reported.[57,64,66] However, the significant potential for injury to the ulnar nerve with closed manipulation leads most contemporary authors to consider entrapment of the epicondyle an absolute indication for surgery.[47,48,53,55]

Evidence of ulnar nerve dysfunction manifested by hyperaesthesia, paraesthesia or paralysis has been considered a relative indication for surgical intervention in medial epicondyle fractures.[67] Wilkins advocates exploration only in the presence of motor dysfunction. In his experience minor paraesthesia or small sensory deficits subside rapidly without exploration.[55] Transposition of the nerve anteriorly to prevent late ulnar neuritis from rubbing on the raw fracture surface of the epicondyle or encasement in scar tissue has been advocated.[64] However, it is probably only indicated in patients with evidence of nerve compression not relieved by lysis of adhesions, and release of the cubital tunnel.[29] In Smith's series of 116 patients with displaced medial epicondylar fractures only one developed late ulnar nerve symptoms. This was attributed to overly aggressive physical therapy including weight carrying and push-ups. An excellent functional result following neurolysis and transposition was obtained.[51]

The controversy in the treatment of medial epicondyle injuries centres on significantly displaced fractures not associated with incarceration or ulnar neuropathy. Literature exists to support either non-operative or operative treatment.

The most convincing argument for closed treatment comes from the 1986 study of Josefsson and Danielsson from Sweden.[68] They reviewed the results of closed treatment in 56 patients between 1930 and 1962 with an average of 35 years follow-up. Despite the fact that 31 patients had developed a pseudarthrosis, no increased frequency of elbow symptoms or decreased range of motion was present compared with those patients with bony union. The only difference between the groups was the presence of mild ulnar nerve symptoms in three patients in the pseudarthrosis group. Based on their findings, Joseffsson and Danielsson felt that very

good function and range of elbow motion could safely be expected, even in the face of a high frequency of pseudarthroses.[68]

In contrast, Hines *et al.* evaluated the results of operative treatment in medial epicondyle fractures displaced more than 2 mm:[48] 23 of 24 patients (96%) had good results with operative treatment. The single poor result was attributed to a technical error in which the epicondylar fragment was inadequately fixed with the production of a non-union. The high incidence of good results was believed to be due to proper fracture reduction and of solid bony union.[48]

Both studies suffered from the lack of a control group. In 1975 Bede *et al.* reviewed their experience with 50 medial epicondylar fractures in children.[46] In 22 cases the fracture was isolated; 13 of these were treated with immobilisation alone with 90% good results. Of the nine treated with open reduction 75% were rated good. In the 28 patients who had a fracture dislocation 72% had good results when treated with closed reduction alone, while only 50% had good results when treated with closed followed by open reduction. Based on their results they supported the traditional criteria of the presence of an intra-articular fragment or ulnar neuritis as indications for open reduction.

Wilson found a statistically significant difference between non-operatively and operatively treated patients in his study.[53] Nineteen of 20 (95%) patients treated closed were asymptomatic compared with 14 of 23 (61%) patients treated surgically.[53] This study concurred with Josefsson and Danielsson's findings that the presence of fibrous union does not cause significant symptoms. Additionally, none of the 12 patients with a fibrous union had any instability. It was concluded that 'the place of operative treatment has been overstated' and Wilson recommended reserving surgery for failure to remove an intra-articular fragment with closed manipulation.[53]

AUTHORS' PREFERRED MANAGEMENT

Undisplaced and minimally displaced fractures are treated with a short period of immobilisation as described previously. Emphasis is placed on instituting an early active range of motion.

Based on the literature available to date, we feel three indications for operative intervention exist. Entrapment of the medial epicondyle in the joint remains an absolute indication. Closed manipulation runs too great a risk of injuring the ulnar nerve. Removal of the fragment with visualisation of the nerve to ensure that it too is free of the joint is recommended.

Exploration of the nerve followed by fragment fixation is indicated if more than minor ulnar sensory neuropathy is present.

In those patients with fragment displacement who do not meet the above criteria we agree with Wilkins that a third indication for surgery exists.[55] This stems from the realisation that some patients will require a rigidly stable elbow for the performance of their work or athletic activities. Examples of these are the dominant arm of a baseball pitcher, tennis player or quarterback. Additionally, those who also depend on their non-dominant arm such as wrestlers, gymnasts and labourers should also be considered for operative intervention.[29]

SURGICAL TECHNIQUE

As Rang points out, operating with the patient prone with the arm in the 'half-nelson' position behind the back will eliminate much unnecessary struggling to see the fragment and hold it in place prior to fixation.[69] A tourniquet will also greatly aid visualisation. A medial incision is made. The ulnar nerve is identified and protected. The medial epicondylar fragment is located and reduced to its bed which is somewhat posterior on the medial column of the distal humerus. Providing the fragment is of sufficient size compression of the fragment is best achieved with a small cancellous screw. This has the added advantage of allowing early motion. Failing this, two smooth pins will provide adequate fixation and control rotation. Resumption of motion may be delayed by binding of the skin by the pins. Since they will be extra-articular, the pins can be placed percutaneously after the fragment has been openly reduced provided, of course, that the ulnar nerve is visualised and protected. This will allow removal in the clinic after 4 weeks. The necessity for a second general anaesthetic, is therefore avoided.

COMPLICATIONS

The major complications associated with medial epicondylar fractures results from failing to recognise that the apophyseal fragment is trapped in the joint. The elbow is stiff and painful with persistent subluxation of the olecranon.[64,70] Associated ulnar nerve dysfunction may also be present. Patrick observed that forceful removal of the fragment would expose eroded articular cartilage on the coronoid. He also believed that the elbow would remain persistently subluxed after fragment removal due to stretching of the capsule and ligaments.[64] Based on these observations he recommended leaving the epicondyle incarcerated in the joint. Blount concurred

with this recommendation if more than 6 weeks had elapsed from the injury.[71] Fowles *et al.* challenged this position based on their experience treating six children an average of 14 weeks after injury.[72] They demonstrated that surgical treatment of the incarceration accompanied by either excision of the fragment with reattachment of the muscles or reattachment of the fragment itself lead to a fivefold increase in range of motion and relief of pain and ulnar nerve dysfunction.[72] The best treatment, of course, remains early recognition and appropriate treatment. Surgical intervention should not, however, be withheld, in the late case.

The other major complication associated with medial epicondyle fractures is ulnar neuropathy. Granger's original description in 1818 included three patients with motor and sensory deficit.[73] In Bede *et al.*'s series the ulnar nerve was injured in 17% of patients with this fracture.[46] Nerve injury should be ruled out in all cases, especially those associated with elbow dislocation and entrapment of the fragment in the joint with treatment as outlined previously. Fortunately, ulnar neuropathy characteristically spontaneously resolves with little long-term sequelae.[51,64,73]

In at least one case, the median nerve has been found encased in a bony foramen in the distal humerus presumably after becoming entrapped between the apophyseal fragment and the distal humerus at the time of the injury.[29]

Granger was the first to observe stiffness as a common complication following medial epicondylar fracture '... the stiffness of the joint is of so obstinate a nature that ... exercise ... must constitute the *principal occupation* of the patient for several weeks'.[73] Smith noted a 20% incidence of a 5–10 degree loss of terminal elbow extension in his 143 patients.[51] Fortunately, little functional deficit results from this loss of elbow motion. Avoidance of prolonged immobilisation and institution of early elbow range of motion remain the best solution to this problem.

After injury the medial epicondylar physis usually closes. This does not create a growth or alignment problem.[49,62]

Other radiographic findings after medial epicondylar injuries have been described. These probably do not constitute a clinical problem. Chief among these is the development of a fibrous union. This has been noted to occur in up to 60% of cases in some series.[68] As Joseffsson and Danielsson discovered, this was not associated with decreased range of motion or function.[68] Wilson detected no instability in 12 patients with a fibrous union.[53]

In addition to fibrous union, at least four other radiographic deformities following medial epicondylar injury have been identified. Development of an ulnar sulcus, a double-contoured epicondyle, hypoplasia and hyperplasia of the medial epicondyle are also described.[50,59,68,74] None of these has been noted to interfere with elbow function. In at least one patient, however, a narrow and deep ulnar sulcus was thought to contribute to the development of ulnar neuritis.[74]

Medial condyle fractures

Fractures of the medial condyle of the distal humerus are very rare. Kilfoyle considered it a fracture which is seen 'once in a lifetime'.[49] Medial condyle fractures constitute only 1–2% of paediatric elbow fractures.[44,45,75,76] Experience with these uncommon fractures has slowly accumulated from isolated case reports.[45,50,67,75–83] The largest series reported to date included 27 cases collected over a 20-year period.[75]

Medial condyle fractures tend to occur in late childhood. A review of 38 patients from nine series showed a range of ages from 8 to 14 years. The youngest reported patients, however, were only 6 months, an age at which the lack of medial condylar ossification makes diagnosis exceedingly difficult.[75,80] In Cheng and Shen's review of 3413 paediatric fractures, medial condyle fractures occurred in less than 1% of children under 7 years old increasing to 4% in the 12- to 16-year-old group.[76] Boys made up 70% of the 27 cases reported in one series.[75]

Despite their rarity, medial condylar fractures deserve a thorough discussion since failure to recognise them and initiate appropriate treatment can lead to disastrous results.

The ossification centre of the trochlea begins to appear between 7 and 10 years of age. It is the third of the four epiphyseal centres of the distal humerus to develop (Chapter 1).

In the seventh edition of his classic: *A practical treatise on fractures and dislocations* Stimson described two distinct fracture patterns of the adult 'internal condyle'.[11] He hypothesised that 'the common cause appears to be violence acting from below upward upon the trochlea, as in a fall upon the flexed elbow...' (Fig. 8.10).[11] This mechanism is described by many patients in several series.[60,67,75,77] It is hypothesised that the sharp edge of the semilunar notch of the olecranon splits the trochlea directly like a wedge. The articular surface is then rotated posterolaterally by the action of the forearm flexors.

A second described mechanism involves a fall onto an outstretched arm with the elbow extended and the wrist dorsiflexed. This avulses the medial

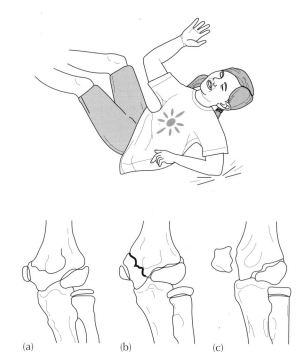

Fig. 8.10 Top: Medial condyle fracture-mechanism of injury: fall onto point of flexed elbow. Bottom: Kilfoyle classification: (a) type I – Incomplete fracture; (b) type II – Fracture extends into articular surface but no fragment displacement; (c) type III – Complete displacement with rotation. Redrawn after Ref. 49 with permission from JB Lippincott Co, Philadelphia.

condyle with a combination of muscular and ligamentous forces accentuated by the valgus alignment of the elbow. The presence of an associated valgus greenstick fracture of the olecranon in at least one case lends support to this theory.[81]

Kilfoyle classified medial condyle fractures based on the amount of displacement (Fig. 8.10).[49] Type I fractures consist of a greenstick fracture or crush of the medial condylar metaphysis extending down to the physis without associated displacement. These may represent an incomplete or abortive supracondylar fracture. Type II injuries are a fracture of the entire condyle extending across the epiphysis into the trochlear fossa. Again, no displacement is present. In type III fractures the entire medial condyle is displaced with moderate to severe rotation of the fragment.[49] Subsequent investigators utilising this scheme found that the age of the patient played an important role in the type of fracture produced. Type I fractures were seen in young patients up to 5 years of age. Type II fractures showed no age preference, while type III fractures predominated in older children.[75] The Kilfoyle classification scheme has been found useful in guiding treatment.[50]

CLINICAL PRESENTATION

Medial condyle fractures are easily confused with much more frequent medial epicondyle fracture. Clinical examination will demonstrate swelling and tenderness over the medial aspect of the elbow. Valgus instability may be present in both. The presence of associated varus instability, however, suggests that an intra-articular fracture of the medial condyle has occurred.

Knowledge of the injuries associated with these entities and the age group in which they occur is helpful in distinguishing them. Medial epicondyle fractures are often associated with elbow dislocations and tend to occur in late childhood and early adolescence. Elbow dislocations rarely occur before the second decade and are infrequent before ossification of the medial condylar epiphysis.[29] The elbow typically dislocates posterolaterally in association with medial epicondyle fractures, while in fractures with trochlear instability the elbow tends to subluxate posteromedially due to the loss of the medial buttress of the trochlea.[78]

ASSESSMENT/INVESTIGATION

Radiographically, differentiation between a fracture of the medial epicondyle and the medial condyle can be very difficult in the young child prior to ossification of the trochlea or medial epicondyle. Harrison *et al.* have described radiographic clues to help sort out this dilemma.[60] Given that the medial epicondyle is largely excluded from the elbow joint, the presence of a positive posterior fat pad sign signifying intrarticular effusion and or haemorrhage suggests the presence of a medial condyle fracture. Corbett found no fat pad displacement in any of the five fractures limited to the medial epicondyle.[84] The presence of a flake of medial metaphysis has also been considered to be indicative of a medial condyle fracture. The larger the metaphyseal flake the greater the likelihood of a more extensive fracture. Metaphyseal flakes have also been described in association with medial epicondyle fractures; however, particularly in younger patients without evidence of trochlear ossification, the presence of a metaphyseal flake should raise the suspicion of a fracture of the medial condyle and be ruled out by an arthrogram or ultrasound.

MANAGEMENT OPTIONS

As with all intra-articular physeal fractures the goal of treatment is to restore anatomic alignment of the growth plate and joint surface. In Kilfoyle type I fractures, which tend to occur in children under the age of 5 years, no displacement is present. These injuries can therefore be treated closed with initial close follow-up to observe for subsequent displacement. Immobilisation for 4–6 weeks was required in the 12 patients in Bensahel's series with a type I fracture. All achieved a good result.[75]

In type II fractures the fracture line extends down into the trochlear fossa without displacement of the fragment. These can also be treated closed provided no intrarticular step-off is present. As with lateral condyle fractures, articular incongruity is difficult to assess prior to ossification of the trochlear epiphysis. An arthrogram may be necessary to correctly characterise the nature of the fracture. Union may be delayed given the intrarticular nature of this fracture and it is best followed until complete healing is present to rule out the presence of a non-union.[49] Bensahel modified Kilfoyle's classification of type II fractures to include marked medial and proximal displacement without rotation of the fragment. Of the nine type II fractures in his series, four had closed reduction and were pinned percutaneously while five underwent open reduction with good results in those fractures treated acutely. No iatrogenic ulnar nerve injuries were described.[75]

In type III fractures displacement and rotation are present. Open reduction and rigid internal fixation are required to prevent subsequent non-union and malalignment.

Results in the treatment of medial condyle fractures are good provided an early diagnosis is made and anatomic reduction is achieved.[54,75,81]

AUTHORS' PREFERRED TREATMENT/SURGICAL TECHNIQUE

Non-displaced (Kilfoyle type I) fractures are treated closed in a fibreglass cast. Radiographs are obtained at weekly intervals initially to rule out late displacement. The cast is removed at 3–4 weeks when periosteal new bone is present. Patients are then followed until complete radiographic union is demonstrated. If close follow-up is not possible, pinning as described below is recommended.

Type II fractures are assessed with an arthrogram under general anaesthesia. Truly non-displaced fractures can be treated by cast immobilisation. In order to prevent late displacement, however, we perform a limited open pinning. A medial incision is made to identify the medial epicondyle and to insure that the ulnar nerve is away from the operative field. Two pins are then inserted under direct vision. True percutaneous pinning is not performed due to the risk of damage to the ulnar nerve. This structure is difficult to identify by palpation and to protect in the face of the significant soft tissue swelling which accompanies these fractures.

Type II fractures, in which an articular step-off is demonstrated, are managed with the limited open technique described above provided an anatomic closed reduction can be obtained. Open reduction is performed if any suspicion of persistent articular step-off remains after attempted closed reduction.

All type III fractures, which are both displaced and rotated, are treated with open reduction and pinning. An anteromedial approach as recommended by Wilkins is used.[29] The ulnar nerve is identified and protected. Care should be taken to avoid dissecting near the posterior surface of the condylar fragment and the medial aspect of the medial crista in order to preserve the already tenuous blood supply to these structures. The joint surface is visualised to ensure that an anatomic reduction has been obtained. Two parallel Kirschner wires are then inserted. These provide good fixation and prevent subsequent rotation of the fragment. The pins are cut short and buried beneath the skin to prevent development of an intra-articular infection. They are removed at 3 or 4 weeks under general anaesthesia treating the patient as a day-case admission.

COMPLICATIONS

The major source of complications in medial condyle fractures is failure of recognition, particularly in the younger child prior to ossification of the trochlear epiphysis (Fig. 8.11). Most commonly, an erroneous diagnosis of medial epicondyle fracture is made, the medial condylar displacement goes unrecognised and inadequate treatment is instituted. In Bensahel's series of 27 medial condyle fractures a delay in diagnosis of up to 3 years was present in eight patients.[75] These patients presented with limited elbow motion, non-unions, cubitus varus and in one case avascular necrosis of the medial condyle. Similar findings have been reported by Papavasiliou, Fowles and Kassab.[54,81] Attempts at late reduction did not improve upon the patient's preoperative status.[75,81] Based on their experience with two late reductions Fowles and Kassab recommended not intervening in fractures more than 3–4 weeks old.

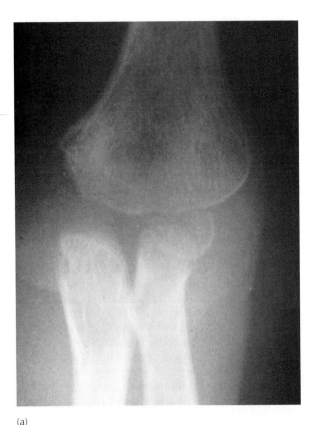

(a)

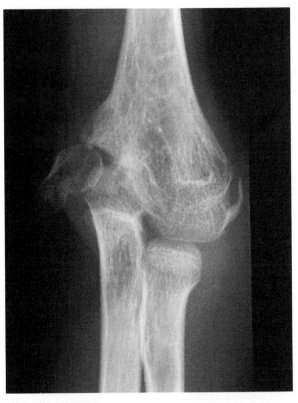

(b)

Fig. 8.11 Medial condyle non-union. (a) A 3-year-old female child, 3 weeks after fall onto elbow; (b) 6 years after injury.

There is a high risk of medial condylar avascular necrosis, even in fractures promptly and correctly treated.

As Haraldsson demonstrated in 1959, the blood supply to the medial elbow ossification centre is tenuous. At the time of trochlear ossification two sets of vessels enter the medial crista. The lateral vessels supply the apex of the trochlea and the lateral aspect of the medial crista. The medial vessels enter through the non-articulating portion of the trochlea and supply the medial aspect of the medial crista. No anastomoses appear to exist between these two sets of vessels.[85]

Injury to this terminal blood supply can lead to significant consequences for the normal growth and development of the elbow. Necrosis of the medial condyle can lead to severe cubitus varus which relentlessly progresses as the arm grows.[81,83] Cubitus varus can also be due to medial physeal growth arrest as well as persistent fracture displacement.[75] Papavasiliou recommends performing a lateral closing wedge osteotomy in patients who develop cubitus varus.[54]

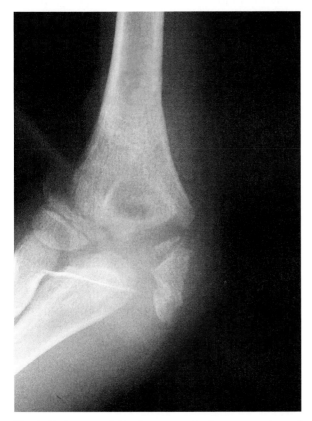

Fig. 8.12 Intercondylar fracture; 90 degree rotation of trochlear fragment is present.

T-Intercondylar fractures

'T' or 'Y' intercondylar fractures of the distal humerus are rare in children. This injury consists of a Salter–Harris type IV fracture of both condyles with the fracture line extending down through the articular surface of the trochlear apex (Fig. 8.12). It tends to occur in older children and adolescents. Maylahn and Fahey reported only six in their series of 300 consecutive paediatric elbow fractures, all of which occurred near skeletal maturity.[44]

It is thought that T-intercondylar fractures are due to an axially directed force driving the sharp edge of the olecranon up through the trochlea.[86] The common flexor and extensor tendons act to rotate the condylar fragments outward. The most commonly cited mechanism of injury involves a fall from a height on to the point of the semi-flexed elbow with the forearm pronated.[87]

Based on their experience with 16 T-intercondylar fractures, Jarvis and D'Astous proposed the following classification scheme: type I – undisplaced; type II – articular surface displacement of greater than 1 mm and type III – fracture-dislocation. In their series there were no type I, 15 type II and 1 type III fractures.[88]

CLINICAL PRESENTATION

The cardinal findings in patients presenting with T-intercondylar fractures are significant soft tissue swelling and an extended position of the elbow. On this basis this injury can easily be confused with an extension type supracondylar fracture.[29] Given the high energy aetiology of the fracture and the resultant displacement of the fracture fragments neurovascular complications can occur and should be ruled out with a careful examination. Subsequent monitoring of the neurovascular status of the forearm in the face of the characteristic massive swelling is mandatory.

ASSESSMENT/INVESTIGATION

Careful scrutiny of the plain x-rays is necessary to distinguish the T-intercondylar fracture from a comminuted supracondylar fracture. As Wilkins points out, the key differential is the presence of a vertical fracture line extending down to the apex of the trochlea.[29] In younger children it may be difficult to correctly characterise the fracture pattern prior to the appearance of the trochlear epiphysis.

The presence of a small medial metaphyseal flake in conjunction with an apparent lateral condyle fracture may be the only clue. Beghin *et al.* recommend performing routine preoperative stress radiographs in any child under 4 years of age in whom an isolated displaced fracture of the lateral or medial condyle is suspected.[89] Arthrography, ultrasound and MRI may also prove useful in this setting.[25,90]

MANAGEMENT OPTIONS

In his classic textbook: *Fractures in Children* Blount argued that permanent limitation of motion resulted from 'ill-advised' open reduction and internal fixation in T-intercondylar fractures.[71] He advocated right angle elbow traction following closed reduction for a period of 4–5 weeks. However, since they are extremely unstable injuries and characteristically involve an articular step-off, most current authors recommend open reduction and internal fixation. In the younger child the articular surface may remain intact despite apparent displacement of the radiographically visible fragments. The fracture line, however, always transects the physeal plate. Anatomic reduction of the fragments and obliteration of the gap in the growth plate is therefore necessary to restore the potential for normal growth and development of the distal humerus.[86] In addition, restoration of early motion is essential to at least partially counteract the high probability of stiffness caused by the significant soft tissue injury which accompanies these fractures. In general, these goals can only be achieved by open reduction and internal fixation.

In the rare fracture with an intact articular surface Wilkins recommends a trial of traction to see if a satisfactory reduction can be obtained.[29] If so, traction is maintained for 2 weeks followed by 2 weeks cast immobilisation.

In the very rare minimally displaced T-intercondylar fracture with an intact articular surface an acceptable closed reduction may be obtainable. Multiple percutaneous pins may then be inserted to hold the reduction.

AUTHORS' PREFERRED MANAGEMENT

Our overriding goal in treating T-intercondylar fractures is to restore articular and physeal congruity with sufficient stability to allow an early active range of motion. Rarely, this can be achieved by closed manipulation and percutaneous pinning. We have not had occasion to use olecranon trac-

tion. Our preferred management is usually open reduction and internal fixation.

SURGICAL TECHNIQUE

The patient is positioned in the lateral decubitus position on the operating table with a pneumatic tourniquet placed high on the arm. Prophylactic intravenous antibiotics are given. Either a posterior triceps splitting approach or olecranon osteotomy is used as this offers the most direct visualisation of both condyles. If the fracture is minimally displaced then either a lateral or medial approach may be used. For badly displaced fractures we prefer the olecranon osteotomy approach. The ulnar nerve is identified and protected. Periosteal stripping is minimised as much as possible to prevent avascular necrosis. The three-part fracture is converted into two parts by reducing the condylar fragments and securing them with a cancellous screw in older children or Kirschner wires in younger children. This combined epiphyseal fragment is now reduced to the humeral shaft and pinned in place similar to a supracondylar fracture. Reconstruction plates, contoured to the lateral and medial columns may be useful in adolescents to obtain more stable fixation and earlier motion. A posterior slab splint along with a stirrup splint about the elbow are applied with the arm in moderate flexion. The neurovascular status is closely monitored postoperatively. If inserted, percutaneous pins are removed at 3 weeks with active movements beginning at that time. No formal physiotherapy is instituted.

COMPLICATIONS

It is known that T-intercondylar fractures cause serious injury to the articular surface of the distal humerus as well as the surrounding soft tissue. Even with optimal treatment limitation of motion both in flexion and extension should be expected.[29,44,87,88] Both patient and parent need to know this in advance. Fortunately, the majority of patients have a satisfactory functional outcome.[87,88]

The few neurovascular complications reported in the literature include radial nerve injury and absence of the radial pulse which was restored by longitudinal traction on the forearm with the elbow extended.[88,91] Given the serious nature of this injury the actual incidence is probably similar to that of completely displaced extension supracondylar fractures.[29]

No long term sequelae, such as post-traumatic arthritis, have been reported.

Lateral epicondyle fractures

Fractures of the lateral epicondyle are exceedingly rare. No series of patients of an appreciable size with this injury has been published. In Maylahn and Fahey's series, only three of 300 consecutive paediatric elbow fractures involved the lateral epicondyle.[44] They are most likely to occur in association with an elbow dislocation and are characteristically seen in children approaching skeletal maturity.[92]

The lateral epicondyle is ossified by extension from the capitellar epiphysis with a small separate centre of ossification appearing about the age of 12 or 13. Fusion to the main epiphysis occurs within a year.[10]

The mechanism of injury most probably involves a varus strain on the elbow with avulsion of the fragment by the common extensor tendon and the lateral collateral ligament.[10,11] In adults, trauma from a direct blow has also been described.[29]

CLINICAL PRESENTATION

Examination will disclose soft tissue swelling and tenderness to palpation about the lateral aspect of the elbow. Elbow range of motion should be assessed to rule out the possibility of incarceration of the lateral epicondyle between the radial head and capitellum. Three cases of this have been reported.[93,94]

ASSESSMENT/INVESTIGATION

Ossification of the lateral epicondyle typically begins at a considerable distance from the humerus on the outer edge of the epiphysis in a characteristic sliver shape. This results in an apparent separation of the epiphysis from the metaphysis and is easily confused with an avulsion fracture.[61] The radiographic key to diagnosis is thus not osseous but rather attention to the presence of soft tissue swelling adjacent to the lateral epicondyle. The radiocapitellar articulation should be examined carefully to rule out interposed osteochondral fragments particularly if the injury has occurred in association with an elbow dislocation.

MANAGEMENT OPTIONS/AUTHORS' PREFERRED TREATMENT

As Stimson observed in 1912, good results can be expected simply with rest.[11] Immobilisation in a sling for comfort is all that is generally required.

The patient is encouraged to advance their activity as tolerated. Open reduction is reserved for intra-articular incarceration of the lateral epicondyle. After removing the fragment it is pinned with two Kirschner wires which are removed at 3–4 weeks.[93]

COMPLICATIONS

Few complications have been reported in this injury. The biggest potential complication is failure to recognise the presence of an incarcerated fragment but this has not been reported to date.

Healing of the lateral epicondyle in a displaced location, or development of a fibrous non-union has not been associated with significant disability.[29,92,96]

Given that this fracture tends to occur near skeletal maturity the risk of growth arrest is minimal.[92]

Lateral condyle fractures

Fractures of the lateral condyle have a deservedly sinister reputation. A host of potential complications are possible if this fracture is not recognised and treated with appropriate respect and attention to detail. Fortunately, accurate diagnosis and appropriate treatment produce consistently good results.

Lateral condyle fractures constitute approximately 17% of all distal humeral fractures in children. It is the most common injury to the distal humeral physis, comprising 54% of the fractures to this growth centre.[97]

Lateral condyle fractures characteristically occur between the ages of 2 and 14 years with a peak occurring around the age of 6 years.[98–100] In Thonell et al.'s series of 356 children boys outnumbered girls by a ratio of 2 to 1.[100]

The capitellar ossification centre is the first growth centre in the elbow to appear (Chapter 1). Ossification usually occurs between the 1st and 24th months, with fusion to the trochlear epiphysis, taking place between 11 and 13 years of age. This combined epiphysis, representing the entire distal humeral epiphysis, fuses to the humeral shaft at age 13–14 years.[101]

As a consequence, during the period of peak incidence of lateral condyle fractures at age 6 years the majority of the epiphysis remain cartilaginous and therefore radiolucent to x-ray examination. Invariably, the radiographically visible fracture fragment represents only a small portion of the involved epiphysis.

In 1956, Milch described the anatomic basis for lateral condyle fracture production and introduced the classification system which pertains to this day.[102] Milch hypothesized that the trochlear groove and the capitulotrochlear sulcus 'while . . . increasing the congruence and therefore the stability of the elbow . . . act as perfect wedges in the event that force is directed axially along either the radius or ulna'.[102] The critical factor in differentiating a type I from a type II injury in Milch's scheme is the integrity of the lateral wall of the trochlea. Forces directed longitudinally along the radius cause the radial head to impact on the capitulotrochlear sulcus with a simple lateral condyle fracture resulting. The fracture line may pass through the capitellar ossification centre. The lateral wall of the trochlea remains intact and serves as a buttress to prevent associated lateral forearm dislocation. This is a Milch type I fracture and is a Salter–Harris type IV physeal injury. According to Rang, this fracture pattern occurs in only 5% of lateral condyle fractures.[69]

Forces directed upward and outward along the ulna cause impaction of the olecranocoronoid ridge against the trochlear groove with the fracture occurring at or medial to the trochlear groove. The lateral portion of the trochlea will be included in the distal fragment. Without this buttress an associated lateral elbow dislocation occurs. This is a Milch type II fracture of the lateral condyle and a Salter–Harris type II fracture with the lateral condyle representing the Thurston–Holland metaphyseal fragment.

Jakob *et al.* proposed a different mechanism of injury based on cadaver studies.[103] Forced varus angulation with the elbow extended and the forearm supinated produced lateral condyle fractures in four of seven specimens. A bridge of cartilage remained in three of the four and acted as a hinge guiding the fragment back into position. When the hinge was divided the fracture became unstable with free rotation and displacement possible. Based on the observation that the fracture line began on the lateral aspect of the condyle Jakob hypothesised that the fragment was avulsed by the lateral collateral ligament and common extensor origin.[103]

Lateral condyle injuries have also been classified by the degree of displacement of the fracture fragment (Fig. 8.13).[103] In type I fractures the fracture line extends from the lateral column of the humerus to the junction between the capitellum and trochlea separating a thin portion of radioopaque metaphysis. The fracture does not penetrate the articular cartilage, is incomplete and remains non-displaced. In type II fractures the fracture line extends through the articular surface. The fragment may be moderately displaced but is not rotated. Type III fractures are displaced and rotated with disruption

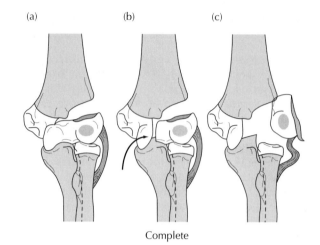

(a)   (b)   (c)

Complete

Fig. 8.13 Classification of lateral condyle fractures: (a) type I; (b) type II – articular hinge is disrupted; (c) type III – complete displacement. Rotation is commonly present. Redrawn after Ref. 103 with permission from *Journal of Bone and Joint Surgery.*

of the normal relationship of the capitellum to the radial head (Fig. 8.14a).

CLINICAL PRESENTATION

Children with lateral condyle fractures will typically present with soft tissue swelling and tenderness concentrated on the lateral aspect of the elbow. Evidence of an associated elbow dislocation may be present if a Milch type II injury is present.[104] In contrast to the marked malalignment which is common in supracondylar fractures lateral condyle fractures have a surprisingly benign appearance.[29] Neurovascular examination will only rarely reveal an acute deficit.

ASSESSMENT/INVESTIGATION

In addition to standard anteroposterior and lateral radiographs of the elbow, oblique views should be obtained in all children suspected of having a lateral condyle fracture. The internal rotation oblique will best demonstrate the amount of displacement and rotation of the lateral condyle fragment.[97]

Given that the peak incidence of lateral condyle fractures occurs prior to trochlear ossification, understanding the true extent of the fracture can be difficult. Often only a thin metaphyseal fragment is visible radiographically. Differentiating the fracture pattern and predicting the stability of the distal fragment is crucial to instituting appropriate treatment. Type I incomplete fractures, in which the

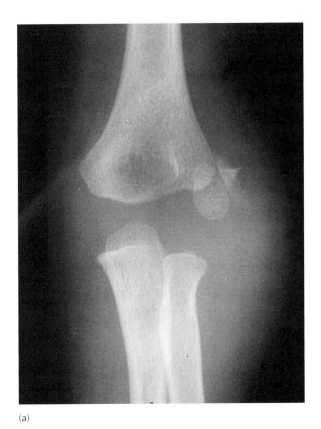 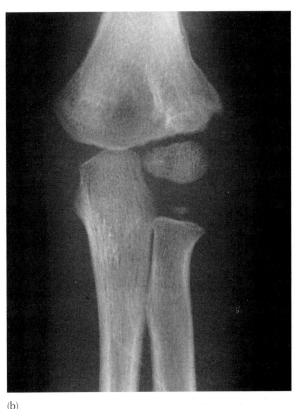

(a)   (b)

Fig. 8.14 (a) Type III lateral condyle fracture: significant rotation of capitellar fragment is present; (b) 8-week follow-up: a small lateral spur is present.

intact articular cartilage hinge resists displacement, can usually be treated closed. Type II fractures in which the articular surface is disrupted may also appear minimally displaced on plain films. They are inherently unstable and subject to further displacement and thus require open reduction and stable fixation.[105,106]

Thonell *et al.* proposed radiographic criteria for predicting the stability of minimal displaced fractures treated conservatively.[100] They divided into three groups, 159 lateral condyle fractures. In group A the fracture line could not be followed to the epiphyseal cartilage. These were classified as stable. Group B fractures were wider laterally than medially and could be followed down to the epiphyseal cartilage. These were classified as indeterminate. Group C fractures were as wide medially as laterally and were classified as unstable. All fractures were closely observed for subsequent displacement while immobilised in plaster. In group A 2.6% subsequently displaced, in group B 24% displaced and in group C 44% eventually displaced. Based on these results Thonell and his co-workers felt their

criteria was useful in selecting high-risk cases for prophylactic internal fixation. Flynn and Richards demonstrated that lateral condyle fractures with an initial displacement of the distal fragment of 3 mm or more always developed further displacement and were at high risk for development of non-union.[107]

Another tool available to guide treatment is elbow arthrography. Assessment of articular incongruity as a measure of fragment stability has proven useful in deciding which patients require open reduction versus closed reduction and percutaneous pinning or simply cast immobilisation. In one series of 16 lateral condyle fractures arthrography influenced the management in 11 cases.[105] In the majority of these the arthrogram confirmed the preoperative diagnosis and treatment plan; however, in two patients arthrography revealed previously undiagnosed articular incongruity. In three patients an unnecessary operation was avoided.[105]

Arthrography can also be useful in identifying the rare patient with more than 2 mm displacement but no articular incongruity in which percutaneous pinning is an effective option.[106]

MANAGEMENT OPTIONS

Treatment of lateral condyle fractures is guided by the amount of displacement present. Type I fractures which are minimally displaced and have an intact articular surface can be treated closed. Close follow-up to avoid missing subsequent displacement is mandatory. One option is to place the child in a posterior slab splint with the elbow in 90 degrees flexion and the forearm supinated to relax the pull of the extensors on the fragment. This is removed at the initial clinic visit 3–5 days after the injury to allow repeat radiographs without the confounding presence of overlying plaster. Alternatively, an initial fibreglass cast may be used. If increased displacement has occurred the child is prepared for surgery. Otherwise, a circumferential cast is applied for an additional 3 weeks. Close follow-up should be continued until radiographs confirming union are obtained. Flynn has emphasised the necessity of maintaining immobilisation until union is present with radiographic follow-up continuing until it is certain the union is solid.[108] In his end-result study of slightly displaced fractures of the lateral condyle Flynn and Richards identified a group of patients with less than 2 mm of initial displacement who required up to 12 weeks to heal. Removal of the cast too early in this group can lead to non-union.[107]

Type II fractures, which include the articular surface, and are moderately displaced may be amenable to a single closed reduction attempt utilising hyperflexion, pronation and direct pressure over the fragment followed by percutaneous pinning. A small subgroup of patients with more than 2 mm of radiographic displacement but an arthrographically demonstrated congruent joint surface can also be treated by percutaneous pinning alone.[106]

Irreducible type II fractures and type III fractures, which are significantly displaced and rotated, require open reduction in order to restore articular and physeal congruity.

Treatment of patients presenting late is controversial. At issue is whether elbow function can be improved by a late open reduction and internal fixation. Osteonecrosis of the capitellum is a frequent result of late attempts at open reduction which requires extensive dissection and soft tissue stripping to reduce the fragment, particularly if the dissection extends posteriorly. In addition, significant scar formation can occur which will restrict elbow motion postoperatively.[104] Dhillon *et al.* found that patients operated on 6 weeks or more after their injury did no better than those left alone.[109] Jakob *et al.* had poor results with delayed open reduction and fixation after three weeks.[103]

Other authors advocate treatment at the time of delayed diagnosis and report good results. Roye *et al.* reported on three patients treated with functional reduction and postoperative continuous passive motion. All united and had improved range of motion and function postoperatively.[110] Flynn and Richards advocated intervening as soon as the diagnosis of non-union is established in order to preserve the growth potential of the physis of the distal fragment and prevent late angulatory deformity.[107] In those patients with closed physes, bone grafting and fixation to achieve union along with varus osteotomy and or medial epiphyseodesis is recommended.[111]

Given the risk of avascular necrosis the likely decreased range of motion and the observation that the average onset of tardy ulnar palsy is 22 years after surgery most authors recommend delaying operative treatment in those patients seen 6 weeks or more after injury until skeletal maturity or onset of symptoms.[104,109,112]

AUTHORS' PREFERRED MANAGEMENT

Type I fractures are treated closed in a fibreglass cast provided oblique x-rays have confirmed that only minimal displacement is present. Weekly clinic follow-up with serial x-rays are obtained to rule out late displacement. The cast is removed at 3–4 weeks and the patients followed until radiographic union is demonstrated. If any concern exists regarding the possibility of non-compliance with the requirement for close follow-up or uncertainty regarding the amount of displacement the patient is treated with percutaneous pinning. We have a low threshold for proceeding to pinning as this eliminates a great deal of worry.

Type II fractures are treated with an attempted closed reduction. If flouroscopy suggests that an acceptable reduction has been obtained a confirmatory arthrogram is performed following provisional fixation with a percutaneous pin.

Irreducible type II and all type III injuries are treated by open reduction.

SURGICAL TECHNIQUE

Under general anaesthesia the patient is positioned supine with the shoulder moved to the edge of the operating table and the arm on a radiolucent arm board. The arm is prepped and draped. A sterile tourniquet is applied. In questionably displaced type I fractures an arthrogram is performed by injecting contrast diluted at least 50% laterally into the elbow via the soft spot formed by the olecranon, radial head and lateral epicondyle. Provided the articular surface is intact, two pins are placed percutaneously in a divergent pattern attempting to avoid the lateral physis. This is not always possible. This usually results in one pin nearly parallel to the joint with the other directed superior to the olecranon fossa. Ideally, the pins cross just inside the lateral metaphyseal border with the widest possible divergence at the fracture site.

In those fractures requiring open reduction a longitudinal incision is made slightly anterior to the lateral condylar ridge with dissection proceeding between the brachioradialis and extensor carpi radialis. Characteristically, the fracture has disrupted these muscle fibres and a haematoma is encountered just deep to the subcutaneous tissue. This can be followed to the fracture site. The wound is irrigated and the haematoma evacuated. Care is taken to avoid posterior dissection in order to protect the posterior vessels which are the sole blood supply to the capitellar epiphysis. Long, thin-bladed retractors, such as those used in rectal surgery, are ideal to allow a view across the entire distal elbow. A headlight may also prove useful. The joint surface must be visualised in order to ensure that articular congruity is restored. This will also assist in obtaining physeal congruity. As there is often plastic deformation of the metaphysis restoring articular congruity is the key to a successful reduction and good outcome. Having the assistant place a valgus stress on the arm may aid reduction by decreasing the pull of the extensor musculature. Once reduced the fragment is fixed with Kirschner wires postioned as described above. These are placed through separate stab incisions. The pins are cut short and buried beneath the skin to prevent development of an intra-articular infection. Occasionally, the distal fragment will be amenable to fixation with a cancellous screw. This has the advantage of creating compression at the fracture site. If possible, the periosteum is closed to prevent lateral spur formation (Fig. 8.14b).

The arm is splinted with a back slab and sugar-tong stirrup splint with the elbow flexed 90 degrees and the forearm in neutral. The pins are removed under general anaesthesia at 4 weeks if adequate healing is evident radiographically. Active range of motion of the elbow is started. No formal physiotherapy is prescribed.

COMPLICATIONS OF SURGERY

In lateral condyle fractures treated with acceptable reduction and maintenance with solid fixation good results can be expected. A host of complications, however, are possible in lateral condyle fractures

not diagnosed or treated with inappropriate attention to detail. The fracture type most susceptible to complications tend to be those which appear minimally displaced and are therefore treated less aggressively.

Delayed union most often occurs in fractures treated non-operatively. The fragments are well aligned but a delay in the union of the condylar fragment to the metaphysis is present. Flynn and Richards identified three patterns of healing in lateral condyle fractures.[107] In those fractures with displacement of 2 mm or less, 49% healed within 6 weeks with abundant metaphyseal callus and periosteal new bone formation. 38% took 8–12 weeks to heal. These healed by endosteal union with little early callus and no periosteal new bone. In the third group, initial displacement of 2–4 mm was present. Progressive displacement occurred within 2 weeks of injury and these fractures were ultimately treated with open reduction and internal fixation. Based on these observations Flynn and Richards recommended long-term immobilization in this slower healing group with follow-up until radiographic union was demonstrated.[107] Wilkins, however, recommends follow-up until the patient is asymptomatic and progressive displacement is not occurring.[29]

Flynn and Richards defined an established non-union as a fracture which had not healed by 12 weeks (Fig. 8.15).[107] They distinguished between a non-union in good position and a non-union in poor position. In non-unions in which the condylar fragment is in good position and the physis is open they strongly advised operative intervention. By procrastinating, a golden opportunity to salvage the condylar fragments growth potential prior to physeal closure would be missed. Their operative technique included minimal soft tissue stripping, placement of a peg bone graft and internal fixation without disturbing the non-union.[107] Wilkins recommends placement of a compressive screw across the metaphysis without application of bone graft. When the condylar fragment is in an acceptable position and does not require manipulation this can be accomplished percutaneously with a cannulated screw (Fig. 8.16).[42] This technique has the added advantage of allowing early resumption of motion.

Appropriate treatment in those patients with an established non-union in a poor position is controversial. Flynn and Richards felt that the attempt to replace the condylar fragment anatomically when it is significantly rotated and displaced would traumatise the physis with a resultant growth arrest and development of a progressive valgus deformity with little having been gained from surgery.[107] Others have emphasised the risk of avascular necrosis of

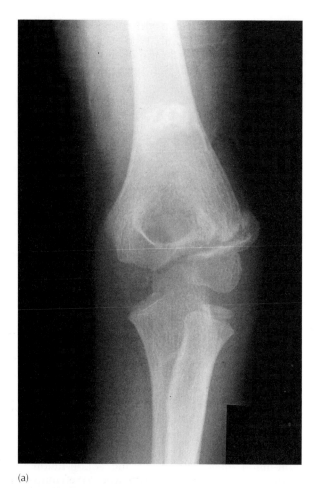

(a)

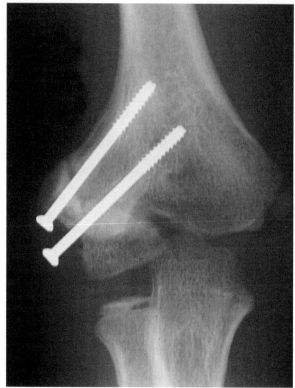

Fig. 8.16 Percutaneous treatment of established lateral condyle non-union with cannulated screws.

(b)

Fig. 8.15 (a, b) Lateral condyle non-union. Sclerosis is present as is persistence of fracture line lucency.

the condylar fragment if extensive dissection, particularly posteriorly, is performed.[29,44] The likelihood of surgical scarring causing postoperative stiffness has also been described.[103,108,113]

Advocates of osteosynthesis for established non-union seek to alter the relentless natural history of this condition. The characteristic clincial course of an established non-union is one of progressive migration proximally and laterally of the condylar fragment producing a developmental cubitus valgus. The associated elbow instability and stretch of the ulnar nerve due to the valgus alignment of the arm leads to pain and the development of a tardy ulnar nerve palsy.[104,114–116] In Gay and Love's series of 57 patients from the Mayo Clinic, however, the onset of the ulnar nerve palsy was delayed an average of 22 years after the original elbow injury.[112] For this reason, most authors currently recommend delaying osteosynthesis until skeletal maturity or until the patient becomes symptomatic.[104,114]

In those patients with evidence of a tardy ulnar nerve palsy without associated instability, treatment should consist of neurolysis and anterior transfer of the ulnar nerve with or without a distal humeral osteotomy.[114]

Although cubitus valgus is the classic angulatory deformity encountered in lateral condyle fractures, cubitus varus can also occur. So *et al.* reported development of cubitus varus in 10 of 24 patients.[117] This occurred in undisplaced as well as displaced fractures. Based on their observations hyperaemic overgrowth was implicated as the cause. Malunion has also been cited as a cause of cubitus varus following lateral condyle fractures.[109]

Cubitus varus following elbow fracture has traditionally been considered solely a cosmetic deformity. Davids *et al.* however, have reported on six patients with post-traumatic cubitus varus who sustained lateral condyle fractures. Their biomechanical analysis suggested that the shear stress across the capitellar physis in a routine fall was increased by varus malalignment. This therefore predisposes these patients to lateral condyle fractures.[118]

A 'fishtail' deformity of the distal humerus is sometimes seen in follow-up radiographs. This is thought to be a result of a loss of the ossific link between the trochlear and capitellar centres with a resultant deficiency of the lateral lip of the trochlea.[109,119] In Rutherford's series he found that this deformity occurred only in those fractures that were inadequately reduced.[120] It has also been hypothesised that the fishtail deformity is due to an injury to the lateral trochlear vessel and represents avascular necrosis of the lateral portion of the medial crista of the trochlea.[29] Little functional disability results and treatment is generally not required.[98]

References

1. Akbarnia BA, Silberstein MJ, Rende RJ, Graviss E, Luisiri A. arthrography in the diagnosis of fractures of the distal end of the humerus in infants. *J Bone Joint Surg* 1986; **68A:** 599–601.
2. Macafee A Infantile supracondylar fracture. *J Bone Joint Surg* 1967; **49B:** 768–70.
3. DeLee J Transverse divergent dislocation of the elbow in a child. *J Bone Joint Surg* 1981; **63A:** 322–3.
4. Barrett W, Almquist E, Staheli L Fracture separation of the distal humeral physis in the newborn. *J Pediatr Orthop* 1984; **4:** 617–9.
5. DeJager L, Hoffmann E Fracture-separation of the distal humeral epiphysis. *J Bone Joint Surg* 1991; **73B:** 143–6.
6. Dias J, Lamont A, Jones J Ultrasonic diagnosis of neonatal separation of the distal humeral epiphysis. *J Bone Joint Surg* 1988; **70B:** 825–8.
7. Downs D, Wirth C Fracture of the distal humeral chondroepiphysis in the neonate. *Clin Orthop* 1982; **169:** 155–8.
8. McIntyre W Supracondylar fractures of the humerus. In: *Management of pediatric fractures.*
9. Paige M, Port R Separation of the distal humeral epiphysis in the neonate. *Am J Dis Child* 1985; **139:** 1203–5.
10. Siffert R Displacement of the distal humeral epiphysis in the newborn infant. *J Bone Joint Surg* 1963; **45A:** 165–9.
11. Stimson L *A practical treatise on fractures and dislocations* (7th edn). New York, Philadelphia: Lea and Febiger, 1912.
12. Smith F Displacement of medial epicondyle of humerus into the elbow joint. *Ann Surg* 1946; **124:** 410–25.
13. Berman J, Weiner D Neonatal fracture-separation of the distal humeral chondroepiphysis: A case report. *Orthopedics* 1980; **3:** 875–9.
14. Chand K Epiphyseal separation of distal humerus in an infant. *J Trauma* 1974; **14:** 521–6.
15. Hansen P, Barnes D, Tullos H Arthrographic diagnosis of an injury pattern in the distal humerus of an infant *J Pediatr Orthop* 1982; **2:** 569–72.
16. Holda M, Manoli A, LaMont R Epiphyseal separation of the distal end of the humerus with medial displacement. *J Bone Joint Surg* 1980; **62A:** 52–7.
17. Kaplin S, Reckling F Fracture separation of the lower humeral epiphysis with medial displacement. *J Bone Joint Surg* 1971; **53A:** 1105–8.
18. Marmor L, Bechtol C Fracture separation of the lower humeral epiphysis. *J Bone Joint Surg* 1960; **42A:** 333–6.
19. Mizuno K, Hirohata K, Kashiwagi D Fracture-separation of the distal humeral epiphysis in young children. *J Bone Joint Surg* 1979; **61A:** 570–3.
20. Rogers L, Rockwood C Separation of the entire distal humeral epiphysis. *Radiology* 1973; **106:** 393–9.
21. Yngve D Distal humeral epiphyseal separation. *Orthopedics* 1985; **8:** 100–3.
22. Peterson H Physeal injuries of the distal humerus. *Orthopedics* 1992; **15:** 799–808.
23. Bright RW, Burstein AH, Elmore SM Epiphyseal plate cartilage. *J Bone Joint Surg* 1974; **56A:** 688–703.
24. Silberstein M Some Vagaries of the capitellum. *J Bone Joint Surg* 1979; **61A:** 244–7.
25. Davidson R, Markowitz R, Dormans J, Drummond D Ultrasonographic evaluation of the elbow in infants and young children after suspected trauma. *J Bone Joint Surg* 1994; **76A:** 1804–13.
26. Roback D Elbow arthrography: brief technical considerations. *Clin Radiol* 1979; **30:** 311–12.
27. Gartland J Management of supracondylar fractures of the humerus in children. *Surg Gynecol Obstet* 1959; **109:** 145–54.
28. Culp Osterman A, Davidson R, Skirven T, Bora F Neural injuries associated with supracondylar fractures of the humerus in children. *J Bone Joint Surg* 1990; **72A:** 1211–15.
29. Wilkins K Residuals of elbow trauma in children. *Orthop Clin North Am* 1990; **21:** 291–314.
30. Cramer K, Green N, Devito D Incidence of anterior interosseous nerve palsy in supracondylar humerus

Letts R (ed) New York: Churchill Livingstone, 1994.

fractures in children. *J Pediatr Orthop* 1993; **13:** 502–5.

31. Camp J, Ishizue K, Gomez M, Gelberman R, Akeson W Alterations of Bauman's angle by humeral position: implications for treatment of supracondylar humerus fractures. *J Pediatr Orthop* 1993; **13:** 521–5.
32. McIntyre W, Wiley J, Charette R Fracture-separation of the distal humeral epiphysis. *Clin Orthop* 1984; **188:** 98–102.
33. Bhende H Clinical measurement of varus-valgus deformity after supracondylar fracture of the humerus. *J Bone Joint Surg* 1994; **76B:** 329–31.
34. Kasser J Percutaneous pinning of supracondylar fractures of the humerus. *Instr Course Lect* 1992; **XLI:** 385–90.
35. Wilkins K Fractures of the medial epicondyle in children. *Instr Course Lect* 1991; **XL:** 3–10.
36. Boyd D, Aronson D Supracondylar fractures of the humerus: A prospective study of percutaneous pinning. *J Pediatr Orthop* 1992; **12:** 789–94.
37. Mehserle W, Meehan P Treatment of the displaced supracondylar fracture of the humerus (type III) with closed reduction and percutaneous cross-pin fixation. *J Pediatr Orthop* 1991; **11:** 705–11.
38. Kurer M, Regan M Completely displaced supracondylar fracture of the humerus in children. *Clin Orthop* 1990; **256:** 205–14.
39. Sutton W, Greene W, Georgopoulos G, Dameron T Displaced supracondylar humeral fractures in children. *Clin Orthop* 1992; **278:** 81–7.
40. Zionts L, McKellop H, Hatahaway R Torsional strength of pin configurations used to fix supracondylar fractures of the humerus in children. *J Bone Joint Surg* 1994; **76A:** 253–6.
41. Bostman O, Makela E, Sodergard J *et al.* Absorbable polyglycolide pins in internal fixation of fractures in children. *J Pediatr Orthop* 1993; **13:** 242–5.
42. Wilkins K (ed) *Operative management of upper extremity fractures in children.* Rosemont: American Academy of Orthopedic Surgeons, 1994: 66–70.
43. Royce R, Dutkowsky J, Kasser J, Rand F Neurologic complications after K-wire fixation of supracondylar humerus fractures in children. *J Pediatr Orthop* 1991; **11:** 191–4.
44. Maylahn D, Fahey J Fractures of the elbow in children: Review of three hundred consecutive cases. *J Am Med Assoc* 1958; **166:** 220–8.
45. Fahey J Fractures of the elbow in children. *Instr Course Lect* 1960; **XVII:** 13–46.
46. Bede W, Lefebvre A, Rosman M Fractures of the medial humeral epicondyle in children. *Can J Surg* 1975; **18:** 137–42.
47. Fowles J, Slimane N, Kassab M Elbow dislocation with avulsion of the medial humeral epicondyle. *J Bone Joint Surg* 1990; **72B:** 102–4.
48. Hines R, Herndon W, Evans J Operative treatment of medial epicondyle fractures in children. *Clin Orthop* 1987; **223:** 170–4.
49. Kilfoyle R Fractures of the medial condyle and epicondyle of the elbow in children. *Clin Orthop* 1965; **41:** 43–50.

50. Papavasiliou V Fracture-separation of the medial epicondylar epiphysis of the elbow joint. *Clin Orthop* 1982; **171:** 172–4.
51. Smith F, Joyce J Fractures of the lateral condyle of the humerus in children. *Am J Surg* 1954; **87:** 324–9.
52. Wilson N, Ingram R, Rymaszewski L, Miller J Treatment of fractures of the medial epicondyle of the humerus. *Injury* 1988; **19:** 342–4.
53. Wilson P Fracture of the lateral condyle of the humerus in childhood. *J Bone Joint Surg* 1936; **18:** 301–18.
54. Papavasiliou V, Kirkos J Dislocation of the elbow joint associated with fracture of the radial neck in children. *Injury* 1991; **22:** 49–50.
55. Wilkins K Residuals of elbow trauma in children. *Orthop Clin North Am* 1990; **21:** 269–89.
56. Brogdon B Little leaguer's elbow. *Am J Roentgenol* 1960; **83:** 671–5.
57. Schwab G, Bennett J, Wood G, Tullos H Biomechanics of elbow instability: The role of the medial collateral ligament. *Clin Orthop* 1980; **146:** 42–52.
58. Woods G, Tullos H Elbow instability and medial epicondyle fractures. *Am J Sports Med* 1977; **5:** 23–30.
59. Smith F Medial Epicondyle injuries. *J Am Med Assoc* 1950; **142:** 396–402.
60. Harrison R, Keats T, Frankel C, Anderson R, Youngblood P Radiographic clues to fractures of the unossified medial humeral condyle in young children. *Skeletal Radiol* 1984; **11:** 209–12.
61. Silberstein M, Brodeur A, Graviss E Some vagaries of the lateral epicondyle. *J Bone Joint Surg* 1982; **64A:** 444–8.
62. Chessare J, Rogers L, White H, Tachdijan M Injuries of the medial epicondylar ossification center of the humerus. *Am J Roentgenol* 1977; **129:** 49–55.
63. Fahey J, O'Brien E Fracture-separation of the medial humeral condyle in a child confused with fracture of the medial epicondyle. *J Bone Joint Surg* 1971; **53A:** 1102–4.
64. Patrick J Fracture of the Medial epicondyle with displacement into the elbow joint. *J Bone Joint Surg* 1946; **28:** 143–7.
65. Harvey S, Tchelebi H Proximal radio-ulnar translocation. *J Bone Joint Surg* 1979; **61A:** 447–9.
66. Roberts N Displacement of the internal epicondyle into the elbow joint. *Lancet* 1934; **2:** 78–9.
67. Potter C Fracture-dislocation of the trochlea. *J Bone Joint Surg* 1954; **36B:** 250–3.
68. Josefsson P, Danielsson L Epicondylar elbow fracture in children. *Acta Orthop Scand* 1986; **57:** 313–5.
69. Rang M *Anthology of orthopaedics.* Edinburgh: Churchill Livingstone, 1966.
70. Schmier A The internal epicondylar epiphysis and elbow injuries. *Surg Gynecol Obstet* 1945; **80:** 416–21.
71. Blount W *Fractures in children.* Baltimore: Williams and Wilkins, 1955.
72. Fowles J, Kassab M, Douik M Untreated posterior dislocation of the elbow in children. *J Bone Joint Surg* 1984; **66A:** 921–6.

73. Granger B On a particular fracture of the inner condyle of the humerus. *Edin Med Surg J* 1818; **14:** 196–201.

74. Skak S, Grossmann E, Wagn P Deformity after internal fixation of fracture separation of the medial epicondyle of the humerus. *J Bone Joint Surg* 1994; **76B:** 297–302.

75. Bensahel H, Csukonyi Z, Badelon O, Badaoui S Fractures of the medial condyle of the humerus in children. *J Pediatr Orthop* 1986; **6:** 430–3.

76. Cheng J, Shen W Limb fracture pattern in different pediatric age groups: A study of 3350 children. *J Orthop Trauma* 1993; **7:** 15–22.

77. Chacha P Fracture of the medial condyle of the humerus with rotational displacement. *J Bone Joint Surg* 1970; **52A:** 1453–8.

78. Cothay D Injury to the lower medial epiphysis of the humerus before development of the ossific centre. *J Bone Joint Surg* 1967; **49B:** 766–7.

79. Dangles C, Tylkowski C, Pankovich A Epicondylotrochlear fracture of the humerus before appearence of the ossification center. *Clin Orthop* 1982; **171:** 161–3.

80. DeBoeck H, Castelyn P, Opdecam P Fracture of the medial humeral condyle. *J Bone Joint Surg* 1987; **69A:** 1442–4.

81. Fowles J, Kassab M Displaced fractures of the medial humeral condyle in children. *J Bone Joint Surg* 1980; **62A:** 1159–63.

82. Ghawabi M Fracture of the medial condyle of the humerus. *J Bone Joint Surg* 1975; **57A:** 677–80.

83. Varma B, Srivastava T Fracture of the medial condyle of the humerus in children: A report of 4 cases including late sequelae. *Injury* 1972; **4:** 171–4.

84. Corbett R Displaced fat pads in trauma to the elbow. *Injury* 1978; **9:** 297–8.

85. Haraldsson S, Osteochondrosis deformans juvenilis capituli humeri including investigation of intraosseous vasculature in distal humerus. *Acta Orthop Scand* 1959; **38**(Supp).

86. Zimmerman H *Treatment of fractures in children and adolescents.* In: Weber B, Brunner C, Freuler F, (eds) Berlin: Springer-Verlag, 1980.

87. Papavasiliou V, Beslikas T T Condylar fractures of the distal humeral condyles during childhood: An analysis of six cases. *J Pediatr Orthop* 1986; **6:** 302–5.

88. Jarvis J, D'Astous J The pediatric T-supracondylar fracture. *J Pediatr Orthop* 1984; **4:** 697–9.

89. Beghin J, Bucholz R, Wenger D Intercondylar fractures of the humerus in young children. *J Bone Joint Surg* 1982; **64A:** 1083–7.

90. Beltran J, Rosenberg Z, Kawelblum M *et al.* Pediatric elbow fractures: MRI evaluation. *Skeletal Radiol* 1994; **23:** 277–281.

91. Grantham S, Tiejen R Transcondylar fracture-dislocation of the elbow. *J Bone Joint Surg* 1976; **58A:** 1030–1.

92. Ogden J *Skeletal injury in the child* (2nd edn). Philadelphia: WB Saunders Co, 1990.

93. McLeod G, Gray A, Turner M Elbow dislocation with intra-articular entrapment of the lateral epicondyle. *J Roy Coll Surg Edinb* 1993; **38:** 112–3.

94. Watson-Jones R *Fractures and joint injuries* (4th edn). Edinburgh: ES Livingstone, 1956.

95. Silberstein M, Brodeur A, Graviss E, Luisiri A Some vagaries of the medial epicondyle. *J Bone Joint Surg* 1981; **63A:** 524–8.

96. Sharrard W *Pediatric orthopaedics and fractures* (2nd edn). Oxford: Blackwell Scientific Publications, 1979.

97. Frymoyer J (ed.) *Orthopaedic knowledge update 4.* Rosemont: American Academy of Orthopedic Surgeons, 1993: 328.

98. Foster D, Sullivan J, Gross R Lateral humeral condylar fractures in children. *J Pediatr Orthop* 1985; **5:** 16–22.

99. Smith RW Observations on disjunction of the lower epiphysis of the humerus. *Dublin Quart J Med Sci* 1850; **9:** 63–74.

100. Thonell S, Mortensson W, Thomasson B Predication of the stability of minimally displaced fractures of the lateral humeral condyle. *Acta Radiol* 1988; **29:** 367–70.

101. Wilson J The treatment of fractures of the medial epicondyle of the humerus. *J Bone Joint Surg* 1960; **42B:** 778–81.

102. Milch H Fractures of the external humeral condyle. *J Am Med Assoc* 1956; **160:** 641–6.

103. Jakob R, Fowles J, Rang M, Kassab M Observations concerning fractures of the lateral humeral condyle in children. *J Bone Joint Surg* 1975; **57B:** 430–6.

104. Wilkins K In: *Fractures in children* (3rd edn). Rockwood C, Wilkins K, King R (eds) Philadelphia: JB Lippincott Co, 1991.

105. Marzo J, d'Amato C, Strong M, Gillespie R Usefulness and accuracy of arthrography in management of lateral humeral condyle fractures in children. *J Pediatr Orthop* 1990; **10:** 317–321.

106. Mintzer C, Waters P, Brown D, Kasser J Percutaneous pinning in the treatment of displaced lateral condyle fractures. *J Pediatr Orthop* 1994; **14:** 462–5.

107. Flynn J, Richards. J Non-Union of minimally displaced fractures of the lateral condyle of the humerus in children. *J Bone Joint Surg* 1971; **53A:** 1096–101.

108. Flynn J Nonunion of slightly displaced fractures of the lateral humeral condyle in children: An update. *J Pediatr Orthop* 1989; **9:** 691–6.

109. Dhillon K, Sengupta S, Singh B Delayed management of fracture of the lateral humeral condyle in children. *Acta Orthop Scand* 1988; **59:** 419–24.

110. Roye D, Bini S, Infosino A Late surgical treatment of lateral condylar fractures in children. *J Pediatr Orthop* 1991; **11:** 195–9.

111. Flynn J, Richards J, Saltzman R Prevention and treatment of non-union of slightly displaced fractures of the lateral humeral condyle in children. *J Bone Joint Surg* 1975; **57A:** 1087–92.

112. Gay J, Love G Diagnosis and treatment of tardy paralysis of the ulnar nerve. *J Bone Joint Surg* 1947; **29:** 1087–97.

113. Hardacre J, Nahigian S, Froimson A, Brown J Fractures of the lateral condyle of the humerus in children. *J Bone Joint Surg* 1971; **53A:** 1083–95.

114. Masada K, Kawai H, Kawabata H, Masatomi T, Tsuyuguchi Y, Yamamoto K Osteosynthesis for old established non-union of the lateral condyle of the humerus. *J Bone Joint Surg* 1990; **72A:** 32–40.
115. McGowan A The results of transposition of the ulnar nerve for traumatic ulnar neuritis. *J Bone Joint Surg* 1950; **32B:** 293–301.
116. Miller E Late ulnar nerve palsy. *Surg Gynecol Obstet* 1924; **38:** 37–46.
117. So Y, Fang D, Leong J, Bong S Varus deformity following lateral humeral condylar fractures in children. *J Pediatr Orthop* 1985; **5:** 569–72.
118. Davids J, Maguire M, Mubarak S, Wenger D Lateral condyle fracture of the humerus following posttraumatic cubitus varus. *J Pediatr Orthop* 1994; **14:** 466–70.
119. Wadsworth T Prematrue epiphyseal fusion after injury of the capitellum. *J Bone Joint Surg* 1964; **46B:** 46–9.
120. Rutherford A fractures of the lateral humeral condyle in children. *J Bone Joint Surg* 1985; **67A:** 851–6.
121. DeLee J *et al.* Fracture separation of the distal humeral epiphysis. *J Bone Joint Surg* 1980; **62A:** 46–51.

CHAPTER 9

Fractures of the proximal ulna and radius in children

MATTHEW EVANS, H KERR GRAHAM

Introduction

In children, fractures of the proximal radius and ulna are much less common than injuries to the distal radius and ulna. They make up between 5% and 8% of paediatric elbow fractures in most series.[1-4] This relative rarity means that few surgeons have extensive experience in management and may feel less than confident when confronted with one of the more unusual combination of injuries affecting this area. However, most injuries managed by simple closed means, heal rapidly and have a good prognosis. A few more severe isolated injuries, segmental fractures or fracture dislocation combinations are more difficult to manage and have a less predictable outcome. The growth centres of the proximal radius and ulna contribute only about 20% to the longitudinal growth of the forearm bones.[5] The more active centres near the wrist contribute the remainder. Consequently remodelling is slower and less complete in the proximal radius and ulna than in the distal radius and ulna, with obvious implications for fracture management.

CLASSIFICATION

Proximal radius and ulna fractures can be classified as shown in Table 9.1.

Table 9.1 Classification of proximal radius and ulna fractures

1. Fractures of the proximal ulna
    Epiphyseal (apophyseal) and physeal injuries
    Metaphyseal (olecranon) fractures
    Fractures of the coronoid process
    Pathological fractures – mainly osteogenesis
      imperfecta
2. Injuries affecting the proximal radius
    Radial head fractures
    Radial neck fractures
    Dislocations of the radial head, the Monteggia lesion
3. Fractures of the proximal radius and/or ulna, in
      association with ipsilateral elbow fractures.
4. Fractures of the proximal radius and/or ulna, in
      association with ipsilateral forearm fractures

GROWTH AND DEVELOPMENT

At birth, the olecranon apophysis extends distally in the semilunar notch and is perpendicular to the long axis of the ulna. With growth it migrates proximally and lies more obliquely (Fig. 9.1a,b,c). The primary ossification centre appears at 9 years and fuses at 15 years.[2] The disc-shaped radial head is entirely cartilaginous at birth, the ossification centre appears at 5 years and fuses at about 15 years (Fig. 9.1d,e,f). Throughout most of childhood the thick cartilage cushions the radial head against injury. The metaphyseal 'beak' seen on an x-ray of the immature elbow may be misdiagnosed as a fracture when 10–15 degrees of angulation of the proximal metaphysis to the diaphysis is normal (Fig. 9.1d).

The blood supply of the radial head epiphysis is via small retinacular vessels which are entirely subperiosteal. These are vulnerable in completely displaced fractures when the radial head is dislocated from the annular ligament. By contrast, there is a rich network of vessels supplying the proximal ulna from both sides of the apophysis. Traumatic avascular necrosis is unknown.

BIOMECHANICS AND PATHOMECHANICS

The elbow joint in children is highly congruent with no tolerance for intra-articular deformity without loss of motion in the flexion–extension plane. In addition, the unique nature of the proximal radioulnar joint allows for no displacement of the centre of rotation without producing a rotating cam effect and consequent loss of forearm rotation.[6] Under normal circumstances the proximal radioulnar joint fulfils exacting requirements of close to 180 degrees of rotation combined with stability. Loss of motion and instability are frequent clinical problems as seen in post-traumatic stiffness and the prevalence of instability problems such as the Monteggia lesion and 'pulled elbow'.

The proximal radius and ulna are vulnerable to indirect injury as the result of a fall on the outstretched hand. The multiplicity of fracture patterns reflect the variety of positions in which the outstretched hand may be placed when breaking a fall. Therefore valgus-extension injuries greatly outnumber varus-flexion injuries. Direct violence injuries result from a backward fall onto the point of the flexed elbow or from a direct blow in sporting activity.[1–3] They are much less common than indirect violence injuries and dogmatic classifications of fracture patterns based on conjectured direct violence injury are questionable. Few parents or children can give a detailed account of how these injuries occur. Even when the injury happens in full view of a watchful parent, the accident is quickly over and parents are more concerned with the consequences than the cause. Another pattern of injury is chronic repetitive stress, encountered in juvenile athletics and certain throwing sports. There is often a single line of failure through the proximal radius and ulna or distal humerus and ulna. This gives an excellent guide as to the direction of the deforming force with obvious implications as to the direction of forces to be applied in a closed reduction manoeuvre. Looking for the 'single line of failure' should alert the surgeon to associated injuries and help in management (Figs 9.2, 9.3).

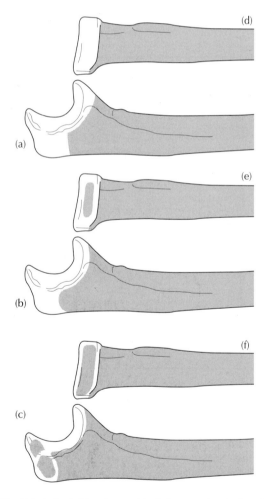

Fig. 9.1 (a,b,c) Development of the proximal ulna from infancy to late childhood. Note the proximal migration of the metaphysis and multcentric apophyseal ossification. (d,e,f,) Development of the proximal radius from infancy to late childhood. Note the cartilaginous radial head, gradually replaced by bone.

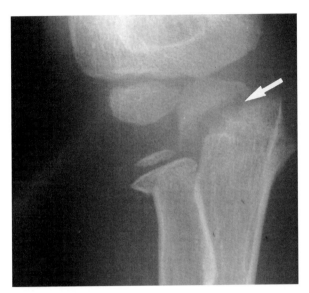

Fig. 9.2 Probable valgus extension elbow injury with angulated metaphyseal radial neck fracture and oblique olecranon fracture showing a 'single line of failure'.

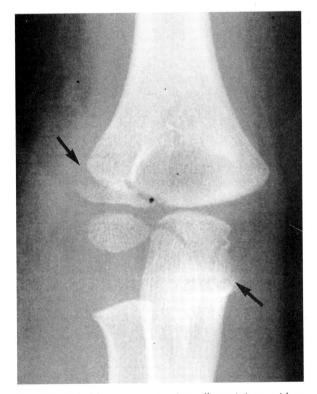

Fig. 9.3 Probable varus extension elbow injury with a fracture separation of the lateral condylar physis and greenstick olecranon fracture. Note the 'single line of failure' a guide to the forces producing the injury and the direction in which reduction forces should be applied.

EPIDEMIOLOGY

In general, elbow injuries are more common in boys than in girls, affect the dominant side more than the non-dominant and each injury has a characteristic age distribution. In countries of northern and southern latitudes with marked seasonal changes in daylight and temperature elbow fractures in children are more frequent in summer than in winter. The series of radial neck fractures which we have previously reported follows this general pattern although those described by others do not.[1,7,8]

CLINICAL FEATURES

The history is usually of a child aged 4–12 years who sustains a fall on the outstretched hand and complains of elbow pain and loss of function. Fractures of the proximal radius and ulna are usually less striking in presentation than for example a displaced supracondylar fracture. Incomplete, greenstick fractures may present with subtle physical signs and relatively well preserved function. Careful assessment of the range of forearm rotation is particularly important. In late presenting cases swelling and bruising may guide as to the site of injury. The Monteggia lesion in younger children is often missed because the ulna fracture is a minor greenstick injury or associated with plastic bowing. Unless the radial head dislocation is considered and sought on x-ray the diagnosis may be delayed.

Fractures of the proximal radius and ulna are rarely complicated by neurovascular compromise.[4,8–13] Traction injury to the radial or posterior interosseous nerves may be seen in up to 10% of Monteggia lesions and less frequently with radial neck fractures.[6,7,9,12] Ulnar nerve palsy is occasionally seen with olecranon fractures.[1] Other nerve lesions may result from the effects of secondary swelling or the pressure from a cast. Compartment syndrome is more likely to be the result of swelling within an unyielding cast than as the direct result of the injury. The dangers of complete casts around a swollen elbow are well recognised but not always avoided. Volkmann's ischaemia has been reported after immobilisation of an undisplaced olecranon fracture in a complete cast.[11]

RADIOLOGY

Good quality anteroposterior and lateral radiographs remain the mainstay of diagnosis in paediatric elbow fractures. These are not always easily obtained in the Emergency Room with an apprehensive child; preliminary (translucent) splintage

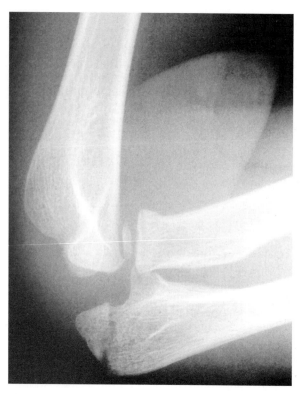

Fig. 9.4 The oblique or coronoid view of the proximal ulna. The olecranon fracture is clearly seen and the radial head is almost clear of the coronoid.

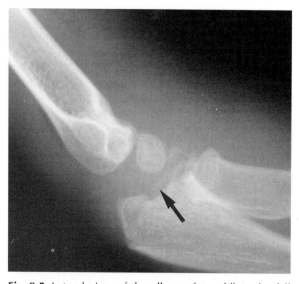

Fig. 9.5 Lateral view of the elbow of a toddler who fell on his outstretched hand. There is a slightly displaced fracture of the olecranon extending along the joint as far as the coronoid. Is the position acceptable? What is the status of the articular surface?

and analgesia may be required. The lateral oblique (coronoid) view can be helpful to separate the normal overlap of radial head and olecranon and is also useful to diagnose or assess displacement in lateral condylar physeal injuries (Fig. 9.4). Comparison views of the uninjured side should not be requested routinely but can on occasions be very helpful to the most experienced surgeons. Special investigations include arthrography, computed tomography and magnetic resonance imaging. Only arthrography is useful in the acute situation. A small amount of water soluble contrast injected into the child's elbow at the time of operative management (under general anaesthesia and using fluoroscopy) can give invaluable information relevant to management (Figs 9.5, 9.6, 9.7).

MANAGEMENT

As with all children's fractures, the majority of fractures affecting the proximal radius and ulna are managed conservatively. The options include:

1. No treatment required, apart from reassurance and analgesia.
2. Simple immobilisation in a backslab or collar and cuff. This gives pain relief and should rarely be continued for longer than 3 weeks.
3. Closed reduction and cast immobilisation.
4. Percutaneous reduction.
5. Closed reduction and percutaneous fixation.
6. Open reduction and internal fixation.

Fractures of the proximal ulna

APOPHYSEAL INJURIES

Apophyseal injuries are rare. Multicentric or irregular ossification may be confused with fracture and can sometimes be recognised by comparison views.[2,14] Some injuries are incomplete, undisplaced and stable. These can be managed by a short period of immobilisation.

Examination under fluoroscopy will demonstrate incongruity or instability, when present, and the need for reduction and fixation. Some injuries will be more stable and congruous in extension. Extension casts are awkward and the child's elbow should not be immobilised in extension for more than 3 weeks. Few displaced injuries reduce fully in extension and this method of treatment should not be accepted without careful scrutiny of the radiographs to ensure that a complete reduction has

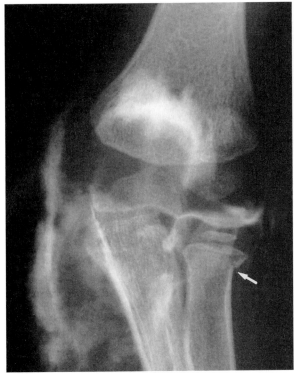

Fig. 9.6

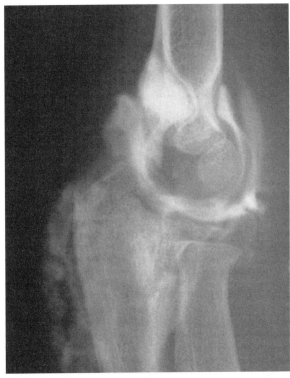

Fig. 9.7

Figs 9.6 and 9.7 Contrast arthrography demonstrates the integrity of the articular cartilage in anteroposterior and lateral projections. The elbow was screened fluoroscopically and satisfactory stability and congruence was demonstrated in both flexion and extension. We refer to this procedure as 'dynamic elbow arthrography'. In the anteroposterior arthrogram note the radial neck fracture and the small ossification centre in the radial head surrounded by thick articular and physeal cartilage. This is why children suffer radial neck fractures much more frequently than radial head fractures. The injury was managed conservatively with a good result.

been achieved. The early penalty for malunion is stiffness and later, the possibility of degenerative changes (Figs 9.8, 9.9).

Open reduction is accomplished via a posterior approach, limiting periosteal stripping to a minimum. The periosteum is densely adherent to the apophysis and over vigorous mobilisation may affect the blood supply and growth. Using limited exposure, it is wise to check the reduction intraoperatively by radiological means.

The fixation technique of choice is tension band-suture. This consists of two longitudinally orientated Kirschner wires with a tension band loop of No. 1 polydioxanone suture, which is slowly absorbed over a few months. Hardware removal is simplified to a stab incision to recover the Kirschner wires instead of a tedious dissection through callus and under periosteum for the wire loop – the difference between an office/local anaesthetic/day case procedure and something much more extensive.

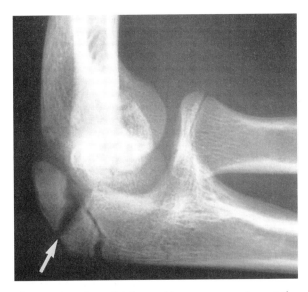

Fig. 9.8 Apophyseal injury with some separation at the joint surface.

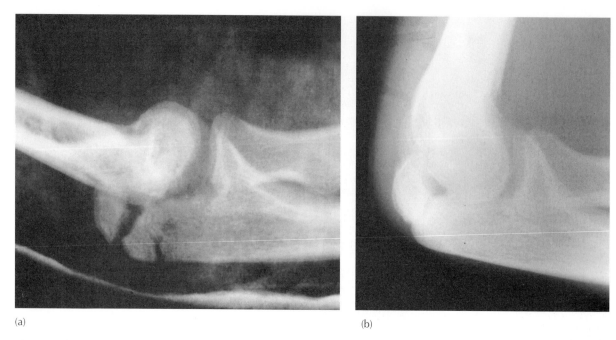

(a)

(b)

Fig. 9.9 This injury was treated conservatively in extension (a) but it did not reduce and healed with displacement (b). Loss of motion was minimal but incongruity may predispose to arthrosis in later life. Open reduction would have been a better option.

The tension band suture and longitudinal Kirschner wires do not seem to disturb growth, which is mostly appositional.

Screw fixation should be reserved for adolescents when the risk of growth disturbance is minimal.

OLECRANON FRACTURES

There are two main types of metaphyseal olecranon fractures in children, the juxtaphyseal or sleeve fracture and the metaphyseal fracture proper (Fig. 9.10). Both injury patterns are characterised by associated ipsilateral elbow injuries in at least 50% of cases.[4] Paradoxically the associated injury is often more difficult to diagnose but is more likely to require operative intervention and may be the determining factor in prognosis. Complex segmental forearm fractures may be accompanied by olecranon and/or proximal radial fractures. Pathological olecranon fractures in children are frequently seen in children with type 1 osteogenesis imperfecta.

Olecranon fractures may be further classified according to fracture configuration and the degree of displacement. Classification by the mechanism of injury must be questionable because x-rays alone are inadequate and the history may not be helpful. The fracture configuration is usually transverse and usually much less comminuted than adult pattern olecranon fractures. The cartilaginous apophysis

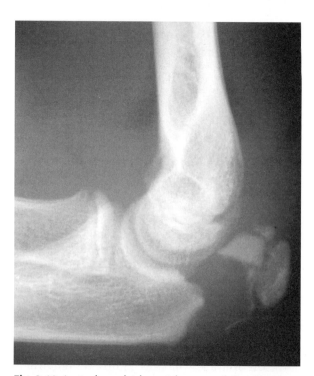

Fig. 9.10 Juxtaphyseal 'sleeve' fracture of the olecranon with an extension along both the articular surface and posterior aspects of the elbow. With this displacement (Group C) of the articular surface and disruption of the extensor mechanism open reduction and fixation with a tension band suture was used.

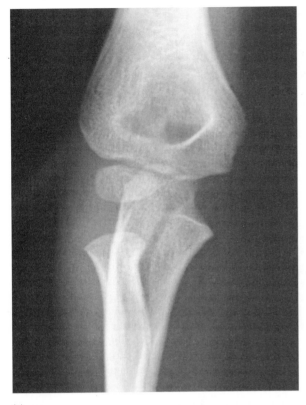

(a)

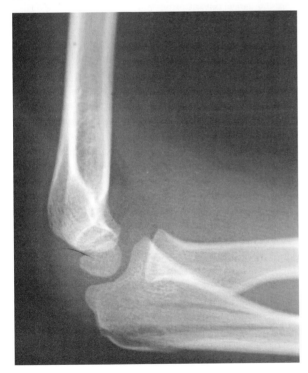

(b)

Fig. 9.11 (a,b) Longitudinal split fracture of the olecranon with Group A displacement, managed conservatively.

and dense periosteum seem to be protective. Oblique and longitudinal fracture patterns are also common[4,11,15] (Figs 9.11a,b). Grading of fracture displacement as a guide to management has received considerable prominence in the literature.[1,4,10] However, it is illogical to suggest a single cut-off point to determine which fractures require open versus closed management. Articular involvement, age and associated injuries are also important factors. When the joint surface is involved it is important to distinguish between a step in the articular surface and separation of the articular surface. Intuitively it would be expected that separation of 3 mm would carry a different prognosis than a step of 3 mm.

Stability may be as important as displacement and can be assessed by fluoroscopic examination.

We therefore consider fracture displacement in three groups which gives a practical guide as to management.

FRACTURE DISPLACEMENT AT THE ARTICULAR SURFACE

Group A: <2 mm conservative management;
Group B: 2–4 mm displacement 'grey zone';
Group C: >4 mm displacement – closed treatment unlikely to be successful, open reduction preferred for the majority.

If the articular surface is not involved the determining factor is the integrity of the extensor mechanism. This may also need to be tested by fluoroscopic examination to supplement clinical findings. Static x-ray films may not be adequate.

Fractures which occur close to the physeal line may extend along the articular/growth plate cartilage and on the extensor aspect of the olecranon, analogous to the sleeve fracture of the patella. Articular involvement may be underestimated on plain films and more information can be gained by arthrography or inspection at open operation.

MANAGEMENT

Group A

The majority of olecranon fractures in children are undisplaced or minimally displaced and stable. These are easily managed conservatively by immobilisation in a long arm plaster slab for 3 weeks. In children stiffness is not a risk and a backslab is safe in the presence of swelling. The long arm plaster slab gives better pain relief than a collar and cuff or triangular sling (Figs 9.2, 9.3).

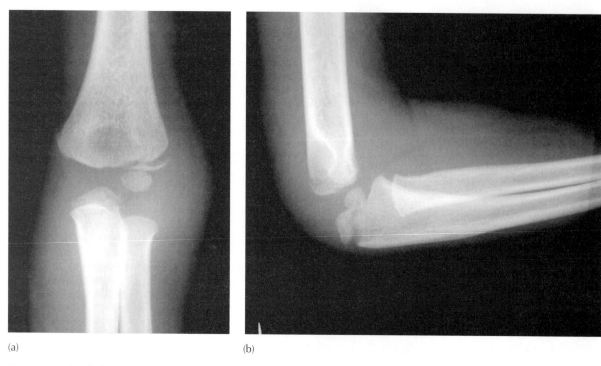

(a)   (b)

Fig. 9.12 (a,b) Slightly displaced fractures of the lateral condylar physis and olecranon – a common combination. Can this combination be managed conservatively? What position should be used in plaster?

Group B

These fractures constitute the second largest group and are a 'grey zone'. A careful examination under anaesthesia with fluroscopic screening to determine congruency and stability may be necessary. Some can be managed closed, usually in extension. Occasionally closed reduction is possible but the reduction in unstable and percutaneous Kirschner wire fixation is indicated. Some Group B fractures will require open reduction and fixation (Figs 9.12a, b; 9.13, 9.14).

Group C

Very displaced and unstable fractures require open reduction and internal fixation (20% of total). The fixation constructs include:

1. Kirschner wires alone.
2. Tension band suture.
3. Tension band wire.
4. Screw fixation, with a tension band suture or wire (Fig. 9.15).

These constructs are listed in increasing order of stability. Kirschner wires alone are unstable and have no place in current management, except for stabilisation after closed reduction of a minimally

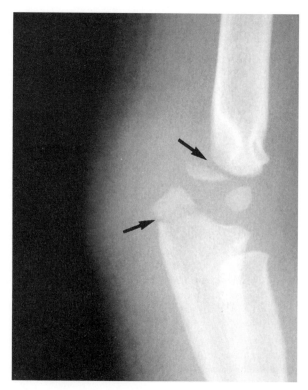

Fig. 9.13 Many advise extension for these types of olecranon fractures but in this case the extended position results in displacement of the lateral condylar fracture.

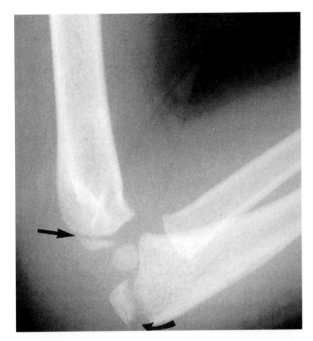

Fig. 9.14 In flexion the lateral condyle is reduced but the olecranon fracture is displaced with a 'step' in the articular surface. With the elbow flexed the lateral condyle was fixed with percutaneous Kirschner wires. The elbow was then extended and the olecranon was also fixed with percutaneous Kirschner wires. A backslab was used with the elbow at 90 degrees of flexion for 4 weeks. More than one fracture is a relative indication for fixation of one or both fractures.

displaced fracture (Fig. 9.16a). Selection is made according to age and fracture stability. Younger children usually have a simple separation of the fracture which can be managed by a tension band suture technique (Fig. 9.16b). In this age group early mobilisation is neither desirable nor necessary. Adolescents and children with osteogenesis imperfecta are more appropriately managed by tension band wiring or screw/tension band wire fixation,which is the most stable construct[17] (Figs 9.16c,d).

Although kangaroo tendon has been used in the past for the repair of olecranon fractures, it is no longer popular, even in Australia.[18]

Ipsilateral elbow fractures most commonly associated with olecranon fractures are fractures of the radial neck, lateral condyle, medial epicondyle and radial head dislocation (Figs 9.2, 9.3). However, olecranon fractures may be associated with any other fracture variants and the radiographs must be scrutinised carefully in all cases. There are also serious segmental forearm fracture patterns in which widely displaced distal fractures may detract

(a) Pins and suture

(b) Pins and wire

(c) Screw only

(d) Screw only and wire

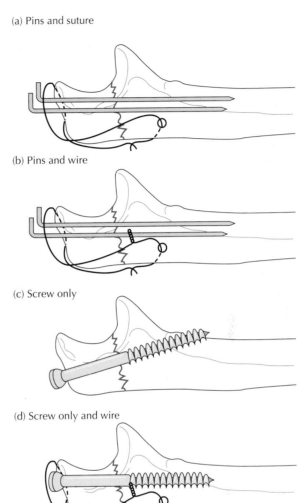

Fig. 9.15 (a,b,c,d) Fixation constructs for paediatric olecranon fractures. (a) Tension band suture is ideal for most olecranon fractures, offering sufficient stability and ease of hardware removal. (b) Standard tension band wiring is better for older children, very unstable fractures and pathological fractures e.g. osteogenesis imperfecta. (c) Bicortical screw fixation may not require removal but may affect apophyseal growth and should therefore be used only in older children. (d) Tension band wire with an intramedullary screw is probably the most stable construct but should only be used in adolescents.

attention from an apparently innocuous olecranon fracture. The olecranon fracture may be the only intra-articular fracture, the only one requiring open reduction and the only one with an uncertain prognosis (Figs 9.17a,b,c). In general multiple upper limb fractures, in association with olecranon fractures, should be treated by open or closed reduction and Kirschner wire fixation (Figs 9.18a,b).

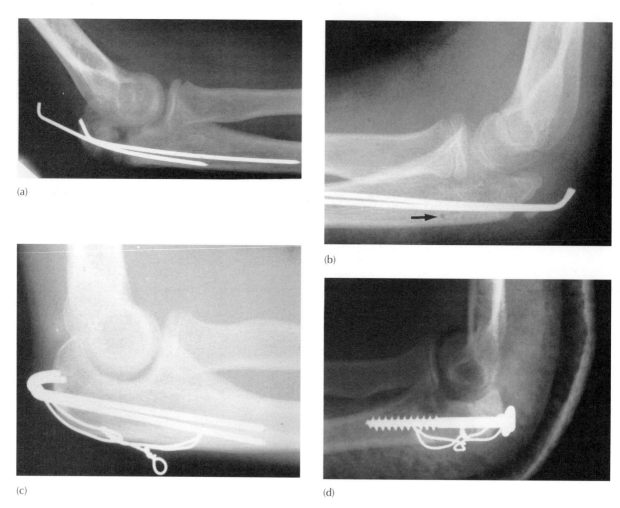

Fig. 9.16 (a) Longitudinal Kirschner wires are unstable and should not be used alone. A tension band suture or wire should be added. (b) Tension band suture. Note the drill hole for the suture which is placed in the same manner as the standard tension band wire construct. It is easier to tighten than wire, offers sufficient stability for most fractures if plaster fixation is used and only the Kirschner wires need to be removed. (c) The most frequent problem with tension band wire is skin irritation over prominent wire loops. (d) The most stable construct is a screw and wire loop but this is not advised except in adolescents.

OUTCOME

The majority of olecranon fractures in children heal rapidly, in good position with full return of function. Significant loss of motion is unusual when the elbow has not been immobilised for more than 3 weeks. The majority of isolated Group A and B injuries, managed conservatively will recover a full range of elbow motion. In Group C injuries, managed by open reduction and fixation, 20 degrees or more loss of motion is common.

The exception to this favourable scenario is in children with osteogensesis imperfecta where failure of fixation and revision surgery is not uncommon. Hence we recommend more robust primary fixation of these injuries.

Disabling stiffness is rare, the exception being as the result of radioulnar synostosis. The posterior approach incision often results in a wide, keloid scar in children. Meticulous subcuticular closure is mandatory.

Poor results are more frequently the result of associated injuries.

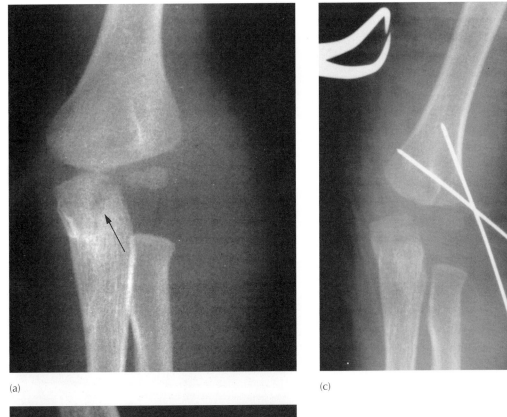

(a)

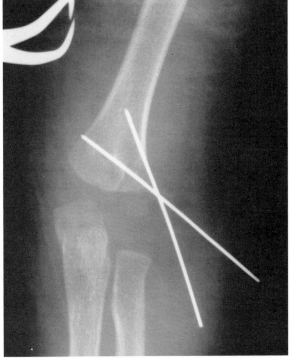

(c)

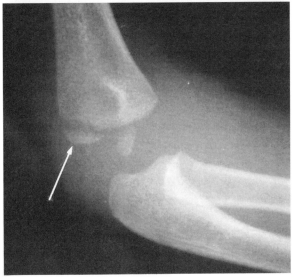

(b)

Fig. 9.17 (a) Greenstick olecranon fracture in a very young child – could be managed conservatively. (b) The oblique view shows a minimally displaced lateral condylar fracture. (c) Managed by percutaneous Kirschner wire fixation. At least 50% of paediatric olecranon fractures are accompanied by ipsilateral elbow fractures. These must be evaluated carefully and some will require operative management.

COMPLICATIONS

The most common complication is failure to recognise and adequately treat an accompanying injury. Minimally displaced, conservatively managed fractures usually heal rapidly with restoration of full range of motion and full function.[4,10,11,15,16] Operatively managed fractures are by definition more severe and problems with hardware over the subcutaneous ulna is a frequent problem, solved by

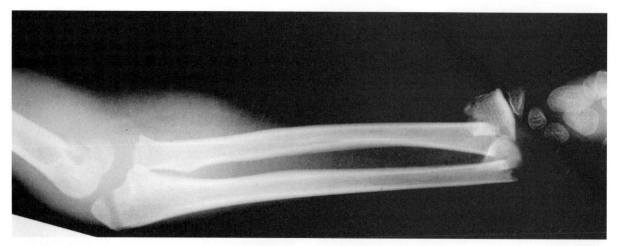

(a)

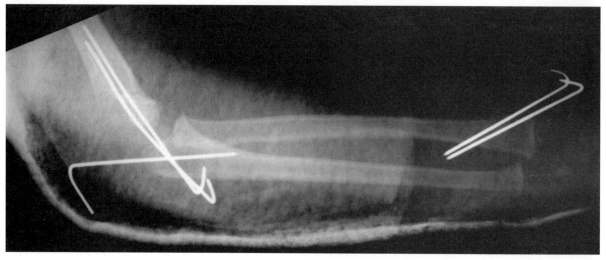

(a)

Fig. 9.18 (a,b) Multiple upper limb fractures including completely displaced metaphyseal distal radius and ulna fractures, displaced and unstable olecranon fracture and minimally displaced lateral condylar physeal injury. All were managed by closed reduction and percutaneous Kirschner wire fixation.

hardware removal. We have seen failure of fixation and the need for revision surgery only in children with osteogenesis imperfecta.

Proximal radioulnar synostosis is a rare but serious complication which usually follows severe injuries to both radius and ulna requiring open management of both fractures. However, it may be seen after apparently trivial injuries managed by closed treatment.[1,4,7]

Persistent stiffness, usually loss of terminal extension, is common but not usually severe or disabling. Stiffness can be minimised by appropriate manage-

ment of associated injuries and limiting immobilisation to 3 weeks.

CORONOID FRACTURES

Coronoid fractures are rare in children and it is exceptional for them to require open reduction or fixation. In the very young they may pose diagnostic dilemmas. Coronoid fractures may co-exist with sleeve fractures which involve the articular surface of the olecranon. When doubt exists as to the degree of displacement of the articular surface and hence the need for open reduction, arthrography can be very helpful (Figs 9.5, 9.6, 9.7).

Fractures of the proximal radius

In younger children the radial head is largely or entirely cartilaginous, well able to withstand forces in compression and angulation resulting from falls on the outstretched hand. Hence fractures affect the metaphysis and proximal growth plate much more frequently than the radial head. This is the reverse of the adult pattern.[1,4,7]

Controversy exists regarding many aspects of proximal radial fractures in children, including classification and management. In recent years two new methods of management have been described and are gaining in popularity. These are closed intramedullary pinning (CIMP) and reduction by percutaneous Kirschner wire leverage (PKWL). From these recent advances it is possible to construct a management algorithm (see Table 9.3).

CLASSIFICATION

Fractures of the proximal radius are most logically classified according to anatomical site and displacement.

In the growing child the anatomical classification is straightforward – metaphyseal injuries and the Salter–Harris classification for growth plate injuries. In our published series, metaphyseal injuries predominated, closely followed by Salter–Harris types I and II.[7] Types III and IV fractures, i.e. involving the radial head are quite rare[1,4,7] and were not seen in our series. Salter–Harris type V may not exist as a primary injury in this anatomical site but types I and II injuries are often associated with premature closure of the proximal radial growth plate and mild cubitus valgus.

RADIAL HEAD–NECK FRACTURES

1. Metaphyseal
2. Salter–Harris I–V (types I and II predominate)
3. Fracture dislocation
4. Monteggia lesions

FRACTURE DISPLACEMENT

As with fractures of the proximal ulna, approximately 50% of radial neck fractures are associated with other injuries, including fractures of the olecranon, medial epicondyle, lateral condyle, supracondylar fractures and complex segmental forearm fractures.[4,7] The associated injuries may be the determining factor in prognosis and dictate management.

Isolated radial head and neck fractures are first classified according to their anatomical site and secondarily according to displacement. Metaphyseal fractures and Salter–Harris types I and II injuries comprise more than 95% of the total and are managed along similar lines.[4,6,7,9] Steele and Graham introduced a practical classification according to angulation and displacement which serves as a guide to management.[7] This classification is similar to that described by Metaizeau but is preferred because it includes both angulation and displacement of the fracture.[19] A radial head fracture which unites with displacement will result in restricted forearm rotation because of the rotating 'cam' effect even in the absence of angular malunion.[6] Displacement is therefore more important than angulation and must be considered in grading these fractures. Grading displacement in percentage terms of the diameter of the radial metaphysis builds in an automatic correction for age/size and is preferred to expressing displacement in millimetres. It should be noted that the radial shaft is sometimes displaced or translocated in relation to the displaced head and neck of the radius and capitellum. Such translocation must be recognised and is easily reduced by closed manipulation or by PKWL.

Table 9.2

Grade	Displacement (%)	Angulation (degrees)	Management	Prognosis
I:	0–10	0–30	Symptomatic	Excellent
II:	11–50	31–60	Closed reduction/PKWL	Good
III:	51–90	61–90	PKWL, rarely CIMP	Good/fair
IV:	>90	>90	open replacement	Uncertain/poor

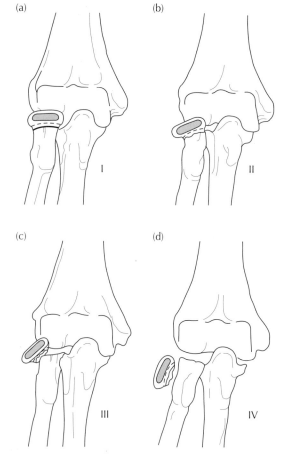

Fig. 9.19 Classification of paediatric radial neck fractures by Steele and Graham. This can be applied to metaphyseal fractures and Salter–Harris type I and II injuries which comprise 95% of the total. Redrawn with permission from *Journal of Bone and Joint Surgery*.

MANAGEMENT

Regarding the outcome of displaced radial head and neck fractures in children, Rang observes 'The imperfect results were much more common in the operated cases than in the conservatively treated cases. . . .' The lesson to be learned is that you should not give up closed reduction until you have tried every trick you know.[3] Most authorities agree with this conservative approach to open reduction.[1,2,6] Fortunately there are some 'new tricks' to aid closed reduction.

- Grade I fractures are managed symptomatically.
- Grade II fractures are usually managed by closed reduction but some will require PKWL for failed closed reduction.

- Grade III fractures will usually require PKWL but a few will reduce fully by closed manipulation; CIMP is an alternative for reducible but unstable injuries.
- Grade IV injuries are usually caused by dislocation of the elbow and are managed by open replacement, sometimes including annular ligament repair and occasionally including Kirschner wire fixation.

The technique of closed reduction has been well described and illustrated by previous authors.[1-4] The outcome of closed reduction is unpredictable. The fracture may be fully reduced, incompletely reduced, or the position may remain unchanged. If the fracture is incompletely reduced the precise displacement/angulation should be noted, the range of forearm rotation checked and a decision reached as to whether the position should be accepted or an alternative management strategy employed.

Closed intramedullary pinning is one of a number of elegant intramedullary fixation techniques described in the French paediatric orthopaedic literature[19,20] and more recently in English[19,20] (Fig. 9.20). A pin of 1.2–2.00 mm diameter is inserted into the medullary canal via the distal radial metaphysis and the displaced radial neck is manipulated back into position by a rotational movement. It has been described as a method of reduction and fixation in the management of more severely displaced radial neck fractures. However, it is an unnecessarily complex and invasive technique for most radial neck fractures. Crossing an open physis with a pin which then circumscribes a circular motion during the manipulation procedure must carry a risk of growth disturbance. Direct reduction by closed manipulation or by PKWL is simpler and just as effective. We have demonstrated that PKWL is an effective method of reduction for the majority of radial neck fractures which are not dislocated outside the annular ligament. Furthermore, fixation is not required for the majority of these injuries, because the risk of losing position after reduction is negligible. The only scenario in which CIMP offers an advantage over PKWL is a reducible but unstable fracture. The majority of fractures which are reducible are also stable. Unstable reductions are usually incomplete and require open reductions. It is of note that those who use CIMP reserve PKWL as an ancillary means of reduction for their more difficult cases.[19,20] It would seem more logical to use PKWL after failed closed reduction and thereby avoid the need for retained hardware.

Percutaneous Kirschner wire leverage (PKWL) is an old technique,[21] undergoing something of a renaissance in terms of interest and published reports.[7,22,23] It is applicable for the majority of displaced radial

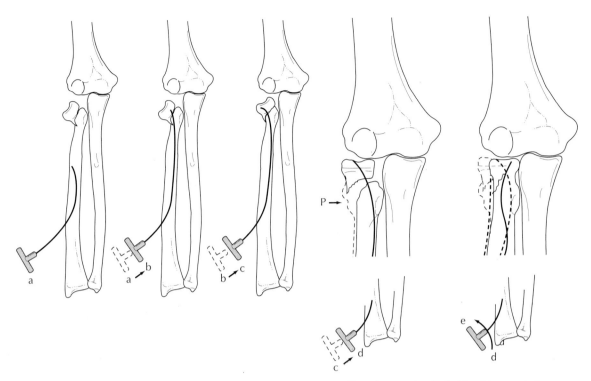

Fig. 9.20 Closed intramedullary pinning as described by Metaizeau.[19] Redrawn after Ref. 19 with permission.

neck fractures when closed reduction has failed and there is some remaining contact between the radial head and neck, no matter how tenuous.

After failure of closed reduction the range of forearm rotation is recorded and the elbow is screened fluoroscopically to ascertain the position of forearm rotation in which the angulation/displacement is maximal. This probably corresponds to the position of rotation at the time of injury. A long smooth Kirschner wire or Steinman pin (1.2–1.8 mm) is used in a T-handled chuck. The diameter of the wire is chosen according to the age of the patient and size of the elbow. Using a flimsy wire runs the risk of breaking a wire within the joint, necessitating an arthrotomy for removal. A long wire and good chuck keeps the operator's hand out of the x-ray field (Figs 9.21a,b,c).

Others have used a purpose-designed two-pronged instruments or 'bident'[24] but we find a single wire perfectly satisfactory.[7]

The point of the Kirschner wire is inserted into the fracture under fluoroscopic control from an anterolateral approach, taking care to stay proximal and avoid the posterior interosseous nerve. The point of the instrument is advanced across the fracture as far as the far cortex and the fracture is reduced by a cephalad sweep of the operator's hand, levering the radial head and neck against the

capitellum. Overreduction is impossible and redisplacement is rare because there is usually enough annular ligament intact to retain the radial head in the reduced position. The range of forearm rotation is reassessed and is usually dramatically improved by the reduction. The stability of reduction is also checked by fluoroscopic screening of the proximal radius during a full range of forearm rotation. In the unlikely event of the fracture being reducible but unstable, stability can be achieved by CIMP or percutaneous Kirschner wire fixation of the radial head to the proximal ulna. Instability is almost always because of inadequate reduction – if the fluoroscopic record is inadequate obtain formal radiographs. Transcapitellar fixation of a malreduced fracture will always give a poor result.

After PKWL the elbow is immobilised for 3 weeks in an above-elbow backslab plaster with the forearm in neutral rotation and the elbow flexed to 90 degrees. At 3 weeks new radiographs are obtained out of plaster and a gentle active range of motion exercises are commenced, no matter what the x-rays show.

The management of the grade IV completely displaced or dislocated fracture is controversial. These injuries are usually the result of dislocation of the elbow; the radial head is knocked off anteriorly during the dislocation or posteriorly during the

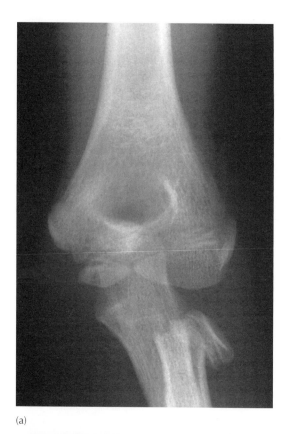

(a)

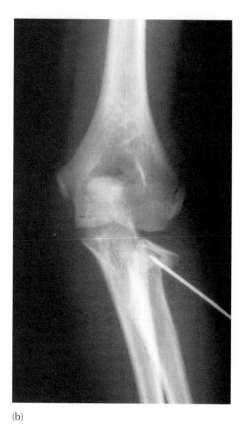

(b)

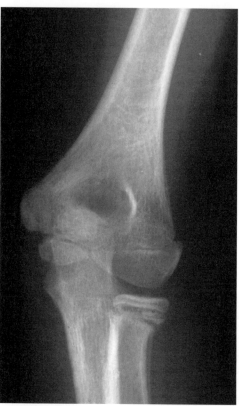

(c)

Fig. 9.21 Percutaneous Kirschner wire leverage (PKWL) for radial neck fractures in children. (a) Grade III fracture, 70 degrees of angulation and 70% displaced. (b) Intraoperative percutaneous wire leverage after failed closed reduction. (c) The position at cast removal after 3 weeks.

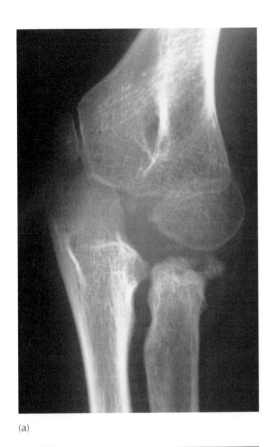

(a)

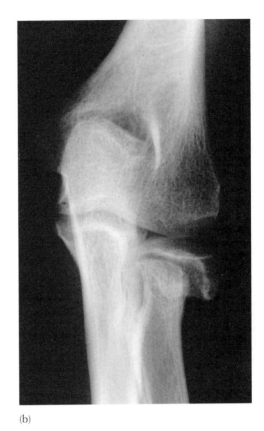

(b)

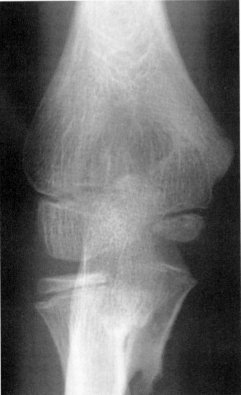

(c)

Fig. 9.22 Complications of grade IV completely displaced radial neck fractures include: (a) avascular necrosis – usually results in pain and stiffness; (b) non-union or in this case a stable fibrous union with a near normal range of motion and no pain; (c) radiounlar synostosis: synostosis is more common after severe injuries to both radius and ulna and after open reduction; it may also be seen after minor injuries managed by closed means.

Table 9.3 Radial neck fractures in children – management algorithm

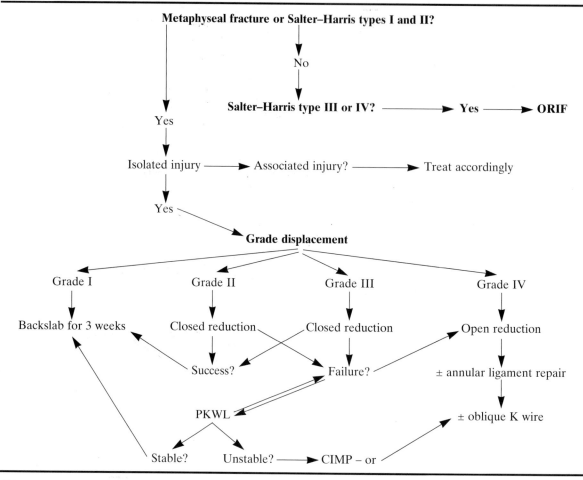

ORIF: open reduction, internal fixation; PKWL: percutaneous Kirschner wire leverage; CIMP: closed intramedullary pinning.

reduction. Occasionally a closed reduction of the dislocation will reduce the radial head and nothing else is required. More often the dislocation reduces easily, leaving the radial head and neck dislocated out of the torn annular ligament.

The numbers in reported series are too small to base definitive statements on management or prognosis. Some facts are reasonably clear. The prognosis is uncertain because the displaced head/neck fragment has lost all or most of its blood supply. Avascular necrosis, non-union, late displacement and malunion are all reported complications (Figs 9.22a,b,c).

Fixation of the fracture results in frequent hardware problems and should be avoided, when possible. It is not possible to retain stable fixation such as a transcapitellar Kirschner wire until revascularisation and union is complete. It is therefore doubtful whether fixation has anything to add in

management and we prefer simple open replacement and repair of the annular ligament. This is followed by 3 weeks of cast immobilisation, 3 weeks in a collar and cuff and then a range of motion exercises, no matter what the x-rays show. There seems little point in adding immobilisation stiffness to an already difficult situation. The least invasive method of fixation is an oblique Kirschner wire; rarely is the metaphyseal fragment large enough to accept a screw (Fig. 9.23a,b).

Transcapitellar wires are liable to fracture and should never be used because there are better alternatives with fewer risks.

PROGNOSIS

Grade I fractures and grade II and III fractures which are managed successfully by closed means

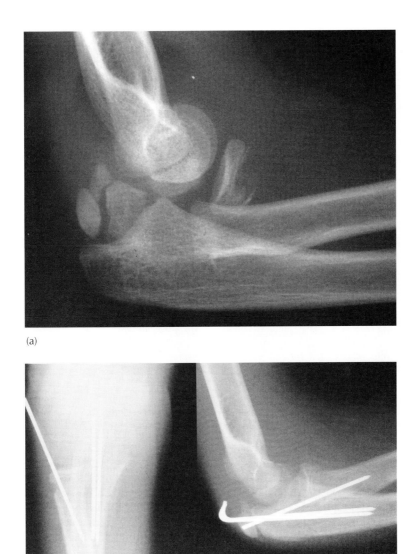

(a)

(a)

Fig. 9.23 (a) Anterior dislocation of the elbow has knocked off the radial head and pulled off the olecranon. (b) The olecranon fracture was managed by open reduction and tension band suture and the radial head by open reduction and oblique Kirshner wire fixation. This wire was easily removed after 3 weeks and is safer than tran-scapitellar wire fixation.

have an excellent prognosis. Proximal radioulnar synostosis is a rare but devasting complication.[1,4,7] Minor degrees of residual displacement and angulation are accepted in preference to open reduction. The intraoperative range of motion is a useful guide as to the acceptability of the reduction. Elbows which have 70% of forearm rotation after closed reduction are likely to regain a full or adequate range of motion with growth and remodelling. As skeletal maturity approaches, the quality of the reduction is more critical. Up to the age of 6 years, 45 degrees of angulation or 20% displacement can

be accepted. Between 7 and 12 years up to 30 degrees of angulation and 10% displacement can be accepted in preference to open reduction. Over the age of 12 years anatomic reduction is preferred (Fig. 9.24a,b).

COMPLICATIONS

The most common complication is failure to diagnose and treat an associated injury. Incomplete reduction or slight loss of position is common but

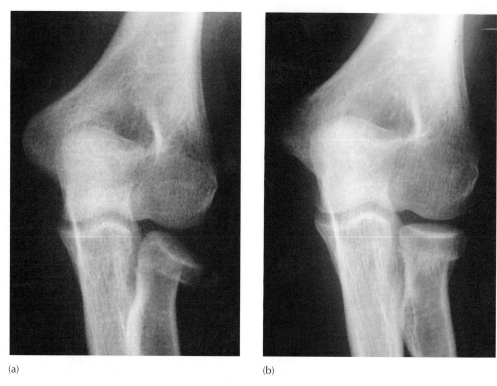

(a)   (b)

Fig. 9.24 In the skeletally mature adolescent anatomic reduction of radial fractures is required because there will be little or no remodelling. In this example reduction was achieved by PKWL.

rarely seems to result in stiffness or long-term problems.[7,9,22-24] The degree of displacement or angulation is sometimes underestimated in the Emergency Room and the patient is not referred for reduction. This is because the direction of angulation varies according to the position of the hand in space in relation to the body when it strikes the ground to break the fall. It is only possible to assess the precise degree of angulation/displacement by intraoperative fluoroscopy. It is not possible to make the fracture look more displaced than it is in reality but some radiological projections will seriously underestimate fracture displacement. Premature closure of the proximal radial physis is common and may result in a mild cubitus valgus. Shortening rarely exceeds 5 mm and proximal migration resulting in wrist symptoms is unknown, so long as the radial head is retained until maturity. Enlargement of the radial head as a result of hyperaemia is also frequent and of little consequence.

It is the completely displaced fracture, requiring open replacement and fixation which has a predictably poor outcome. Avascular necrosis is the result of expulsion of the radial head out of the annular ligament at the time of injury and is not the result of open replacement. It is associated with delayed union and late displacement of the fracture,

resulting in severe stiffness and sometimes pain. Fibrous union can be stable and allow near normal function. In elbows demonstrating these complications, the x-ray appearances do not always correlate with symptoms. Patients should be managed on a symptomatic basis; little can be done to improve the radiological appearances. The temptation to resort to early excision of the radial head should be resisted. It is a better option at skeletal maturity and few children will need this type of salvage surgery.

Monteggia lesion

In children, the Monteggia lesion is much more common than the Galeazzi lesion, the reverse of the adult pattern. Furthermore, the majority of injuries can be managed by closed means whereas the majority of Monteggia fracture-dislocations in adults require open management. The mechanism of injury is usually indirect violence as the result of a fall on the outstretched hand, similar to most other injuries around the elbow. The pathomechanics of the various types of Monteggia lesions are the subject of conjecture, dogma and disagreement in the literature.

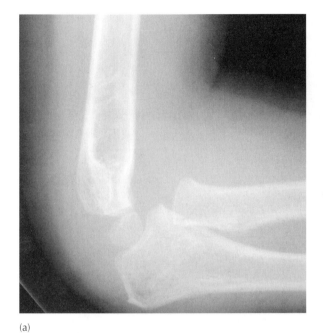
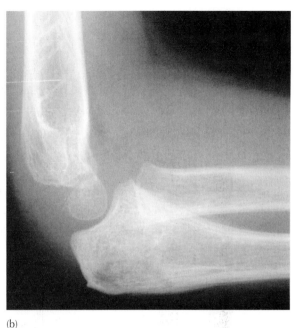

(a)   (b)

Fig. 9.25 A In young children a type I Monteggia lesion with a greenstick olecranon fracture does not present with dramatic physical signs. As an acute injury it is easily managed by closed reduction and immobilisation in flexion and supination. (b) The appearance at 6 weeks, following cast removal.

The Monteggia lesion is easily overlooked and diagnosis may be delayed in up to 20% of children resulting in increased difficulty in management, compromised outcome and litigation.[25] The rules are simple; an isolated displaced fracture of a forearm bone must of necessity be accompanied by a displacement of the proximal or distal radioulnar articulation. The proximal or distal joint must therefore always be x-rayed, not as part of a long view of the whole forearm but by a true lateral view of the wrist or elbow.[1]

CLINICAL FEATURES

The child presents after a fall on the outstretched hand. Soft tissue swelling and an associated deformity may be seen. The clinical picture is more influenced by the ulnar fracture than the radial head dislocation, the signs of which may be subtle. It is not surprising therefore that the most commonly missed Monteggia lesion is a type I injury associated with plastic bowing or a greenstick fracture of the ulna (Fig. 9.25a,b). Neurovascular compromise is uncommon but should be noted. Radiological examination may reveal an apparently isolated fracture of the ulna but the elbow and wrist joints must be carefully examined. A line drawn along the

radial shaft through the radial neck should bisect the capitellum in a true anteroposterior or lateral view and in most – but not all – oblique views.[1]

BADO CLASSIFICATION[26]

Type I: Anterior dislocation of the radial head; fracture of the ulnar diaphysis at any level with anterior angulation.
Type II: Posterior or posterolateral dislocation of the radial head; fracture of the ulnar diaphysis with posterior angulation.
Type III: Lateral or anterolateral dislocation of the radial head; fracture of the ulnar metaphysis.
Type IV: Anterior dislocation of the radial head; fracture of the proximal one-third of the radius and ulna.

Bado's classification, based on an analysis of adult cases, requires modification for children's Monteggia lesions. The direction of radial head displacement is usually compound, for example, anterolateral displacement is most common (Fig. 9.26a,b). Posterior displacement is always posterolateral. The radial head cannot dislocate directly posteriorly; as it dislocates from the radial notch of the ulna, there is always some lateral displacement. The type IV injury is excessively rare and does not

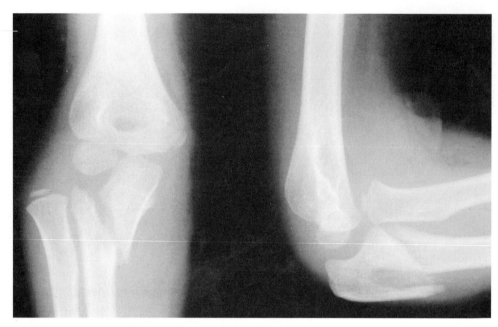

Fig. 9.26 (a,b) Most Monteggia lesions demonstrate displacement in a compound direction, in this case anterolateral.

merit a separate group but should be considered as a Monteggia equivalent. The Monteggia equivalents are common in children and must be given greater prominence but isolated radial neck fracture does not deserve inclusion. 'Pulled elbow' should not be included as a Monteggia equivalent; it is a distinct clinical syndrome. Finally, the direction of displacement of the radial head in respect of the ulna can only be demonstrated with precision by computed tomography examination soon after injury. This is neither necessary nor practical in the management of the majority of Monteggia injuries. Classifications based on retrospective study of two oblique x-rays are less than accurate!

We suggest as an alternative that displacement is considered as a continuum from anterior, through anterolateral, then direct lateral, to posterolateral. When viewed as a continuum in this way it is self-evident that the reduction manoeuvre and position of immobilisation must be individualised and not based on a rigid classification which implies a specific management strategy.

In addition there are a number of Monteggia equivalent lesions, originally described by Bado and clarified amongst others by Olney and Menelaus.[12,26] These include anterior dislocation of the radial head with anterior plastic bowing of the ulna. The majority of 'isolated' radial head dislocations fall into this category and are Bado type I equivalents. An anteriorly angulated fracture of the radial neck (without dislocation) in combination with an anteriorly angulated fracture of the ulna is another type I equivalent. There are similar types II and III equivalents.

The final type I equivalent is anterior dislocation of the radial head in combination with a segmental fracture of the ulna (olecranon and diaphysis).

MANAGEMENT

Monteggia lesions can usually be managed by closed reduction and plaster immobilisation. Good quality anteroposterior and lateral x-rays of the elbow and the forearm fracture are required. When necessary, administer analgesia and apply temporary (radiolucent) splintage before requesting definitive x-rays.

Under general anaesthesia, proceed to clinical and fluoroscopic examination of the injured elbow. The radial head is usually reducible by a combination of direct pressure over the radial head combined with realignment of the ulnar fracture, flexing the elbow and rotating the forearm into supination[12] (Fig. 9.27a,b,c,d). The majority of Monteggia lesions are anterior or anterolateral and are most stable in supination and flexion. A few posterolateral injuries may require extension for a few weeks; in our experience this is rare. Radial heads which are unstable in flexion are usually unstable in extension. Irreducibility or instability after reduction are the result of interposition of soft tissues or dis-

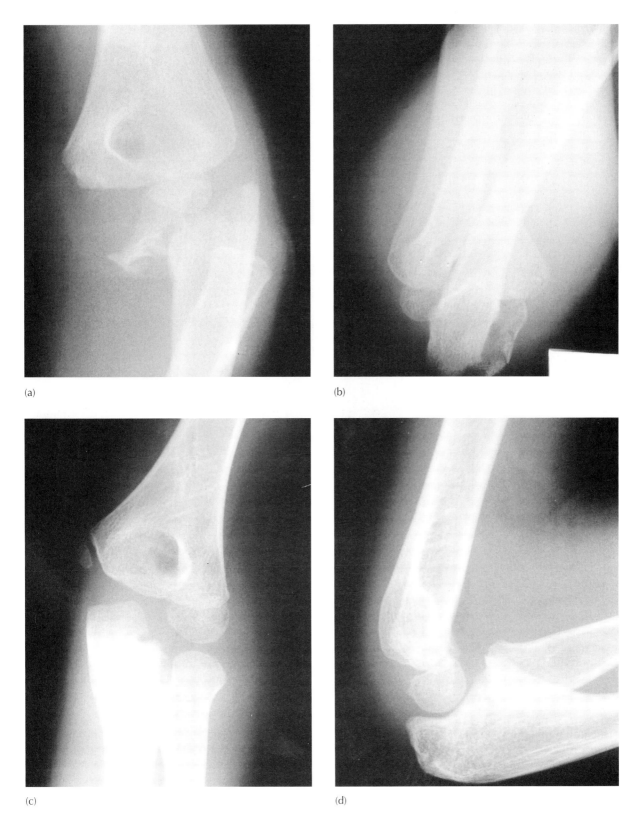

(a)

(b)

(c)

(d)

Fig. 9.27 The majority of Monteggia lesions in children can be managed by closed means. Note the type I Monteggia fracture dislocation (a) The reduction in flexion and supination (b) of both the radial head and olecranon fracture. The appearance at 6 weeks after cast removal (c,d) There is slight residual deformity of the olecranon which will remodel in time.

Fig. 9.28 Severely displaced open type II Monteggia fracture dislocation, combined with displaced fractures of the distal radius and ulna (a,b). The radial head reduced closed but was very unstable because of instability of the ulnar fracture. After debridement the ulnar fracture was reduced and held with a narrow dynamic compression plate (c,d).

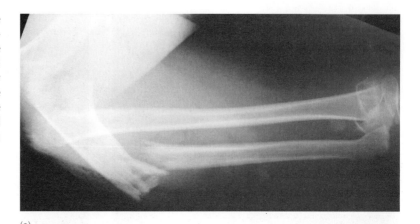

(a)

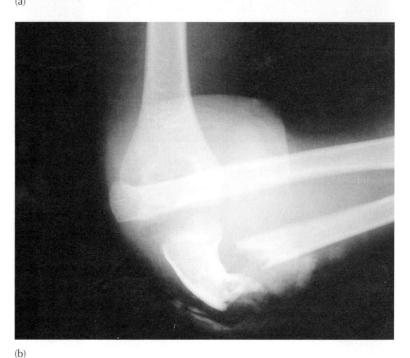

(b)

placement of the ulnar fracture. In acute injuries open reduction of the radial head to remove interposed soft tissue is usually all that is required but additional steps including annular ligament repair or reconstruction, temporary Kirschner wire stabilisation and open reduction of the ulnar fracture (usually combined with internal fixation) may all have a role.[1,2,12,25,27,28]

Fixation of the ulna can be achieved by an intramedullary Kirschner wire or Steinman pin or with plate and screw fixation (Fig. 9.28a,b,c,d). Late displacement is well recognised and dictates a policy of careful follow up with a lateral x-ray of the elbow weekly, for 2 weeks.[1,25] Immobilisation is advised for a total of 6 weeks.

Delay in diagnosis causes delay in management which increases the difficulties in closed management. Up to 3 weeks from injury closed reduction is possible but the reduction is less likely to be stable. Temporary Kirschner wire fixation is indicated if the reduction is complete but unstable. An oblique wire through the radial neck into the proximal ulna is much safer and just as effective as a transcapitellar wire.[13]

Chronic dislocations require careful analysis before management. Many are worth reconstructing using a combination of open reduction, annular ligament repair or reconstruction and ulnar osteotomy.[28] Complications of late reconstruction include neurological and vascular injuries as well as

Fig. 9.28 (*Continued*)

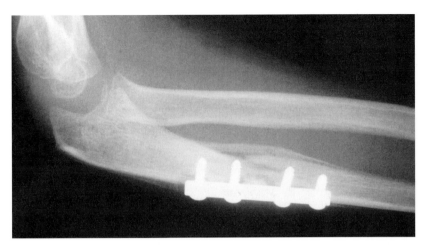

(c)

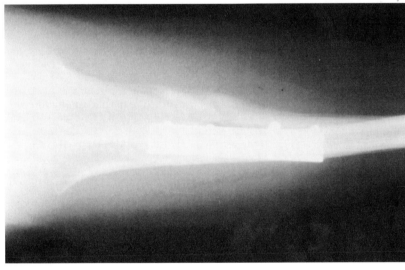

(d)

pain, stiffness and early degenerative changes.[25] Although there are no studies which demonstrate conclusively the superiority of reconstruction over conservative treatment, the results in Melbourne are sufficiently encouraging to favour the former.

The lesson is clear, early diagnosis and prompt closed management is the key to a good result.

COMPLICATIONS

The most common complication is delay in diagnosis and management. The ulnar fracture is open in 5–10% of cases. Nerve injuries occur in 10% of Monteggia lesions and are almost all radial or posterior interosseous nerve palsies.[12] The majority recover quickly and completely. An expectant policy is advised.

Loss of reduction after closed reduction may require subsequent open treatment. Malunion of the ulna may lead to redislocation of the radial head and require osteotomy. Non-union of the ulna and synostosis are rare.

Compartment syndrome and Volkmann's contracture are also rare and are probably caused by swelling within a complete cast.

References

1. Wilkins KE Fractures and dislocations of the elbow region. In: *Fractures in children.* Rockwood CA, Wilkins KE, King RE (eds) Philadelphia: Lippincott, 1991: 509–828.
2. Ogden JA *Radius and ulna in skeletal injury in the child* (2nd edn). Philadelphia: WB Saunders Co, 1990: 451–526.
3. Rang M *Elbow in children's fractures* (2nd edn) Philadelphia: JB Lippincott Co., 1983: 152–96.
4. Dormans JP, Rang M Fractures in the olecranon and radial neck in children in operative management of children's fractures. *Orthop Clin North Am* 1990; **21:** 257–68.
5. Pritchett JW Growth and development of the distal radius and ulna. *J Pediatr Orthop* 1996; **16:** 575–7.
6. Wedge JH, Robertson DE Displaced fractures of the neck of the radius. *J Bone Joint Surg* 1982; **64B:** 256.
7. Steele JA, Graham HK Angulated radial beck fractures in children: A prospective study of percutaneous reduction. *J Bone Joint Surg* 1992; **74B:** 760–4.
8. Newman JH Displaced radial neck fractures in children. *Injury* 1977; **9:** 114–21
9. D'Souza S, Vaishya R, Klenerman L Management of radial neck fracture in children: A retrospective analysis of 100 patients. *J Pediatr Orthop* 1993; **13:** 232–8.
10. Graves S, Canale T Fractures of the olecranon in children: Long-term follow-up. *J Pediatr Orthop* 1993; **1:** 239–41.
11. Matthews JG Fractures of the olecranon in children. *Injury* 1980; **12:** 207–12.
12. Olney BW, Menelaus MB Monteggia and equivalent lesions in childhood. *J Pediatr Orthop* 1989; **9:** 219–23.
13. Letts M, Locht R, Wiens J Monteggia fracture-dislocations in children. *J Bone Joint Surg* 1985; **67B:** 724–7.
14. Silberstein MJ, Brodeur AE, Gravis ER, Luisiri A Some vagaries of the olecranon. *J Bone Joint Surg* 1981; **76A:** 722–5.
15. Newell RLM Olecranon fractures in children. *Injury* 1975; **7:** 33–6.
16. Papavasiliou VA, Beslikas TA, Nenopoulos S Isolated fractures of the olecranon in children. *Injury* 1987; **18:** 100–2.
17. Wainwright D Fractures of the olecranon process. *J Bone Joint Surg* 1941; **29B:** 403–6.
18. Murphy DF, Greene WB, Dameron TD Displaced olecranon fractures in adults. *Clin Orthop* 1987; **224:** 215–23.
19. Metaizeau JP, Lascombes P, Lemelle L-L *et al.* Reduction and fixation of displaced radial neck fractures by closed intramedullary pinning. *J Pediatr Orthop* 1993; **13:** 355–60.
20. Sessa S, Lascombes J, Prevot J, Gagneux E Fractures of the radial head and associated elbow injuries in children. *J Pediatr Orthop* 1996; **5:** 200–9.
21. Bohler J Die Konservative Behandlung von Bruchen des Radiushalse. *Chirurg* 1950; **21:** 687–8.
22. Rodriguez CE Percutaneous reduction of displaced radial neck fractures in children. *J Trauma* 1994; **37:** 812–4.
23. Bernstein SM, McKeever P, Bernstein L Percutaneous reduction of displaced radial neck fractures in children. *J Pediatr Orthop* 1993; **13:** 85–8.
24. Angelov A A New method for treatment of the dislocated radial neck fracture in children. In: *Fractures in children.* Chapchal G (ed) New York: Georg Thieme Verlag, 1981: 192–4.
25. Rodgers WB, Waters PM, Hall JE Chronic Monteggia lesions in children. *J Bone Joint Surg* 1996; **78A:** 1322–7.
26. Bado JL The Monteggia lesion. *Clin Orthop* 1967; **50:** 71–86.
27. Wiley JJ, Galey JP Monteggia injuries of the children. *J Bone Joint Surg* 1985; **67B:** 728–31.
28. Best TN Management of old unreduced Monteggia fracture dislocations of the elbow in children. *J Pediatr Orthop* 1994; **14:** 193–9.

CHAPTER 10

Dislocations of the elbow in children

BRUCE L GILLINGHAM, DOUGLAS M HEDDEN

Introduction

Elbow dislocations in children are unusual. In Maylahn and Fahey's series of 300 consecutive paediatric elbow injuries, only six pure elbow dislocations occurred.[1] In a larger consecutive series from Sweden, elbow dislocations represented only 45 of 1579 (3%) elbow injuries in children.[2] Although infrequent, the elbow is the joint most often dislocated in children under the age of 10 years.[3] The majority of elbow dislocations occur in association with a fracture[4] of which the radial head and neck, lateral condyle and medial epicondyle are the most common. Elbow dislocations are an injury of adolescence with the peak incidence occurring between 13 and 14 years of age when the physes are beginning to close[2,5] and 71% occur in boys.[4]

The elbow has little inherent osseous stability. As Ogden has pointed out it is essentially a hinge joint constrained by soft tissues.[6] Schwab et al. demonstrated the preeminent role of the medial collateral ligament in elbow stability, particularly the anterior oblique portion in 1980.[7]

Mechanism of injury

Dislocation of the elbow is generally produced by a fall onto the outstretched hand with the elbow incompletely flexed. It may also occur secondary to a hyperextension injury.[6]

Sojbjerg et al. could only produce posterior elbow dislocations in cadavers with a combined valgus and external rotatory torque with the elbow flexed to 30 degrees. Varus and internal rotation torque did not produce a dislocation. Simultaneous disruption of the anterior portion of the medial collateral ligament and annular ligament was the most frequent finding.[8]

In the overwhelming majority of elbow dislocations the proximal radius and ulna are displaced as a unit posteriorly in relation to the distal humerus with the majority of these accompanied by lateral displacement.[6] Posteromedial, lateral and anterior dislocations have also been reported.[3,9,10]

Rarely, disruption of the proximal radioulnar joint will occur causing a divergent dislocation. These occur in a transverse fashion with the olecranon

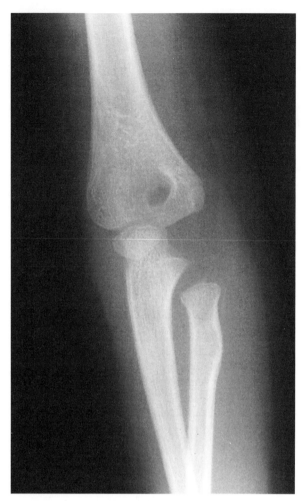

Fig. 10.1 Convergent dislocation. Translocation of the proximal radius and olecranon has occurred.

displaced posteromedially and the radial head posterolaterally. Due to the extensive ligamentous disruption that accompanies these injuries closed reduction is easily accomplished.[11–19]

Rarer still is an elbow dislocation associated with translocation of the radius and ulna (Fig. 10.1). In this condition, which has only been reported in seven patients, the radial head articulates with the trochlea and the olecranon with the capitellum. This is thought to occur because of pronation of the forearm after severe disruption of the proximal radioulna soft tissue restraints. This condition, also termed a convergent dislocation, is easily missed because on cursory inspection of the radiograph the elbow appears reduced. Treatment usually requires open reduction.[63]

Elbow dislocation

CLINICAL PRESENTATION

The deformity produced by dislocation of the elbow is generally quite obvious. The forearm will appear foreshortened. Significant soft tissue swelling will be present owing to the associated ligamentous and periarticular injury. Marked muscle spasm may be manifest. Palpation will reveal loss of the normal triangular relationship of the olecranon and humeral condyles. In the common posterolateral dislocation the radial head will be palpable in the subcutaneous tissues. A dimple may overlay the olecranon fossa.[20] Neurological and vascular injuries frequently occur as a result of elbow dislocation. A careful neurovascular examination is therefore mandatory prior to performing any intervention.

ASSESSMENT/INVESTIGATION

Radiographs should be obtained prior to reducing the elbow unless a vascular deficit warrants immediate reduction. These will not only define the nature of the dislocation but will identify any associated fractures. It is particularly important to rule out the commonly associated medial epicondyle fracture as well as fractures of the coronoid process, radial neck and lateral epicondyle.[21–23] Fractures of the medial condyle, lateral condyle and an intra-articular flap fracture of the olecranon have also been reported.[6,24,25] In children under 2 years of age transphyseal fracture-separation of the distal humerus should be ruled out as this is often confused with elbow dislocation in this age group. The treatment in these two conditions are significantly different.

MANAGEMENT OPTIONS

Only the treatment of isolated elbow dislocations will be discussed here. Treatment of fractures associated with elbow dislocation are covered in the sections in Chapter 8 detailing treatment of the specific fracture.

The majority of elbow dislocations are reducible by closed means. In Carlioz and Abols review only six of 58 posterior dislocations in children were unreducible.[4] A trapped medial epicondyle was present in two, two were subsequently found to have osteochondral flap fractures of the olecranon and the remaining two had interposed ligaments.[4]

The fundamental goal underlying elbow reduction is to overcome, as Stimson observed in 1912,

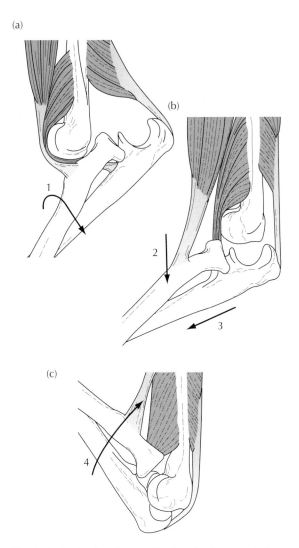

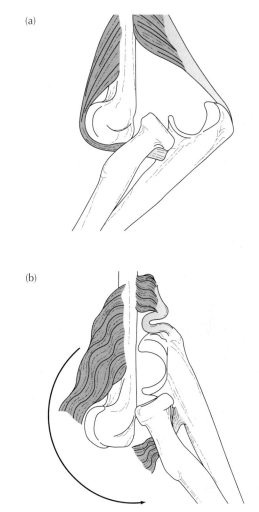

Fig. 10.2 Reduction forces. (a) First the forearm is hyper-supinated (arrow 1) to unlock the radial head. (b) Simultaneous forces must be applied distally along the axis of the humerus (arrow 2) and distally along the axis of the forearm (arrow 3). (c) Once the coronoid is manip-ulated distal to the humerus, the elbow is then flexed (arrow 4) to stabilise the reduction. Redrawn after Ref. 55 with permission from JB Lippincott Co, Philadelphia.

Fig. 10.3 Hyperextension forces. (a) Normally, the brachialis is stretched across the distal humerus. (b) Hyperextending the elbow before it is reduced greatly increases the arc of motion and leverage placed across the brachialis. This can result in rupture of large portions of the muscle. Redrawn after Ref. 33 with permission from Excerpta Medica, New Jersey.

'the muscles spasmodically contracted on all sides of the joint'.[26] As Wilkins has demonstrated the reduction forces must be exerted along the long axis of the humerus to overcome the contracted biceps and brachialis anteriorly and triceps posteriorly.[20] Once this is accomplished, the proximal ulna and radius must be passed from posterior to anterior. A second force is therefore required along the long axis of the forearm. Countertraction for both of the above forces is required (Fig. 10.2).

A number of reduction manoeuvers have been described.[26-30] Ambroise Pare' described a method with the patient seated. The affected arm was placed around a post with the operator supplying traction on the wrist while simultaneously flexing the elbow on the post.[31]

Crosby devised a supine method involving three slings pulling in four directions to provide the nec-essary forces and counterforces.[32] Stimson recom-mended initial elbow hyperextension to lever the coronoid past the distal humerus.[26] This has been shown, however, to generate forces up to five times normal on the already traumatised brachialis muscle and capsule (Fig. 10.3).[33] In addition, pronating the forearm while hyperextending the elbow has been implicated as a cause of median nerve entrapment during elbow reduction.[34]

The majority of authors favour initial hyper-supination of the forearm to unlock the radial head from the posterolateral aspect of the lateral distal humerus.[20] Following this the proximal forearm is either pulled or pushed back into place. In Parvin's method the patient is placed prone with the arm hanging freely off the side of the table. Without prior sedation or anaesthesia, gentle traction is applied by grasping the wrist over a period of 1 to 10 minutes. Simultaneously, the humerus is lifted laterally to produce approximately 20 degrees of elbow flexion until reduction is complete.[30] One advantage of this manoeuvre is that it can be performed by one person. The table provides the necessary counter forces on the humerus.

In the method described by Meyn and Quigley the patient is also prone and the wrist is grasped to provide distal forearm traction.[35] However, in contrast to Parvin's technique the olecranon is directly guided back into place with the operator's thumb and index finger.[35] A similar technique performed with the patient's arm draped over the back of a chair has been described by Lavine.[28]

Hankin has described an unassisted method in which the patient is positioned supine and the surgeon grasps the patients hand, aligns his forearm along the patient's and places his elbow in the patient's antecubital fossa.[27] The surgeon's elbow is then used as both the fulcrum of a longitudinal distracting lever and countertraction as the patient's elbow is gradually flexed. Flexion is continued until the coronoid is brought anterior to the distal humerus.[27]

Following successful closed reduction most authors recommend a short period of immobilisation in a posterior splint ranging from 5 to 7 days to 3 weeks.[27,36]

Open reduction in a fresh dislocation is reserved for the rare irreducible dislocation, open dislocations and when dictated by the treatment for an associated fracture such as an incarcerated medial epicondyle.

The presence of associated ligamentous disruption and post-reduction instability is not an indication for surgical repair. Josefsson and Nilsson demonstrated in a prospective randomised trial that surgical treatment did not lead to a statistically significant improvement in outcome in isolated elbow dislocations which had been reduced closed.[37]

AUTHORS' PREFERRED TREATMENT

Closed reduction is performed after carefully assessing the neurovascular status of the patient's arm and obtaining radiographs to rule out associated fractures. As the primary block to reduction is muscular spasm, younger children and apprehensive older children and adolescents are manipulated under general anaesthesia. Cooperative older children are sometimes treated in the emergency room under intravenous sedation. We prefer the prone position and grasp the wrist to exert gradual longitudinal forearm traction while gripping the olecranon and lifting it away from and guiding it anterior to the humerus as described by Meyn and Quigley.[35] We find that this technique helps unlock the coronoid from the olecranon fossa and decreases the risk of fracturing the coronoid during reduction. Control of medial and lateral displacement is also possible with this method. A thorough neurovascular examination is performed post-reduction. Anteroposterior and lateral radiographs are obtained to document reduction prior to application of the splint. This is essential as the associated soft tissue swelling may lead to a false impression that reduction has been achieved.[6] This also identifies the presence of a previously occult fracture or one produced during reduction. A posterior splint with the elbow flexed 90 degrees is applied for comfort. This is removed after resolution of the acute inflammatory phase at approximately 7–10 days. Active range of motion is encouraged but assisted passive movement is not allowed. If the elbow is unstable after reduction, the use of a cast brace which allows only flexion and extension is useful.

Open reduction is performed for the rare irreducible dislocation, open dislocation, or when an associated fracture requires surgical stabilisation.

COMPLICATIONS

The most common complication is stiffness. Characteristically, children will lose roughly 10 degrees of extension. This is thought to be due to the significant capsular tearing which accompanies elbow dislocation. Generally, no cosmetic or functional difficulties result. Immobilisation longer than 3 weeks and forced passive range of motion exercises will only compound the loss of motion. Children are generally their own best physiotherapists and should be allowed to pursue activities as desired. Swimming should be recommended. Up to a year may be required before maximum range of motion is obtained.[6]

The most worrisome complication is arterial injury. Fortunately, this is uncommon in isolated dislocations. In fact, a recent review of the English literature disclosed only six children under 15 years with elbow dislocations associated with brachial artery lesions.[38] Four of these were in patients who had sustained open injuries.

Evidence of distal ischemia is generally present when a complete arterial rupture occurs. A pulse obtained by Doppler, however, does not guarantee patency of the artery and if doubt exists regarding the vascular status of the limb an arteriogram should be performed.[39]

Although a well developed system of collateral vessels is present about the elbow, Louis *et al.* demonstrated consistent disruption of this collateral circulation between the inferior ulnar collateral artery and the anterior ulnar recurrent artery in posterior elbow dislocations.[40] Thus, in the absence of brachial flow, compensation with collateral flow is unlikely. Evidence of distal ischaemia should, therefore, be thoroughly investigated and repair or reconstruction of the brachial artery performed if indicated.

Neurological complications are more frequent than vascular. In Linscheid and Wheeler's series of elbow dislocations in all age groups, vascular injury occurred in eight of 110 while neurologic complications occurred in 24.[3] Sixteen of these involved the ulnar nerve, three the median and four both nerves. The remaining patient sustained a brachial plexus injury.[3] Fortunately, most nerve injuries associated with elbow dislocation are transient paraesthesias and resolve completely.

In Carlioz and Abols series of 58 elbow dislocations confined to children, the only neurological complications encountered were two transient ulnar nerve injuries.[4] The ulnar nerve can become trapped in the elbow in association with incarceration of a medial epicondyle fracture (Chapter 8).

Median nerve injury, although rare, can have serious sequelae. Hallett described in 1981 a case of entrapment of the median nerve in the elbow and reviewed the 13 previously reported cases.[34] Based on this he proposed three different ways in which the median nerve could become trapped in the elbow (Fig. 10.4). In type 1 the nerve is caught between the humerus and ulna. In type 2 the nerve runs through a bony tunnel at the site of a healed medial epicondyle fracture. In type 3 the nerve is looped into the front of the elbow.

Median nerve entrapment is particularly worrisome because it can be difficult to detect. Little pain is produced directly by the entrapment, sensory examination is difficult in younger children and progression of motor deficit can be subtle.[41] If more than mild hyperaesthesia is present entrapment of the nerve should be suspected. Pronation of the forearm while the elbow is hyperextended may predispose the nerve to entrapment.[34] Early removal of the nerve is the treatment of choice. Late diagnosis, however, is not uncommon given the subtlety of

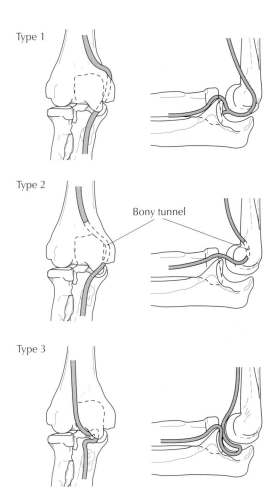

Fig. 10.4 The three ways in which the median nerve can be trapped after posterior dislocation of the elbow. Type 1 – median nerve passes through trochleoulnar joint. Type 2 – median nerve passes through a bony tunnel at the site of the healed fracture. Type 3 – median nerve looped into the front of the elbow. Redrawn after Ref. 34 with permission from *Journal of Bone and Joint Surgery.*

its presentation. Matev[41] described a radiographic sign of late entrapment consisting of a depression in the cortex of the medial metaphysis with interruption of the local periosteal reaction corresponding to the course of the median nerve at the humerus (Chapter 13). Resection of the entrapped portion of the nerve with end-to-end reanastomosis may be required in these late cases if no electrical conduction across the damaged section is present. The results in these cases have been surprisingly good.[42]

Recurrent dislocation is rare but as Wilkins points out, is confined to the paediatric age group.[20] Our current understanding of this condition is based on the landmark article written by Osborne and Cotterill in 1966.[29] They demonstrated that the essential pathological deficit is failure of the posterolateral ligamentous and capsular structures which were torn or stretched at the time of the original dislocation to become reattached. The head of the radius slides off the capitellum into a pocket of capsule created by the stripped soft tissues. The lateral liagment that would normally prevent this is stripped away from the lateral column and is incompetent.[29] Based on this understanding of the pathologic lesion Osborne and Cotterill designed a posterolateral capsular plication and reattachment procedure which has proven effective. They and other authors recommend, however, non-operative treatment if the dislocations are infrequent in order to allow the normal developmental tightening of the capsule and ligaments to take place.[29,43,44]

Unreduced dislocations have become increasingly rare. Most published reports have included patients from remote areas without access to up-to-date medical care.[21,45] Open reduction is generally required if more than 2–3 weeks have elapsed from the original injury. The significant shortening of the soft tissues about the elbow which takes place makes closed reduction impossible.

Speed described the Campbell triceps tongue approach in 1925.[46] This affords excellent exposure and allows triceps lengthening, ulnar nerve transposition and internal fixation if required.[21,46] Fowles *et al.* reported a fourfold improvement in motion after open reduction in 11 children. He recommended an interval of conservative treatment in those children seen from 3 weeks to 2 months after injury since some of these patients will regain a functional range of motion and not require surgery.[21]

Myositis ossificans is fortunately rare in association with elbow dislocations. Thompson and Garcia found a 3% incidence in simple dislocations increasing to 18% in dislocations associated with fractures.[47] Although it can cause significant limitation of motion it should be distinguished from the more common heterotopic ossification which occurs in the collateral ligaments and posterior capsule and rarely limits motion.[6]

Myositis is thought to be related to injury within the relatively thin brachialis muscle during the initial dislocation and exacerbated by hyperextension during reduction (Fig. 10.3). Overly vigorous passive range of motion during the rehabilitative phase is also thought to contribute by causing recurrent inflammation and haematoma within the previously injured muscle.[6] Children tend to resorb ectopic calcification and ossification before it matures and thus surgical treatment is rarely required. If resorption does not occur, excision may become necessary. This, however, should be delayed until the bone matures as evidenced by well defined peripheral sclerosis on x-ray.[6]

Despite the litany of complications which are possible, most children who sustain a simple elbow dislocation have a favourable outcome. Josefsson and Danielsson performed follow-up examinations and radiographs on 52 patients an average of 24 years after injury.[48] Among the patients who had sustained the injury when they were less than 16 years old there were few with residual symptoms, signs or radiographic changes.[48]

Subluxation of the radial head (nursemaid's elbow)

Pulled elbow is a very common injury in young children which occasionally leads to difficulty in diagnosis but rarely in treatment.

CLINICAL PRESENTATION

The child is unwilling to use the elbow and holds it in the flexed position. There is often a history of a traction injury to the extremity. There may be a past history of a similar problem as recurrence is relatively common. As the child grows this will stabilise and the injury is quite uncommon after the age of 3 years.

ASSESSMENT/INVESTIGATION

Radiographic assessment is often unnecessary and x-rays will be normal as this is a subluxation and not a true dislocation. Radiographs may, however, be useful to rule out other injuries. Kosuwon *et al.* reported the use of ultrasound to document this condition and showed that the distance between the radial head and capitellum was increased. Although scientifically valuable, in clinical practice ultrasonic assessment is usually not required.[49]

AUTHORS' PREFERRED MANAGEMENT

With the elbow flexed the forearm is firmly and steadily supinated with a thumb over the radial neck. Resistance will initially be met but the forearm will then fully supinate often with a palpable click over the radial neck. If the time interval between subluxation and reduction is short the child will often immediately start using the elbow. However, if there has been a time delay it may take

24 hours or so before the child starts using the elbow normally. If it takes longer than this the parents are asked to return the child for assessment, otherwise follow-up is not necessary. If the child has a recurrent problem the parents may be taught the reduction manoeuvre and told to seek help only if the child does not quickly recover.

Dislocation of the radial head

Isolated dislocation of the radial head is not uncommon; however, most are either congenital or they are the residual deformity of a missed Monteggia lesion.

Any patient presenting with a dislocated radial head should undergo examination of the contralateral elbow in order to assess whether the condition is bilateral and therefore likely to be congenital. Agnew and Davis reported six cases in which they believed the diagnosis was unilateral congenital dislocation.[50] This is exceedingly rare and represented only 0.16% of their new cases.[50]

In the presence of a unilateral dislocation of the radial head without a history of trauma it is still most likely that the child sustained a mild injury to the arm which resulted in a greenstick fracture of the ulna and dislocation of the radial head. The other more common scenario is that the child was treated for a forearm fracture which healed but range of motion never returned. In this case the ulnar fracture has healed and the dislocated radial head has gone unrecognised. Careful examination of the ulna will reveal an abnormal bow with volar angulation.

Lincoln and Mubarak do not believe that isolated traumatic dislocation of the radial head exists.[51] In their series an identifiable ulnar injury was present in all cases. They describe the ulnar bow sign which is helpful to pick up these subtle injuries (Fig. 10.5).

Dislocation of the radial head associated with a fracture of the proximal ulna (Monteggia fracture dislocation)

The Monteggia lesion is an important topic as it often goes unrecognised. Treated early the results are excellent. Poor results, however, are common when only late treatment is possible.

Monteggia described the lesion which bears his name in 1814.[64] He reported a fracture of the proximal ulna accompanied by an anterior dislocation of the radial head which was only appreciated when the initial cast was removed. The injury is usually caused by hyperextension to the elbow which results in either a complete or incomplete volarly angulated fracture of the proximal ulna. Rather than causing a similar fracture in the radius the radial head dislocates either tearing the annular ligament or avulsing it from its attachment to the ulna. The ulnar fracture may in fact be anywhere along the ulna shaft and still result in a dislocation of the radial head.

Bado added to the understanding of these lesions and classified them according to the direction of the radial head dislocation.[52] The type I injury is an anterior dislocation of the radial head associated with an anteriorly angulated ulna fracture (Fig. 10.6). The type II injury is a posterior dislocation of the radial head with a posteriorly angulated ulnar fracture (Fig. 10.7). The type III injury consists of a lateral dislocation of the radial head with a laterally angulated ulnar fracture (Fig. 10.8). Type IV injuries are the same as type I but with an associated proximal radial fracture (Fig. 10.9). Several Monteggia equivalents are described and these are thought to be more associated with pronation injuries.

(a)

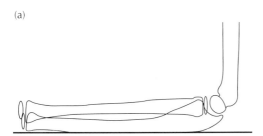

(b)

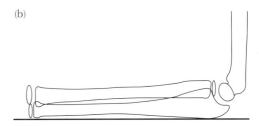

Fig. 10.5 (a) Line shows normal straight border of ulna demonstrated by ulnar bow line. (b) Line shows bowing of ulna: minimal Monteggia fracture-dislocation with radial head subluxation and positive ulnar bow sign. Redrawn after Ref. 51 with permission from Raven Press Ltd, New York.

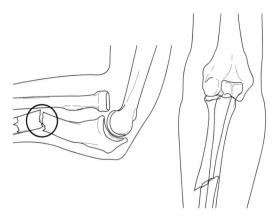

Fig. 10.6 Type I Monteggia fracture-dislocation. Volarly angulated ulna fracture with anterior radial head dislocation.

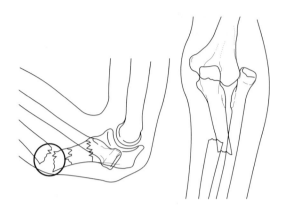

Fig. 10.7 Type II Monteggia fracture-dislocation. Posteriorly angulated ulna fracture with posterolateral dislocation of the radial head.

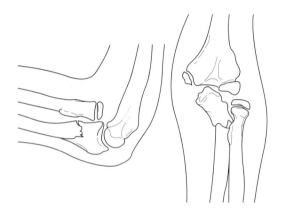

Fig. 10.8 Type III Monteggia fracture-dislocation. Fracture of the olecranon metaphysis with lateral dislocation of the radial head.

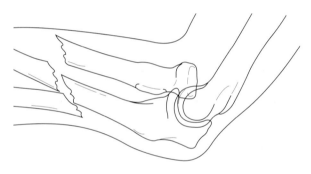

Fig. 10.9 Type IV Monteggia fracture-dislocation. Fractures of both radial and ulnar shafts with anterior dislocation of the radial head. Figures 10.6–10.9 redrawn after Ref. 52 with permission from JB Lippincott Co, Philadelphia.

Monteggia lesions are infrequent and account for a small percentage of elbow injuries in children. However, with such a significant potential for morbidity with delayed treatment early recognition is crucial to a good outcome.

CLINICAL PRESENTATION

Following a fall onto the arm or the outstretched hand the child will present with a swollen painful forearm with tenderness about the elbow. The degree of deformity is often great and there may be puckering of the skin on the volar aspect of the forearm. The late presentation is usually due to loss of motion and not pain.

ASSESSMENT/INVESTIGATION

Careful clinical examination is important when examining a child with a forearm fracture. Tenderness about the elbow must be specifically sought in order to appreciate the extent of the injury. A palpable lump anteriorly at the elbow will often be felt. The child will resist elbow movement. A marked limitation of motion is often present.

Careful neurological examination is also important. With anterior dislocation of the radial head the posterior interosseous nerve is at risk. With anterior angulation of the ulnar fracture injuries to the ulnar, median or anterior interosseous nerves may occur.

With significant displacement of the ulnar fracture, damage to the forearm musculature may simulate a nerve injury as some of the flexor muscles may be torn or contused. Indeed with even more force the ulna may perforate the skin and small puncture wounds on the volar surface should be looked for as this will dictate the management.

Careful interpretation of the radiographs is vital. It must be remembered that an isolated fracture of a forearm bone is rare and usually due to a direct blow. If one bone is fractured then the other should be as well. If it is not, dislocation of the joint proximal or distal to the bone must be excluded. This necessitates good radiographs showing both the elbow and wrist joints. Nothing less should be accepted. In addition plastic deformation of the ulna may be present, especially if the ulnar border is bowed rather than straight.

On the lateral view of the elbow it is important to remember that a line drawn along the radius should bisect the capitellum in any projection regardless of the flexion or extension of the elbow joint. If there is any doubt a radiographs of the opposite side should be undertaken.

MANAGEMENT OPTIONS

For acute injuries closed reduction is almost universally successful except in some of the Monteggia equivalent injuries. If the reduction is unstable intramedullary rodding of the ulna is usually all that is necessary.[53] If the radial head does not reduce then open reduction should be performed. At the time of open reduction the annular ligament must be repaired if possible either by direct suture of the torn ligament or by reattachment of the avulsed ligament.

For those very unstable injuries which require further internal fixation there is no agreement on how the radius should be pinned. King advocates and Letts condems the use of a radiocapitellar pin.[55,56]

The position of immobilisation will depend on the fracture pattern. Type I fractures are immobilised in flexion with the arm in supination, whereas type II and III injuries are usually best managed in extension.

The management of old unreduced Monteggia lesions is much more controversial. Blount states that: 'Malunited and unreduced Monteggia fractures that are 3 months old should be allowed to go untreated'.[57]

Many options exist for the missed lesion. If it is early, attempted closed reduction is possible but as the time from injury increases the likelihood for success significantly decreases. Open reduction may be performed with the addition of other procedures. These include:

1. reconstruction of the annular ligament;
2. correction of the ulnar deformity with ulnar osteotomy;
3. radial shortening.

The other option is to leave the radial head dislocated and perform a radial head excision when the child is mature.

Ulnar osteotomy with open reduction of the radial head with or without annular ligament reconstruction has gained acceptance.[58–60] Good results may be expected from this approach. Best had one patient who was treated 5 years 7 months after the injury. The result was very good with normal function, full flexion, extension, and pronation and only a 20 degree loss of supination.

AUTHORS' PREFERRED MANAGEMENT

Management at the time of injury

For type I fractures closed reduction of the ulna and spontaneous reduction of the radial head is the management of choice. Occasionally pressure over the radial head is needed to aid reduction. A cast should then be used with the elbow in 90 degrees of flexion and full supination. If the reduction is very unstable then a small intramedullary rod is placed down the ulna percutaneously from the olecranon. If the radial head will not reduce (an extremely unlikely event) then open reduction through a lateral approach and direct repair of the annular ligament is recommended. The elbow is immobilised for 3 weeks after which a protected range of motion is permitted.

Type II injuries are treated in a similar fashion but with the elbow in extension.

Type III injuries are treated similarly but while many prefer to cast these in flexion we prefer extension as we find it easier to mold the cast into valgus with the elbow locked in extension.

Type IV and other equivalents may also be treated by closed means. As the number of sites of injury increase so does our tendency to use intramedullary fixation. With a radial neck fracture, ulnar fracture and radial head dislocation an ulnar intramedullary rod placed through the olecranon plus a radial intramedullary rod placed through the radial metaphysis proximal to the growth plate provides stabilisation (Fig. 10.10). This makes closed reduction of the radial head easier.

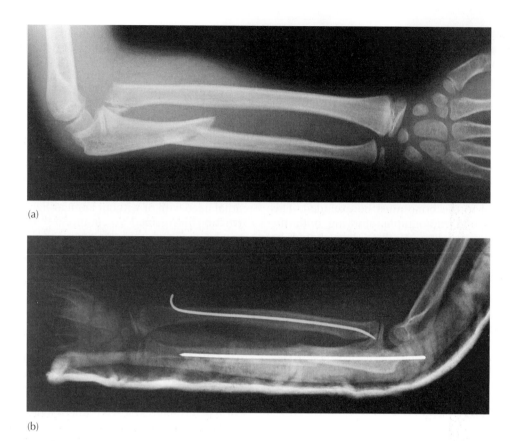

(a)

(b)

Fig. 10.10 (a) Monteggia equivalent with radial neck fracture and proximal ulna fracture. (b) Use of intramedullary wires to stabilise ulna and reduce and hold radial neck fracture.

Late injuries

We prefer surgical management in this situation. Open reduction of the radial head through a Boyd approach (Chapter 7) is used and unless reduction of the radial head is stable an ulnar osteotomy is performed through the same approach. We prefer to internally fix the osteotomy with a plate so that redisplacement of the head is less likely. Reconstruction of the annular ligament is then undertaken through an extension of the same incision using a lateral strip of triceps tendon. This is left intact at its ulnar insertion and then wrapped around the radial neck and brought through a drill hole in the ulna. Fixation of the radiocapitellar joint is avoided if possible but if necessary we prefer a transcapitellar pin of good size to minimise the possibility of breakage. This is removed at 3 weeks, after which protected movement is commenced.

For very late presentations, radial head excision to relieve pain is useful. This should be performed after skeletal maturity, in order to prevent subsequent distal radioulnar joint instability.

SURGICAL TECHNIQUE

Placement of an ulnar intramedullary rod

Once reduction of the ulnar fracture is obtained the arm is prepared and draped. A power drill is then used to insert a K-wire directly into the intramedullary canal through the olecranon. Once in the canal the wire may either be drilled or gently tapped down the canal in order to stabilise the fracture. Tapping or pushing is safer than drilling and is less likely to perforate the cortex. The pin should then be bent over but left protruding through the skin so as to allow removal in the outpatient clinic.

If the ulna fracture cannot be reduced, a K-wire with a bent tip is passed into the distal intramedullary canal and then rotated to obtain the reduction.

Placement of a radial intramedullary rod

The entry site is on the radial border of the distal forearm at least 1 cm proximal to the growth plate. An image intensifier is used to verify the correct insertion point. A small incision is made and the soft tissues are spread with a haemostat so as to decrease the risk of injury to the recurrent branch of the radial nerve. Using a tissue protector a bone awl or drill is used to make an oblique hole in the radial cortex. As with the ulna, the wire is then advanced until stability of the fracture is obtained.

Approach for the late Monteggia lesion

A Boyd approach (Chapter 7) is used, taking care to protect the posterior interosseous nerve. The radial head is usually encased in scar tissue which requires excision. The space for the radial head is then cleared. Following this the incision is extended along the ulna in order to allow a corrective osteotomy. This is performed using a small oscillating saw at the previous fracture site or proximal to it if it is a very distal fracture. The osteotomy site is then plated. Stability is assessed and if the radial head is still unstable an annular ligament reconstruction is performed. The incision is extended proximally and a lateral strip of the triceps tendon about 8 mm wide and as long as possible is harvested leaving it attached to the ulna distally. This strip is then passed around the radial neck from posteriorly to anteriorly and then through a drill hole in the ulna where it is sutured to itself.[61] This usually stabilises the radial head but if it still has a tendency to sublux it is important to check whether the ulnar deformity has been appropriately corrected. If it has, a transcapitellar pin of at least 2 mm diameter should be inserted. A cast is applied with the elbow at 90 degrees and the forearm in full supination. It is removed at 3 weeks and an active range of motion started.

COMPLICATIONS

The biggest complication of the Monteggia fracture-dislocation is failure of diagnosis. The missed injury will lead to stiffness but often little pain. It may also lead to a cosmetic deformity with valgus at the elbow and a palpable and visual lump. Heterotopic bone formation may occur but is usually benign and does not seem to limit function. Nerve injuries have been discussed. These are of course at risk with surgical intervention. Synostosis

of the radius and ulna has been reported and theoretically this may be increased with open reduction.[62] Surgery brings the added risk of infection and if utilised breakage of the transcapitellar pin.

References

1. Maylahn D, Fahey J Fractures of the elbow in children: review of three hundred consecutive cases. *J Am Med Assoc* 1958; **166:** 220–8.
2. Henrikson B Supracondylar fracture of the humerus in children. *Acta Chir Scand Suppl* 1966; **369:** 1–72.
3. Linscheid R, Wheeler D Elbow dislocations. *J Am Med Assoc* 1965; **194:** 1171–6.
4. Carlioz H, Abols Y Posterior dislocation of the elbow in children. *J Pediatr Orthop* 1984; **4:** 8–12.
5. Josefsson P, Gentz C, Johnell O, Wendeberg B Surgical versus non-surgical treatment of ligamentous injuries following dislocation of the elbow joint. *J Bone Joint Surg* 1987; **69A:** 605–8.
6. Ogden J *Skeletal injury in the child* (2nd edn). Philadelphia: WB Saunders Co, 1990.
7. Schwab G, Bennett J, Woods G, Tullos H Biomechanics of elbow instability: The role of the medial collateral ligament. *Clin Orthop* 1980; **146:** 42–52.
8. Sojbjerg J, Helmig P, Kjaersgaard-Andersen P Dislocation of the elbow: An experimental study of the ligamentous injuries. *Orthopedics* 1989; **12:** 461–3.
9. Neviaser J, Wickstrom J Dislocation of the elbow: A retrospective study of 115 patients. *South Med J* 1977; **70:** 172–3.
10. Roberts PH Dislocation of the elbow. *Brit J Surg* 1969; **56:** 806–15.
11. DeLee J, Wilkins K, Rogers L, Rockwood C Fracture-separation of the distal humeral epiphysis. *J Bone Joint Surg* 1980; **62A:** 46–51.
12. Holbrook J. Green N Divergent pediatric elbow dislocation. *Clin Orthop* 1988; **234:** 72–4.
13. Sovio O, Tredwell S Divergent dislocation of the elbow in a child. *J. Pediatr Orthop* 1986; **6:** 96–7.
14. Vicente P, Orduna M Transverse divergent dislocation of the elbow in a child. *Clin Orthop* 1993; **294:** 312–3.
15. Carey R Simultaneous dislocation of the elbow and the proximal radio-ulnar joint. *J Bone Joint Surg* 1984; **66B:** 254–6.
16. Carl A, Prada S, Teixeira K Proximal radioulnar transposition in an elbow dislocation. *J Orthop Trauma* 1992; **6:** 106–9.
17. Eklof O, Nybonde T, Karlsson G Luxation of the elbow complicated by proximal radioulnar translocation. *Acta Radiol* 1990; **31:** 145–6.
18. Harvey S, Tchelebi H Proximal radio-ulnar translocation. *J Bone Joint Surg* 1979; **61A:** 447–9.
19. MacSween W Transposition of radius and ulna associated with dislocation of the elbow in a child. *Injury* 1979; **10:** 314–6.
20. Wilkins K Residuals of elbow trauma in children. *Orthop Clin North Am* 1990; **21:** 291–314.

21. Fowles J, Kassab M, Moula T Untreated intra-articular entrapment of the medial humeral epicondyle. *J Bone Joint Surg* 1984; **66B:** 562–5.

22. Papavasiliou V, Nenopoulos S, Venturis T Fractures of the medial condyle of the humerus in childhood. *J Pediatr Orthop* 1987; **7:** 421–3.

23. Woods G, Tullos H Elbow instability and medial epicondyle fractures. *Am J Sports Med* 1977; **5:** 23–30.

24. Blasier R Intra-articular flap fracture of the olecranon in a child. *J Bone Joint Surg* 1989; **71A:** 945–7.

25. Saraf S, Tuli S Concomitant medial condyle fracture of the humerus in a childhood posterolateral dislocation of the elbow. *J Orthop Trauma* 1989; **3:** 352–4.

26. Stimson L A *Practical treatise on fractures and dislocations* (7th edn). New York, Philadelphia: Lea and Febiger, 1912.

27. Hankin F Posterior dislocation of the elbow. *Clin Orthop* 1984; **190:** 254–6.

28. Lavine L A simple method of reducing dislocations of the elbow joint. *J Bone Joint Surg* 1953; **35A:** 785–6.

29. Osborne G, Cotterill P Recurrent dislocation of the elbow. *J Bone Joint Surg* 1966; **48B:** 340–6.

30. Parvin R Closed reduction of common shoulder and elbow dislocations without anesthesia. *Arch Surg* 1957; **75:** 972–5.

31. Pare' A In: *Ten books of surgery.* Linker R, Womack N (eds) with the magazine of the instruments necessary for it. Athens: University of Georgia Press, 1969.

32. Crosby E Dislocation of the elbow reduced by means of traction in four directions. *J Bone Joint Surg* 1936; **18:** 1077.

33. Loomis L Reduction and after-treatment of posterior dislocation of the elbow. *Am J Surg* 1994; **63:** 56–60.

34. Hallett J Entrapment of the median nerve after dislocation of the elbow. *J Bone Joint Surg* 1981; **63B:** 408–12.

35. Meyn M, Quigley T Reduction of posterior dislocation of the elbow by traction on the dangling arm. *Clin Orthop* 1974; **103:** 106–8.

36. Hassman G, Brunn F, Neer C Recurrent dislocation of the elbow. *J Bone Joint Surg* 1975; **57A:** 1080–4.

37. Josefsson P, Nilsson B Incidence of elbow dislocation. *Acta Orthop Scand* 1986; **57:** 537–8.

38. Manouel M, Minkowitz B, Shimotsu G *et al.* Brachial artery laceration with closed posterior elbow dislocation in an eight year old. *Clin Orthop* 1993; **296:** 109–2.

39. Hofammann K, Moneim M, Omer G, Ball W Brachial artery disruption following closed posterior elbow dislocation in a child-assessment with intravenous digital angiography. *Clin Orthop* 1984; **184:** 145–9.

40. Louis D, Ricciardi J, Spengler D Arterial injury: A complication of posterior elbow dislocation. *J Bone Joint Surg* 1974; **56A:** 1631–6.

41. Matev I. A radiological sign of entrapment of the median nerve in the elbow joint after posterior dislocation. *J Bone Joint Surg* 1976; **58B:** 353–5.

42. Green N Entrapment of the median nerve following elbow dislocation. *J Pediatr Orthop* 1983; **3:** 384–6.

43. Beaty J Fractures and dislocations about the elbow in children. *Instr Course Lect* 1992; **XLI:** 373–84.

44. Herring J, Sullivan J Recurrent dislocation of the elbow. *J Pediatr Orthop* 1989; **9:** 483–4.

45. Allende G, Freytes M Old dislocation of the elbow. *J Bone Joint Surg* 1944; **26:** 691–706.

46. Speed J An Operation for unreduced posterior dislocation of the elbow. *South Med J* 1925; **18:** 193–8.

47. Thompson H, Garcia A Myositis ossificans: Aftermath of elbow injuries. *Clin Orthop* 1967; **50:** 129–34.

48. Josefsson P, Danielsson L Epicondylar elbow fracture in children. *Acta Orthop Scand* 1986; **57:** 313–5.

49. Kosuwon W, Mahaisavariya B, Saengnipanthkul S *et al.* Ultrasonography of the pulled elbow. *J Bone Joint Surg* 1993; **75B:** 421–2.

50. Agnew D, Davis R Congenital unilateral dislocation of the radial head. *J Pediatr Orthop* 1993; **13:** 526–8.

51. Lincoln T, Mubarak S 'Isolated' traumatic radial-head dislocation. *J Pediatr Orthop* 1994; **14:** 454–7.

52. Bado J The Monteggia lesion. *Clin Orthop* 1967; **50:** 71–86.

53. Dormans J, Rang M The problem of Monteggia fracture-dislocations in children. *Orthop Clin North Am* 1990; **21:** 251–6.

54. Kalamchi A Monteggia fracture-dislocation in children. *J Bone Joint Surg* 1986; **68A:** 615–9.

55. King R. In: *Fractures in children.* Rockwood C, Wilkins K, King R (eds) Philadelphia: JB Lippincott Co, 1991.

56. Letts M, Locht R, Weins J Monteggia fracture-dislocation in children. *J Bone Joint Surg* 1985; **67B:** 724–7.

57. Blount W *Fractures in children.* Baltimore: Williams and Wilkins, 1955.

58. Best T Management of old unreduced Monteggia fracture dislocations of the elbow in children. *J Pediatr Orthop* 1994; **14:** 193–9.

59. Oner F Diepstraten A Treatment of chronic post-traumatic dislocation of the radial head in children. *J Bone Joint Surg* 1993; **75B:** 577–81.

60. Stoll T, Willis R, Paterson D Treatment of the missed Monteggia fracture in the child. *J Bone Joint Surg* 1992; **74B:** 436–40.

61. Bell-Tawse A The treatment of malunited anterior Monteggia fractures in children. *J Bone Joint Surg* 1965; **47B:** 718–23.

62. Bruce H, Harvey JJ Monteggia fractures. *J Bone Joint Surg* 1974; **56A:** 1563–76.

63. Gillingham B, Wright J Convergent dislocation of the elbow. *Clin Orthop* 1997; **340:** 198–201.

64. Monteggia A *Inst Chirurg* 1814; **5:** 130.

CHAPTER 11

Fractures of the distal humerus in adults

AH CRENSHAW JR

Introduction

Although injuries to the adult elbow historically have not received as much attention as similar injuries at the knee, they often result in considerable impairment. A fracture of the lower extremity may heal with contracture, some loss of motion of the adjacent joints, and other soft-tissue compromise but still yield a good functional result. The outcome in the upper extremity, however, may result in a severe functional impairment in both occupational and daily living activities.

Fractures involving the elbow joint often produce extensive soft-tissue damage in addition to the bony injury. The forearm musculature arising from the distal humerus tends to produce rotational displacement and results in condylar malalignment in the anteroposterior plane. This changes the arch of rotation of one condyle to the arc of rotation of the other condyle, limiting both flexion and extension (Fig. 11.1).

Early careful assessment of the patient's radiographs is necessary after these fractures in order to allow appropriate treatment to be instituted. When open reduction is delayed by indecision or follows

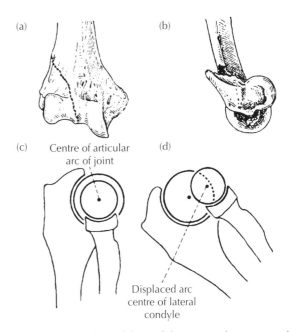

Fig. 11.1 Effects of condylar malalignment. The centres of the articular arc of the separate condyles are located on the same horizontal line through the distal humerus (a,c). When one condyle is malaligned with another (b,d), flexion and extension of the elbow are blocked.

failure of closed methods, the best time for surgery may be lost, and soft-tissue contractures, myositis ossificans, and a more difficult reconstructive procedure are likely. However, soft-tissue damage, skin abrasions, open wound, multiple injuries, or poor general condition of the patient may on occasions necessitate postponement of surgery.

Limitation of elbow movement is the most common complication after these fractures and has several causes (Table 11.1).

Classification of distal humeral fractures

Distal humeral fractures can be classified by anatomical site of injury:

Epicondylar fractures
    medial or lateral
Supracondylar fractures
Transcondylar fractures
Intercondylar fractures
Condyle fractures
    medial or lateral
Fractures of the articular surface
    capitellum and trochlea

Epicondylar fractures

In adults isolated fractures of the medial and lateral epicondyle are rare.

MEDIAL EPICONDYLAR FRACTURES

Medial epicondylar fractures are thought to result from direct trauma and may be undisplaced, displaced, or become incarcerated in the joint if the fracture is associated with an elbow dislocation.[1] In all cases because of the proximity of the ulnar nerve a careful neurological examination is mandatory.

Undisplaced or minimally displaced fractures can be treated conservatively with 2 weeks sling immobilisation followed by active elbow exercises. Displaced fractures and those incarcerated in the joint require open reduction and internal screw fixation.

LATERAL EPICONDYLAR FRACTURES

Lateral epicondylar fractures are seen less frequently, and can almost always be managed conservatively.

Table 11.1 Causes of limited elbow movement following distal humeral fractures

1. Mechanical block
    a. An inverted V deformity of the humeral condyles after T and Y fractures
    b. Bony offset after unreduced shearing fractures of the articular surface
    c. Generalised joint irregularity after unreduced comminuted condylar fractures
2. Obliteration of the olecranon fossa
    a. Displacement of the humeral condyles
    b. Exuberant callus
    c. Fibrous tissue
3. Periarticular fibrosis
    a. Trauma of injury
    b. Poor surgical technique
    c. Excessive bulky or poorly placed fixation implants (plates, screws, pins)
4. Infection
5. Inappropriate rehabilitation
    a. Repeated stretching
    b. Tearing of adhesions by forceful manipulation

The elbow should be immobilised for 2 weeks in a sling following which active elbow exercises should be performed.

Supracondylar fractures

Adult supracondylar fractures are encountered less frequently than in children. They occur through the extra-articular portions of the medial and lateral distal humeral columns at the level of the coronoid and olecranon fossae.[2,3]

MECHANISM OF INJURY

Extension forces, such as that produced by a fall on the outstretched hand, produce posterior displacement of the distal fragment. A fall on the posterior aspect of the flexed elbow or a direct blow produces the anterior displacement of the distal fragment seen in the flexion-type supracondylar fracture. Flexion-type fractures are rare and constitute less than 5% of all supracondylar fractures.

CLINICAL PRESENTATION

Patients with supracondylar fractures commonly present with marked swelling, especially when the fracture is of the extension-type and displaced. The medial and lateral epicondyles are in the appropriate relationship to the olecranon, forming an isosceles triangle, distinguishing this injury from a posterior elbow dislocation.

Careful neurovascular examination of the arm is essential, especially in extension-type fractures. Laceration of the brachial artery by the proximal fracture fragment can occur either at the time of injury or during reduction, with development of a compartment syndrome. In addition neurological damage may occur to any of the three major nerves that cross the elbow joint, although it is the radial nerve that is most commonly injured.[4,5]

TREATMENT OPTIONS

Non-operative treatment

Undisplaced or minimally displaced supracondylar fractures can be treated with posterior long-arm splint immobilisation for 2 to 3 weeks, followed by motion exercises.[6] Displaced fractures can be satisfactorily treated with a traction hanging-arm cast or a coaptation splint if the patient's condition or functional capacity so warrants.

Displaced extension-type supracondylar fractures can be treated by closed reduction under anaesthesia and immobilisation in flexion. The amount of flexion necessary to maintain an adequate reduction, however, may occlude venous return or the brachial artery. For this reason percutaneous pinning of the fracture is preferred. This allows the elbow to be immobilised in less flexion and decreases the danger of postoperative vascular complications. If this is not undertaken extremely close observation is necessary to detect the development of vascular compromise. Often, a good reduction is lost as swelling decreases if the medial and lateral columns of the distal humerus are not stabilised.

Displaced flexion-type supracondylar fractures are often unstable and difficult to manage by non-operative means. Closed reduction and percutaneous fixation or open reduction and internal fixation are preferred.

If operative treatment is contraindicated because of severe swelling, skin conditions, or the patient's overall condition, displaced supracondylar fractures can be treated satisfactorily with side-arm (Dunlop) or overhead olecranon pin traction until the patient's condition allows operative treatment.[7] Lengthy hospitalisation is necessary if traction treatment is the definitive therapy.

Operative treatment

The operative treatment options in the management of adult supracondylar fractures are either closed reduction and percutaneous fixation (Kirschner wires, Steinmann pins, or screws) or open reduction and internal fixation. Indications for surgery include the inability to achieve or maintain an adequate reduction, brachial artery injury, nerve entrapment, ipsilateral forearm fracture, multiple injuries, pathological fracture, and the delayed treatment of compound fractures following wound debridement and irrigation.

Closed reduction and percutaneous fixation

Jones[8] reported the use of closed reduction and percutaneous Kirschner wire or Steinmann pin fixation of supracondylar fractures in adults. This technique still requires a period of immobilisation, but less flexion of the elbow is necessary and vascular compromise from swelling is less of a problem. This technique requires an adequate closed reduction after which the medial and lateral columns should be stabilised. The fixation device should engage the far cortex of the bone opposite the column stabilised.

We prefer screw fixation with overdrilling of the distal fragment in order to allow compression of the fracture site. Two lateral Kirschner wires will not prevent rotational displacement. The ulnar nerve can be easily avoided if care is taken with pin or wire placement.

Open reduction and internal fixation

When closed reduction cannot be obtained or when vascular injuries are present, open reduction and internal fixation of both the medial and lateral columns with screws or hand-contoured plates and screws should be performed. This can either be undertaken through medial and lateral approaches or via a posterior approach. Contoured plates and screws are preferred when comminution of one or both columns is present. Waddell and others[9,10] have pre-contoured DuPont plates which they state can be applied solely to the lateral column if the medial column is not comminuted. Rigid internal fixation is necessary if early elbow motion is to be attempted. If open reduction is performed, the goal should be stable, rigid internal fixation; otherwise, non-operative treatment should be selected.

AUTHOR'S PREFERRED MANAGEMENT

Undisplaced and minimally displaced fractures can be immobilised with a long-arm posterior splint for 2–3 weeks, followed by active motion exercises.

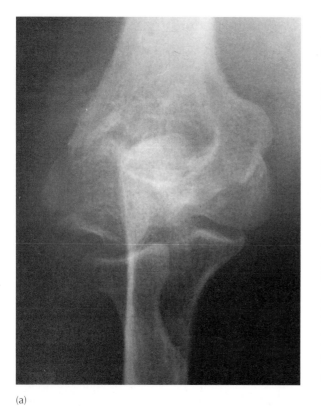

(a)

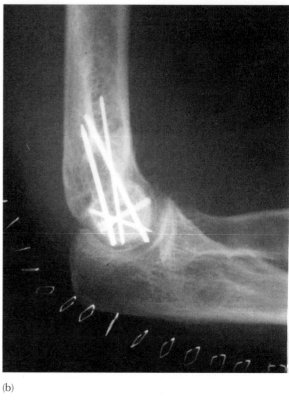

(b)

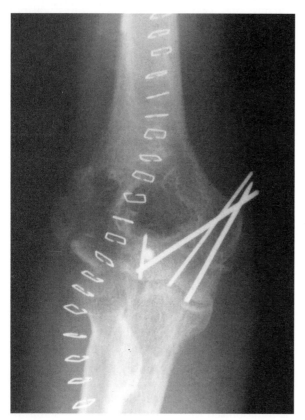

(c)

Fig. 11.2 (a) Comminuted transcondylar fracture of the distal humerus. (b) The trochlear fragment was fixed with smooth Kirschner wires left below the articular cartilage surface. (c) The wires were left prominent proximally and removed at 6 weeks. The capitellar fragment required excision. Threaded pins are preferable, as they will not migrate.

Displaced supracondylar fractures are unstable, and open reduction through a posterior approach, with rigid internal fixation using a double-plating technique is preferred. Helfet and Hotchkiss[11] have shown this to provide the most stable fixation configuration. Hand-contoured dynamic compression plates or malleable pelvic reconstruction plates fitted 90 degrees to each other on both columns are preferred, especially if comminution is present. Bone grafting can be performed at the time of initial fixation. Active exercises are started at 1–2 weeks.

Traction treatment is rarely indicated for displaced supracondylar fractures. Occasionally, a patient's overall condition or severe swelling may prevent early operative treatment. Overhead olecranon pin traction is preferred, and if the shoulder is not injured, overhead traction can be rigged to allow the patient to assume a 'chest upright' position to improve pulmonary function.

COMPLICATIONS

Non-union of supracondylar fractures fortunately is rare and primarily due to the inability to achieve stable, rigid fixation combined with insufficient immobilisation.

Malunion can result in an unsightly cubitus varus ('gun stock') deformity,[12,13] seen after supracondylar fractures in children. Cubitus valgus secondary to malunion can create ulnar nerve sensory and motor dysfunction. A normal shoulder can compensate for rotational malunion providing it is not severe. Malunion in the anteroposterior plane is well tolerated as long as a function range of motion (30–130 degrees of flexion) is maintained.

Unrecognised injuries of the brachial artery, or a delay in treatment, can lead to disasterous limb loss. The risk of compartment syndrome after open or closed reduction of supracondylar fractures is always present. Unremitting pain or numbness in the extremity should immediately alert the surgeon to this possible diagnosis and immediate corrective action, including forearm fasciotomy should be performed.

Postoperative stiffness is probably the most common complication. Prolonged immobilisation after an anatomic reduction and rigid internal fixation may result in fibrous ankylosis of the elbow. Protected early active and active-assisted motion approximately 2 weeks after surgery is preferred.

Heterotopic ossification is always a potential complication of elbow injuries, and its severity appears to be proportional to the severity of the injury.[14,15] There is some evidence to suggest that indomethacin may be useful in this situation.[16]

Transcondylar fractures

Transcondylar fractures are often grouped with supracondylar fractures, but they are rare injuries and require special consideration. The fracture line usually extends transversely across the condyles and is often intra-articular. These fractures frequently are quite unstable and unite slowly when treated conservatively. A hanging arm cast requires the elbow to be immobile. When union is delayed, elbow function is often significantly compromised. Exuberant callus in this location invariably leads to significant reduction in joint motion. These fractures can often be reduced and fixed with percutaneous threaded Steinmann pins inserted through the lateral and medial condyles into the distal humeral metaphysis (Fig. 11.2). Alternatively lag screws may be inserted through a small incision without the need for extensive dissection.

AUTHOR'S PREFERRED MANAGEMENT

Newer cannulated screw systems allow provisional pin fixation, followed by screw fixation without removal of the provisional pins. Cancellous screws can be easily inserted through the medial and lateral columns to secure the intra-articular distal fragment. The screws are placed beneath the subchondral bone surface (Fig. 11.3). This method produces suf-

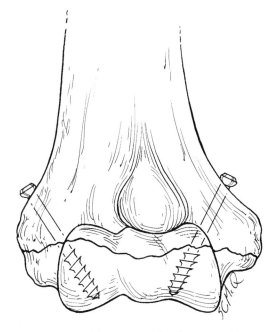

Fig. 11.3 Fixation of transcondylar fracture with 4 mm partially threaded cancellous screws.

ficient fixation for early protected motion and leads to union with more nearly normal joint mobility.

COMPLICATIONS

Transcondylar fractures are often intra-articular and may unite slowly. Longer immobilisation is therefore necessary if secure fixation is not achieved. The potential for non-union is greater if the fracture is intra-articular. Malunion of intra-articular fractures can lead to disabling post-traumatic arthritis. Failure to keep fixation devices extra-articular can also lead to severe disability.

The potential for other complications is similar to that after supracondylar fractures.

Intercondylar T and Y fractures

MECHANISM OF INJURY

As the name implies, these fractures have a component that separates the articular surface of the distal humerus between the medial and lateral condyles. They may result from a fall on the outstretched hand or a direct blow to the posterior aspect of the elbow can create this fracture pattern.[17] Bickel and Perry[18] suggested that the wedge shape of the olecranon articular surface impacting into the trochlear groove splits the condyles of the distal humerus apart. Associated soft-tissue injuries are usually significant.

Good quality anteroposterior and lateral radiographs are often sufficient to enable evaluation of this injury although in undisplaced fractures tomography may be required in order to detect the vertical component of the fracture. In displaced injuries, the fracture is usually worse than the films indicate.

CLASSIFICATION

Although Desault in 1811[19] was the first to appreciate the articular separation that occurred with this type of fracture it was not until 1936 that T and Y shaped fracture patterns were described by Reich.[20] More recently Riseborough and Radin[21] have extended the classification such that four groups based on radiographic assessment of fracture, separation, rotation, and comminution of the distal articular surface are described. These groups are:

1. undisplaced fractures extending between the capitellum and trochlea;

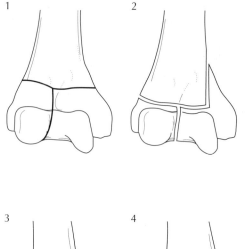

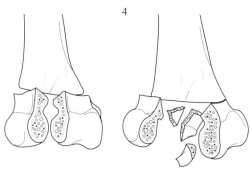

Fig. 11.4 Classification of intercondylar fractures of distal humerus. Types 2 and 3 fractures are treated by open reduction and internal fixation. Most type 4 fractures are treated non-operatively unless reconstruction is technically possible

2. displaced T or Y fractures with the fracture extending from the groove on the articular surface of the trochlea, proximally between the condyles, and the fracture line extending transversely or obliquely across the shaft. The condyles are separated from each other and from the shaft, although on the anteroposterior radiograph they do not appear appreciably rotated;
3. fractures with rotational displacement of the condyles;
4. fractures with severe comminution of the articular surface and wide separation of the condyles (Fig. 11.4).

TREATMENT OPTIONS

Non-operative treatment

Until the last 20 years or so non-operative management has been the accepted method of treatment for these difficult fractures. This has included closed reduction and immobilisation, traction, and for the severely comminuted fracture treatment as 'a bag of bones'.

Following closed reduction, immobilisation is often necessary for between 4 and 6 weeks in order to allow adequate fracture union before mobilisation is permitted. This period of immobility is often deleterious as regards the final range of elbow movement.

Traction also requires a significant period of immobilisation. It is achieved using either Dunlop or olecranon pin traction for 2 weeks following which a further 2–3 weeks immobilisation in a splint or cast is usually necessary.

Eastwood[22] advocated fracture reduction by compressive manipulation of the fracture fragments followed by collar and cuff immobilisation in flexion for the severely comminuted distal humeral fractures. Active elbow movement was permitted after 2 weeks.

Operative treatment

Miller in 1939[23] advocated blind nailing of T-shaped fractures of the distal humerus. The technique was considered to avoid additional damage to the already traumatised soft tissues. Although this procedure has little application today the development of cannulated screw systems does permit percutaneous fixation of certain fractures (or fracture components) with minimal additional soft tissue damage.

More commonly T- and Y-shaped fractures require rigid internal fixation.[24-28] This should be undertaken by firstly anatomically reconstructing the T or Y component of the fracture. Following this the reconstructed articular surface should be securely fixed to the humeral shaft by repair of the humeral columns (Fig. 11.5). Reconstruction of the articular surface is best accomplished by Kirschner wire provisional fixation, followed by permanent screw fixation. Newer cannulated screws are useful in that the screws can be simply placed over the provisional Kirschner wires. Care must be taken to avoid screw placement in the olecranon fossa, coronoid fossa, and articular surface (Fig. 11.6). If significant bone loss is present between the capitellum and trochlea a corticocancellous graft should be interposed to help reconstruct the distal articular anatomy (Fig. 11.7).

Fixation of the articular component to the humeral shaft is best accomplished by repair of both the lateral and medial columns with hand-contoured reconstruction plates fitted 90 degrees to each other. If the medial column is not severely comminuted, a rigid pre-contoured DuPont plate can be fitted to repair the lateral column (Fig. 11.8).

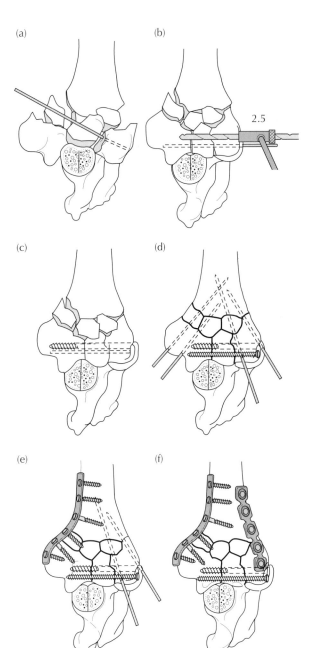

Fig. 11.5 Sequence of reconstruction of the distal humerus. (a,b,c) The articular portions are reassembled with Kirschner wire fixation followed by screw fixation. (d) Kirschner wires can then be used to provide provisional fixation of the distal humerus. (e) Hand-contoured one-third tubular plate is attached to the medial side. (f) A 3.5 pelvic reconstruction plate is applied on the posterolateral border. Redrawn after Ref. 49 with permission from Springer-Verlag, Berlin.

This device is much more rigid than either a single semi-tubular or pelvic reconstruction plate.

Once rigid fixation is achieved, active motion can be started in 1 to 2 weeks. Henley[29] reported 75%

(a)

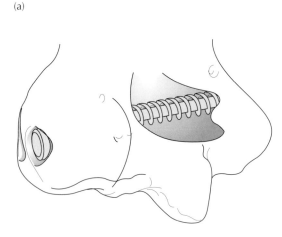

(b)

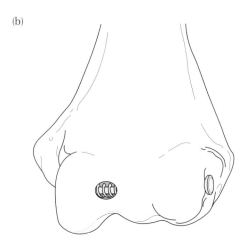

Fig. 11.6 Placement of screw across distal humerus. (a) Transverse screw across condyles of distal humerus traversing olecranon fossa would markedly restrict elbow extension. (b) Transverse screw traversing distal humeral condyles encroaching on articular surface of trochlea.

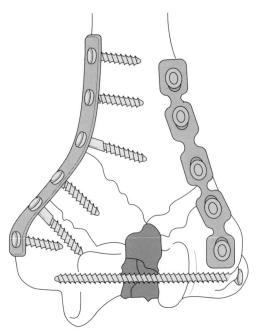

Fig. 11.7 If bone is missing in the intercondylar portion, a corticocancellous bone graft can be interposed to re-establish the anatomic proportions

good or excellent results in 33 intercondylar humeral fractures treated with open reduction and internal fixation. Letsch *et al.*[30] obtained 81% good or very good results in 104 intra-articular distal humeral fractures treated with open reduction and internal fixation. Gabel *et al.*[31] obtained 90% good or excellent results in 10 fractures fixed with dual contoured plates. These studies indicate that good results can be obtained even in selected type 4 fractures if rigid fixation is achieved using AO/ASIF principles and early postoperative rehabilitation.

In patients with gross fracture comminution Ciullo and Melanokos,[32] and Bolano[33] have used an Ilizarov type external fixator. Their early results

indicate that hinged-type distraction external fixators that allow early motion can be a good treatment option for these severe fractures (Fig. 11.9).

AUTHOR'S PREFERRED MANAGEMENT

Type 1 undisplaced fractures should be splinted at 90 degrees of elbow flexion. The splint is supported with a collar and cuff sling. An active range of motion exercises is begun at 2–3 weeks.

For minimally displaced type 2 fractures closed reduction and percutaneous cannulated screw fixation of the intercondylar and supracondylar portions of the fracture is preferred providing an anatomical reduction can be achieved. If this is not possible or the type 2 fracture is more significantly displaced open reduction and rigid internal fixation is required. This should be performed via a Campbell triceps splitting or Van Gorder posterior approach. If, however, there is concern as to the degree of articular comminution a transolecranon approach should be used (Fig. 11.10). This enables excellent visualisation of the humeral articular surfaces.

Postoperatively the arm is immobilised in a posterior splint at 90 degrees of elbow flexion with the forearm in neutral rotation for 1 to 2 weeks. An

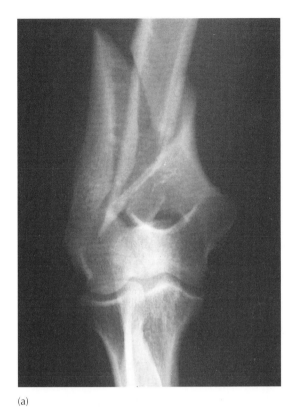

(a)

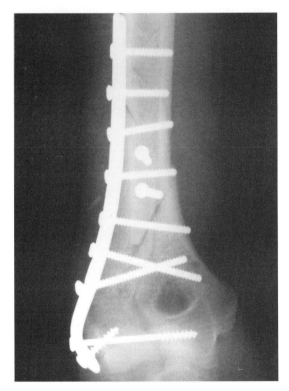

(b)

Fig. 11.8 Fixation of comminuted T-condylar humeral fracture with DuPont plate.

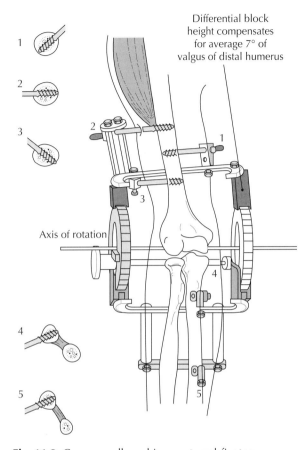

Fig. 11.9 Compass elbow hinge external fixator.

active range of motion exercises is then begun. Full extension is the most difficult to achieve. Dynamic splinting with a turnbuckle device can be useful if extension has reached a plateau at 6–8 weeks.

In type 3 fractures the condyles are rotated by the pull of the flexor and extensor muscle insertions. All of these fractures require open reduction with reconstruction of the intercondylar component of the injury and rigid internal fixation. Reconstruction of both the medial and lateral columns with hand-contoured plates is the procedure of choice. Postoperative management of type 3 fractures is similar to that for type 2 fractures.

The management of type 4 fractures must be individualised and the age and functional expectations of the patient should be considered.

Reconstruction of at least the condylar component of the injury should be attempted. If following this, rigid fixation to the humeral shaft is impossible, traction or distraction external fixation should be undertaken. Gentle early motion can be commenced while the patient is in olecranon pin traction or in a hinged distraction fixator.

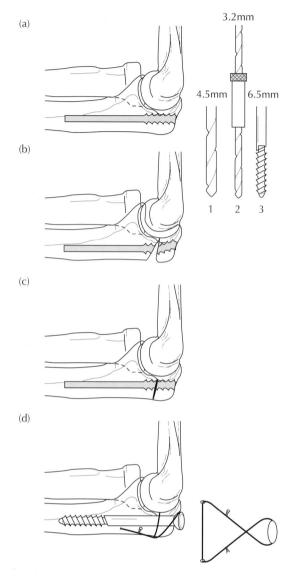

Fig. 11.10 Osteotomy of olecranon. (a) Preparation of hole for 6.5 mm cancellous screw. (b) Incomplete osteotomy made with thin saw or osteotome. (c) Osteotomy completed by cracking bone. (d) Lag screw (6.5 mm) and tension ban wire fixation. Redrawn after Ref. 50 with permission from Mosby Year-Book Inc, St Louis.

In elderly patients with limited functional ability open reduction and internal fixation is best avoided. Treatment should consist of initial immobilisation in a posterior splint or long-arm traction cast with collar and cuff sling until the fracture is stable enough to begin motion.

Compound intercondylar fractures should always be individually assessed since management is influenced by the type of wound, time of surgery, associated vascular injury and the environment in which the wound occurred. When all factors are optimal rigid internal fixation is advised for fractures associated with grade I or grade II wounds. For patients with grade III open wounds irrigation and debridement of the wound is recommended together with application of a rigid external fixator with the elbow at 90 degrees. If the condylar component of the fracture is grossly disrupted limited fixation of this part of the fracture complex may be advisable depending on the individual features of the injury. The wound should be left open and the patient returned to the operating room every 48 hours for repeated debridement until the wound is ready for closure.

In the presence of arterial injury, rapid rigid internal fixation after debridement is preferred. The elbow can then be safely extended and vascular repair performed.

COMPLICATIONS

Non-union of intercondylar fractures is rare, even in irreparable type 4 fractures treated without surgery.[34]

Malunion of the intercondylar portion of these fractures can lead to condylar malalignment, with limitation of both flexion and extension. Malunion of an articular surface can cause post-traumatic arthritis.

Postoperative stiffness is the most common complication of this injury, with full extension being the most difficult to regain. Rigid internal fixation is necessary to allow active and active-assisted motion at 1–2 weeks after surgery. Prolonged immobilisation can lead to fibrous ankylosis (Fig. 11.11). Vigorous stretching by a therapist, forced motion whether active or passive, and manipulation under anaesthesia are forbidden. Stretching and forced motion usually result in increased periarticular haemorrhage and fibrosis, increased joint irritability, and decreased rather than increased motion.

Fractures of the condyles of the humerus

Isolated fractures of the medial or lateral condyle of the humerus are uncommon in adults. Knight[35] found that fractures of a single condyle accounted for only 5% of distal humeral fractures in adults. The lateral condyle is fractured more frequently than the medial condyle.[36–38]

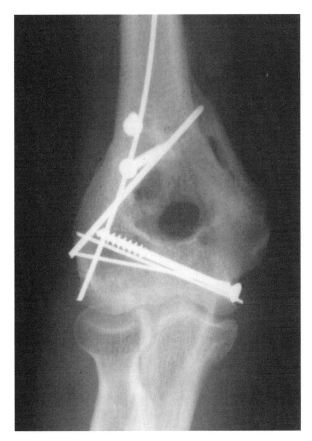

Fig. 11.11 Intercondylar humeral fracture was anatomically repaired and held in long-arm cast for 2 months. The result was a 5 degree arc of motion after months of physical therapy. Operative lysis of adhesions, triceps advancement, and extensive active exercises were necessary to overcome this near ankylosis of the joint.

MECHANISM OF INJURY

The mechanism of injury of condylar fractures of the humerus has been studied in detail by Milch.[36,37] Lateral condylar fractures result from impaction of the radial head between the capitellum and trochlea, whilst medial condylar fractures result from the longitudinal groove of the sigmoid notch of the olecranon compressing and fracturing the trochlea.

CLASSIFICATION

Milch[36,37] has classified unicondylar fractures into two types depending on whether the lateral wall of the trochlea remains attached to the humerus or is part of the fracture fragment. In type I fractures the

lateral wall of the trochlea is attached to the humerus and these injuries Milch suggested could be managed conservatively. In type II fractures the lateral wall of the trochlea is attached to the fracture fragment. Milch considered these to represent fracture dislocations since the radius and ulna displace with the fracture fragment. This type of injury requires internal fixation.

TREATMENT OPTIONS

Non-operative treatment

Undisplaced unicondylar fractures can be satisfactorily treated with splint or cast immobilisation for 4 weeks providing that the fracture is carefully monitored to exclude fracture displacement.

Displaced type I medial or lateral condylar fractures can be treated by closed manipulation and splintage. However having reduced the fracture it is preferable to hold the reduction by percutaneous screw fixation.

Operative treatment

Displaced type I fractures that cannot be anatomically reduced and all type II fractures require internal fixation. This should be undertaken either through a lateral Kocher approach (lateral condyle fracture) or via a transolecranon approach (medial condyle fracture) in order to allow adequate visualisation of the articular surfaces. Screw fixation of the fracture is usually adequate and will permit early active motion.

AUTHOR'S PREFERRED MANAGEMENT

Undisplaced type I fractures are treated non-operatively with cast immobilisation for 4 weeks together with careful supervision. Displaced type I fractures are manipulated and providing an anatomical reduction is achieved percutaneous screw fixation is undertaken. If closed reduction is unsuccessful then operative reduction and fixation is performed. All type II fractures are treated by open reduction and screw fixation.

COMPLICATIONS

Inadequate reduction or loss of fixation of displaced lateral condyle fractures may result in cubitus valgus deformity and late ulnar nerve symptoms.[38] Inadequate reduction or loss of fixation of displaced medial condyle fractures may restrict joint motion and produce a cubitus varus deformity.

Non-union or malunion of a condyle fracture may also result in elbow deformity and instability. However, as Holdsworth and Mossad[39] have shown, excellent elbow function despite deformity is likely in the presence of a unicondylar non-union. Degenerative change whilst to be expected does not usually occur until the sixth or seventh decade.[39]

Fractures of the capitellum

Fractures of the capitellum are one of the most frequent purely intra-articular fractures that occur about the elbow. They account for 6% of all fractures of the distal humerus.[40] Although the injury may occur in isolation it is more frequently seen in association with radial head fractures and posterior elbow dislocations.[41,42]

MECHANISM OF INJURY

Fractures of the capitellum usually result from a fall onto the outstretched upper extremity with the radial head impacting against the capitellum and resulting in a varying sized shear fracture. They may also occur as the result of direct elbow trauma.

CLASSIFICATION

Classification of fractures of the capitellum depends on the size of the articular fragment and its comminution. Type I is a large fragment of bone and articular cartilage; type I is a small shell of bone and articular cartilage, and type I is a comminuted fracture (Fig. 11.12).

DIAGNOSIS

The diagnosis of capitellar fractures depends on good quality lateral radiographs. Often the antero-posterior radiograph will not define the fracture particularly if it is type II and small. Small fragments lying in the superior part of the joint may be confused with fragments from the radial head although it is uncommon to find radial head fragments in this proximal position. As such therefore if a fragment lies superior to the capitellum and proximal to the radial head it will more commonly be from an anterior capitellar fracture than from a radial head fracture. Tomography sometimes is necessary for correct fracture definition.

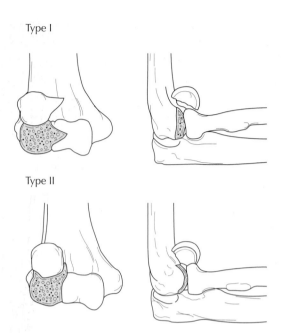

Type I

Type II

Fig. 11.12 In a type I capitellar fracture, a portion of the trochlea may be involved. In type II capitellar fractures, very little subchondral bone is attached to the capitellar fragment. There is no fracture through the lateral condyle in the sagittal plane in either type I or II fracture.

TREATMENT OPTIONS

Methods of treatment include closed reduction,[43,44] open reduction with and without internal fixation[45,46] or excision of the fragments.[44,47] Advocates of excision claim the operation is a simple definitive procedure, allows early range-of-motion exercises, avoids avascular necrosis of the fragment, and avoids non-union. Furthermore, fixation of the fragment is frequently difficult. On the other hand, advocates of open reduction and internal fixation claim that a raw, bony articulating surface is avoided and that late valgus deformity and possible instability are prevented. Closed reduction is almost never successful.

AUTHOR'S PREFERRED MANAGEMENT

Type I fractures without trochlea involvement or in older patients should be treated by excision of the fragment. If the trochlea is involved or if the fragment is large and in a young patient, open reduction and internal fixation should be performed.

A lateral approach usually is sufficient, regardless of fracture type. The joint is inspected for small pieces of cartilage and bone, then thoroughly irrigated of all

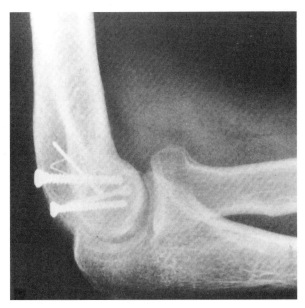

Fig. 11.13 Isolated fracture of capitellum following open reduction and internal fixation using cortical screws.

debris. When a large portion of the articular surface is displaced and the fragment contains sufficient bone to allow internal fixation, anatomic reduction and internal fixation are indicated. This can either be undertaken using small lag screws inserted from posterior to anterior or preferably using Herbert screws inserted from anterior to posterior and buried beneath the articular cartilage[48] (Fig. 11.13).

Type II and type III fractures should be treated by excision of the fragments followed by early range-of-motion exercises.

Fractures of the trochlea

Isolated fractures of the trochlea are extremely rare. Usually when present they are associated with intercondylar humeral fractures and elbow dislocations. As such treatment should be directed to the more severe injury and depending on the size of the trochlea fragment this should either be excised or reattached depending on which is the more appropriate.

References

1. Patrick J Fracture of the medial epicondyle with displacement into the elbow joint. _J Bone Joint Surg_ 1946; **28:** 143–7.
2. Horne G Supracondylar fractures of the humerus in adults. _J Trauma_ 1980; **20:** 71–4.
3. Siris IE Supracondylar fractures of the humerus. _Surg Gynecol Obstet_ 1939; **68:** 201–22.
4. Holstein A, Lewis CB Fractures of the humerus with radial nerve paralysis. _J Bone Joint Surg_ 1963; **45A:** 1382–8.
5. Packer JW, Foster RR, Garcia A, Grantham SA The humeral fracture with radial nerve palsy: is exploration warranted? _Clin Orthop_ 1972; **88:** 34–8.
6. Smith L Supracondylar fractures of the humerus treated by direct observation. _Clin Orthop_ 1967; **50:** 37–42.
7. Prietto CA Supracondylar fractures of the humerus: a comparative study of Dunlop's traction versus percutaneous pinning. _J Bone Joint Surg_ 1979; **61A:** 425–8.
8. Jones KG Percutaneous pin fixation of fractures of the lower end of the humerus. _Clin Orthop_ 1867; **50:** 53–69.
9. Waddell JP Supracondylar fractures of the humerus. _Tech Orthop_ 1986; **1:** 44.
10. Waddell JP, Hatch J, Richards RR Supracondylar fractures of the humerus: results of surgical treatment. _J Trauma_ 1988; **28:** 1615–21.
11. Helfet DL, Hotchkiss RN Internal fixation of the distal humerus: A biomechanical comparison of methods. _J Orthop Trauma_ 1990, **4:** 260–4.
12. Smith L Deformity following supracondylar fractures of the humerus. _J Bone Joint Surg_ 1960; **42A:** 235–52.
13. D'Ambrosia RD Supracondylar fractures of the humerus - prevention of cubitus varus. _J Bone Joint Surg_ 1972; **54A:** 60–6.
14. Buxton St JD Ossification in the ligaments of the elbow joint. _J Bone Joint Surg_ 1938; **20:** 709–14.
15. Thompson HC III, Garcia A Myositis ossificans: aftermath of elbow injuries. _Clin Orthop_ 1967; **50:** 129–34.
16. Ritter MA, Gioe JJ The effect of indomethacin on para-articular ectopic ossification following total hip arthroplasty. _Clin Orthop_ 1982; **167:** 113–7.
17. Helfet DL Bicondylar intraarticular fractures of the distal humerus in adults: their assessment, classification and operative management. _Adv Orthop Surg_ 1985; **8:** 223–35.
18. Bickel WH, Perry RE Comminuted fractures of the distal humerus. _J Am Med Assoc_ 1963; **184:** 553–7.
19. Desault PJ _A treatise on fractures, luxations and other affections of the bones_ (2nd edn). Philadelphia: Kimber and Conrad, 1811.
20. Reich RS Treatment of intercondylar fractures of the elbow by means of traction. _J Bone Joint Surg_ 1936; **18:** 997–1004.
21. Riseborough EJ, Radin EL Intercondylar T fractures of the humerus in the adult: A comparison of operative and non-operative treatment in twenty-nine cases. _J Bone Joint Surg_ 1969; **51A:** 130–41.
22. Eastwood WJ The T-shaped fracture of the lower end of the humerus. _J Bone Joint Surg_ 1937; **19:** 364–9.
23. Miller OL Blind nailing of the T fracture of the lower end of the humerus which involves the joint. _J Bone Joint Surg_ 1939; **21:** 933–8.

24. Cassebaum WH Operative treatment of T and Y fractures of the lower end of the humerus. *Am J Surg* 1952; **83:** 265–70.
25. Kelly RP, Griffin TW Open reduction of T-condylar fractures of the humerus through an anterior approach. *J Trauma* 1969; **9:** 901–14.
26. Cassebaum WH Open reduction of T and Y fractures of the lower end of the humerus. *J Trauma* 1969; **9:** 915–25.
27. Johansson H, Olerud S Operative treatment of intercondylar fractures of the humerus. *J Trauma* 1971; **11:** 836–43.
28. Bryan RS, Bickel WH 'T' condylar fractures of the distal humerus. *J Trauma* 1971; **11:** 830–5.
29. Henley MB Intra-articular distal humeral fractures in adults. *Orthop Clin North Am* 1987; **18:** 11–23.
30. Letsch R, Schmit-Neuerburg KP, Sturmer KM, Walz M Intraarticular fractures of the distal humerus: surgical treatment and results. *Clin Orthop* 1989; **241:** 238–44.
31. Gabel GT, Hanson G, Bennett JB, Noble PC, Tullos HS Intraarticular fractures of the distal humerus in the adult. *Clin Orthop* 1987; **216:** 99–108.
32. Ciullo JV Melanokos AE Hinged external fixation of the elbow: A salvage procedure. Presented at the 61st Annual Meeting of the American Academy of Orthopaedic Surgeons, New Orleans, Louisiana, 24 February–1 March, 1994.
33. Bolano LE Ilizarov Hinge/distraction external fixation of the elbow: an adjunct to post traumatic reconstruction. Presented at the 61st Annual Meeting of the American Academy of Orthopaedic Surgeons, New Orleans, Louisiana, 24 February–1 March, 1994.
34. Ackermann G, Jupiter JB Non-union of fractures of the distal end of the humerus. *J Bone Joint Surg* 1988; **70A:** 75–83.
35. Knight RA Fractures of the humeral condyles in adults. *South Med J* 1955; **48:** 1165–73.
36. Milch H Fractures and fracture-dislocations of the humeral condyles. *J Trauma* 1964; **4:** 592–607.
37. Milch H Fractures of the external humeral condyle. *J Am Med Assoc* 1956; **160:** 641–6.
38. Jupiter JB, Neff U, Regazzoni P, Allgower M Unicondylar fracture of the distal humerus. An operative approach. *J Orthop Trauma* 1988; **2:** 102–9.
39. Holdsworth BJ, Mossad MM Fractures of the adult distal humerus. Elbow function after internal fixation. *J Bone Joint Surg* 1990; **72B:** 362–5.
40. Knight RA The management of fractures about the elbow in adults. In: *American Academy of Orthopaedic Surgeons: Instructional Course Lectures* Vol. 14. Ann Arbor: JW Edward, 1957: 123.
41. Alvarez E, Patel MR, Nimberg G, Pearlman HS Fracture of the humeri capitellum. *J Bone Joint Surg* 1975; **57A:** 1093–6.
42. Dushuttle R, Coyle M, Zawadsky J, Bloom H Fractures of the capitellum. *J Trauma* 1985; **25:** 317–21.
43. Nicholson JT Compound comminuted fractures involving the elbow joint. *J Bone Joint Surg* 1946; **28:** 565–75.
44. Lansinger O, Mare K Fractures of the humeri capitellum. *Acta Orthop Scand* 1981; **52:** 39–44.
45. Milch H Unusual fracture of the capitulum humeri and capitellum radii. *J Bone Joint Surg* 1931; **13:** 882–6.
46. Collert S Surgical management of fracture of the capitulum humeri. *Acta Orthop Scand* 1977; **48:** 603–6.
47. Fowles JV, Kassab MT Fractures of the capitulum humeri: treatment by excision. *J Bone Joint Surg* 1974; **56A:** 794–8.
48. Simpson LA, Richard RR Internal fixation of a capitellar fracture using Herbert screws. A case report. *Clin Orthop* 1986; **209:** 166–8.
49. Heim U, Pfieffer KM *Internal fixation of small fractures* (3rd edn) Berlin: Springer-Verlag, 1986.
50. Crenshaw AH Fractures of the shoulder girdle, arm, and forearm. In: *Campbell's operative orthopaedics* (8th edn). St Louis: Mosby Year Book Inc, 1992.

CHAPTER 12

Fractures of the proximal ulna and proximal radius in adults

AH CRENSHAW JR

Fractures of the olecranon

Fractures of the olecranon in adults are comparable with those of the patella; when the fragments are separated, open reduction and internal fixation is usually necessary. The only occasional exception to this approach is an olecranon fracture in an elderly patient with low functional demands.[1] In this situation conservative treatment with early active movements can often be instituted. For the majority when surgery is performed reduction must be exact, since any residual irregularity of the articular surface will cause limited motion, delayed recovery, and post-traumatic arthritis. The fixation should be strong enough to allow gentle active exercises even before there is radiographic evidence of complete union.

MECHANISM OF INJURY

Fractures of the olecranon may be caused by either direct trauma such as a fall onto the tip of the elbow or by indirect trauma following a fall onto a partially flexed elbow. In this situation indirect forces generated by the triceps muscle avulse the olecranon.

CLINICAL PRESENTATION

Patients who sustain olecranon fractures usually present with a painful swollen elbow supported by the unaffected arm or a makeshift sling. If the fracture has been caused by direct trauma there may be grazing or a laceration over the tip of the elbow. A careful neurological examination should be performed with particular reference to the ulnar nerve because of its close proximity to the olecranon. In addition the vascular status of the arm should be carefully assessed. Anteroposterior and lateral radiographs should be performed in order to determine the complexity of the fracture.

CLASSIFICATION OF OLECRANON FRACTURES

Colton in 1973[2] proposed a classification of adult olecranon fractures which he stated could be used

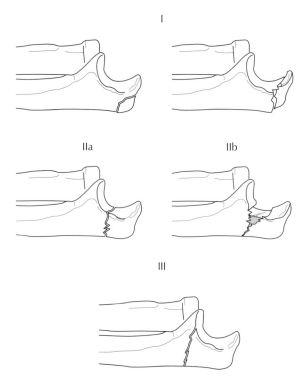

I

IIa   IIb

III

Fig. 12.1 Classification of olecranon fractures based on extent of articular involvement (see text). Redrawn after Ref. 54 with permission from Mosby Year-Book, St Louis.

as a basis for treatment. The classification is still widely used and consists of four groups (Fig. 12.1):

Avulsion group

In this group a transverse fracture line separates a small proximal fragment of the olecranon process from the rest of the ulna. The fracture may be undisplaced or distracted by the pull of the triceps muscle.

Oblique group

The fracture in this group begins near the deepest part of the trochlear notch and passes to the subcutaneous surface of the ulna. Varying degrees of comminution may be present.

Fracture dislocation (Monteggia) group

The olecranon fracture occurs at or fractionally proximal to the level of the tip of the coronoid process. This results in a plane of instability through the fracture and radio humeral joint producing a fracture dislocation of the elbow.

Unclassified group

This group includes severely comminuted fractures of the olecranon process which may also be associated with distal humeral and radial and ulna shaft fractures. The injury is usually the result of high energy trauma.

TREATMENT OPTIONS

Non-operative treatment

Although the majority of olecranon fractures require operative treatment a small number can be treated non-operatively. Within this group are patients with undisplaced olecranon fractures who can be treated with a long-arm posterior splint for between 2 and 3 weeks followed by early protected motion. These patients must be carefully supervised to be certain the fracture does not displace.

Elderly patients with low functional demands can also be treated conservatively. These patients should be provided with a sling and allowed to mobilise the elbow as comfort allows. Early active movement should be encouraged.

Operative treatment

Several operative procedures are available for the treatment of olecranon fractures. The most commonly used are:

1. open reduction and fixation with a figure-of-8 wire loop;[2,3]
2. intramedullary fixation;[2,4]
3. hand-contoured plate and screws;[3,5]
4. external fixation;[6]
5. excision of the proximal fragment.[7,8]

The choice of technique depends upon the nature and location of the fracture, the amount of comminution, and the bone stock of the patient. Advocates of fracture reduction and fixation claim that this method provides an anatomic reduction of the bony fragment and a congruous articular surface. Rigid fixation allows early movement; elbow stability is preserved and the extensor power of the triceps muscle is maintained. Advocates of excision of the olecranon fragment claim that by so doing the possibility of an incongruous articular surface is eliminated since the fragment is removed. In addition, fixation device failure cannot occur and no fixation device requires subsequent removal. Excision of the fragment does not impair elbow stability or extensor power, and the operation permits the institution of early elbow motion.

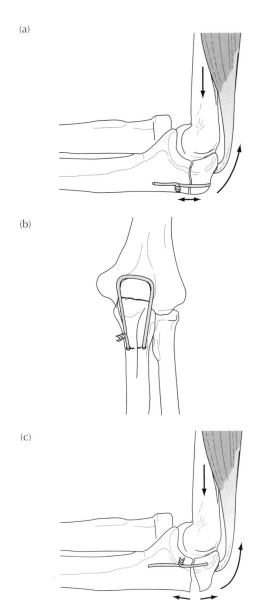

Fig. 12.2 (a,b) Simple loop is not as satisfactory as figure-of-8 loop for fixing fracture of the olecranon. (c) It is insufficient when its long axis is in or is anterior to the long axis of the olecranon. Redrawn after Ref. 55 with permission.

The indications, principles of fixation and biomechanical advantages of the operative methods are discussed for each treatment type.

Open reduction and fixation with a figure-of-8 wire loop

This method of fixation is applicable to fractures of the olecranon that are not comminuted and that are well proximal to the coronoid process. The technique is most commonly used for avulsion and transverse fractures and is usually combined with intramedullary fixation in comminuted fractures and fracture-dislocations. A simple loop is not as satisfactory as a figure-of-8 loop (Fig. 12.2a,b). The tension surface of the bone is the superficial surface, and a figure-of-8 wire placed on this surface produces compression along the olecranon fracture line with the trochlea functioning as a fulcrum. If a simple wire loop is used, particularly when it is anterior to the axis of the olecranon, the pull of the triceps will tend to separate the fragments posteriorly (Fig. 12.2c) and tilting of the proximal fragment will result in limited extension. Use of the tension band principle requires early active motion of the elbow so that compression across the fracture line can occur (Fig. 12.3). When using this method it is important to place the figure-of-8 wire loop between the deep surface of the triceps and the olecranon. If the wire loop is superficial to the triceps active motion of the elbow will produce loosening of the fixation.

Biomechanically fixation using a figure-of-8 tension band provides secure fixation for non-comminuted olecranon fractures.[9] The wiring technique should be performed in classical AO fashion using two tightening knots (Fig. 12.4).[10]

Wolfgang et al.[11] reported good or excellent results in 29 of 30 displaced olecranon fractures fixed with medullary Kirschner wires and tension band wiring using AO principles. They noted migration in only two fractures.

Intrameduallary fixation

Intramedullary fixation has been used for simple transverse and oblique fractures and also for comminuted olecranon fractures. Most frequently screws or threaded pins have been used and at times a figure-of-8 tension band wire has also been added.[2,4,12] The problem with the technique is that adequate fixation may not be obtained proximally and the screw thread may not engage sufficiently in the distal fragment to prevent distraction at the fracture site by the pull of the triceps muscle. In addition with comminuted fractures care must be exercised to avoid diminishing the articular arch of the olecranon.[13]

A biomechanical analysis by Murphy et al.[14] found that a long medullary 6.5 mm AO cancellous screw combined with a 16–gauge figure-of-8 wire was stronger than a screw or figure-of-8 wire fixation alone (Fig. 12.5). Clinical evaluation of 37 fractures treated by open reduction and several methods of internal fixation showed superior results with this technique. By contrast Fyfe et al.[9]

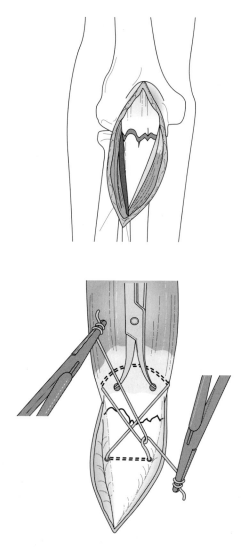

Fig. 12.3 Repair of fracture of the olecranon by wire loop. Wire is passed through hole drilled in distal fragment and through triceps aponeurosis adjacent to bone. Figure-of-8 loop adds stability to the fracture and prevents distraction and posterior bowing. Redrawn after Ref. 54 with permission from Mosby Year-Book, St Louis.

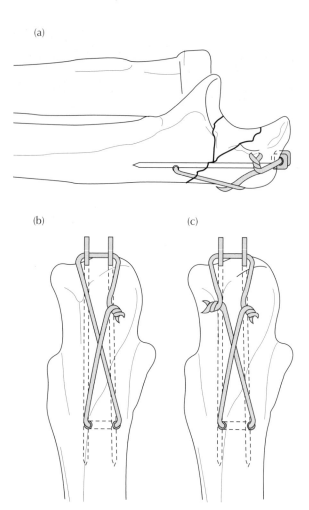

(a)

(b)   (c)

Fig. 12.4 Weber–Vasey traction-absorption wiring technique for olecranon. (a) Side view. (b) Posterior view. (c) Double twist modification of wiring suggested by Weber. Modified from Ref. 2 with permission.

found tension band wiring stronger than screw fixation combined with a figure-of-8 wire unless the fracture was such as to allow compression of the fracture surfaces. In this situation the screw and wire technique was preferable.

Plate fixation

Fractures with marked comminution are difficult to treat using a tension band wire since the compression that the device produces is likely to produce shortening of the olecranon. In this situation the use

of a hand contoured semi-tubular plate and screws will provide rigid fixation[3] (Fig. 12.6). The plate should be contoured such that proximally it curves around the olecranon and fits snugly to the posterior surface of the bone. In the region of the articular surface the plate holding screws should be unicortical. Bone graft may be added if there are any bony defects.

On rare occasions with severe comminution of the mid-portion of the olecranon process a satisfactory reconstruction may be impossible. For these cases Barford advised excision of the comminuted section with the formation of a shortened olecranon with a radius of curvature consistent with that of the trochlear.[2] This reconstruction is technically difficult and as such it is always better to err on the side of making the radius of the notch too large rather

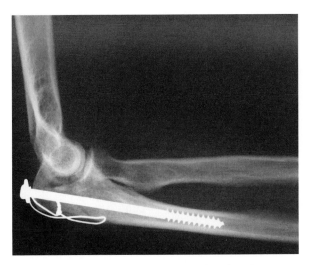

Fig. 12.5 Olecranon fracture repaired with a long 6.5-mm AO cancellous screw and figure-of-8 tension-band wire loop. Screw must engage cortex of diaphysis of ulna.

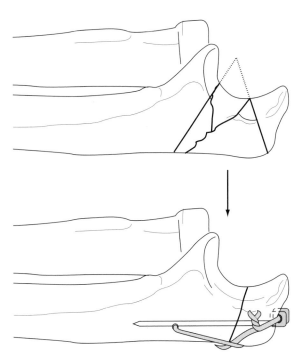

Fig. 12.7 Technique of excision of central third of olecranon process, as described by Barford.

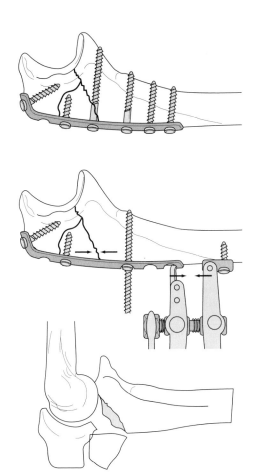

Fig. 12.6 Plate fixation can be used to stabilise comminuted fracture of the olecranon. (Redrawn after Ref. 56 with permission from Springer-Verlag, Berlin.)

than too small. Fixation of the reconstructed olecranon may be undertaken using intramedullary Kirschner wires and a figure-of-8 tension band wire (Fig. 12.7) or by the use of a contoured semi-tubular plate.

Biomechanical studies undertaken by Fyfe *et al.*[9] and Horner *et al.*[15] have shown that semi-tubular plates provide more rigid fixation of olecranon fractures than tension band wiring or intramedullary devices.

External fixation

The use of external fixation in the management of open and closed olecranon fractures has been reported by Burghele and Serban.[6] The technique involves the transverse passage of Kirschner wires through the proximal and distal olecranon fragments. These are then connected externally producing a frame fixator. Elbow movement is permitted after 2–3 days and the reported clinical results are excellent. External fixation of fractures is, however, associated with a risk of pin track infections and since these pins are placed in close proximity to the elbow joint the risk of intra-articular sepsis must always be borne in mind if this method of fracture fixation is undertaken.

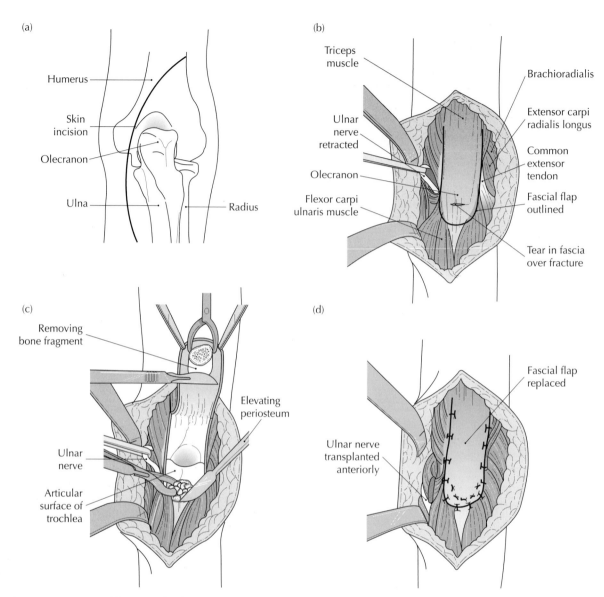

Fig. 12.8 Excision of fragment for fracture of the olecranon process. (a) With the arm across the chest skin incision is shown. (b) U-shaped flap of triceps aponeurosis to be turned proximally. (c) Fragment of bone is excised by sharp dissection, and distal fragment is reshaped. (d) With the elbow held in extension; (f) aponeurosis is sutured. The elbow is immobilised in moderate flexion.

Excision of proximal fragment

Excision of the proximal fragment eliminates the risk of fracture non-union and minimises the possibility of post-traumatic arthritis resulting from irregularity of the articular surface.[7,8] Effective function of the elbow, however, is dependant on secure anchorage of the triceps tendon to the distal fragment. The technique can only be used when enough of the olecranon is left to form a stable base for the trochlea. Thus it is not indicated when a comminuted fracture extends as far distally as the coronoid process. Even when used correctly, the method may be criticised because the elbow is less efficient without the proximal end of the ulna and because the olecranon projection of the posterior aspect of the elbow joint is lost. McKeever and Buck[7] introduced this form of treatment and advocated it for old ununited fractures, fractures that were extensively comminuted, fractures in the very elderly, and any fracture not involving the trochlea notch. They stated that up to 80% of the olecranon could be excised without appreciably affecting the stability of the elbow joint (Fig. 12.8). MacAusland and Wyman[16] have also advocated excision of the olecranon if the fracture is an isolated injury; however, they note that, in the presence of any evidence of injury to the anterior bony or soft tissue structures, excision of the olecranon is contraindicated for fear of producing elbow instability. They have stated that the entire olecranon process can be excised if the coronoid and the anterior structures are undamaged. Gartsman *et al.*[17] have found that excision of even large fragments of the olecranon with repair of the triceps results in 20% fewer operative complications than open reduction and internal fixation techniques.

It is essential that the anterior structures of the elbow joint be intact. If the coronoid is fractured or severe soft tissue injury is present, excision of the olecranon will result in elbow instability.

Since the ulnar nerve can be more easily traumatised after excision of the olecranon, McKeever and Buck,[7] as well as MacAusland and Wyman,[16] recommend anterior transposition of the nerve at the time of olecranon excision.

AUTHOR'S PREFERRED MANAGEMENT

Undisplaced olecranon fractures are treated with a long-arm posterior splint for 2 weeks followed by early protected motion.

Fractures involving the proximal tip of the olecranon are best treated by excision or tension-band wiring.

Simple transverse and oblique fractures should be treated by either an intramedullary 6.5 mm cancellous screw plus tension-band wiring or intramedullary Kirschner wires plus tension-band wiring. Combinations of Kirschner wires and screws are used if the major fracture line is oblique. Oblique fractures are also easily treated with a cancellous 6.5 mm screw plus a tension-band wire. Both limbs of the tension-band wire are twisted, as suggested by Weber, to give more even compression at the fracture site (Fig. 12.4 c).

If following a comminuted olecranon fracture the articular surface can be reconstructed fixation using a hand-contoured semi-tubular plate and screws applied to the posterior surface of the bone should be undertaken. Supplementary interfragmentary fixation with screws or Kirschner wires can also be used if necessary. Where fracture comminution makes reconstruction impossible a Barford procedure (Fig. 12.7) is preferable to excision of the olecranon.

Excision of the olecranon is recommended only in the following circumstances:

1. severely comminuted fractures in which open reduction and internal fixation is not technically possible;
2. non-articular fractures;
3. failed previous open reduction and internal fixation;
4. non-unions;
5. when treatment is delayed 10–14 days;
6. in severe open fractures or when local soft tissue conditions are precarious – in such instances the subcutaneous location of the internal fixation devices might present a problem.

Damage severe enough to the olecranon that leaves more than 50% of the articular surface and supporting bone unreconstructable has probably damaged anterior structures sufficiently to cause elbow instability if the proximal olecranon is excised. Excision can always be performed later when the anterior structures have healed.

Once rigid internal fixation has been performed, or the olecranon fragment excised and the triceps muscle reattached, a posterior long arm splint is applied for between 1 and 2 weeks. Following this active guarded motion is commenced.

Compound olecranon fractures, providing the wound is small and fracture not contaminated, are best treated by debridement, irrigation and rigid internal fixation using intrameduallary Kirschner wires and tension band wiring. More severe compound wounds require debridement, irrigation and return to surgery at 48 hours for delayed fracture fixation and wound closure. In all cases the original compound wound should be left open and closed as a delayed procedure. If available, external fixation may be an appropriate alternative option.

COMPLICATIONS

Loss of elbow range of movement is a common complication of olecranon fractures. Flexion is rarely reduced but some loss of extension may occur in between 50% and 75% of patients.[18,19] Between 81% and 94% lose less than 30 degrees[19,20] and thus functional disability is uncommon. Eriksson *et al.*[18] noted that only 3% of patients were consciously aware of restricted movement.

A 10% incidence of ulnar neuropathy has been reported following olecranon fractures.[18] This may result from direct damage to the nerve or its blood supply at the time of the fracture, poor surgical technique or postoperative scarring.

Following olecranon fractures there is a risk of post-traumatic degenerative arthritis occurring within the elbow joint. Helm *et al.*[13] had a 2% incidence following internal fixation whilst others have reported an incidence of 20%.[17,20] Inadequate fracture reduction and the severity of the fracture are factors more likely to be associated with degenerative change.

Non-union has been reported in up to 5% of olecranon fractures.[21] Where possible simple excision and triceps advancement should be undertaken and would be expected to give good results.[22] At times revision surgery with rewiring or replating together with bone grafting may be more appropriate.

Problems with the internal fixation device such as a painful subcutaneous location may also occur. Olecranon bursitis is a common problem secondary to the proximal ends of Kirschner wires or large screw heads. Tapping bent-over Kirschner wires deeply into the bone or making sure screw heads are placed beneath the triceps tendon can eliminate this problem. The twisted ends of wire loops should be kept on either side of the proximal ulna and never left directly over the posterior surface. If symptoms are persistent removal of the fixation device should be undertaken once the fracture has united.

Fractures of the coronoid process of the ulna

CLASSIFICATION

The largest reported series of coronoid process fractures is that by Regan and Morrey.[23] They reviewed 35 patients with this fracture and from their assessment of the radiographs advocated the following classification:

Type I - avulsion of the tip of the process (14 cases).
Type II - fracture of 50% or less of the process (16 cases)
Type III - fracture of more than 50% of the process (5 cases)

A total of 28% of type I fractures were found to be associated with dislocations of the elbow compared with 37% of type II and 80% of type III injuries.

TREATMENT

Regan and Morrey[23] advised treatment of coronoid process fractures based on their fracture classification:

Type I fractures

These fractures are managed in association with other injuries to the elbow. Thus if the elbow has been dislocated, the dislocation is treated and the type I coronoid process fracture is managed conservatively.

Type II fractures

Providing the elbow is stable early motion of the elbow is advised. If the elbow is unstable Regan and Morrey advocate the use of a distraction external fixation device until the soft tissues heal.

Type III fractures

These injuries are usually unstable and should be managed using a distraction external fixation device.

The results of treatment as might be expected are more successful for type I injuries and least successful for type III injuries.

Fractures of the head and neck of the radius

Fractures of the head and neck of the radius are common injuries and account for approximately one-third of all elbow fractures.[24] They occur at any age but most frequently are seen during the fourth decade of life.

MECHANISM OF INJURY TO RADIAL HEAD AND NECK

Most radial head fractures result from a fall onto the outstretched hand with the elbow partially flexed and the forearm pronated. Occasionally they follow direct trauma.

CLINICAL PRESENTATION

At presentation patients have a painful swollen elbow which becomes more painful on forearm rotation. At times particularly if the fracture is comminuted crepitus may be detected on pronation and supination. Confirmation of the diagnosis can often be made on anteroposterior and lateral radiographs, although sometimes the only abnormality visible may be elevation of the fat pads in the presence of a haemarthrosis. In this situation radial head oblique views should be undertaken in order to reveal the fracture (Chapter 5).

CLASSIFICATION

Although several classifications have been suggested based on the amount of fracture fragments displacement or comminution of the radial head,[25,26] the most useful classification is that proposed by Mason.[24] This classifies radial head fractures into three types (Fig. 12.9):

Type I - undisplaced segmental (Marginal) fracture
Type II - displaced segmental fracture
Type III - comminuted fracture.

A type IV fracture has been added to this classification and consists of a comminuted fracture together with dislocation of the elbow. The classification is of value since it gives a guide to treatment and prognosis.

TREATMENT OPTIONS

Non-operative treatment

Undisplaced or minimally displaced fractures of the head of the radius can be successfully treated non-operatively. Aspiration of the elbow to remove the haemarthrosis is effective in reducing pain and should be performed soon after injury whenever possible. Fleetcroft[27] found the long-term results permanently improved following aspiration of the joint whereas Holdsworth *et al.*[28] whilst confirming the improvement in pain relief were unable to show any difference in long-term results in those undergoing elbow aspiration compared with those not having this treatment.

Following aspiration a collar and cuff sling may be required for 7–10 days but the patient should be encouraged during this period to begin active elbow movements.

Operative treatment

Several operative procedures have been advocated for the treatment of radial head fractures:

1. excision of the fracture fragment;[29,30]
2. excision of the radial head;[24,31]
3. open reduction and internal fixation;[32,33,34]
4. insertion of a radial head prosthesis.[35,36]

Excision of the fracture fragment

For displaced segmental fractures of the radial head excision of the fracture fragment has been advocated.[30] This can be undertaken through a lateral Kocher incision.

Excision of the radial head

In adults excision of the radial head rather than excision of the fracture fragment has been advised when the fragment involves more than one-third of the articular surface, or when the fracture fragment is displaced by more than 3 mm. In addition, excision should be undertaken for severely comminuted radial head fractures or if there are multiple loose fragments within the joint. It should also be considered in patients with restricted forearm rotation.

The timing of surgery remains controversial and although the consensus opinion would be for early radial head excision[24,37,38] (1–14 days), some have suggested it is preferable to allow the acute injury to settle prior to operative treatment. Surgery should be performed through a lateral Kocher incision.

Open reduction and internal fixation

The advent of mini AO screw fixation systems and more recently the Herbert screw[32,33] has enabled radial head fractures that would previously have

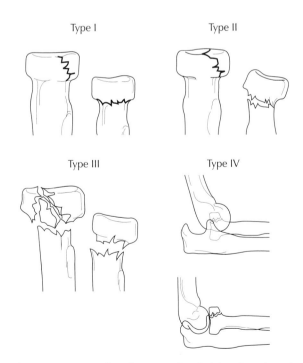

Fig. 12.9 Mason classification of radial head and neck fractures. Redrawn after Ref. 57 with permission.

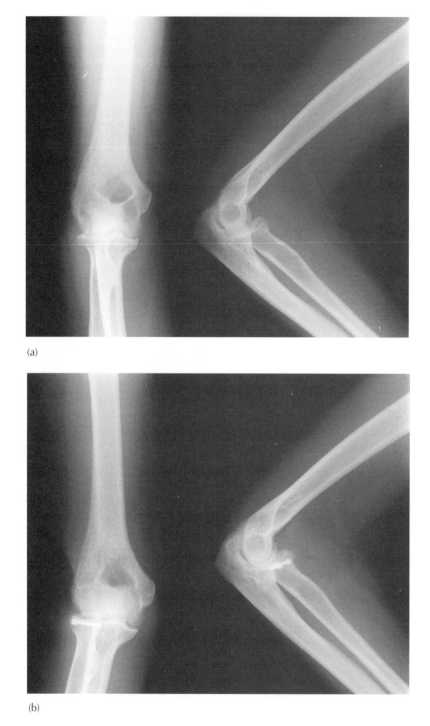

(a)

(b)

Fig. 12.10 Fixation of a radial head fracture using Herbert screws. (a) The initial injury is seen to be a type II fracture. (b) Following fixation an anatomical reconstruction has been obtained.

required excision to be reduced and internally fixed (Fig. 12.10). This technique is most appropriate for anterolateral radial head fractures since this part of the head clearly presents itself when a lateral Kocher approach to the elbow is performed. In addition this segment does not articulate with the ulna at the proximal radioulnar joint. Reconstruction of comminuted radial head fractures has been advocated[39] although technically this is significantly more demanding.

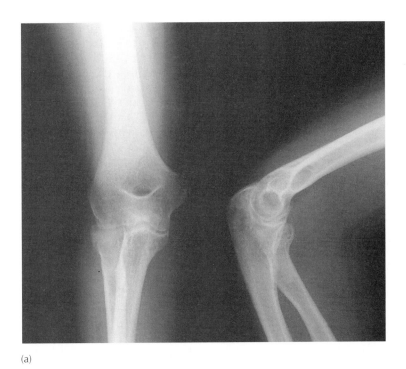

(a)

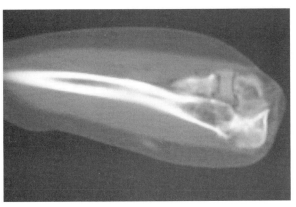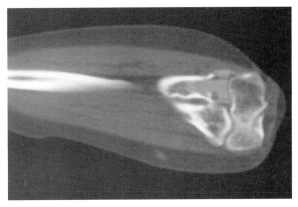

(b)

Fig. 12.11 A radial head arthroplasty was inserted in this case when reconstruction proved impossible. (a) Radiography (anteroposterior and lateral). (b) CT scan.

Insertion of a radial head prosthesis

This technique was popularised by Swanson *et al.*[36] using silicone implants. It can be useful for the treatment of comminuted radial head fractures in the presence of elbow instability (Fig. 12.11). Surgery should be performed through a lateral Kocher incision. A titanium implant available from Wright Medical avoids silicone particle synovitis.

AUTHOR'S PREFERRED MANAGEMENT

The management of radial head fractures should be determined by a careful analysis of the radiographs. In addition, aspiration and infiltration of the radio humeral joint with local anaesthetic followed by assessment of the arc of pronation and supination may also be valuable. MacAusland and Wyman[16] suggest that, if 70 degrees of active pronation and

(a)

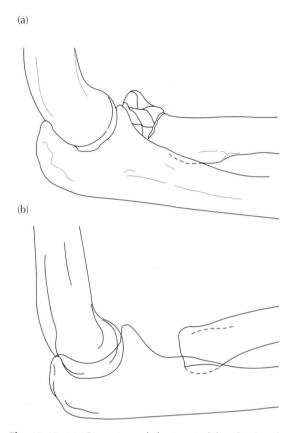

(b)

Fig. 12.12 (a) Comminuted fracture of head of radius involving articular surface. (b) After excision. Many fractures of this type are followed by proliferative changes with subsequent limitation of motion, especially if excision of radial head is delayed.

70 degrees of active supination are obtainable, surgery should not be performed, regardless of what is seen on the radiographs.

When the radial head fracture is comminuted, or forearm rotation significantly limited, excision of the head of the radius is usually the treatment of choice (Fig. 12.12). The procedure should be done early, preferably within the first 24–48 hours, and will usually result in a useful but rarely normal elbow.

Isolated large uncomminuted fractures of the radial head can be treated by open reduction and fixations with a mini AO screw or Herbert screw.[32–34]

In the absence of an elbow dislocation or ligamentous injury radial head fractures that require excision are not usually associated with postoperative elbow joint instability, significant cubitus valgus, proximal displacement of the radius or distal radioulnar joint abnormality. A few patients complain of weakness in the extremity and mild discomfort in the distal radioulnar joint with heavy activities, but these are not sufficiently common or of sufficient magnitude to suggest the routine use of a spacer type of radial head replacement prosthesis. Coleman *et al.*[40] found good functional results with no deterioration over time in their long-term follow-up of 17 patients who underwent excision of the radial head for isolated fractures.

One exception to total excision at the initial operation is the association of a fracture of the head of the radius with a dislocation of the elbow and fracture of the coronoid process. In this situation the elbow is extremely unstable, and, if the head is totally excised, the elbow will probably redislocate. Thus in these type IV fracture-dislocations, the status of the coronoid process should be used to determine how to treat the radial head fracture. If the coronoid process is intact and the radial head fracture is displaced, the dislocation should be reduced and the radial head fracture treated by early excision of the head. If the coronoid process is fractured and is a large intact fragment, open reduction and internal fixation of the coronoid fragment should be performed and the radial head excised. If the coronoid process is fractured and is comminuted, reduction of the elbow should be undertaken but excision of the radial head delayed until the coronoid process fracture and soft tissues have healed. This will usually require 3–6 months. In such circumstances inserting a radial head prosthesis may salvage some degree of elbow stability if none of the radial head can be preserved.

The results of partial excision of the head of the radius are poorer than those of total excision and therefore this is not recommended.

COMPLICATIONS

Loss of full extension and decreased pronation and supination are the most common complications of radial head fractures.

The valgus carrying angle increases after radial head excision by on average 8 degrees.[29] This, however, is not associated with elbow instability providing that the ulnar collateral ligament is intact.[41] Instability does, however, occur if the radial head is excised in the presence of an unrecognised ulnar collateral ligament injury.[41]

Proximal migration of the radius occurs commonly after radial head excision although the amount of migration is often small (2–3 mm).[38,42,43] The relationship of this complication to wrist symptoms is variable.

Heterotopic ossification and proximal radioulnar synostosis are rare complications and are associated with severe elbow trauma and delayed radial head excision.

The complications of radial head arthroplasties are similar to those seen with silastic joints at other sites.[44] Synovitis[45] and implant failure,[46,47] both of which require removal of the arthroplasty, occur most frequently.

Fractures of the neck of the radius

Fractures of the neck of the radius are classified into types I, II, and II in a fashion similar to fractures of the radial head as described by Mason.[24] Ebraheim *et al.*[48] described repair of the displaced radial head to the intact radial neck using a small T-plate and 2.7 mm screws as an alternative to radial head excision in unstable elbow fracture-dislocations. Long oblique neck fractures can be repaired with small cortical screws using an interfragmentary technique (Fig. 12.13).

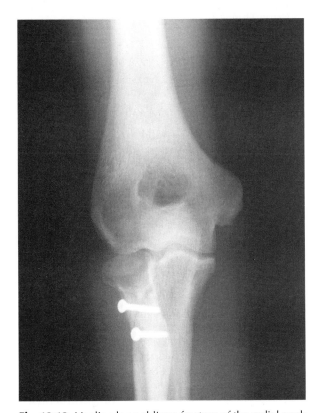

Fig. 12.13 Healing long oblique fracture of the radial neck fixed with 3.5-mm cortical screws using interfragmentary technique. Pronation and supination arc is almost normal.

Essex–Lopresti fracture-dislocations

A severe fall on the outstretched hand can result in a fracture of the radial head or neck, disruption of the distal radioulnar joint, and tearing of the interosseous membrane for a considerable distance proximally (Fig. 12.14). The tethering effect of the proximal-radial oriented fibres of the interosseous membrane is lost and if the radial head is resected, rapid proximal migration of the radius can occur. This can result in wrist pain because of ulna–carpal impingement and elbow pain because of radiocapitellar impingement. Late reconstruction once migration has occurred is unsatisfactory. Disruption of the distal radioulnar joint must be recognised early before radial migration occurs. Pain at the distal radioulnar joint in conjuction with a displaced fracture of the radial head or neck should alert the surgeon to the possibility of this injury combination. Open reduction

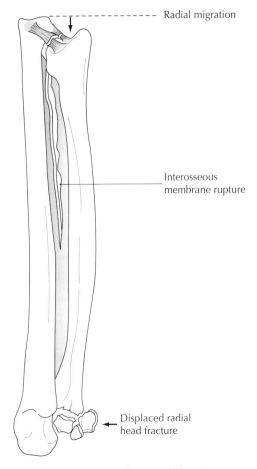

Radial migration

Interosseous membrane rupture

Displaced radial head fracture

Fig. 12.14 Essex–Lopresti fracture-dislocation.

and internal fixation of the proximal radial fracture, plus pinning of the distal radioulnar joint, should be performed; the pin is left in place for 6 weeks. Edwards and Jupiter[49] advise replacement of the radial head if the radial head fracture is irreparable. Pinning of the distal radioulnar joint is still necessary to allow healing of the interosseous membrane because a silastic radial head spacer alone will not completely restore axial stability.

Fractures of the proximal third of the ulna with dislocation of the radial head (Monteggia fracture-dislocation)

The combination of injuries known as the Monteggia fracture-dislocation is often treacherous to treat. It consists of a fracture of the ulna with dislocation of the proximal end of the radius with or without a fracture of the radius.

Bado[50] classified the injury into four types:

I. fracture of the middle or proximal third of the ulna with anterior dislocation of the radial head and a characteristic apex anterior angulation of the ulna;
II. fracture of the middle or proximal third of the ulna (usually apex posteriorly angulated) with posterior dislocation of the radial head and often a fracture of the radial head;
III. fracture of the ulna just distal to the coronoid process with lateral dislocation of the radial head, and
IV. fracture of the proximal or middle third of the ulna, anterior dislocation of the radial head and fracture of the proximal third of the radius below the bicipital tuberosity (Fig. 12.15).

In all series type I far exceeds all others in frequency. Several mechanisms of injury probably exist, including direct blows to the ulnar aspect of the forearm and a fall with hyperpronation or hyperextension, with the strong supinating force of the biceps pulling the radial head anteriorly as the fracture of the ulna is produced by the compression forces of the fall.

TREATMENT OPTIONS

Treatment of this injury, especially of the dislocation of the radial head, is controversial. Bohler[51]

stated that all Monteggia fracture-dislocations could be treated non-operatively. Speed and Boyd[52] surveyed the results of 52 of these injuries treated before 1940 and found that the best results were obtained when open reduction of the radial head with repair or reconstruction of the annular ligament was performed together with internal fixation of the ulna. Boyd and Boals[53] in 1969 reported 159 Monteggia-type injuries and recommended rigid internal fixation of the fractured ulna with either a compression plate or a medullary nail and closed reduction of the radial head. Most of the dislocated radial heads in this later series could be reduced by manipulation, and almost 80% of their results were excellent to good when acute injuries were so treated.

Careful diagnosis and prompt adequate treatment are recommended for this potentially hazardous combination of injuries. In long bone fractures radiographic evaluation must always include the joints proximal and distal. The radial head must always line up with the capitellum on all radiographs no matter in what position the extremity is placed. Benign-appearing minimally displaced fractures of the proximal third of the ulna must be followed closely for increasing angulation of the ulna and subsequent radial head subluxation or dislocation (Fig. 12.16).

AUTHOR'S PREFERRED MANAGEMENT

For acute injuries in which the dislocation of the radial head can be reduced by closed methods, open reduction of the dislocation is not indicated, but the fracture of the ulna requires rigid fixation. In the proximal third of the ulna, where the medullary canal is large, a compression plate should be used. In the middle third, where the meduallary canal is small, either a compression plate or a medullary nail is appropriate. Careful intraoperative radiographic analysis of the radiocapitellar joint must be made after fixation of the ulnar shaft fracture. Subluxation of the radial head requires open reduction.

For acute injuries in which interposition of the annular ligament or capsule prevents reduction of the radial head, open reduction of the dislocation, repair or reconstruction of the annular ligament, and rigid internal fixation of the fracture of the ulna as just described should be performed through the Boyd approach (Figs 12.17, 12.18) (Chapter 17).

For injuries older than 6 weeks in which the dislocation of the radial head has never been reduced or in which insufficient fixation of the fracture of the ulna has allowed angulation of this fracture and redislocation of the radial head, the radial head

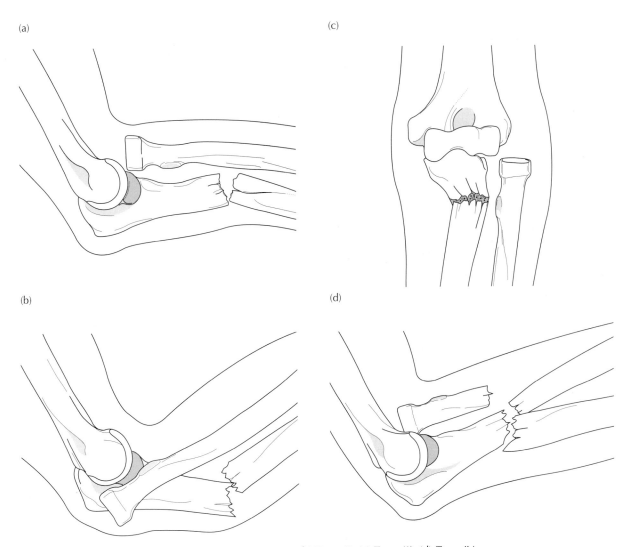

Fig. 12.15 Monteggia fracture-dislocations. (a) Type I. (b) Type II. (c) Type III. (d) Type IV.

should be excised. If the ulna is sufficiently angulated or is ununited, it should be rigidly fixed (usually with a compression plate) and supplemented by cancellous bone grafts.

Closed reduction of the radial head and internal fixation of the ulna

The dislocation of the radial head should be reduced by traction on the forearm and countertraction on the arm, followed by flexion of the elbow to 120 degrees. Intraoperative radiographs should then be performed to confirm that the reduction of the radial head is congruent. Open reduction and internal fixation of the ulna fracture is then performed by exposing the ulna along its subcutaneous border.

The fracture is fixed with either an intramedullary nail or a compression plate. Bone graft applied at the fracture site encourages union.

After wound closure, the elbow is held flexed at 120 degrees in a long-arm splint to prevent redislocation of the radial head. Repeat radiographs are necessary to confirm continued reduction of the radial head. At 2 weeks the posterior plaster splint is windowed and the sutures removed. During the first 6 weeks the elbow must be maintained at between 110 and 120 degrees of flexion using a long-arm cast for 4 weeks and a collar and cuff sling for the last 2 weeks. Once the cast has been removed gentle pronation and supination is permitted, but extension is not allowed below 90 degrees until 6 weeks after injury.

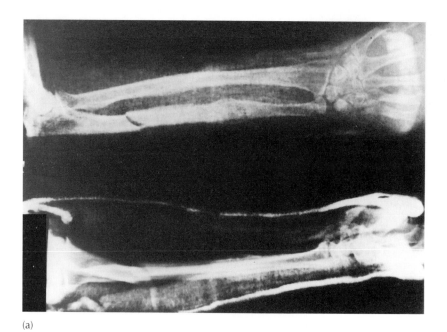

(a)

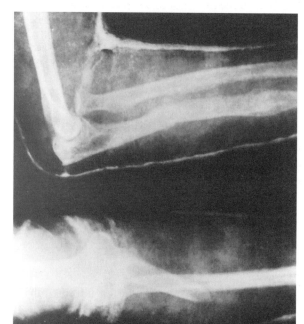

(b)

Fig. 12.16 (a) Roentgenograms after application of a long-arm cast for what was thought to be a minimally displaced fracture of the ulna. (b) One week later, dislocation of the radial head and increased angulation of the ulnar fracture.

Open reduction of the radial head and internal fixation of the ulna

When reduction of the radial head is prevented by interposition of the annular ligament or capsule the fracture of the ulna and the dislocation of the radial head should be exposed through the Boyd approach (Fig. 12.17a). If the annular ligament is intact, it should be incised and retracted to allow reduction of the radial head. More commonly, it is torn or avulsed and displaced into the sigmoid notch of the ulna. If the ligament is not excessively frayed, repair with fine non-absorbable sutures may be possible. More commonly this is impossible and reconstruction using a 1–1.5 cm wide fascia strip approximately 12 cm long dissected from the forearm fascia from distal to proximal is required.

(a)

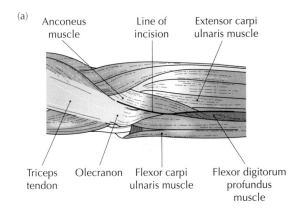

Anconeus muscle   Line of incision   Extensor carpi ulnaris muscle

Triceps tendon   Olecranon   Flexor carpi ulnaris muscle   Flexor digitorum profundus muscle

(b)

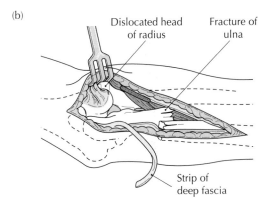

Dislocated head of radius   Fracture of ulna

Strip of deep fascia

(c)

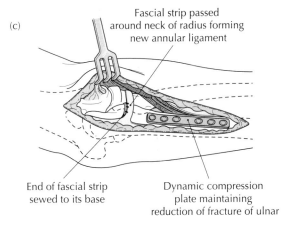

Fascial strip passed around neck of radius forming new annular ligament

End of fascial strip sewed to its base   Dynamic compression plate maintaining reduction of fracture of ulnar

Fig. 12.17 Speed and Boyd procedure for Monteggia fracture-dislocations. (a) Dislocation of the head of the radius and fracture of the ulna are exposed through one incision (Boyd). (b) Exposure has been completed. Strip of deep fascia, its base level with radial neck, has been freed. (c) Dislocation of proximal radius has been reduced, and new annular ligament has been sutured about radial neck. Ulnar fracture has been fixed with compression plate.

The proximal end of the fascia is left attached to the proximal ulna where the deep fascia blends with the periosteum of the olecranon (Fig. 12.17b). The fascia strip is then passed posterior to the radial neck, proximal to the biceps tuberosity of the radius, and then around the neck of the radius. The ulnar fracture is rigidly fixed and the new annular ligament is sutured around the radial neck (Fig. 12.17c). The ligament should be snug but not tight enough to restrict pronation and supination.

When a significant fracture of the radial head or neck occurs, the radial head should be excised at the time of repair of the ulnar fracture.

After wound closure, the arm is immobilised in a long-arm splint with the elbow at 120 degrees of flexion. Postoperative management is as described for closed reduction of the radial head.

COMPLICATIONS

The most common complication of Monteggia fracture-dislocations is failure to diagnose the injury in a timely fashion. Benign-appearing fractures of the proximal ulna should be followed closely for subluxation or dislocation of the radial head (Fig. 12.16). Although late dislocation and malunion of the ulna can be corrected, the results are less satisfactory than when these are treated as acute injuries.

As immobilisation for 6 weeks with the elbow flexed as much as 120 degrees is necessary to maintain reduction of the radial head, postoperative stiffness is common and extensive rehabilitation necessary to obtain functional extension.

SIDESWIPE FRACTURES

Sideswipes fractures are similar clinical entities only in that the mode of injury is the same for all: an elbow protruding from a car window is struck by a car passing in the opposite direction or strikes a fixed object. Aside from the seriousness of the injury, all similarity ceases. Grotesque combinations of fractures may be produced. The accompanying soft tissue injuries vary from minor lacerations and abrasions to massive grade 3 open wounds.

AUTHOR'S PREFERRED METHOD

The most common combination consists of an open fracture of the olecranon at the level of the coronoid process, anterior dislocation of the head of the radius and of the distal fragment of the ulna, and a

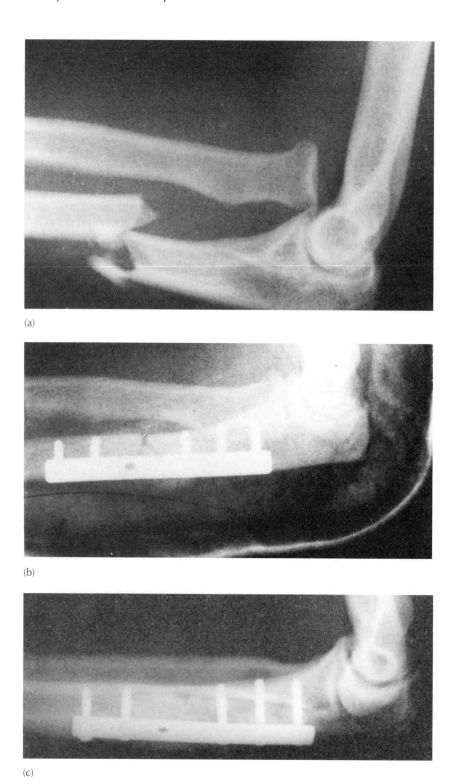

(a)

(b)

(c)

Fig. 12.18 (a) Type I Monteggia fracture-dislocation in which the intact annular ligament held the radial head dislocated. (b) Two weeks after surgery in which the annular ligament was excised, the radial head was reduced, and the ulnar fracture was fixed with a compression plate, iliac grafts were applied because of comminution, and annular ligament was repaired. (c) Two years after surgery, function is full except for 10 degrees loss of extension. From Ref. 54 with permission from Mosby Year-Book, St Louis.

comminuted fracture of the lower third of the humerus. This combination is treated by reduction of the anterior dislocations and fixation of the comminuted fracture of the olecranon with a intramedullary pin and tension band wiring. An external fixator is frequently used to stabilise the entire fracture complex.

To this basic combination any or all of these fractures may be added:

1. Fracture of the shaft of the ulna. The medullary nail used to fix the comminuted fracture of the olecranon also immobilises this fracture of the ulna. The nail should be inserted in a retrograde manner from the shaft fracture to avoid carrying contaminated material down the medullary canal.
2. Comminuted fracture of the radial head. The Boyd approach gives sufficient exposure of the fractures of the olecranon and radial head. Treatment of the radial head fracture is excision.
3. Fracture of the shaft of the radius. This fracture is not usually compound. If the fracture of the ulna is securely fixed, delaying open reduction of the radial fracture for 10–12 days is preferable. A compression plate or an intramedullary nail should then be used to fix the radius.
4. Comminuted fracture of the condyles of the humerus. Fixation of this fracture is described in the previous section on fractures of the distal humerus.

Not every fracture caused by a sideswipe injury can receive full attention immediately. Attention is directed primarily to the care of the open wound and restoration of the elbow joint. If necessary, treatment of fractures of the shafts of the long bones may be delayed. When so many injuries occur in the same extremity, loss of position, infection, or non-union may be anticipated. Trauma to the elbow joint is usually so severe that residual disability is certain. Results vary from complete ankylosis to a fairly serviceable range of motion. Calcification in the soft tissues around the joint is often so extensive that only a few degrees of motion are possible. Even so, restoration of the contour of the elbow joint to as near normal as possible may allow arthroplasty of the joint at a later date.

References

1. Rowe CR The management of fractures in elderly patients is different. *J Bone Joint Surg* 1965; **47A:** 1043–59.
2. Colton CL Fractures of the olecranon in adults: Classification and management. *Injury* 1973; **5:** 121–9.
3. Muller ME, Allgower M, Schneider R, Willenegger H *Manual of internal fixation: techniques recommended by the AO group* (2nd edn). New York: Springer-Verlag, 1979.
4. Harmon PH Treatment of fractures of the olecranon by fixation with stainless-steel screws. *J Bone Joint Surg* 1945; **27:** 328–9.
5. Weseley MS, Barenfeld PA, Eisenstein AL The use of the Zuelzer hook plate in fixation of olecranon fractures. *J Bone Joint Surg* 1976; **58A:** 859–63.
6. Burghele N, Serban N Fractures of the olecranon: Treatment by external fixation. *Ital J Orthop Traumatol* 1982; **8:** 159–61.
7. McKeever FM, Buck RN Fracture of the olecranon process of the ulna: Treatment by excision of fragment and repair of triceps tendon. *J Am Med Assoc* 1947; **135:** 1–5.
8. Adler S, Fay GD, MacAusland WR Jr Treatment of olecranon fractures: Indications for excision of the olecranon fragment and repair of the triceps tendon. *J Trauma* 1962; **2:** 597.
9. Fyfe IS, Mossad MM, Holdsworth BJ Methods of fixation of olecranon fractures: An experimental mechanical study. *J Bone Joint Surg* 1985; **67B:** 367–72.
10. Weber BG, Vasey H Osteosynthese BEI Olecranon Fraktur. *Rev Accid Trav Mal Prot* 1963; **56:** 90.
11. Wolfgang G, Burke F, Bush D Surgical treatment of displaced olecranon fractures by tension band wiring technique. *Clin Orthop* 1987; **224:** 192.
12. MacAusland WR Treatment of fractures of the olecranon by longitudinal screw or nail fixation. *Ann Surg* 1942; **116:** 293.
13. Helm RH, Hornsby R, Miller SWM The complications of surgical treatment of displaced fractures of the olecranon. *Injury* 1987; **18:** 48–50.
14. Murphy DF, Green WB, Gilbert JA, Dameron TB Displaced olecranon fractures in adults: Biomechanical analysis of fixation methods. *Clin Orthop* 1987; **224:** 210.
15. Horner SR, Sadasivan KK, Lipka JM, Saha S Analysis of mechanical factors affecting fixation of olecranon fractures. *Orthopaedics* 1984; **12:** 1469.
16. MacAusland WR Jr, Wyman ET Fractures of the adult elbow. In: *American Academy of Orthopaedic Surgeons: Instructional Course Lectures* Vol 24. St Louis: CV Mosby Co, 1975: 169.
17. Gartsman GM, Sculco TP, Otis JC Operative treatment of olecranon fractures. *J Bone Joint Surg* 1981; **63A:** 718–21.
18. Eriksson E, Sahlen O, Sandahl U Late results of conservative and surgical treatment of fracture of the olecranon. *Acta Chir Scand* 1957; **113:** 153–6.
19. Holdsworth BJ, Mossad MM Elbow function following tension band fixation of displaced fractures of the olecranon. *Injury* 1984; **16:** 182–7.
20. Kiviluoto O, Santavirta S Fractures of the olecranon. *Acta Orthop Scand* 1978; **49:** 28–31.
21. Wolfgang G, Burke F, Bush D Surgical treatment of fracture of the olecranon. *Acta Chir Scand* 1987; **113:** 153–6.

22. Waldram MA, Porter KM Late treatment of nonunion of fracture of the olecranon. *Injury* 1987; **18:** 419–20.

23. Regan W, Morrey BF Fractures of the coronoid process of the ulna. *J Bone Joint Surg* 1989; **71A:** 1348.

24. Mason ML Some observations on fractures of the head of the radius with a review of one hundred cases. *Brit J Surg* 1954; **42:** 123–32.

25. Murray RC Fractures of the head and neck of the radius. *Brit J Surg* 1940; **28:** 106–18.

26. Paulsen JO, TopHoj K Fracture of the head and neck of the radius. *Acta Orthop Scand* 1974; **45:** 66–75.

27. Fleetcroft JP Fractures of the radial head: Early aspiration and mobilisation. *J Bone Joint Surg* 1984; **66B:** 141–2.

28. Holdsworth BJ, Clement DA, Rothwell PNR Fractures of the radial head – The benefit of aspiration. *Injury* 1987; **18:** 44–7.

29. Carstam N Operative treatment of fractures of the head and neck of the radius. *Acta Orthop Scand* 1950; **19:** 502–26.

30. Wexner SD, Goodwin C, Parkes JC II *et al.* Treatment of fractures of the radial head by partial excision. *Orthop Rev* 1985; **14:** 83–6.

31. Key J Treatment of fractures of the head and neck of the radius. *J Am Med Assoc* 1931; **96:** 101–4.

32. Bunker TD, Newman JH The Herbert differential pitch bone screw in displaced radial head fractures. *Injury* 1985; **16:** 621–4.

33. McArthur RA Herbert screw fixation of fracture of the head of the radius. *Clin Orthop* 1987; **224:** 79–87.

34. Khurana JS, Kattapuram SV, Becker S *et al.* Injury with an associated fracture of the radial head. *Clin Orthop* 1988; **234:** 70–1.

35. MacKay I, Fitzgerald B, Miller JH Silastic Replacement of the head of the radius in trauma. *J Bone Joint Surg* 1979; **61B:** 494–7.

36. Swanson AB, Jaeger SH La Rochelle D Comminuted fractures of the radial head: The role of silicone-implant replacement arthroplasty. *J Bone Joint Surg* 1981; **63A:** 1039–49.

37. Jacobs J, Kernodle H Fractures of the head of the radius. *J Bone Joint Surg* 1946; **28:** 616–22.

38. Bakalim G Fractures of the radial head and their treatment. *Acta Orthop Scand* 1970; **41:** 320–31.

39. Sanders RA, French HG Open reduction and internal fixation of comminuted radial head fractures. *Am J Sports Med* 1986; **14:** 130–5.

40. Coleman DA, Blair WF, Shurr D Resection of the radial head for fracture of the radial head. *J Bone Joint Surg* 1987; **69A:** 385–92.

41. Morrey BF, An KN Articular and ligamentous contributions to the stability of the elbow joint. *Am J Sports Med* 1983; **11:** 315–9.

42. Taylor TKF, O'Connor BT The effect upon the inferior radio-ulnar joint of excision of the head of the radius in adults. *J Bone Joint Surg* 1964; **46B:** 83–8.

43. Levin PD Fracture of the radial head with dislocation of the distal radio-ulnar joint: Case report. Treatment by prosthetic replacement of the radial head. *J Bone Joint Surg* 1973; **55A:** 837–40.

44. Stanley D, Herbert TJ The Swanson ulnar head prosthesis for post-traumatic disorders of the distal radio-ulnar joint. *J Hand Surg* 1992, **17B:** 682–8.

45. Gordon M, Bullough PG Synovial and osseous inflammation in failed silicone – rubber prostheses. *J Bone Joint Surg* 1982; **64A:** 574–40.

46. Morrey BF, Askew L, Chao EY Silastic prosthestic replacement for the radial head. *J Bone Joint Surg* 1981; **63A:** 454–8.

47. Mayhall WST, Tiley FT, Paluska DJ Fractures of silastic radial head prostheses. *J Bone Joint Surg* 1981; **63A:** 459–60.

48. Ebraheim NA, Skie MC, Zeiss J *et al.* Internal fixation of radial neck fractures in a fracture-dislocation of the elbow: A case report. *Clin Orthop* 1992; **276:** 187–91.

49. Edwards GS J, Jupiter JB Radial head fractures with acute distal radioulnar dislocation: Essex-Lopresti revisited. *Clin Orthop* 1988; **234:** 61–9.

50. Bado JL The Monteggia lesion. *Clin Orthop* 1967; **50:** 71–86.

51. Bohler L *The treatment of fractures* (English 5th edn) (translated from German 13th edn by Hans Tretter *et al.*), 3 vols. New York: Grune and Stratton, 1956–58.

52. Speed JS, Boyd HB Treatment of fractures of the ulna with dislocation of the head of radius (Monteggia fracture). *J Am Med Assoc* 1940; **115:** 1699–705.

53. Boyd HB, Boals JL The Monteggia lesion: A review of 159 cases. *Clin Orthop* 1969; **66:** 94–100.

54. Crenshaw AH Jr Fractures of the shoulder girdle, arm, and forearm. In: *Campbell's operative orthopaedics* (8th edn). St Louis: Mosby Year-Book, 1992.

55. Knight PA The management of fractures about the elbow in adults. *Instr Course Lect* 1957; **14:** 123.

56. Heim U, Pfeiffer KM *Internal Fixation of Small Fractures* (3rd edn). Berlin: Springer-Verlag, 1988.

57. Broberg MA, Morrey BF Results of treatment of fracture-dislocations of the elbow. *Clin Orthop* 1987; **216:** 109.

CHAPTER 13

Dislocations of the elbow in the adult

PER OLOF JOSEFSSON

Introduction

In adults the elbow is second only to the gleno-humeral joint for frequency of dislocation whilst in children under the age of ten years it is the most commonly dislocated major joint.[1] Although dislocations may occur throughout life they are most frequent during the first two decades[2] (Fig. 13.1).

Classification of elbow dislocations

Stimson's 1890 classification of elbow dislocations is most commonly used to describe these injuries.[3] It is based on the direction of dislocation which is determined by the position of the distal half of the joint.

Posterior and posterolateral dislocation of the radius and ulna is the most frequent injury pattern.[1-5] Genuine lateral dislocations are rare.[1] Anterior dislocation is always associated with a fracture of the olecranon and has also been referred to as transolecranal dislocation.[6] Even more unusual are divergent and convergent dislocations[7] (Chapter 9).

MECHANISM OF INJURY

A dislocation of the elbow is almost always caused by a fall on the outstretched hand. Two primary theories for the mechanism of dislocation exits. According to one theory the dislocation takes place when the elbow is slightly flexed and is due to a

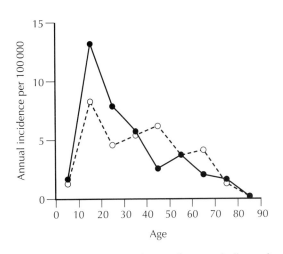

Fig. 13.1 Age and sex-specific incidences of elbow dislocations in Malmo. ●----● men, o---o women. Redrawn after Ref. 1 with permission from Scandinavian University Press, Stockholm.

direct force acting along the forearm together with a reflex triceps muscle contraction.[8,9] This axial force was suggested to be combined with external rotatory (supination) and valgus moments.[10] In the other theory hyperextension is suggested to be the cause of the dislocation.[1,11,12] There are also several studies showing the preponderance for left-sided dislocations – about 60%.[1,2,4,5] The more frequent involvement of the non-dominant elbow in dislocations may have several causes including the reduced dexterity of the non-dominant upper limb compared with the dominant limb, activities being undertaken with the dominant arm at the time of injury, or perhaps an unconscious protection of the dominant arm when the fall occurs.

Clinical presentation and acute treatment

The reduction of the dislocated elbow is assumed often to take place spontaneously and is followed by findings of swelling, haematoma and sometimes typical fractures from the coronoid process or avulsed fragments from the epicondyles. If at presentation the elbow is dislocated, immediate closed reduction should be performed. This may be possible under intravenous sedation but in many cases general anaesthesia will be necessary. It is usually easiest to reduce the elbow in approximately 45 degrees of flexion. The technique involves the principle of countertraction on the humerus, together with pulling on the forearm in the direction of reduction or pushing with the thumb on the olecranon. Radiographic assessment prior to reduction is not necessary in typical cases. However, after the reduction, radiographs of the elbow should be performed in order to be certain the reduction is congruent and also to look for fracture fragments. It is very important to check the pulse in the wrist and the neurological status of the hand after reduction.

The further treatment of an acute dislocation of the elbow will, depending on the presence or absence of displaced intra-articular fractures, be discussed from two points of view – simple dislocations and complex dislocations.

Simple dislocations

A dislocation of the elbow will result in extensive soft tissue injuries with complete rupture of the medial and lateral-collateral ligaments at their proximal attachments, rupture of the anterior capsule with injury to the brachialis muscle and in most cases ruptures of the muscular origins on the epicondyles.[13,14] These injuries are therefore unstable, when examined under general anaesthesia, and compared with the contralateral side. The instability is obvious on the medial side of the joint when the elbow is stressed in valgus but only slight or no instability is detected on the lateral side of the joint when a varus stress is applied[14] (Fig. 13.2). The anatomical configuration of the joint surface with a ball and socket joint laterally and a hinge joint medially is probably the explanation for the difference in varus–valgus instability despite bilateral, total ligament rupture. Approximately one-third of elbows, when examined under general anaesthesia following reduction, are easily redislocatable. These redislocations will occur most easily in the semiflexed position at about 45 degrees. This tendency to redislocate has been correlated to extensive muscular injuries.

No benefit is gained from primary surgical ligament and muscular repair in these simple dislocations[13,15] and therefore, following closed reduction, the elbow should be immobilised at a right angle (or more acute angle if there is no vascular compromise) in a posterior plaster splint. If the elbow is also immobilised in full pronation the stability of the reduced elbow will increase according to studies by O'Driscoll *et al*.[10] Prolonged immobilisation correlates strongly with unsatisfactory results and immobilisation for more than 4 weeks appears to be critical.[16,17] Immobilisation for 0–1 week is appropriate for elbows which appear to be well retained in the reduced position otherwise 2–3 weeks is advisable.

Complex dislocations

The success of non-surgical treatment for simple dislocations of the elbow is explained by the osseous articulation of the joint, which makes the elbow inherently stable during the period of soft tissue healing. However, up to 50% of elbow dislocations are combined with fractures of the elbow[2] (Fig. 13.3). The most common fractures are those of the medial epicondyle, the lateral epicondyle, the radial head, the coronoid process, the capitellum and the olecranon.[2] Displaced articular fractures will increase the instability of the joint and extensive fractures of the radial head and the coronoid process are known to result in severe instability with a high risk of redislocation and the development of severe osteoarthritis[18] (Fig. 13.4). Reconstruction of the joint articulation by reduction and fixation of fracture frag-

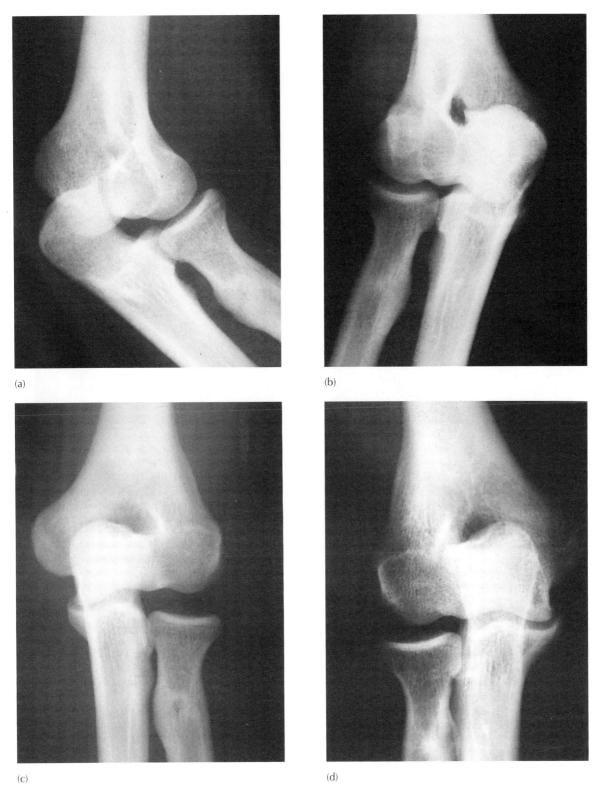

(a)

(b)

(c)

(d)

Fig. 13.2 A 27-year-old man with a posterior dislocation of the left elbow. The dislocation was primarily treated by closed reduction. The stability of the joint under general anaesthesia was assessed and with valgus stress marked instability was noted (a) in comparison with the uninjured elbow (b). No instability was felt with varus stress but the radiograph revealed increased joint space (c) compared with the uninjured side (d).

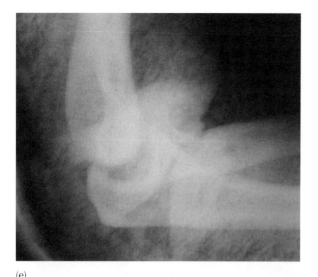

(e)

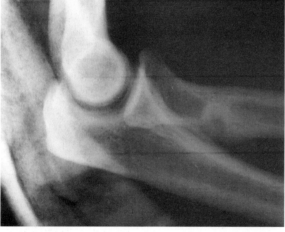

(f)

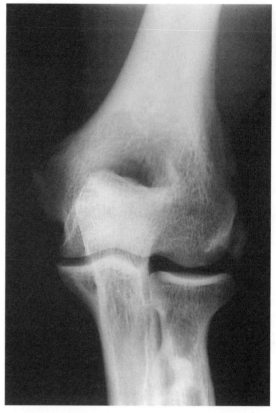

(g)

Fig. 13.2 continued. Also increased joint space was seen in a posterior plaster cast under anaesthesia (e). The joint space was normalised (f) 2 days later. At follow-up 4 years later typical calcifications in the epicondylar areas were seen (g).

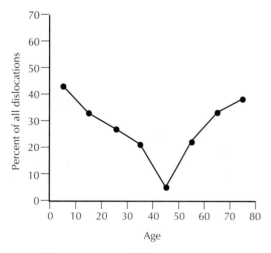

Fig. 13.3 The occurrence of fractures in association with 178 elbow dislocations in relation to age.

ments of the radial head and the coronoid process is therefore important if possible. When severe comminution of the radial head makes removal unavoidable, the medial and lateral collateral ligaments together with the muscle attachments to the epicondyles should all be repaired. The ligaments are usually avulsed at their proximal attachment and the use of osteosutures through drill holes in the bone may be necessary. In these very unstable cases immobilisation at a right angle should be maintained for a relatively long time, i.e. 3–4 weeks. The elbow should also be examined radiographically within a week to check that the joint has not redislocated. For dislocations with comminuted fractures of the radial head together with fractures of the coronoid process a radial head prosthesis may be used as a temporary spacer and stabiliser during the time of soft tissue healing.[19]

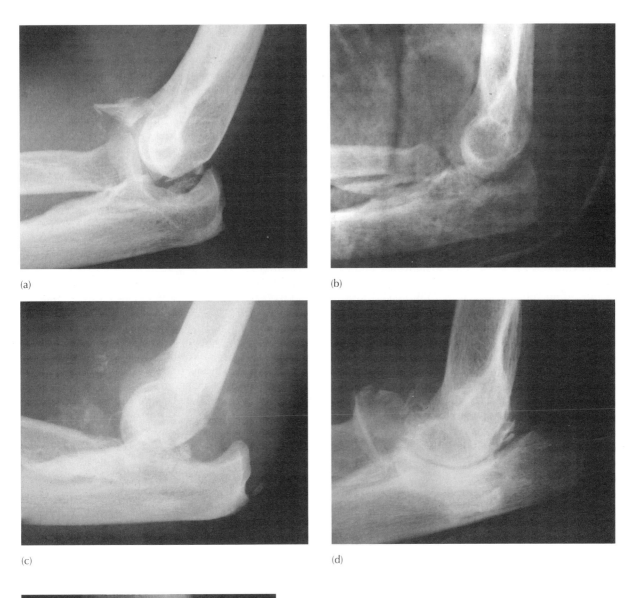

(a)

(b)

(c)

(d)

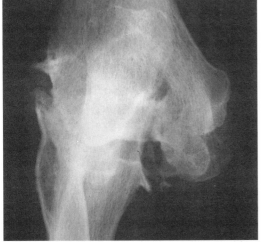

(e)

Fig. 13.4 A 69-year-old man with a posterior dislocation of the right elbow. The dislocation was immediately reduced and displaced fractures of the radial head and the coronoid process were seen (a). The radial head and the displaced fragment of the coronoid process were primarily excised (b). A posterior plaster cast was applied for 14 days. On the 21st day a redislocation was diagnosed (c) and a further closed reduction was performed. No further radiographic examination was performed until 10 years later. The elbow was still dislocated and severe osteoarthritis had developed (d,e).

In anterior–transolecranal dislocations open reduction and rigid internal fixation of the olecranon fracture is necessary.

Results and complications of treatment

SIMPLE DISLOCATIONS

Simple dislocations treated by closed reduction and immobilisation for between 1 and 2 weeks do not usually develop significant complications even at long-term follow-up.[20] However, approximately 50% of adults will have some symptoms referable to the injured elbow with the most common complaint being reduced range of motion and loss of extension. At long-term follow-up (24 years) Josefsson *et al.*[20] noted an average loss of extension in adults of 12 degrees ± 12 degrees (range 0 – 35 degrees).

Elbow movement following simple dislocations improves for between 6 and 12 months after injury but does not appear to progress spontaneously beyond that time.[20] In most cases following simple dislocations calcification and irregularities in the epicondylar regions are noted radiographically and are due to injury to the ligamentous and muscular attachments (Fig. 13.2g).

NEUROVASCULAR COMPLICATIONS

Transient neurovascular complications are often seen in association with elbow dislocations.[1] The radial pulse may initially be absent after injury but return immediately following reduction. Transient impairment of ulnar and median nerve function is common but will usually disappear within a couple of months. Persistent ulnar nerve discomfort may occur due to repetitive anterior dislocation of the nerve over the medial epicondyle when the elbow is flexed.[1,15] The nerve returns to its anatomical position posterior to the medial epicondyle when the elbow is extended.

INTERPOSITION

Interposition of soft tissue or bony fragments may make closed reduction of a dislocated elbow impossible (Fig. 13.5). It should, however, be noted that an increased joint space may be a normal radiographic finding following reduction of a dislocated elbow if the x-rays were taken under general anaesthesia. This appearance results from extensive soft tissue damage[13] and will disappear when the patient is awake and has regained muscle tone. Interposition of osteochondral fragments may at times be difficult to detect, particularly in the skeletally immature[21] (Fig. 13.6). In addition, interposition of the median nerve[22–24] (Fig. 13.7) and the

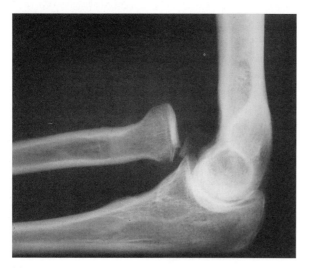

(a)

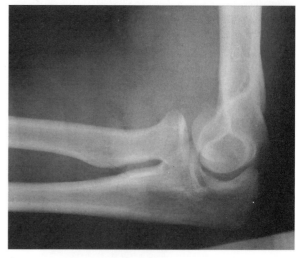

(b)

Fig. 13.5 A 33-year-old man with a dorsal dislocation of the right elbow. After closed reduction the radial head remained dislocated (a). At surgery the biceps tendon was found displaced around the radial head. The biceps tendon was reduced into its normal position and the radial head was easily reduced. Also a displaced fragment of the radial head was excised (b).

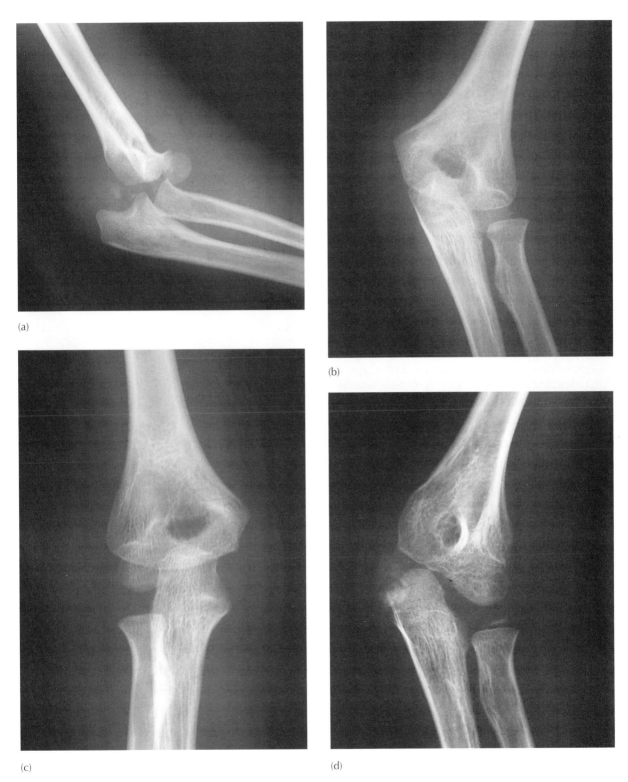

(a)

(b)

(c)

(d)

Fig. 13.6 A 9-year-old boy with a dorsal dislocation (a) of the left elbow. After closed reduction an increased valgus angulation was seen (b) compared with the uninjured elbow (c). On a radiograph 4 months later ossification in the medial part of the joint was seen (d). Not until 13 months after the injury was the entrapped medial epicondyle reduced and pinned into its normal position. An increased valgus angulation and a severely reduced range of motion was present. After surgery rapid improvement occurred.

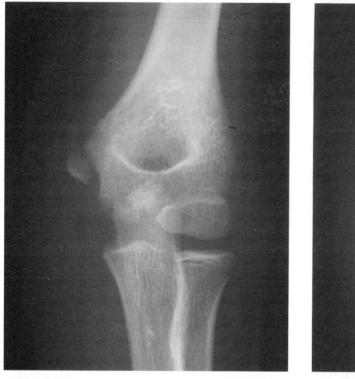
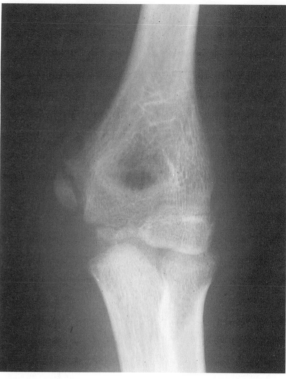

(a)   (b)

Fig. 13.7 An 11-year-old boy with a posterior dislocation of the left elbow. The radiograph after closed reduction appeared normal (a). 14 days after injury impaired function of the median nerve was noted. A radiograph 2 months after injury was considered normal; however, a cortical depression just proximal to the medial apophysis had appeared due to local pressure of an entrapped median nerve (Matev's sign) (b). Due to increasing symptoms the elbow was surgically explored 7 months after the injury and an entrapped median nerve was reduced into its normal position. After surgery rapid improvement occurred.

brachial artery[25] have been observed. These interposed structures should be reduced into their normal position by open surgery without delay.

THE BRACHIAL ARTERY

The brachial artery may be disrupted.[26,27] This must be diagnosed without delay and treated by immediate arterial repair. Particularly in cases with extensive vascular injury there is a risk of developing acute compartment syndrome which, if not decompressed, will result in muscular necrosis and Volkmann's ischaemic contracture.

EXTRA SKELETAL OSSIFICATION

Extra skeletal ossification – myositis ossificans – develops in the brachialis muscle (Fig. 13.8). This is

most common in severe injuries with associated fractures and in cases of delayed primary treatment.[28] Forced passive motion of a stiff elbow is stated to greatly increase the risk of myositis ossificans.[28,29]

RECURRENT DISLOCATION

Recurrent dislocation of the elbow joint is uncommon.[11] Osborne and Cotterill[9] in 1966 stated that surgical treatment is indicated when dislocations occur frequently with trivial violence in the older adolescent or adult patient. They described repair of the capsular and ligamentous damage. They noted at operation that the posterolateral ligamentous and capsular structures were important stabilisers of the elbow and therefore they performed a capsular and ligamentous repair of the lateral side of the joint (Fig. 13.9). When there is much medial

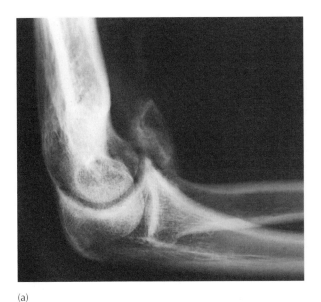
(a)

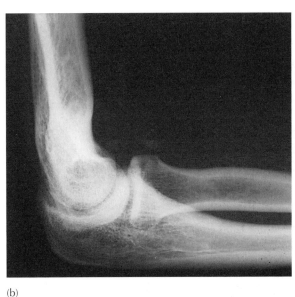
(b)

Fig. 13.8 A 27-year-old man with a dorsal dislocation of the left elbow. A closed reduction followed by immobilisation for 15 days was performed. Range of motion did not improve in a normal way and a radiograph 4 months after the injury showed typical myositis ossificans. The heterotopic bone was excised (b) and the range of motion improved.

ligament laxity, repair of the medial ligaments should also be performed.

RECURRENT SUBLUXATION

Recurrent subluxation of the elbow appearing as posterolateral rotatory instability[30] is difficult to diagnose. This involves a transient rotatory subluxation of the ulnohumeral joint and a secondary posterior dislocation of the radial head. The annular ligament is intact and the cause of the condition is laxity of the lateral ligament. Treatment is operative with repair of the lateral ligament and capsule (Chapter 14).

NEGLECTED POSTERIOR DISLOCATION

Neglected posterior dislocations are described from developing countries.[31-33] According to Fowles *et al.*[32] attempts at closed reduction after 3–4 weeks are hazardous and for older dislocations Mahaisavariya *et al.*[33] recommend open reduction with removal of fibro-osseous tissue from the trochlear notch, the olecranon fossa and the coronoid fossa. In long-standing dislocations (greater than 3 months) contracture of the triceps muscle makes reduction impossible and lengthening of the muscle must be performed. Plaster cast immobilisation for 2–3 weeks has been used, and in very unstable elbows

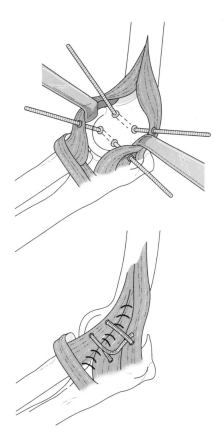

Fig. 13.9 The Osborne and Cotterill operation for lateral capsular and ligamentous damage in recurrent dislocation of the elbow. Redrawn after Ref. 9 with permission from *Journal of Bone and Joint Surgery*.

Kirschner wire transfixation was been performed. With the use of tendon graft stabilisation Arafiles[31] started flexion-extension exercises after 6 days.

References

1. Linscheid RL, Wheeler DK Elbow dislocations. *J Am Med Assoc* 1965; **194:** 1171–6.
2. Josefsson PO, Nilsson BE Incidence of elbow dislocation. *Acta Orthop Scand* 1986; **57:** 537–8.
3. Stimson LA *A treatise on fracture.* Philadelphia: Henry C Lea's Son and Co, 1890.
4. Neviaser J, Wickstrom JK Dislocation of the elbow – a retrospective study of 115 patients. *South Med J* 1977; **70:** 172–3.
5. Roberts PH Dislocation of the elbow. *Brit J Surg* 1969; **56:** 806–15.
6. Guerra A, Innao V Transolecranal dislocations. *Ital J Orthop Traumatol* 1982; **8:** 175–81.
7. Carey RPL Simultaneous dislocation of the elbow and the proximal radio- ulnar joint. *J Bone Joint Surg* 1984; **66B:** 254–6.
8. Johansson O Capsular and ligament injuries of the elbow joint. A clinical and arthrographic study. *Acta Chir Scand* 1962; Suppl 287.
9. Osborne G, Cotterill P Recurrent dislocation of the elbow. *J Bone Joint Surg* 1966; **48B:** 340–6.
10. O'Driscoll SW, Morrey BF, Korinek S, An K-N Elbow subluxation and dislocation. *Clin Orthop* 1992; **280:** 186–97.
11. Hassmann GC, Brunn F, Neer II CS Recurrent dislocation of the elbow. *J Bone Joint Surg* 1975; **57A:** 1080–4.
12. Loomis LK Reduction and after-treatment of posterior dislocation of the elbow. With special attention to the brachialis muscle and myositis ossificans. *Am J Surg* 1944; **LX111:** 56–60.
13. Josefsson PO, Gentz C-F, Johnell O, Wendeberg B Surgical versus non-surgical treatment of ligamentous injuries following dislocation of the elbow joint. A prospective randomised study. *J Bone Joint Surg* 1987; **69A:** 605–8.
14. Josefsson PO, Johnell O, Wendeberg B Ligamentous injuries in dislocations of the elbow joint. *Clin Orthop* 1987; **221:** 221–5.
15. Josefsson PO, Gentz CF, Johnell O, Wendeberg B Surgical versus nonsurgical treatment of ligamentous injuries following dislocations of the elbow joint. *Clin Orthop* 1987; **214:** 165–9.
16. Broberg MA, Morrey BF Results of treatment of fracture dislocations of the elbow. *Clin Orthop* 1987; **216:** 109–19.
17. Mehlhoff TL, Noble PC, Bennett JB, Tullos HS Simple dislocation of the elbow in the adult. *J Bone Joint Surg* 1988; **70A:** 244–9.
18. Josefsson PO, Gentz C-F, Johnell O, Wendeberg B Dislocation of the elbow joint and intra-articular fractures. *Clin Orthop* 1989; **246:** 126–30.
19. Harrington IJ, Tountas AA Replacement of the radial head in the treatment of unstable elbow fractures. *Injury* 1981; **12:** 404–12.
20. Josefsson PO, Johnell O, Gentz C-F Long-term sequelae of simple dislocation of the elbow. *J Bone Joint Surg* 1984; **66A:** 927–30.
21. Fowles JV, Kassab MT, Moula T Untreated intraarticular entrapment of the medial humeral epicondyle. *J Bone Joint Surg* 1984; **66B:** 562–5.
22. Hallet J Entrapment of the median nerve after dislocation of the elbow. A case report. *J Bone Joint Surg* 1981; **63B:** 408–12.
23. Matev I A radiological sign of entrapment of the median nerve in the elbow joint after posterior dislocation. *J Bone Joint Surg* 1976; **58B:** 353–5.
24. Steiger RN, Larrick RB, Meyer TL Median nerve entrapment following elbow dislocation in children. A report of two cases. *J Bone Joint Surg* 1969; **51A:** 381–5.
25. Mains DB, Freeark RJ Report on compound dislocation of the elbow with entrapment of the brachial artery. *Clin Orthop* 1975; **106:** 180–5.
26. Grimer RJ, Brooks S Brachial artery damage accompanying closed posterior dislocation of the elbow. *J Bone Joint Surg* 1985; **67B:** 378–81.
27. Hofammann III KE, Moneim MS, Omer GE, Ball WS Brachial artery disruption following closed posterior elbow dislocation in a child – assessment with intravenous digital angiography. A case report with review of the literature. *Clin Orthop* 1984; **184:** 145–9.
28. Thompson III HC, Garcia A Myositis ossificans. Aftermath of elbow injuries. *Clin Orthop* 1967; **50:** 129–34.
29. Wilson PD Fractures and dislocations in the region of the elbow. *Surg Gynecol Obstet* 1933; **56:** 335–59.
30. O'Driscoll SW, Bell DF, Morrey BF Posterolateral rotatory instability of the elbow. *J Bone Joint Surg* 1991; **73A:** 440–6.
31. Arafiles RP Neglected posterior dislocation of the elbow – a reconstruction operation. *J Bone Joint Surg* 1987; **69B:** 199–202.
32. Fowles JV, Kassab MT, Douik M Untreated posterior dislocation of the elbow in children. *J Bone Joint Surg* 1984; **66A:** 921–6.
33. Mahaisavariya B, Laupattarakasem W, Supachutikul A *et al.* Late reduction of dislocated elbow. *J Bone Joint Surg* 1993; **75B:** 426–8.

This plate section shows in colour, illustrations which appear in the text in black and white. The original figure numbers have been retained.

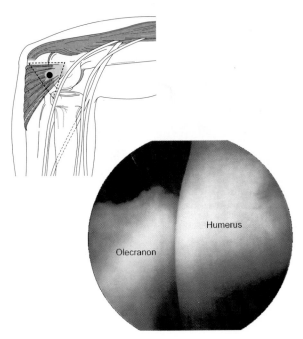

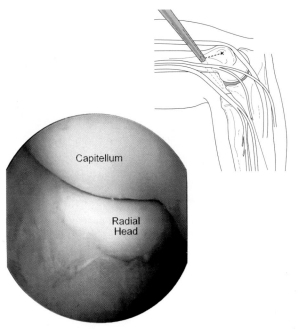

Fig. 6.4 The direct lateral portal is established in the middle of a triangle formed by the lateral epicondyle, the olecranon, and the radial head. Visible structures include the olecranon and humerus in the posterior compartment.

Fig. 6.5 The superomedial portal is established approximately 2 cm proximal to the medial humeral epicondyle. Visible structures include the capitellum and radial head.

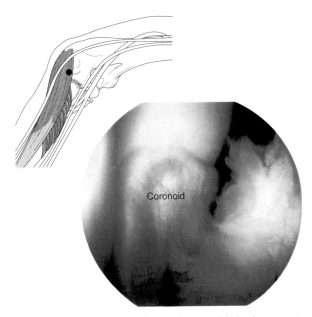

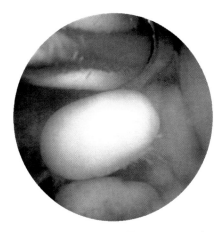

Fig. 6.6 The anterolateral portal is established approximately 3 cm distal and 2 cm anterior to the lateral humeral epicondyle. Visible structures include the coronoid process of the ulna.

Fig. 6.8 A loose body in the elbow as seen through the arthroscope.

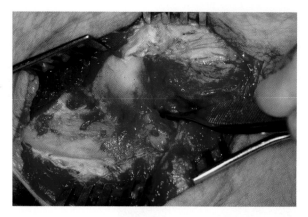

Fig. 14.3 Posterolateral instability – at operation, the forceps indent the lax capsule proximal to the subluxed radial head.

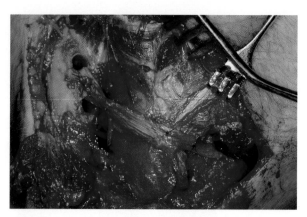

Fig. 14.4 Reconstruction of the lateral ulnar collateral ligament using a tendon graft.

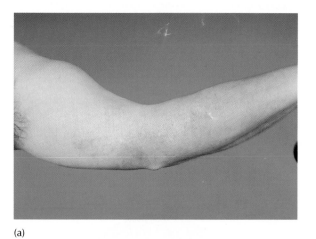

(a)

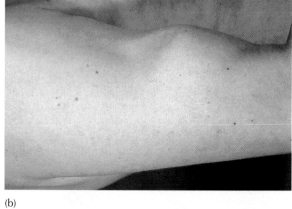

(b)

Fig. 15.1 (a) The proximally retracted belly of biceps in a case of distal tendon avulsion. (b) The distal retraction associated with rupture of the long head of biceps.

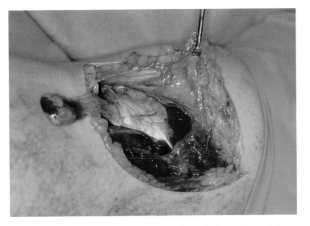

Fig. 15.3 Avulsed tendon exposed and placed on skin.

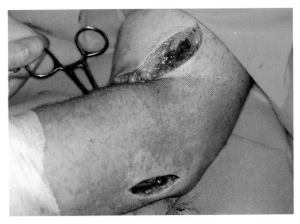

Fig. 15.5 The two incisions with instrument passed along tendon track, through anconeus and overlying skin.

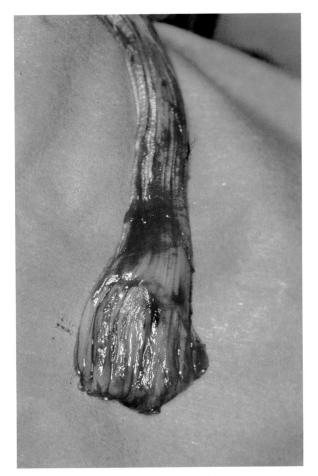

Fig. 15.4 Bulbous end of avulsed tendon.

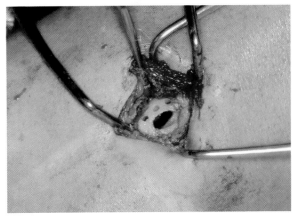

Fig. 15.6 Cavity excavated in bicipital tuberosity with three well spaced drill holes in its anterior rim.

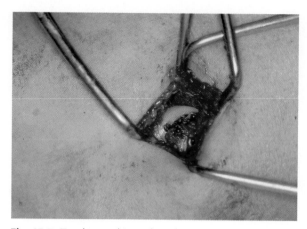

Fig. 15.7 Tendon end introduced into cavity and sutured in place.

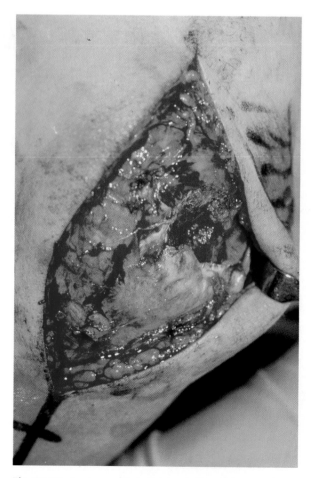

Fig. 15.11 Acute avulsion to triceps insertion.

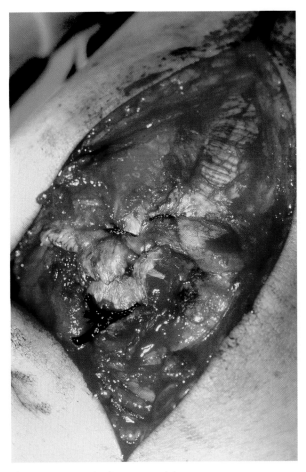

Fig. 15.12 Repaired acute avulsion.

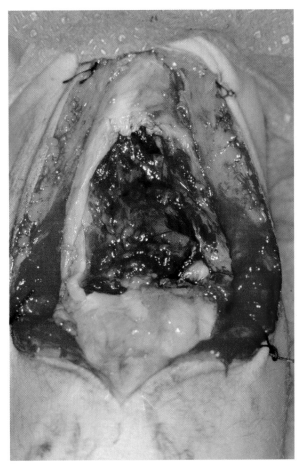

Fig. 15.13 Defect remaining after excision of scar tissue in case presenting late.

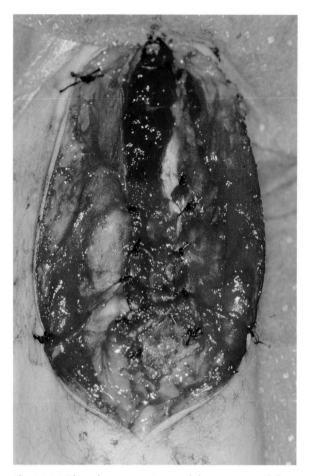 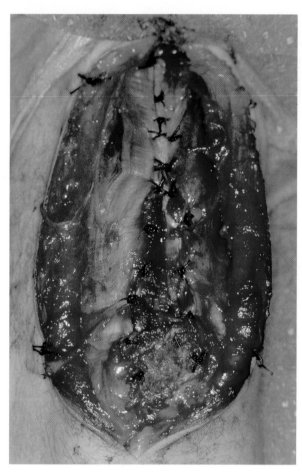

Fig. 15.14 Flap of aponeurosis turned down to cover defect.

Fig. 15.15 Closure of defect from which flap derived.

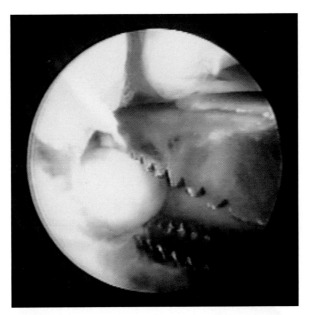

Fig. 17.6 Arthroscopic removal of loose body with grasper.

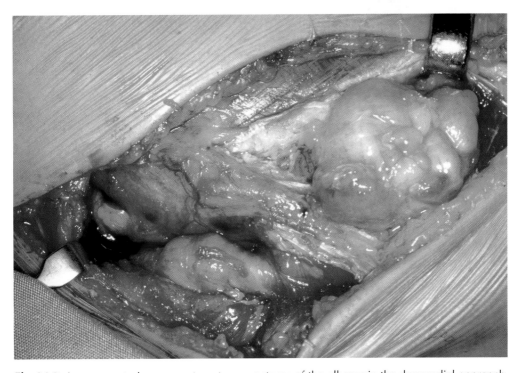

Fig. 24.3 An open anterior compartment synovectomy of the elbow via the dorsoradial approach.

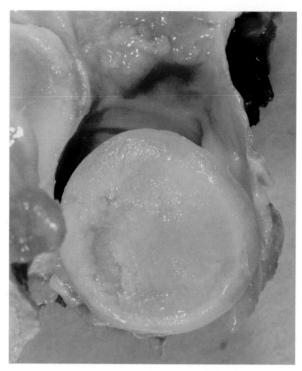

Fig. 28.2 Posteriomedial radial head ulceration.

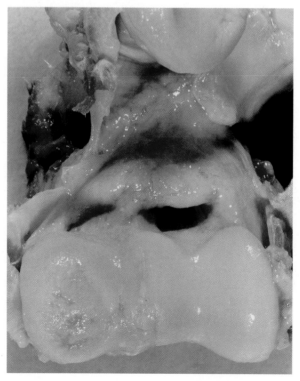

Fig. 28.3 Marked degeneration change affecting the capitellum with preservation of the cartilage over the trochlea.

CHAPTER 14

Chronic elbow instability

ANDY CARR, LECH RYMASZEWSKI

Introduction

The elbow joint is one of the most stable articulations in the body[1] yet despite this it is the second most commonly dislocated major joint in adults. Recurrent dislocation, however, is relatively rare, with the majority initially occurring before the age of 15 years.[2] In this age group surgical treatment may not be required as the elbow tends to become more stable with growth.

The incidence of repeated subluxation of the elbow joint has probably been underestimated in the past and a high index of suspicion is necessary as the diagnosis is often subtle. Symptoms of giving way, snapping or locking may be attributed to calcification or loose bodies seen on x-ray.[3] Clinical examination does not usually reveal instability due to muscle spasm caused by apprehension.[4]

Chronic instability may arise due to a single major traumatic event, usually a dislocation or fracture-dislocation. Medial instability may also result from a chronic overuse injury, particularly in sporting activities involving pitching and throwing, which produce a valgus stress on the elbow.[5] Pain after repetitive throwing is the usual presentation and may be associated with ulnar nerve symptoms and occasionally signs.

Other patterns of instability may also occur and will be discussed in this chapter.

Stability of the elbow

BONY CONSTRAINTS

The elbow joint relies almost equally on bony and soft tissue constraints for its stability.

The ulnohumeral articulation is a complex joint. The main articular surface of the humerus is the trochlea which is located mid-way between the medial and lateral columns. This articular surface is inclined in 7 degrees of internal rotation, 30 degrees of anterior rotation and a valgus tilt of approximately 7 degrees. The proximal ulna wraps around this trochlear articular surface and because of anterior and posterior indentations above the articular surface a considerable amount of flexion and extension is still permitted despite a high degree of capture of the olecranon on the distal humerus. The anatomy of the radiocapitellar joint provides much less bony stability whilst allowing full pronation and supination in all positions of flexion and extension. The radial head is maintained in a constant position relative to the ulna, partly because of the strong annular ligament but also because of the shape of the articular surfaces.

LIGAMENTS AND CAPSULE

The complex arrangement of fibres around the elbow provides considerable stability of the joint. The ligaments are thickenings or condensations within the capsular structure and are divided into medial or ulnar and lateral or radial complexes.

The medial collateral ligament complex

This is usually subdivided into three parts – the anterior, posterior and transverse bands. The anterior band of the medial ligament is the strongest part of this complex and originates from the inferior surface of the medial epicondyle posterior to the axis of rotation and inserts on the medial aspect of the coronoid process.[6]

Biomechanical work has noted recruitment of the fibres of the anterior band of the medial ligament during most of the arc of flexion,[7] implying that it has a stabilising effect for most positions and movements. The anterior part of this band is mostly tight from full extension to 80 degrees of flexion, whereas the posterior part of the anterior band becomes most taut with flexion beyond 55 degrees. The posterior medial collateral ligament is stretched only when the elbow is in a flexed position. The transverse part of the ligament does not appear to confer much stability to the joint.

The lateral collateral ligament complex

This has three components – the radial collateral, annular and lateral ulnar collateral ligaments.

The annular ligament is a substantial structure which envelops the radial head originating and inserting on the anterior and posterior parts of the lesser sigmoid notch of the ulna. The radial collateral ligament is a poorly demarcated fan-shaped ligament which passes from the lateral epicondyle directly onto the annular ligament. Morrey and An[6] have also described a well-defined posterior margin of the radial collateral ligament that inserts onto the ulna at the supinator crest. This is the lateral ulnar collateral ligament. The radial collateral and lateral ulnar collateral ligaments are believed to be taut throughout flexion and extension and are therefore analogous to the anterior band of the medial ligament.

Biomechanics

The main ligamentous restraint to valgus instability is the anterior band of the medial collateral ligament, particularly in the mid-range of flexion. Anatomical studies have shown that when this ligament is divided the maximal increase in laxity is approximately 12 degrees at 70 degrees flexion. Further valgus instability is prevented by the radial head acting as a secondary restraint.[8] Radial head excision in the presence of an intact medial ligament does not significantly affect stability but if the ligament has been divided and the head removed gross instability will occur.[9]

Stability to a varus stress is largely provided by the humeroulnar joint with a contribution from the lateral ligament complex. Olsen *et al*.[10] found that cutting the radial collateral ligament in cadavers and then applying a varus stress produced a maximal laxity of 11.8 degrees at 110 degrees of elbow joint flexion.

Patterns of instability

VALGUS INSTABILITY

This occurs most commonly following trauma or chronic overuse of the elbow. It usually develops after damage to the medial collateral ligament, particularly its anterior band. It may also follow radial head trauma particularly if the head is excised.[11]

Chronic overuse injuries tend to occur in athletes who throw or pitch and this may cause microscopic tears of the medial collateral ligament with eventual attenuation. This gives rise to mild instability and pain when a valgus stress is applied. This presentation is seen much more frequently in North America due to the popularity of baseball, whereas it is uncommon in the UK since there is no equivalent sport.

VARUS INSTABILITY

This usually arises as a result of disruption of the lateral collateral ligament complex following elbow dislocations and fracture-dislocations. Although mild instability can be demonstrated in stress views it is unusual for this to be a significant clinical problem, unless it is associated with posterolateral instability.

ANTERIOR INSTABILITY

Anterior instability is rare but may occur with an olecranon non-union associated with collateral ligament damage. This allows the coronoid process and radial head to subluxate proximally.

POSTERIOR INSTABILITY

This pattern is always associated with fractures of the coronoid process and radial head or neck. The collateral ligaments can be damaged but may be largely intact. Dislocation or subluxation are often associated with these fractures. It is essential that this pattern is recognised in the early management of these injuries because without accurate reduction of the bony elements persistent incongruity may result.

POSTEROLATERAL ROTATORY INSTABILITY

In 1966 Osborne and Cotterill[3] pointed out that recurrent subluxation and dislocation is caused primarily by collateral ligament laxity, especially on the lateral side with secondary damage to the capitellum and radial head.

O'Driscoll *et al.*[4] analysed this further, describing the condition of posterolateral rotatory elbow instability due to laxity of the lateral ulnar collateral ligament. This lesion has become increasingly recognised in patients with recurrent instability. O'Driscoll *et al.*[12] demonstrated on cadavers that posterolateral rotatory instability forms the initial part of a spectrum of injury which can finally result in a complete elbow dislocation. The mechanism involves forced supination, valgus and axial compression of the extended elbow joint which tears the lateral ulnar collateral ligament allowing the radial head to disengage from the capitellum and subluxate posteriorly, followed by dislocation of the coronoid process. The diagnosis depends on a positive 'lateral pivot-shift' test, applying the above forces, to demonstrate the rotatory subluxation of the ulnohumeral joint and secondary dislocation of the radiohumeral joint (Fig. 14.1).

Clinical assessment and management

In order to accurately assess the elbow a detailed clinical history is required from the patient with particular regard to the initial injury and subsequent

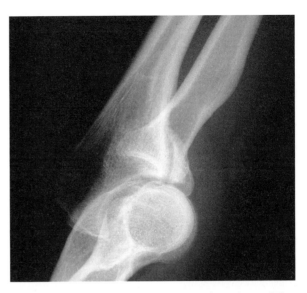

Fig. 14.1 An x-ray confirming posterolateral instability with subluxation of the radial head and widening of the ulnohumeral joint. The subluxation is produced with the lateral 'pivot-shift test' applying a valgus force.

problems. It is important to determine which activities and movements produce the symptoms.

With medial collateral ligament injuries the patient may have ill-defined discomfort and uneasiness on throwing actions. Press-ups may produce similar symptoms in patients with posterolateral rotatory instability.

On examination the elbow often appears normal with no swelling or significant muscle wasting. It usually has a very good range of movement.

Varus and valgus instability can be demonstrated by applying the appropriate force. Confirmation of instability should be obtained by stress radiographs (Fig. 14.2). The elbow must be held in at least 30 degrees of flexion in order to avoid locking the olecranon into its fossa and thus stabilising the joint. It is easy to misinterpret the stress x-ray if it has been taken with the elbow in a slightly different rotation and conclude that a change in the carrying angle has occurred. It is therefore essential to demonstrate that the joint surfaces actually separate.[13]

Posterolateral instability is tested with the patient supine and the shoulder flexed to 70 degrees. The examiner then applies axial compression, supination and a valgus force to the extended elbow as it is flexed to 20-30 degrees. Instability is demonstrated with subluxation of the radial head which becomes considerably more prominent and a dimple in the skin appears just proximal to it. The patient is usually too apprehensive to allow this manoeuvre to be performed and therefore confirmation under a

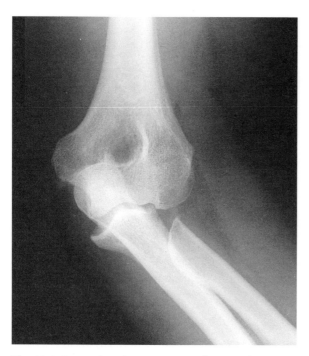

Fig. 14.2 Stress view demonstrating valgus instability due to a lax medial ligament and radial head excision.

general anaesthetic is indicated. Flexion over 40 degrees produces a sudden reduction analogous to the pivot-shift test in the knee.

Arthroscopy

In addition to an examination under anaesthetic, arthroscopy may be of value in aiding the detection

of posterolateral instability and allowing inspection of the joint for loose bodies not detected on x-ray.[14]

Treatment

In general, chronic instability of the elbow is rare and may be treated with modification of activity and muscle strengthening exercises.[15] However, if significant ligamentous disruption has occurred then surgery is likely to be the only solution. Various procedures have been described in the past which presumably caused considerable contracture around the elbow joint. Milch[16] described the use of a tibial bone block to reinforce the tip of the coronoid for recurrent posterior instability.

Osborne and Cotterill[3] successfully treated eight patients with recurrent dislocation by reefing the deficient posterolateral capsule to eliminate the pocket into which the radial head subluxed (Fig. 14.3). Similar results have been reported by Symeonides *et al.*[17] and Hassmann *et al.*[18] This was presumably effective as it restored the functional integrity of the lateral ligament complex.

LIGAMENT RECONSTRUCTION

Although successful direct repair of the lateral collateral and anterior band of the medial ligaments has been reported, reconstruction with a graft is now recommended for most patients with chronic instability. The technique achieves reliable results with marked improvement of symptoms and function.[19, 20]

The palmaris longus tendon is the most commonly used graft and has been shown to be stronger than the elbow ligament complexes.[7] It

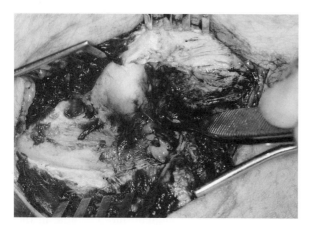

Fig. 14.3 Posterolateral instability – at operation, the forceps indent the lax capsule proximal to the subluxed radial head. This figure is reproduced in colour in the colour plate section.

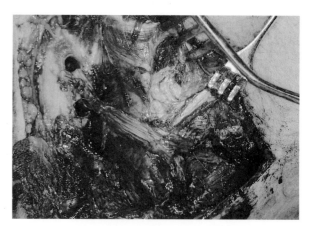

Fig. 14.4 Reconstruction of the lateral ulnar collateral ligament using a tendon graft. This figure is reproduced in colour in the colour plate section.

can be augmented with a prosthetic ligament or a heavy suture. It is essential that these are placed at the isometric points in the medial epicondyle and coronoid process, and the lateral epicondyle and ulna (Fig. 14.4). If this is not done, unnecessary tethering may cause restriction of movement. Jobe[5] now recommends that the ulnar nerve can be left *in situ* rather than transposed.

Postoperative management involves immobilisation for 3–5 weeks and then cast bracing for an additional 6–12 weeks, depending on the degree of instability. If gross instability is noted prior to surgery then consideration should be given to using a distraction device as described by Morrey[21] which should allow protection of the reconstructed ligaments for 2-3 weeks.

A medial ligament reconstruction may well be unsuccessful in cases when the radial head has been excised as it tends to stretch. Theoretically, insertion of a radial head replacement should provide stability on the lateral side of the elbow allowing the scar tissue to heal at the correct length. However, silicone rubber does not function well as a spacer and a metallic radial head is likely to sublux and impinge as the radial shaft is frequently malaligned on the capitellum due to soft tissue contracture.

References

1. Roberts PH Dislocation of the elbow. *Brit J Surg* 1969; **56:** 806-15.
2. Malkawi H Recurrent dislocation of the elbow accompanied by ulnar neuropathy: A case report and review of the literature. *Clin Orthop* 1981; **161:** 270-4.
3. Osborne G, Cotterill P Recurrent dislocation of the elbow. *J Bone Joint Surg* 1966; 48B: 340-6.
4. O'Driscoll SW, Bell DF, Morrey BF Posterolateral rotatory instability of the elbow. *J Bone Joint Surg* 1991; **73A:** 440-6.
5. Jobe FW, Stark H, Lombardo S Reconstruction of the ulnar collateral ligament in athletes. *J Bone Joint Surg* 1986; **68A:** 1158.
6. Morrey BF, An K Functional anatomy of the ligaments of the elbow. *Clin Orthop* 1985; **201:** 84-90.
7. Regan W, Korinek SL, Morrey BF, An K Biomechanical study of ligaments around the elbow joint. *Clin Orthop* 1991; **271:** 170-9.
8. Sojbjerg JO, Ovesen J, Nielsen S Experimental elbow instability after transection of the medial collateral ligament. *Clin Orthop* 1987; **218:** 186-90.
9. Morrey BF, An K, Tanaka S Valgus stability of the elbow. A definition of primary and secondary constraints. *Clin Orthop* 1991; **265:** 187-95.
10. Olsen BS, Vaesel MT, Sojbjerg JO, Helmig P, Sneppen O Lateral collateral ligament of the elbow joint: Anatomy and kinematics. *J Shoulder Elbow Surg* 1996; **5:** 103-12.
11. Norwood LA, Shook JA, Andrews JR Acute medial elbow ruptures. *Am J Sports Med* 1981; **9:** 16-9.
12. O'Driscoll SW, Morrey BF, Korinek S, An K Elbow subluxation and dislocation. *Clin Orthop* 1992; **280:** 186-97.
13. Johanson O Capsular and ligamentous injuries of the elbow joint. A clinical and arthrographic study. *Acta Chir Scand (Suppl)* 1962; 287.
14. O'Driscoll SW, Morrey BF Arthroscopy of the elbow. *J Bone Joint Surg* 1992; **74A:** 84-94.
15. Dryer R, Buckwalter J, Sprague B Treatment of chronic elbow instability. *Clin Orthop* 1974; **148:** 254-5.
16. Milch H Bilateral recurrent dislocation of the ulna at the elbow. *J Bone Joint Surg* 1936; **18:** 777-80.
17. Symeonides PP, Paschaloglou C, Stavrou Z, Pangalides TH Recurrent dislocation of the elbow. Report of three cases. *J Bone Joint Surg* 1975; **57A:** 1084-6.
18. Hassmann GC, Brunn F, Neer CS Recurrent dislocation of the elbow. *J Bone Joint Surg* 1975; **57A:** 1080-4.
19. Conway JE, Jobe FW, Glousman RE, Pink M Medial instability of the elbow in throwing athletes. *J Bone Joint Surg* 1992; **74A:** 67-83.
20. Nestor BJ, O'Driscoll SW, Morrey B Ligamentous reconstruction for posterolateral rotatory instability of the elbow. *J Bone Joint Surg* 1992; **74A:** 1235-41.
21. Morrey BF Distraction arthroplasty. *Clin Orthop* 1993; **293:** 46-54.

CHAPTER 15

Tendon injuries

JAMES RM ELLIOTT

Introduction

Injuries to tendons around the elbow are infrequent but functionally significant. The number of reported cases is increasing and predisposing factors are being suggested in some cases. It is important that the situations in which they may occur are recognised and a careful assessment of the relevant musculotendinous units and associated structures made. There is a tendency for diagnosis to be delayed making the subsequent treatment more difficult.

Incidence

The first publication dealing with any tendon disruption was in 1722 and concerned a rupture of the quadriceps mechanism.[1] A distal biceps tendon avulsion was noted in 1842.[2] The first report of a distal triceps tendon avulsion was made in 1863.[3]

While reports have concentrated on injuries to the distal biceps and triceps tendons, a tear of the tendon of brachialis has been identified using magnetic resonance imaging (MRI)[4] and a single report of rupture of brachioradialis at its musculotendinous junction (well removed from the elbow) has

also been published.[5] Anzel et al. reviewed the Mayo Clinic experience of 1014 disruptions of muscles or tendons in 781 patients between 1945 and 1954.[1] They found that 69 involved the biceps, eight the triceps (four were due to lacerations), five the brachioradialis (all due to lacerations) and two the brachialis (both due to lacerations). The location of the injury within each muscle was not recorded, but the majority of the biceps disruptions probably involved its proximal end.

Pathophysiology

Tendons have the capacity for repair without an extrinsic blood supply. Most of their nutrition is by diffusion from surrounding tissues.[6]

Kannus and Josza[7] studied tendons from 891 patients that had ruptured 'spontaneously'. They defined a spontaneous rupture as one that occurred during movements or activities that did not normally result in damage. Characteristic histopathological features of degeneration were found in 97%. These included hypoxic degenerative tendinopathy, mucoid degeneration, tendolipomatosis and calcifying tendinopathy. In the remainder they found an intratendinous foreign body, rheumatoid tendinitis, a xanthoma and a tumour or tumour-like lesion such as a ganglion. They concluded that degenerative change is common in people over the age of 35. These workers and others had previously established that individuals with blood group O appeared to have an increased risk of first time single or multiple tendon rupture and also of re-rupture.[8]

Chronic renal disease has also been said to predispose to tendon rupture. The chronic acidosis which results produces an increase in fibres within the tendon that take up elastic tissue stains and thus possibly causes tendon weakness.[9] Alternatively, pathological changes in the bone at the site of tendon insertion can be produced by secondary hyperparathyroidism.[10] Primary hyperparathyroidism has also been implicated either as a result of the direct action of parathormone or because of calcium deposits within the tendon.[11]

Other suggested predisposing factors are:

- bursitis
- Marfan's syndrome
- systemic steroid treatment e.g. for systemic lupus erythematosus (SLE)
- anabolic steroids in athletes
- local steroid injection
- osteogenesis imperfecta tarda

In McMaster's rabbit study normal tendon itself did not rupture.[12] Failure occurred instead through the muscle belly or at either end of the tendon (through the musculotendinous junction or at the attachment to bone). These findings were confirmed by his clinical observations.[12] The most common mechanism that produces a partial or complete rupture is the sudden application of a stretching force to a muscle that is contracting. Direct impact trauma either alone or in combination with a stretching force to a contracting muscle, a tetanic contraction or a laceration may also result in rupture.

Distal biceps tendon avulsion

ANATOMY

The distal biceps tendon is composed of elements derived from the bellies of both the long and short heads.[13] Its orientation changes as it descends towards the radius. Initially it is flat in the coronal plane and then passes distally and laterally crossing brachialis obliquely and rotating as it does so.[14] Once it is sagittally orientated it dives posteriorly through the interval between pronator teres and brachioradialis to its insertion onto the posterior

aspect of the bicipital tuberosity. The tendon is separated from the anterior aspect of the tuberosity by a bursa. Inflammation of this bursa may be implicated in some disruptions of the tendon.[15]

The bicipital aponeurosis (lacertus fibrosis) is an expansion that extends medially from the tendon to bend with the flexor fascia of the forearm.[13] It is more likely to be disrupted the greater the retraction of the avulsed tendon.

Seiler *et al.*[16] have shown that the distal tendon's blood supply is mainly at its proximal and distal ends with a relatively hypovascular zone in between. They also demonstrated a substantial reduction in the interval between the lateral border of the ulna and the bicipital tuberosity when the forearm is pronated. They suggested that these are potential factors in the pathogenesis of tendon disruption. While the reduced space on pronation may predispose to tendon attrition, failure usually occurs at its insertion where vascularity is good.

SITE OF INJURY

Biceps disruption can occur at any level:

- the long head
- rarely the short head
- the upper and lower musculotendinous junctions
- the muscle belly
- the insertion into the bicipital tuberosity of the radius.

Avulsion of the distal tendon accounts for only 3–10% of all biceps disruptions.[17–19]

INCIDENCE

Gilcreest[2] noted that Storks had seen a distal biceps tendon avulsion at necropsy in 1842. These injuries have been more frequently reported than distal triceps injuries but are still not often seen by individual surgeons. The largest series is by Jodzewitch and Ejubs who reported on their 30-year experience of 61 patients.[20] Dobbie's useful literature review in 1941[18] suggested that the number of reported cases was probably not a true reflection of the actual incidence.

The injury tends to occur in middle-age. Reported cases range in age from 16 to 80 years with a mean of 45. While the great majority are in males, two reviews each include one partial rupture in a female.[21, 22] Two other studies, which have looked at MRI evaluation, include males and females but the pathology in each is not specified.[4,14] Injury is a little more common on the dominant side.

MECHANISM OF INJURY

Most injuries occur during forceful flexion of the elbow e.g. while lifting a heavy weight. The risk of injury seems to be greater if a counterforce is suddenly and simultaneously applied e.g. catching a falling heavy weight. Sporting activities that involve sudden flexion of the elbow such as handball and tennis or weightlifting have also been responsible.

PRESENTATION

The patient frequently describes a sudden, painful, tearing or bursting sensation during one of the above activities followed by weakness of both flexion and supination. This is confirmed on examination. There is tenderness in the cubital fossa often with ecchymoses, bruising and swelling. In the case of a complete injury the tendon cannot be palpated and the muscle belly has retracted proximally with a characteristic alteration in its shape. This is different to that following rupture of the long head (Figs 15.1a,b). There has usually been disruption of the bicipital aponeurosis. It has been said that if the tendon has retracted by less than 8 cm with the forearm supinated then avulsion of the aponeurosis is incomplete.[23]

In the case of partial rupture, while the history is similar, the above findings are less definite. There may be no ecchymoses or bruising and a tendon defect may not be evident. There is usually weakness of both flexion and supination with pain and tenderness in the cubital fossa.

INVESTIGATIONS

The clinical findings are frequently characteristic. In cases of doubt various imaging techniques may be helpful.

1. Plain radiography may show irregularity of the bicipital tuberosity but is usually unremarkable.
2. Ultrasonography is being increasingly used to help in the diagnosis of tendon injuries. It is non-invasive and, in experienced hands can be useful in the assessment of the distal biceps tendon. However, it is better at evaluating superficial than deep tendons and can not image through bone. It provides limited anatomical detail.
3. Magnetic resonance imaging is also non-invasive but is better at demonstrating anatomical detail and provides superior contrast resolution of soft tissue than ultrasound (Fig. 15.2). It allows multiplanar imaging.[24]

TREATMENT

Most now accept that surgery is the treatment of choice for the acute avulsion in the otherwise fit individual. Untreated injuries result in long-term symptoms of pain under load as well as reduced strength and endurance of both flexion and supination.[17, 25–28] Strength deficits are of the order of 40–50% and endurance deficits are greater. These symptoms are commonly seen in cases where the diagnosis is missed or delayed.

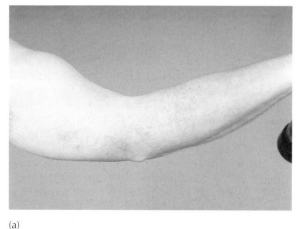

(a)

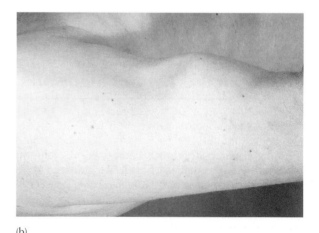

(b)

Fig. 15.1 (a) The proximally retracted belly of biceps in a case of distal tendon avulsion. (b) The distal retraction associated with rupture of the long head of biceps. This figure is reproduced in colour in the colour plate section.

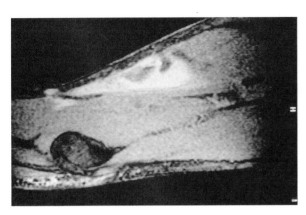

Fig. 15.2 Magnetic resonance image showing retracted avulsed tendon lying within a haematoma.

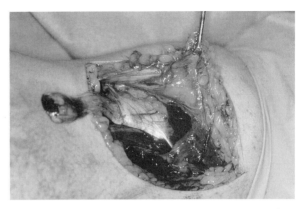

Fig. 15.3 Avulsed tendon exposed and placed on skin. This figure is reproduced in colour in the colour plate section.

The surgical options include attachment of the avulsed tendon to the tendon of brachialis, the ulna, the neck of the radius, or the bicipital tuberosity of the radius.

A virtual restoration to normal strength generally occurs when anatomical reattachment to the bicipital tuberosity is performed, whereas weakness particularly of supination persists with the other techniques. There is debate as to whether the results of reattachment in injured non-dominant limbs are as good as those in injured dominant limbs. The evidence is not consistent and is based on small numbers.[27–30]

There are different techniques for attaching the avulsed tendon to the tuberosity. These include the creation of a cavity and suturing through drill holes,[23,32] the use of anchor sutures and suturing to a periosteal flap.

OPERATIVE TECHNIQUE

The most popular approach is a two-incision technique derived from that of Boyd and Anderson.[31]

The procedure is performed under tourniquet and aseptic conditions. The patient is in the supine position. A curvilinear incision is commenced above the elbow laterally, and passes down to and then medially along the flexor crease, taking care to protect the lateral cutaneous nerve of the forearm (Fig. 15.3). From here it can be extended distally for approximately 5 cm. After division of the deep fascia the avulsed tendon is usually noted to be lying curled proximally within a haematoma. Its end has a somewhat bulbous appearance (Fig. 15.4) and often requires a little trimming so that it will fit into the cavity to be created in the tuberosity. Two heavy non-absorbable Bunnell-type sutures are introduced into the tendon with their ends emerg-

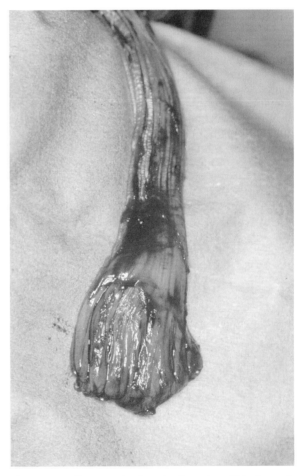

Fig. 15.4 Bulbous end of avulsed tendon. This figure is reproduced in colour in the colour plate section.

ing from its avulsed surface. The tunnel through which the tendon originally passed is identified with a finger. A narrow blunt instrument is passed along it with the elbow in flexion. In order to minimise

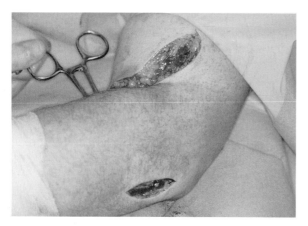

Fig. 15.5 The two incisions with instrument passed along tendon track, through anconeus and overlying skin. This figure is reproduced in colour in the colour plate section.

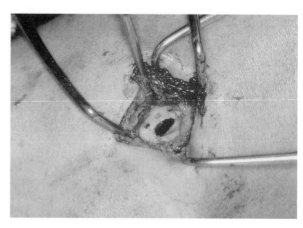

Fig. 15.6 Cavity excavated in bicipital tuberosity with three well spaced drill holes in its anterior rim. This figure is reproduced in colour in the colour plate section.

the risk of heterotopic bone formation that might cause a radioulnar synostosis, it is important to keep away from the ulna and stay against the medial side of the radius, thus avoiding the establishment of a connection between the two.[33] When the bottom of the tunnel is reached, pressure is applied to the blunt instrument and a second incision made by cutting down on it from the extensor surface of the proximal forearm (Fig. 15.5). This incision is developed by blunt dissection and the bicipital tuberosity exposed with the forearm maximally pronated. A cavity is excavated in the tuberosity using a high speed burr and three adequately separated holes are drilled into its posterior rim (Fig. 15.6). The suture ends are carefully led down the tunnel and passed through the drill holes. With the elbow flexed and the forearm now in the mid-prone position the tendon is drawn towards the excavated cavity and into it by traction on the suture. It is necessary to ensure that the tendon end fits snugly into the cavity and is not caught on its edge. The posterior rim is easily seen but the anterior rim is now deep to the tendon and hard to visualise. The sutures are then tied (Fig. 15.7). A suction drain is introduced prior to wound closure.

Cast immobilisation with the elbow at 90 degrees and the forearm supinated is continued for a total of 4 weeks. A dynamic orthosis providing assisted flexion and allowing passive motion from 45 to 145 degrees but maintaining supination is then substituted (Fig. 15.8) and left in place for a further 4 weeks. During this time assisted passive exercises under the supervision of a physiotherapist are undertaken. After this the orthosis is removed and graduated active motion begun. Loads sufficient for the activities of daily living are permitted at 12

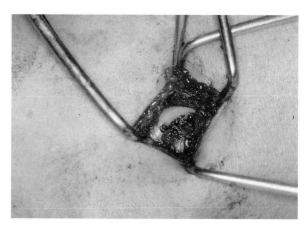

Fig. 15.7 Tendon end introduced into cavity and sutured in place. This figure is reproduced in colour in the colour plate section.

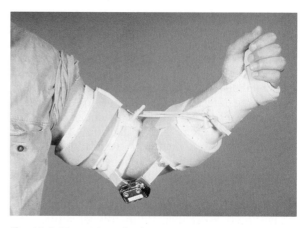

Fig. 15.8 Dynamic orthosis.

weeks but unrestricted loading should be avoided until 6 months following reconstruction.

RESULTS

Prior to the use of objective testing techniques the extent of flexion and in particular, supination weakness in the untreated cases were not always appreciated. Anatomical reattachment has been shown consistently to restore normal or near normal power in the dominant limb.[26,27] A consensus does not exist concerning the results of reattachment in non-dominant limbs. Some feel flexor and supinator power are diminished.[27,29,30] Recovery of endurance seems to be less of a problem.

Reconstruction avoids the persisting pain under load that is characteristic of the conservatively managed case. There do not appear to be any cases of re-rupture in the English language literature despite the evidence that suggests that there is pre-existing tendon degeneration in many cases.

COMPLICATIONS

The main concern about anatomical reattachment is the risk of injury to the radial nerve. It occasionally occurs but usually results in a neuropraxia. In the series of 61 patients presented by Jodzewitch and Ejubs[20] there were three posterior interosseous nerve injuries. They stated that 'complete recovery took place in 6 months' and that the long-term results in 'two cases were good and in one satisfactory'. Permanent damage to the radial nerve is rare. A case of delayed onset posterior interosseous nerve palsy has been reported.[56]

Proximal radioulnar synostosis is a potentially significant complication and has been recorded on a number of occasions. It has been suggested that in order to minimise the risk of it occurring it is important to avoid exposing the ulna and thus prevent the establishment of a direct communication between it and the radius.[26,33] It is unclear whether this actually achieves this goal but it seems logical.

THE LATE CASE

Once 2 or 3 weeks have elapsed from injury, reattachment to the bicipital tuberosity becomes more difficult.[34] Tendon retraction is harder to overcome and the tunnel previously occupied by it is becoming obliterated. Attempts to define the tunnel are associated with a greater risk of radial nerve damage. Attachment of the distal biceps tendon to

that of the brachialis will largely restore flexor power. It is thus a matter of judgement as to whether continuing supination weakness is too high a price to pay for avoiding the possibility of a wrist drop.

If it is felt that anatomical reattachment should be performed, it may be necessary to use a fascia lata autograft or a frozen allograft to augment tendon length. Tendon augmentation devices have also been used.

PARTIAL RUPTURE

Reports of partial rupture of the distal biceps tendon are few.[21,22,35,36] The history of injury and the physical findings are usually similar to those for a complete disruption, but with the tendon remaining palpable. It is important to distinguish a partial rupture from cubital bursitis. If doubt exists about the diagnosis, magnetic resonance imaging can be useful. Only six individual cases have been reported. One of these occurred in a diabetic and was associated with median nerve compression. The status of the bicipital aponeurosis is only recorded in one case. Falchook et al.[14] in a study of the usefulness of magnetic resonance imaging in the evaluation of distal biceps injuries collectively identified six partial ruptures.

Generally, initial management in the above reports was conservative and operative treatment only performed when it was found that pain and weakness persisted. The exception was a case associated with compression of the median nerve where early exploration was carried out.

Surgical treatment consisted of excision of the area of tendon damage followed by anatomical reattachment to the tuberosity as for a complete avulsion.

Distal triceps injuries

ANATOMY

Active extension of the elbow allows the hand to be employed in tasks away from the body such as pushing, thrusting, use of walking aids and providing assistance when rising from a sitting position. Simultaneous contraction of the extensor and flexor musculature stabilises the joint so that it may be used as a secure base in order to allow other prime movers to act.[56]

The triceps is the principle extensor of the elbow joint. The medial head functions during all forms of extension but action of the long and lateral heads is largely confined to resisted extension.[12]

The tendon commences at about the mid-point of the muscle. It consists of two laminae. One is an aponerurosis overlying much of the distal half of the muscle. The deep lamina is derived from the long and lateral heads and is attached to the under-surface of the aponeurosis but lies at right angles to it. Together they are T-shaped in cross-section and are inserted into the olecranon with a lateral band continuing distally over the anconeus to blend with the antebrachial fascia.[13] The bulk of the aponeu-rosis blends with the periosteum of the proximal ulna and attaches via Sharpey's fibres to the dorsal surface of the olecranon. The deep lamina attaches to the medial half of the olecranon's proximal surface.

SITES OF INJURY

Injuries of the triceps apparatus can occur at any level but in the great majority of cases take the form of an avulsion of its insertion into the olecranon process of the ulna. At the time of writing, review of the English language literature reveals 44 cases with the site of injury confirmed at operation. Of these, 33 were distal avulsions, six were intrasub-stance tendon disruptions, two were injuries at the musculotendinous junction, one was a muscle belly rupture and one avulsion injury each occurred at the origins of the medial and lateral heads. There appears to be no recorded injury of the long head.

INCIDENCE

Injury of the distal triceps was first reported in 1868.[3] Fifty to sixty have been reported since. Until 1972 only seven cases had been published in the English language literature. Since 1972 the number of reports has increased but most deal with only one or two cases. The report of Levy *et al.* of 16 cases is the largest collection to date.[37]

The male : female ratio of the reported cases is approximately 3:1. Tendon degeneration appears to play a less significant role than in distal biceps tendon avulsions. This is supported by the younger mean age of the patients (around 33 years in both sexes). Avulsions have been recorded at 7 years of age[38] and at 72.[39]

MECHANISM OF INJURY

Disruption most often occurs when a sudden load is applied to the contracting triceps e.g. a fall on the outstretched hand with the elbow in some flexion. The likelihood of injury is increased if at the same time the muscle receives a direct blow. It has also been recorded as occurring as a result of a fall onto the elbow itself, in a road traffic accident in which the patient braced himself by holding the steering wheel, while weightlifting, receiving a blow over the muscle during martial arts, during an overhand service in a game of volleyball and during a seizure.[40,41] Lacerations have also been recorded[1] but will not be considered further in this chapter.

Reports of local predisposition to tendon disrup-tion are rare.[39] More generally, there have been a number of cases where injury seems to have occurred more easily than usual in those with chronic renal failure.[40] There has been a report of one case of bilateral avulsions in a patient with osteogenesis imperfecta tarda where the bony frag-ment in each case was large and constituted an intra-articular fracture of the olecranon. Systemic and local steroid therapy have also been impli-cated.[42,43]

PRESENTATION

Isolated complete distal triceps tendon avulsion typically presents with a history of a popping or tearing sensation during an incident such as that described above. The patient complains of pain and extension weakness.

Examination in the acute phase reveals an inabil-ity to extend the elbow against gravity, as well as ecchymoses and bruising in the area around the triceps insertion (Fig. 15.9). There may be a dimple over the resulting defect and localised swelling. A defect can often be palpated in the tendon during attempts at resisted extension. In cases where a direct blow has occurred there may be an abrasion

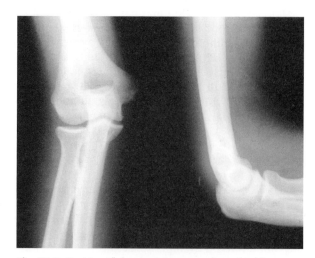

Fig. 15.9 Positive 'flake sign'. Note small avulsed fragment lying posterior to tip of olecranon and lower humerus.

at the site of impact. In one case the presenting symptoms related to the ulnar nerve but the cause was unclear.[42]

Viegas[38] described a modification of the Thompson test (used to help in the diagnosis of Achilles tendon disruption) that can be employed in this situation. The upper segment of the injured limb is supported and the forearm allowed to hang free. The triceps muscle bulk is squeezed. If the distal tendon is intact there should be some passive extension movement of the forearm. Its absence implies a discontinuity of the extensor mechanism.

Identifying the isolated injury should usually be straighforward. Unfortunately awareness that it can occur is not widespread and late diagnosis is common.

In the case that presents late the pain will have persisted but be less severe and the patient is likely to complain of continuing extension weakness which is confirmed on examination. A palpable defect may be noted during attempts at resisted extension. The ecchymoses, bruising and visible dimple are less likely.

The risk of missing this injury is higher when it occurs in combination with a fracture. The largest series of distal triceps tendon avulsions is that by Levy *et al.*[37] who report 16 cases where the tendon injury was associated with bony damage elsewhere. In 15 this took the form of a radial head fracture and in one a fracture of the capitellum. In Tarsney's report one case had a fracture of the radial neck.[44] Goldberg *et al.*[45] in a study of 36 radial head fractures noted radiographic evidence suggestive of injury in the region of the triceps insertion in four. In Lee's single case report there was a concomitant Colles' fracture.[46] In my own experience of three cases one patient had an associated undisplaced marginal fracture of the radial head and a second had an intra-articular effusion but no radiographically evident fracture. In these situations the symptoms and signs arising from the bony damage are liable to be dominant and the triceps injury risks being missed. The most severe pain arises from the fracture and an inability to extend the elbow is often attributed to it. It may therefore be that distal triceps injuries are significantly more common than is currently appreciated. It is thus essential that the distal triceps is assessed in all cases where there is a fracture of the lateral side of the elbow joint (involving the radial head or neck or the capitellum).

INVESTIGATIONS

Plain radiography

A review of the literature shows that in 87% of cases a lateral view of the elbow shows an avulsion

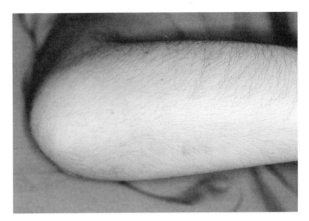

Fig. 15.10 Bruising following distal triceps avulsion.

fracture at the triceps insertion (Fig. 15.10). This is known as the 'flake sign' and essentially represents an extra-articular fracture of the olecranon. The bony fragment is usually small and easy to ignore but its presence is pathognomonic of distal triceps tendon avulsion. The extent of its displacement from the olecranon is variable. A careful search should also be made for evidence of damage to the radial head or neck or the capitellum. The presence of displaced fat pads may help to focus attention.

In the immature skeleton avulsion tends to occur through the junction of the maturing olecranon physis with bone. This produces a larger fragment than in the adult.[38]

Ultrasound

This is being used more frequently to help in the diagnosis of injuries to superficial tendons and can be of value in this location if there is doubt. It provides limited anatomical detail.

Magnetic resonance imaging

The superior detail provided by magnetic resonance imaging enables the distinction between a partial and a complete tear to be made.[47] It also allows occult or subtle associated bony damage to be identified.[48]

TREATMENT

There is general agreement that operative reconstruction is the treatment of choice in the acute complete avulsion injury. Different techniques have been used[49,50] but all aim to reattach the tendon to the olecranon. Most current methods achieve this by using non-absorbable sutures passed through drill holes but in some earlier reports wire was used. Subperisoteal flaps have also been created to form the point of reattachment in some cases.

OPERATIVE TECHNIQUES

The procedure is carried out under tourniquet and aseptic conditions. The patient is in the semi-prone or lateral position and the injured limb is placed over a padded support.

A vertical posterolateral incision is made to avoid the tip of the olecranon. It should be sufficiently long to allow the triceps aponeurosis and olecranon to be comfortably exposed. Provided there are no preoperative neurological signs it is probably not necessary to expose the ulnar nerve but care should be taken to avoid damaging it.

The area of injury is identified and the haematoma evacuated (Fig. 15.11). Non-absorbable sutures are passed into the distal tendon using a criss-cross or Krackow technique.[51] Drill holes are then made in the olecranon so that at least two secure sutures can be passed through from the tendon. These can either be in the form of two crossed or three longitudinal holes. I have not used and am not aware of any reports in the literature concerning the use of anchor sutures in the treatment of this injury but they would seem to be a helpful alternative in non-osteopenic bone. Having passed the sutures, traction is applied to pull the tendon against bone before they are securely tied (Fig. 15.12). Auxillary sutures are used along the sides of the avulsed tissue to secure it to adjacent tendon or muscle thereby augmenting the repair. This can be further reinforced by developing a flap of forearm fascia based at the olecranon and humeral epicondyles and turning it proximally.[50] The tourniquet is deflated and haemostasis achieved. If necessary a suction drain can be used. The wound is closed and a cast applied with the joint in approximately 45 degrees of flexion. This remains in place for 3 weeks.

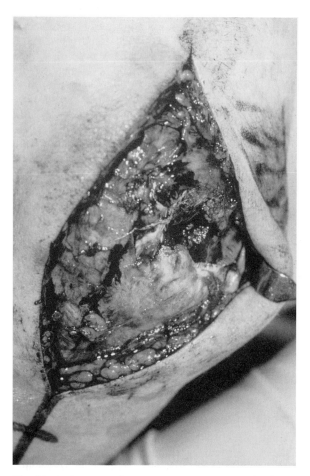

Fig. 15.11 Acute avulsion to triceps insertion. This figure is reproduced in colour in the colour plate section.

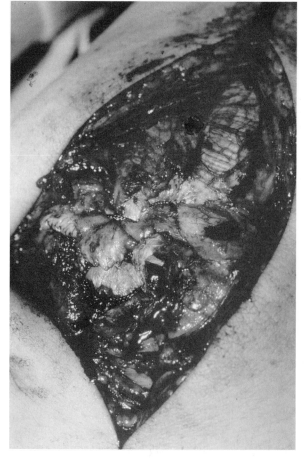

Fig. 15.12 Repaired acute avulsion. This figure is reproduced in colour in the colour plate section.

Gentle active range of motion exercises are then commenced. While normal activity is permissible by 12 weeks, extreme loading should be avoided for 6 months.

As an alternative to using a cast, Levy has recommended that a 4 mm Mersilene band be passed through the triceps aponeurosis proximally and the olecranon distally to take load off the repair and allow early motion.[52] Experience with a similar technique in which wire was used to protect patellar tendon repairs suggests that the detensioning device should be removed routinely at approximately 12 weeks to minimise bone and soft tissue erosion.

Where the bony fragment is large, as in the young teenager, treatment should be by fixation of the fracture fragment with either a screw or by tension band wiring.[38]

RESULTS

Normal or near normal power and function are the usual result even in those that present late. Only one published report has used an objective measurement technique to determine eventual triceps performance following repair.[43] The patient was a bodybuilder and power weight lifter. He had a deficit of 10% for both work and peak torque 18 months following reconstruction. No information regarding endurance is available. A residual fixed flexion deformity of a few degrees is common. The reported experience suggests that recovery has occurred by 8–12 weeks.

COMPLICATIONS

Significant complications are rare. In one case a residual fixed flexion deformity of 20 degrees was noted at 13 years. There are no published instances in the English language literature of re-rupture. Pain is not generally a problem but in one case a small bursa formed over wires used for fixation.[53]

THE LATE CASE

As indicated above there are a significant number of cases where the diagnosis is made late. When the delay exceeds a matter of weeks the aponeurosis has retracted proximally and simple repair is not feasible.

Clayton and Thirupathi[39] have recommended a method for dealing with the problem of tendon retraction. The defect is defined (Fig. 15.13). The technique involves developing and then turning down a flap of the aponeurosis from the area proximal to the tear and suturing it to the olecranon. Anchoring sutures are necessary at the base of the flap to prevent it becoming detached (Fig. 15.14) and a side-to-side closure is made of the defect left at its origin (Fig. 15.15). Postoperative management is the same as in the acute case.

Others have used synthetic tape[54] to bridge the defect.

PARTIAL RUPTURE

The term implies that a portion of the insertion remains intact. Diagnosis requires care and should only be made if extension against resistance is normal by a few days following injury.[55] A magnetic resonance scan helps in evaluation. Some manage this injury conservatively[55] but others recommend treatment as for the complete lesion.[44]

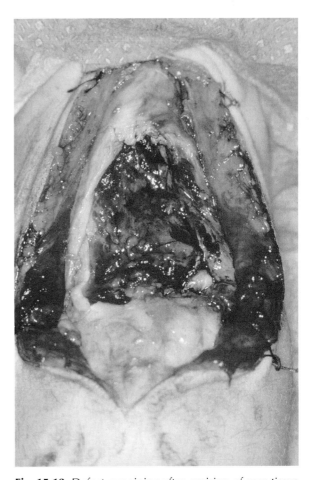

Fig. 15.13 Defect remaining after excision of scar tissue in case presenting late. This figure is reproduced in colour in the colour plate section.

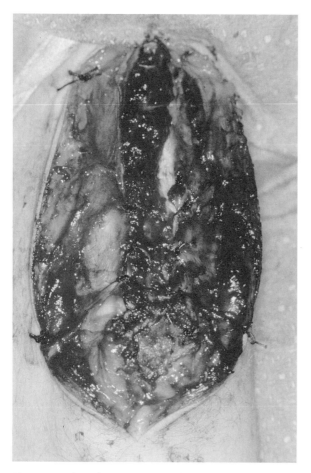

Fig. 15.14 Flap of aponeurosis turned down to cover defect. This figure is reproduced in colour in the colour plate section.

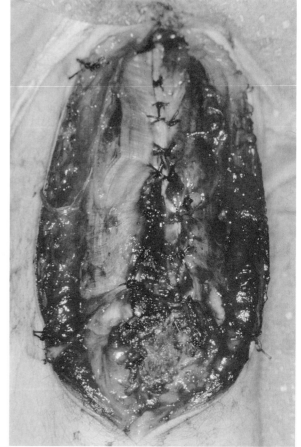

Fig. 15.15 Closure of defect from which flap derived. This figure is reproduced in colour in the colour plate section.

References

1. Anzel SH, Covey KW, Weiner AD, Lipscomb PR Disruption of muscles and tendons. An analysis of 1014 cases. *Surgery* 1959; **45:** 406–14.
2. Gilcreest EL Rupture of muscles and tendons, particularly subcutaneous rupture of the biceps flexor cubiti. *J Am Med Assoc* 1925; **84:** 1819–22.
3. Partridge M A case of rupture of the tendon of the triceps cubiti. *Med Times Gaz* 1968; **1:** 175–6.
4. Fitzgerald SW, Curry DR, Erickson SJ *et al.* Distal biceps tendon injury: MR imaging diagnosis. *Radiology* 1994; **191:** 203–6.
5. Hamilton AT Subcutaneous rupture of the brachioradialis muscle. *Surgery* 1948; **23:** 806–7.
6. Garratt WE Trauma: soft tissue. In: *Orthopaedic knowledge* Update 11. Home Study Syllabus, American Academy of Orthopaedic Surgeons 1987: 90–1.
7. Kannus P, Josza L Histopathological changes preceding spontaneous rupture of a tendon. *J Bone Joint Surg* 1991; **739:** 1507–25.
8. Jozsa L, Balint JB, Kannus P *et al.* Distribution of blood groups in patients with tendon rupture. *J Bone Joint Surg* 1989; **71B:** 272–4.
9. Murphy KJ, McPhee I Tears of major tendons in chronic acidosis with elastosis. *J Bone Joint Surg* 1965; **47A:** 1253–8.
10. Cirincione RJ, Baker BE Tendon ruptures with secondary hyperparathyroidism. *J Bone Joint Surg* 1975; **57A:** 852–3.
11. Preston FS, Adicoff A Hyperparathyroidism with avulsion of three major tendons. Report of a case. *New Engl J Med* 1961; **266:** 968–70.
12. McMaster PE Tendon and muscle ruptures. Clinical and experimental studies on the causes and location of subcutaneous ruptures. *J Bone Joint Surg* 1933; **15:** 705–22.
13. Williams PL, Warwick R, Dyson M, Bannister LH (eds) *Gray's anatomy* (37th edn). Edinburgh: Churchill Livingstone, 1989.
14. Falchook FS, Zlatkin MB, Erbacher GE *et al.* Rupture of the distal biceps tendon: Evaluation with MR imaging. *Radiology* 1994; **190:** 659–63.
15. Karanjia ND, Stiles PJ Cubital bursitis. *J Bone Joint Surg* 1988; **70B:** 832–3.

16. Seiler JG, Parker LM, Chamberland PDC *et al*. The distal biceps tendon. Two potential mechanism in its rupture: Arterial supply and mechanical impingement. *J Shoulder Elbow Surg* 1995; **4:** 149–56.
17. Baker BE, Bierwagen D Rupture of the distal tendon of biceps brachii. *J Bone Joint Surg* 1985; **67A:** 414–7.
18. Dobbie RP Avulsion of the lower biceps brachii tendon. *Am J Surg* 1941; **51:** 661–83.
19. Postacchini F, Puddu, G Subcutaneous rupture of the distal biceps brachii tendon. *J Sports Med* 1975; **15:** 81–90.
20. Jodzewitch H, Ejubs L Surgical treatment of distal biceps tendon injuries. Poster abstract presented at Sixth International Congress on Surgery of the Shoulder, Helsinik, Finland 27 June–1 July 1995.
21. Bourne MH, Morrey BF Partial rupture of the distal biceps tendon. *Clin Orth Rel Res* 1991; **271:** 143–8.
22. Foxworthy M, Kinninmonth AWG Median nerve compression in the proximal forearm as a complication of partial rupture of the distal biceps brachii tendon. *J Hand Surg* 1992; **17B:** 515–7.
23. Le Huec JC, Moinard M, Liquois F *et al*. Distal rupture of the tendon of biceps brachii. *J Bone Joint Surg* 1996; **78B:** 767–70.
24. Mayer DP, Schmidt RG, Ruiz S MRI diagnosis of biceps tendon rupture. *Comput Med Imaging Graph* 1992; **16:** 345–7.
25. Hovelius L, Joseffson G Rupture of the distal biceps tendon. *Acta Orthop Scand* 1977; **48:** 280–2.
26. Morrey BF. Askew LJ, An KN, Dobyns JH Rupture of the bistal tendon of biceps brachii. A biomechanical study. *J Bone Joint Surg* 1985; **67A:** 418–21.
27. D'Allessandro DF, Sheilds CL, Tibone JE, Chandler, RW Repair of distal biceps tendon ruptures in athletes. *Am J Sports Med* 1993; **21:** 114–9.
28. Morrey, BF Tendon injuries about the elbow. In: *The elbow and its disorders* (2nd edn). Morrey BF (ed) Philadelphia: WB Saunders Co, 1993.
29. Agins HJ, Chess JL, Hoekstra DV, Teitge RA Rupture of the distal insertion of the biceps brachii tendon. *Clin Orth Rel Res* 1988; **234:** 34–8.
30. Leighton MM, Bush-Joseph CA, Bach BR Distal biceps brachii repair. Results in dominant and nondominant extremities. *Clin Orthop Rel Res* 1995; **317:** 114–21.
31. Boyd HB, Anderson LD A method for the reinsertion of the distal biceps brachii tendon. *J Bone Joint Surg* 1961; **43A:** 1041–3.
32. Plessas SJ, Mihara K, Holdsworth BJ, Wallace WA Management of early and late ruptures of the distal biceps tendon. Presented at Sixth International Congress on Surgery of the Shoulder in Helsinki, Finland, 27 June–1 July 1995.
33. Failla JM, Amadio PC. Morrey BF, Beckenbaugh RD Proximal radioulnar synostosis after repair of distal biceps brachii rupture by the two-incision technique. *Clin Orth Rel Res* 1990; **253:** 133–6.
34. Le Huec JC, Zipoli B, Liquois F *et al*. A distal rupture of the biceps tendon. MRI evaluation and surgical repair. Presented at Sixth International Congress on Surgery of the Shoulder in Helsinki, Finland, 27 June–1 July, 1995.
35. Nielsen K Partial rupture of the distal biceps brachii tendon. A case report. *Acta Orthop Scand* 1987; **58:** 287–8.
36. Rokito AS, McLaughlin JA, Gallagher MA, Zuckerman JD Partial rupture of the distal biceps tendon. *J Shoulder Elbow Surg* 1996; **5:** 73–5.
37. Levy M, Goldberg I, Meir I Fracture of the head of the radius with a tear or avulsion of the triceps Tendon. *J Bone Joint Surg* 1982; **64B:** 70–2.
38. Viegas SF Avulsion of the triceps tendon. *Orthop Rev* 1990; **19:** 533–6.
39. Clayton ML, Thirupathi RG Rupture of the triceps tendon with olecranon bursitis. A case report with a new method of repair. *Clin Orthop Rel Res* 1984; **184:** 183–5.
40. Searfoss R, Tripi J, Bowers W Triceps brachii rupture. Case report. *J Trauma* 1976; **16:** 244–6.
41. Mont MA, Torres J, Tsao, A.K Hypocalcaemic-induced tetany that causes triceps and bilateral quadriceps tendon ruptures. *Orthop Rev* 1994; **23:** 57–60.
42. Herrick RT, Herrick S Ruptured triceps in a power-lifter presenting as cubital tunnel syndrome. *Am J Sports Med* 1987; **15:** 514–6.
43. Stannard JP, Bucknell AL Rupture of the triceps tendon associated with steroid injections. *Am J Sports Med* 1993; **21:** 482–5.
44. Tarsney FF Rupture and avulsion of the triceps. *Clin Orthop Rel Res* 1972; **83:** 177–83.
45. Goldberg I, Peyland J, Yosipovitch Z Late results of excision of the radial head for an isolated closed fracture. *J Bone Joint Surg* 1986; **68A:** 675–9.
46. Lee MLH Rupture of the triceps tendon. *Brit Med J* 1960; **2:** 197.
47. Tiger E, Mayer DP, Glazer R Complete avulsion of the triceps tendon: MRI diagnosis. *Comput Med Imaging Graph* 1993; **17:** 51–4.
48. Fritz RC Magnetic resonance imaging of the elbow. *Semin Roentgenol* 1995; **30:** 241–64.
49. Anderson JJ, LeCocq JF Rupture of the triceps tendon. *J Bone Joint Surg* 1957; **39A:** 444–6.
50. Bennett BS Triceps tendon rupture. *J Bone Joint Surg* 1962; **44A:** 741–4.
51. Krackow KA, Thomas SC, Jones LC A new stitch for ligament-tendon fixation. Brief note. *J Bone Joint Surg* 1986; **68A:** 764–6.
52. Levy M Repair of triceps tendon avulsions or ruptures. Brief report *J Bone Joint Surg* 1987; **69B:** 115.
53. Pantazopoulos T, Exarchou E, Stavrou Z, Hartofilikidis-Garofilidis G Avulsion of the triceps tendon. *J Trauma* 1975; **15:** 827–9.
54. Sherman OH, Snyder SJ, Fox JM Triceps tendon avulsion in a professional body builder. *Am J Sports Med* 1984; **12:** 328–9.
55. Farrar EL, Lippert FG Avulsion of the triceps tendon. *Clin Orth Rel Res* 1981; **161:** 242–6.
56. Katzman BM, Caligiuri DA, Klein DM, Gorup JM Delayed onset of posterior interosseous nerve palsy after distal biceps tendon repair. *J Shoulder Elbow Surg* 1997; **6:** 393–5.

CHAPTER 16

Arthrolysis of the post-traumatic stiff elbow

NEVILLE RM KAY

Introduction

The ease and rapidity with which the elbow stiffens after trauma has been recognised for many years and surgical attempts to correct this are not new. Wilson in 1944[1] described capsulectomy for the relief of flexure contracture of the elbow following fracture, whilst Bhattacharyya[2] described a combined medial and lateral approach in 1974. Urbaniak et al.[3] in 1985 and Breen et al.[4] in 1988 reported the use of the anterior approach to the elbow. Breen et al.[4] also advocated continuous passive motion postoperatively.

Weizenbluth and his colleagues[5] reported a series of 13 cases, utilising the lateral approach and emphasised the necessity to release all the soft tissues that are seen to interfere with motion. In addition, excision of bone obstacles found during the surgical exposure was advised. These authors also stressed the importance of the appropriate selection of patients but placed little emphasis on the effects of post-traumatic calcification.

With the power of the keyboard changing industrial and domestic life, the disability associated with a stiff elbow is increasingly recognised and interest in arthrolysis of the post-traumatic stiff elbow has acquired greater significance.

The end result of trauma to the elbow still appears to be unpredictable. It is by no means unusual to see patients with 'insignificant' fractures of the radial head ending up with permanently stiff elbows whilst other patients, often with displaced fractures of the radial head achieve a pain free fully mobile joint. Although speculation as to the cause of this significant difference is intriguing, there can be little doubt that natural joint laxity is helpful in preserving joint mobility after trauma. Conversely collagen diathesis (the associated presence of Dupuytren's contracture) is often associated with the tendancy to stiffen.

Classification of post-traumatic stiffness

Morrey[6] classified post-traumatic stiffness of the elbow principally into extrinsic and intrinsic causes but noted that a mixed picture was also possible. Extrinsic causes were stated to be due to contracture of the capsule, muscle or the development of osseous bridges. That ectopic bone can form around both the uninjured and injured elbow in patients with severe burn and central nervous system trauma is well documented.[7] It occurs most commonly in the region of the anterior capsule, and brachialis muscle. Children seem particularly vulnerable to post-traumatic ossification[8] with periosteal stripping and haematoma calcification being frequently incriminated.

Morrey's[6] intrinsic causes of post-traumatic stiffness were stated to be due to intra-articular adhesions, avascular necrosis of comminuted fracture fragments, and displacement of the fracture components.

Although this classification clearly identifies the aetiological factors responsible for post-traumatic stiffness of the elbow, in the author's experience a more useful classification is based on clinical assessment and radiographic analysis:

I   Soft tissue contracture.
II Soft tissue contracture with ossification.
III Undisplaced intra-articular fracture with soft tissue contracture.
IV Displaced intra-articular fracture and soft tissue contracture.
V   Displaced intra-articular fracture soft tissue contracture and ectopic ossification.
VI Post-traumatic bony bars.

The practical significance of such a classification is that groups I, III, and IV may well be amenable to aggressive arthrolysis but as yet the author has met with little success in groups II V and VI.

The role of the collateral ligaments in elbow contracture

The role of the anterior capsule and the brachialis muscle in the production of elbow contracture following trauma is well documented,[8,9] but less attention has been given to the role of the collateral ligaments in maintaining post-traumatic elbow stiffness.

The anterior part of the anterior band of the medial collateral ligament is most taut from full extension to 80 degrees of flexion whilst the posterior part of this band becomes most taut with flexion beyond 55 degrees. On the lateral side of the elbow the radial collateral and lateral ulnar collateral ligaments are taut throughout flexion and extension. Damage to these ligaments with scarring in either the medial or lateral ligament complex is likely therefore to result in elbow stiffness.

The role of the osseous anatomy in elbow contracture

In addition to capsular, ligamentous and muscular damage most elbow injuries are associated with fractures. Failure to reduce the fracture adequately will result in loss of joint congruity and increased elbow stiffness. This situation is further compromised by the development of intra-articular adhesions.[6]

Preoperative patient assessment

In the selection of patients for elbow arthrolysis it is important to have a well motivated patient, since the postoperative rehabilitation regime is often prolonged and may require at least one manipulation of the elbow under general anaesthetic.

Good skin, preferably unscarred, is a further prerequisite and the muscles around the elbow must be essentially normal and able to function once the elbow is released. It serves little value having a mobile elbow but inadequate muscle control. Neurological complications are therefore a contraindication.

Whilst ectopic bone is not an absolute contraindication to surgery the recognition of soft tissue ossification/calcification should increase the pessimism with which arthrolysis is approached. The removal of 'mature' bony bars has, in the author's experience been disappointing and resulted in minimal improvement in range of elbow movement.

During the preoperative assessment the patient should be advised that postoperative analgesia will be provided by means of a brachial plexus block.[10,11] Failure to provide adequate pain relief postoperatively will result in the patient not moving the elbow and thus further stiffness will develop.

The patient should also be told that immediately after the operation movement of the elbow will be commenced by means of a continous passive motion machine.[11] A variety of different machines for the elbow are available but care should be exercised in the use of ambulatory continuous passive motion machines which leave the hand and arm dependant. Troublesome oedema of the hand may occur with the use of this type of appliance.

Preoperative radiographic assessment

A careful preoperative radiographic assessment cannot be overemphasised. However, despite meticulous attention the surgeon must be prepared for surprises. The bedrock of the radiographic assessment are good quality anteroposterior and lateral views of the elbow. These will usually allow identification of loose bodies together with bony and ankylosed fragments. Tomography and computed tomography scanning may also be valuable in determining the contour of the articular surface and whether fragments are attached to bone by bone or by fibrous tissue.

Arthrolysis of the post-traumatic stiff elbow

Arthrolysis of the post-traumatic stiff elbow is not an operation to be undertaken lightly by the occasional elbow surgeon. Weizenbluth *et al.*[5] noted 'arthrolysis of the elbow is not an innocent procedure. Even a badly damaged elbow can be made worse by mismanagement'.

Surgical techniques

Although posterior contractures may occur the commonest abnormality is associated with an anterior capsular contracture. This may be treated surgically either via an anterior approach[3,4] lateral approach[6] or combined lateral and medial approach.[2]

ANTERIOR APPROACH

Urbaniak *et al.*[3] reported their experience of this approach in 15 patients:

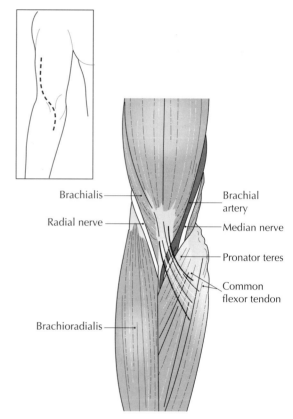

Brachialis — Brachial artery

Radial nerve — Median nerve

Pronator teres

Common flexor tendon

Brachioradialis

Fig. 16.1 The skin incision and surgical anatomy for the anterior approach to the elbow in order to perform an anterior capsulotomy. Redrawn after Ref. 3.

The anterior skin incision begins proximally and laterally, curves across the elbow-flexion crease and continues distally and medially along the forearm (Fig. 16.1). The medial and lateral antebrachial cutaneous nerves, median, radial and musculocutaneous nerves and the brachial artery are all identified and protected.

The interval between the common flexor origin and the biceps tendon is developed (Fig. 16.2) and the brachialis muscle partially released from the joint capsule. The interval between the biceps tendon and the brachioradialis is located which allows further development of the plane between the brachialis muscle and anterior capsule of the joint. By retracting the brachialis the entire anterior capsule is visualised allowing the anterior capsulotomy to extend from the medial collateral ligament to the lateral collateral ligament (Figs 16.3, 16.4). If necessary in order to improve extension a lengthening tenotomy of the biceps and myotomy of the brachialis can also be performed. The wound is closed over suction drainage.

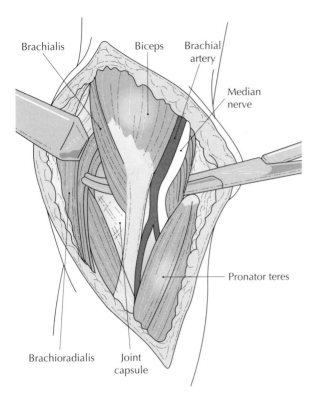

Brachialis   Biceps   Brachial artery   Median nerve   Pronator teres   Brachioradialis   Joint capsule

Fig. 16.2 The medial interval between the biceps and pronator teres is developed to expose the medial part of the capsule. The joint line is located by flexing and extending the elbow. A clamp is passed laterally to identify the lateral portion of the anterior part of the capsule. The brachialis muscle is freed from the anterior capsule. Redrawn after Ref. 3.

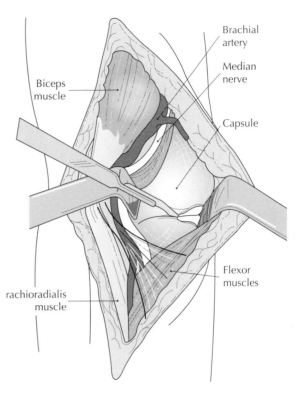

Brachial artery   Median nerve   Capsule   Biceps muscle   rachioradialis muscle   Flexor muscles

Fig. 16.3 The medial portion of the anterior part of the capsule is incised after retracting the brachial artery and median nerve laterally. Redrawn after Ref. 3.

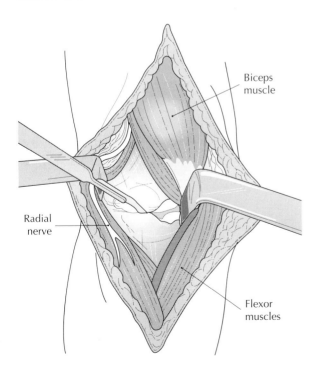

Biceps muscle   Radial nerve   Flexor muscles

Fig. 16.4 The anterior capsulotomy is completed by retracting the biceps tendon medially and the radial nerve laterally. The brachialis muscle can be retracted to either side and is not cut. Redrawn after Ref. 3.

LATERAL APPROACH

Morrey[6] prefers to undertake an anterior capsulectomy through a lateral approach.

With the patient supine and a sandbag beneath the ipsilateral shoulder the forearm is placed across the chest. The skin incision begins at the interval between anconeous and extensor carpi ulnaris and extends proximally beside the lateral aspect of triceps for approximately 15 cm (Fig. 16.5). The anconeus is freed from the ulna. The triceps insertion is reflected subperiosteally from the ulna and the more proximal triceps is released from the distal

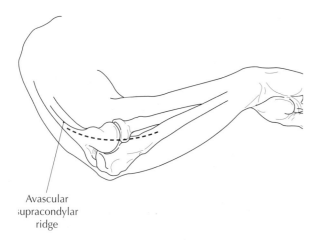

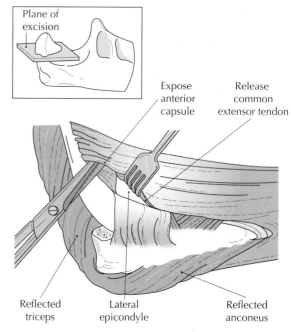

Fig. 16.5 Lateral skin incision. Redrawn after Ref. 12.

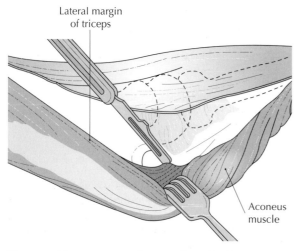

Fig. 16.7 The extensor mechanism of the elbow is reflected medially. The tip of the olecranon is excised. The common extensor origin is released from the lateral epicondyle and elevated to expose the anterior capsule of the elbow. Redrawn after Ref. 12.

Fig. 16.6 The triceps tendon is reflected subperiosteally from the tip of the olecranon. Redrawn after Ref. 12.

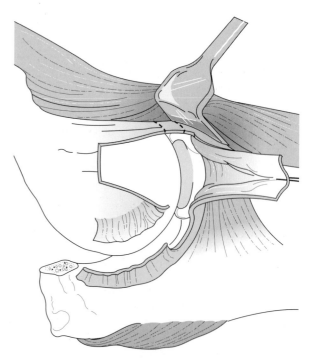

humerus (Fig. 16.6). By careful dissection the elbow joint and olecranon are exposed. The olecranon process and posterior capsule are excised. The extensor origin is released from the lateral epicondyle and the brachialis muscle elevated from the anterior joint capsule (Fig. 16.7). The lateral collateral ligament is identified. If possible it is preserved but if not it is released from the humerus (Fig. 16.8). The brachialis muscle is retracted anteriorly and a segment of the anterior capsule excised. This usually improves elbow extension.

If released, the lateral collateral ligament is reconstructed using non-absorbable sutures placed through drill holes in the humerus and the wound is closed.

Fig. 16.8 The lateral collateral ligament is released as a distally based flap. This allows reattachment following capsulectomy. The anterior capsule is exposed and a segment resected all the way to the medial side (broken lines). Redrawn after Ref. 12.

LATERAL AND MEDIAL APPROACH

Bhattacharyya[2] performed arthrolysis of post-traumatic stiff elbows in 56 patients using lateral and medial incision. In this technique it is wisest to start laterally and then progress to the medial aspect of the joint only if a satisfactory release cannot be obtained through the lateral incision.

The lateral incision is as described above. The medial incision is centred somewhat posterior to the medial epicondyle and extends proximally and distally for approximaterly 5 cm. The ulna nerve is identified, protected and retracted anteriorly allowing the plane to be developed between triceps and flexor carpi ulnaris. The capsule is then opened exposing the elbow joint. By careful dissection the capsule is reflected from the ulna attachment.

This approach enables the anterior capsule to be released safely under direct vision across its entire anterior attachment and also permits release or removal of bony obstacles from the medial aspect of the joint.

Having improved flexion and extension of the elbow the superior radioulnar joint is assessed. The forearm is pronated and supinated and adhesions fibrosis and ankylosis freed.

AUTHOR'S PREFERRED APPROACH

All patients undergoing arthrolysis for post-traumatic stiffness of the elbow are advised to expect lateral and medial incisions. If a satisfactory release can be achieved via a lateral approach then the medial approach is not undertaken. The presence of bony bars on the medial aspect of the joint, however, are in the author's experience best approached from the medial side.

POSTOPERATIVE MANAGEMENT

In order to provide effective pain relief and maximise elbow movement a continuous brachial plexus block is advised.[10–12] This should be continued for approximately 3 days postoperatively.

In order to maintain the improvement in movement obtained by surgery continuous passive motion is advocated. Morrey[12] advises the use of this immediately postoperatively although it is my preference to allow postoperative swelling to settle and commence continuous passive motion once the suction drains have been removed.

Following discharge from hospital night splintage of the arm in extension helps prevent recurrence of the anterior contracture.

Results

Urbaniak et al.[3] in 15 patients undergoing anterior capsulotomy improved the preoperative flexion deformity from a mean of 48 degrees to 19 degrees postoperatively (61%). The improvement was most marked in those patients without preoperative evidence of intra-articular degeneration (improvement 65%) compared with those who did have degenerative change (improvement 50%).

In six patients treated by anterior capsulectomy Morrey[12] reported improvement from an average preoperative arc of total motion of 32 degrees (range 0–65 degrees) to 74 degrees postoperatively (range 40–105 degrees).

Morrey[12] also reported his experience with distraction arthroplasty with and without interposition; techniques which have not been performed by the author. Using an interponant the mean arc of total motion improved from 27 degrees preoperatively (range 0–60 degrees) to 107 degrees postoperatively (70–150 degrees). This was slightly better than when distraction arthroplasty was undertaken without interposition.

Complications

Morrey[6] had only one complication from 13 patients undergoing capsulectomy without distraction whereas in those patients treated using the distraction device the complication rate was approximately 25% with 10% requiring further procedures due to the complication. The main complications were infection, and neuritis involving the ulnar and radial nerves.

In the author's experience of 12 cases without distraction, ulnar neuritis occurred in one patient and troublesome dependant oedema of the hand occurred in another patient using an ambulatory continuous passive motion machine.

References

1. Wilson PD Capsulotomy for relief of flexure contracture of the elbow following fracture. *J Bone Joint Surg* 1944; **26**: 71–86.
2. Bhattacharyya S Arthrolysis – a new approach to surgery of post traumatic stiff elbow. *J Bone Joint Surg* 1974; **56B**: 567.
3. Urbaniak JR, Hansen PE, Beissinger SF, Aitken MS Correction of post-traumatic flexion contracture of the elbow by anterior capsulotomy. *J Bone Joint Surg* 1985; **67A**: 1160–4.

4. Breen TF, Gelberman RH, Ackerman GN Elbow flexion contractures treated by anterior release and continuous passive motion. *J Hand Surg* 1988; **13B:** 286–7.
5. Weizenbluth M, Eichenblat M, Lipskeir E, Kessler I Arthrolysis of the elbow: 13 vases of post-traumatic stiffness. *Acta Orthop Scand* 1989; **60:** 642–5.
6. Morrey BF Post-traumatic stiffness: distraction arthroplasty. In: *The elbow and its disorders.* Morrey BF (ed) Philadelphia: WB Saunders Co, 1993: 476–91.
7. Garland DE A clinical perspective of common forms of acquired aeterotrophic ossification. *Clin Orthop* 1991; **263:** 13–29.
8. Wilson JN Adhesions joint stiffness and traumatic ossification. In: *Watson Jones fractures and joint injuries* (5th edn). Wilson JN (ed) Edinburgh: Churchill Livingstone, 1976: 65–92.
9. Thompson HC, Garcia A Myositis ossificans: – aftermath of elbow injuries. *Clin Orthop* 1967; **50:** 129–34.
10. Gaumann DM, Lennon RL, Wedel DJ Continuous axillary block for postoperative pain management. *Reg Anaesth* 1988; **13:** 77.
11. Rymaszewski L, Glass K, Parikh R Post-traumatic elbow contracture treated by arthrolysis and continual passive motion under brachial plexus anaesthesia. *J Bone Joint Surg* 1996; **78B** (Supp I): 30.
12. Morrey BF Post-traumatic contracture of the elbow. *J Bone Joint Surg* 1990; **72A**: 601–18.

CHAPTER 17

Sports injuries of the elbow

STEPHEN R SOFFER

Introduction

Elbow injuries are common in athletes. Chronic overuse as well as acute problems require accurate diagnosis based on a thorough history and physical examination in order to enable athletes to return to competitive play. Whether the patient is treated operatively or non-operatively, an adjunctive well structured rehabilitation programme with emphasis on sport-specific exercises is extremely helpful.

Return to sports should always be gradual after an injury. An organised interval training programme, such as the interval throwing programme for a baseball pitcher, is very useful. It provides the athlete with a well structured method based on achieving functional goals such that it is possible to return to competitive sports with minimal risk of re-injury.

This chapter will review by anatomical region those elbow injuries most likely to be experienced by athletes.

Medial compartment disorders

MEDIAL COLLATERAL LIGAMENT INJURIES

The primary ligamentous stabiliser of the elbow is the anterior oblique portion of the medial or ulna collateral ligament.[1] This ligament is commonly injured in throwing sports such as baseball. Repetitive valgus stress on the elbow may lead to attenuation of the medial collateral ligament and chronic valgus instability. Eventually, acute rupture of the ligament may occur.[2] Acute rupture may also result from abrupt valgus deviation of the elbow during contact sports such as American football.

The diagnosis of medial collateral ligament insufficiency is based on a thorough history and physical examination. Patients often complain of medial side elbow pain during the late cocking or early acceleration phase of throwing. Decreased ball velocity is another common complaint. They may recall hearing a 'pop' during a particular throw or pitch in the case of acute rupture. Ulnar nerve symptoms may be present from traction or compression of the nerve, or from acute haemorrhage into the ulnar nerve sheath.

Physical examination reveals tenderness and swelling over the medial collateral ligament, medial epicondyle or ligament insertion. Patients with chronic valgus instability will have more subtle symptoms and physical signs and are therefore more difficult to diagnose. Laxity with valgus stress at 30 degrees of flexion may be evident but is often difficult to palpate (Fig. 17.1). Comparison with the uninjured elbow is helpful. Examination of the ulnar nerve should also be performed. Resisted wrist flexion or forearm pronation, may cause pain

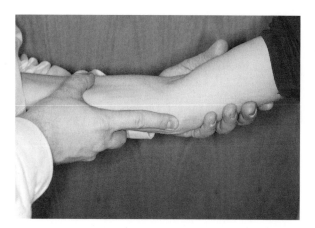

Fig. 17.1 Valgus stress of the elbow at 30 degrees of flexion.

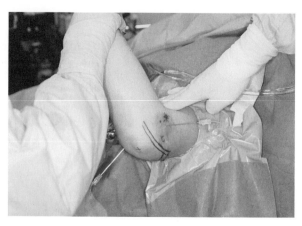

Fig. 17.2 Arthroscopic stress test of the elbow. Valgus stress placed on the elbow during arthroscopy demonstrates medial collateral ligament laxity by distraction of the coronoid from the distal humerus.

over the medial elbow indicating flexor pronator tendon injury. This may mimic medial collateral ligament injury or occur concomitantly.

Imaging studies such as stress radiographs, arthrography, computed tomography arthrography, and magnetic resonance imaging with or without contrast enhancement are helpful in confirming the diagnosis of the medial collateral ligament injury only if they are positive. If negative, the patient may still have medial collateral ligament laxity. Arthroscopy of the elbow employing the Arthroscopic Stress Test[3] will demonstrate even a few millimetres of laxity of the medial collateral ligament (Fig. 17.2).

Conservative treatment of medial collateral ligament injuries is often successful. Rest, ice, anti-inflammatory medications, and a well supervised physical therapy programme will often return the injured athlete to full function, especially those athletes with incomplete ligament ruptures. If the patient is a throwing athlete, rehabilitation using a throwing programme is utilised prior to competitive play. Steroid injection into the medial aspect of the elbow is not recommended as further attenuation of the ligament may occur.

If conservative treatment fails in a throwing athlete with significant valgus instability, surgery is indicated. Surgery may also be indicated in an acute medial collateral ligament rupture in an elite throwing athlete who wants to return to highly competitive play. The elite baseball pitcher with an acute complete rupture of the medial collateral ligament, for example, will often require ligament surgery to return to professional pitching.

Surgery involves repair of the torn medial collateral ligament or reconstruction with autogenous tissue. Results from reconstruction are better than

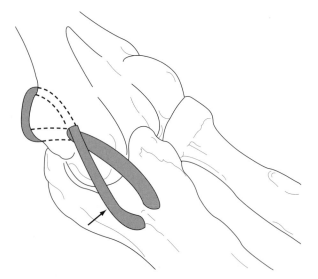

Fig. 17.3 Medial collateral ligament reconstruction.

direct repair and thus a reconstruction is usually the procedure of choice.[4,5] An ipsilateral palmaris longus tendon or a lesser toe extensor tendon is utilised as the tendon graft, and placed through drill holes made in the medial epicondyle and ulna in a figure-of-8 fashion (Fig. 17.3). Most baseball players are able to return to tossing a baseball at 3–4 months and competitive throwing 9–12 months after surgery. However, a return to the pre-injury level of competition for a professional pitcher may require over 18 months.[5,6] Successful return to the previous level of athletic participation can be expected in two-thirds of patients undergoing ligamentous reconstruction.[4]

ULNAR NEURITIS

Athletes may develop inflammation of the ulnar nerve from traction or compression. This is commonly seen in baseball, tennis and racquetball players. Valgus instability in the thrower may lead to stretch injury to the nerve. Also, adhesions from medial collateral ligament irritation, calcific deposits and bony spurs may tether the nerve.[7,8] Compression of the nerve may occur from forearm flexor hypertrophy, cubital tunnel entrapment, medial head of triceps hypertrophy, or the anconeus epithrochlearis muscle.[9,10]

Recurrent ulnar nerve subluxation occurs in 16% of the general population with flexion of the elbow from an extended position.[11] Recurrent subluxation of the ulnar nerve anterior to the medial epicondyle, as occurs with repetitive throwing or racquet sports, can lead to irritation of the nerve.

Patients usually complain of pain, numbness or tingling extending from the medial aspect of the elbow to the ring and little fingers. The hand may feel heavy or 'dead' especially with athletic activity. Patients with recurrent ulnar nerve subluxation may sense a popping or snapping sensation with elbow flexion. Examination may reveal tenderness behind the medial epicondyle of the elbow, a positive Tinel sign over the cubital tunnel or decreased sensation over the ulnar nerve distribution of the hand. Muscle weakness is rare. Electromyographic studies are often normal. Radiographs are usually normal but may show calcium deposits or bony spurs near the ulnar nerve.

Conservative treatment involves rest, ice, anti-inflammatory medications, and occasionally immobilisation in a splint. If conservative treatment fails, surgical ulnar nerve decompression and subcutaneous anterior transposition should be performed.[12]

If ulnar neuritis is associated with medial collateral ligament laxity, ulnar nerve surgery alone is inadequate. The medial collateral ligament must be reconstructed to prevent the valgus laxity that is responsible for the symptoms.[5]

MEDIAL EPICONDYLAR STRESS FRACTURE (APOPHYSITIS)

In skeletally immature throwing athletes, usually between the ages of 9 and 12 years, repetitive valgus stress to the medial side of the elbow may lead to a stress fracture of the medial epicondyle or 'little leaguer's elbow'.[13] Pain with throwing, tenderness over the medial epicondyle and an elbow flexion contracture are common findings. Radiographs of both elbows should be obtained since these will often show fragmentation, separation or enlargement of the injured medial epicondyle. Rest from throwing for 3 weeks, followed by rehabilitation exercises and the introduction of a throwing programme will usually enable the elbow to recover.

MEDIAL EPICONDYLE AVULSION FRACTURE

Avulsion fractures of the medial epicondyle are not uncommon in skeletally immature athletes. They may occur in throwing sports such as baseball or follow direct trauma as in American football when often the elbow is also dislocated. Clinically pain and tenderness is present over the medial epicondyle. Radiographs confirm the diagnosis.

Mild displacement of a medial epicondylar fracture may permit acceptable function in many non-throwing athletes. However, resulting laxity of the medial collateral ligament from even small amounts of rotational displacement will disable a thrower. With time, degenerative changes occur in the radiocapitellar joint from residual valgus laxity. In the throwing athlete, anatomical reduction of displaced medial epicondylar fractures is advocated. This usually requires open reduction and internal fixation of the fracture (Fig. 17.4). Early range of motion may begin after surgery along with a well supervised rehabilitation programme.

FLEXOR PRONATOR STRAIN

Acute overload of the flexor pronator muscle group may occur with valgus stress during throwing. Associated medial collateral ligament laxity must be ruled out. Isolated flexor pronator muscle strains are treated with ice, anti-inflammatories, and physical therapy. Complete ruptures of the flexor pronator origin are rare.

MEDIAL EPICONDYLITIS

Often termed 'golfer's elbow', medial epicondylitis also occurs in athletes subjecting their elbows to repetitive valgus forces such as tennis players, racquetball players, baseball players and javelin throwers.[14,15]

The flexor pronator muscles attempt to decrease the valgus stress placed on the elbow. Poor conditioning, overuse, and improper technique lead to microtrauma and inflammation of the flexor pronator origin.[14]

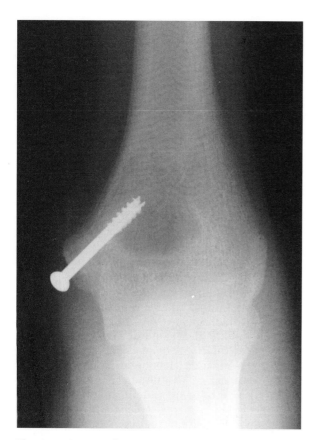

Fig. 17.4 Open reduction internal fixation of a medial epicondyle fracture.

Lateral compartment disorders

LATERAL COLLATERAL LIGAMENT INJURIES

Although in throwing athletes valgus stress on the elbow may cause injury to the medial collateral ligament, the lateral collateral ligament is only rarely injured during sporting activities unless the elbow is dislocated.[17,18] If dislocation occurs injury to the lateral collateral ligament may result in elbow instability. Treatment should be performed by surgical repair if the ligament has been detached from the humerus, or reconstruction, if the ligament has been torn.

LATERAL COMPARTMENT ARTICULAR INJURIES

Compressive forces are generated in the lateral compartment secondary to valgus stress on the elbow during athletics. As the medial side of the elbow experiences tension forces, the lateral side experiences compressive forces leading to articular cartilage damage to the radial head and capitellum. The articular fragments may break off into the joint causing loose bodies. This scenario occurs in baseball players most commonly, but can also occur in javelin throwers, gymnasts, tennis or racquet ball players.

In the skeletally immature, the vascular supply of the capitellum is especially vulnerable to repetitive valgus stress. Subchondral bone necrosis may occur in addition to fragmentation of the articular surface with loose bodies formation.[3,19,20] This process known as osteochondritis dissecans occurs most commonly in the capitellum (Chapter 19). Radial head osteochondritis dissecans is less common.

Patients with articular injuries complain of elbow pain, catching or locking. Flexion contractures of 15 degrees or more are not uncommon. Examination reveals tenderness and crepitus over the radiocapitellar joint. Radiographs may show irregularity of the capitellum or radial head, and perhaps loose bodies. Magnetic resonance imaging clearly defines avascular bone in osteochondritis dissecans (Fig. 17.5).

In the adult, indications for surgery are failure of conservative treatment, loose bodies, and locking of the elbow. In osteochondritis dissecans, treatment is based on the degree of separation of the lesion. If the lesion is not detached, conservative treatment with rest, anti-inflammatory agents and physical therapy to restore range of motion will

Patients usually complain of medial elbow pain during athletic activity such as with a golf swing or tennis serve. The flexor pronator origin is tender and pain is elicited with resisted wrist flexion or forearm pronation. Radiographs are usually normal, but may show calcific deposits or bony spurs. Ulnar nerve and medial collateral ligament examination should also be performed since pathology in these areas may mimic medial epicondylitis.

Non-operative treatment involves rest, ice, anti-inflammatory medications, physical therapy modalities and counter-force bracing. Steroid injection into the medial elbow are not recommended because of the potential deleterious effects on the medial collateral ligament. If after several months, conservative treatment fails, surgery is indicated. This usually involves removal of the degenerative, inflamed tendon with drilling holes into the medial epicondyle to stimulate a healing response.[16] Results are good to excellent in over 90% and return to athletic activities can usually be undertaken within 3–4 months.

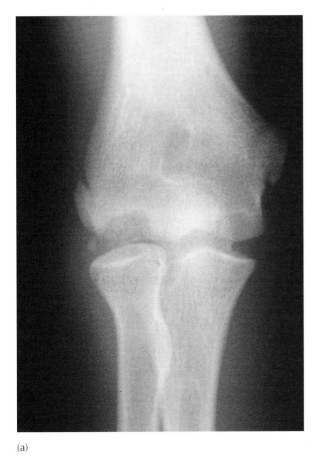

(a)

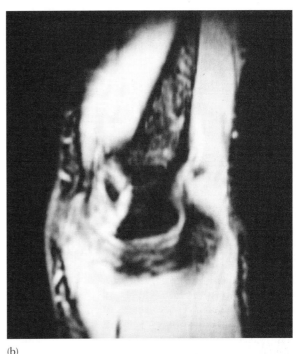

(b)

Fig. 17.5 (a) Anteroposterior x-ray of osteochondritis dissecans of capitellum. (b) Lateral magnetic resonance imaging of osteochondritis dissecans of capitellum.

often be successful. If the lesion is separated or detached, surgery is usually necessary.

Arthroscopic excision of the loose fragment along with either chondroplasty or abrasion arthroplasty of the articular surface affords relief of symptoms and permits return to athletics[3,21–23] (Fig. 17.6).

Occasionally, acute lateral compartment compression will lead to an osteochondral fracture of either the capitellum or radial head. This is seen most commonly in gymnasts. Patients present with acute pain in the elbow, an effusion, and restricted motion. If plain radiographs fail to show the lesion, computed tomography arthrography or magnetic resonance imaging may be helpful. Arthroscopic excision of the small fragment is the treatment of choice.

POSTERIOR INTEROSSEOUS NERVE COMPRESSION

Peripheral nerve injuries of the elbow are fully discussed in Chapter 21. In sports, posterior interosseus

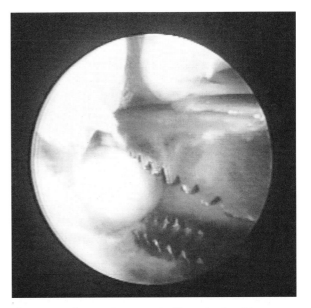

Fig. 17.6 Arthroscopic removal of loose body with grasper. This figure is reproduced in colour in the colour plate section.

nerve compression is uncommon. However, it should be included in the differential diagnosis of patients with lateral sided elbow pain.

LATERAL EPICONDYLITIS

Often termed 'tennis elbow' lateral epicondylitis involves the common extensor origin. It occurs most commonly in tennis, racquetball, squash and fencing. Improper backhand technique, striking the ball off centre (not in the 'sweet spot'), over tightened racquet strings, and inappropriate grip size, have all been implicated as causes of tennis elbow. Nirschl described the pathology as 'angioblastic hyperplasia' of the extensor carpi brevis tendon.[24]

Pain is described as originating in the lateral epicondyle and may radiate into the forearm of the dominant arm. Examination reveals tenderness over the lateral epicondyle. Pain over the lateral epicondyle occurs with resisted finger or wrist extension. Firm gripping of an object, such as in a hand shake, will elicit pain over the lateral side of the elbow. Radiographs are usually normal but may show calcific deposits over the lateral epicondyle.

The initial treatment is usually conservative. This consists of ice, anti-inflammatories, cessation of the causative activity, counter-force bracing (Fig. 17.7) and physical therapy modalities. Appropriate adjustments in terms of stroke mechanics, techinque and equipment are necessary to prevent re-injury. Keeping the wrist locked during the back-hand stroke is advised. Racquets that are lighter in weight and have larger 'sweet spots' will unload the common extensor tendon. String tension

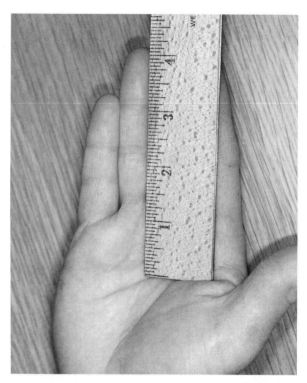

Fig. 17.8 The distance from the proximal palmer crease to the tip of the ring finger approximates racquet grip size.

should be decreased to 55 lb (25 kg). Grip size must not be too small. The distance from the proximal palmar crease to the tip of the ring finger approximates the racquets grip size (Fig. 17.8). If this initial conservative treatment fails, corticosteroid injection may be administered.

Many patients respond to conservative treatment but if after several months symptoms persist surgical treatment should be considered. Although many operative procedures have been described (Chapter 20), the technique described by Nirschl and Pettrone[24] is preferred. This involves excision of the origin of the degenerated extensor carpi radialis brevis tendon with drilling of the bone to stimulate a healing response. Patients usually return to light tennis 8 weeks after surgery.

Posterior compartment disorders

VALGUS EXTENSION OVERLOAD SYNDROME

Olecranon impingement syndrome often termed 'boxer's elbow', is caused by repetitive hyperextension of the elbow.[25,26] In throwing athletes who

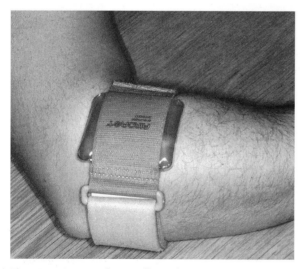

Fig. 17.7 Counter-force elbow brace for lateral epicondylitis.

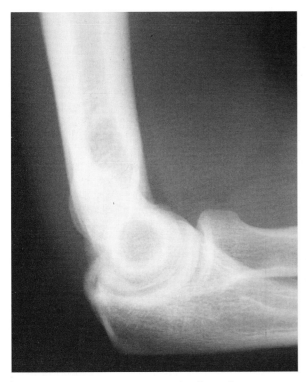

Fig. 17.9 Valgus extension overload syndrome causes posterior osteophyte to form on olecranon tip.

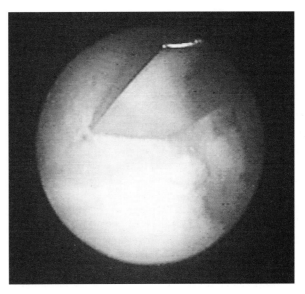

Fig. 17.10 Arthroscopic removal of posterior osteophyte.

develop posterior elbow pain the mechanism of injury is somewhat different. Repetitive throwing, as in pitching a baseball, subjects the posterior compartment of the elbow to excessive valgus and extension forces. Extension overload during the follow-through phase of pitching causes ostephyte formation on the olecranon tip and resultant loose body formation; with further repetitive movements olecranon impingement occurs. Valgus overload during the acceleration phase of pitching causes abutment of the posteromedial olecranon osteophyte on the medial aspect of the olecranon fossa and posterior humeral condyle creating a painful area of chrondromalcia[3,27,28] (Fig. 17.9).

The patient is usually a pitcher who complains of pain during acceleration and follow-through phases of pitching. Ball control is difficult, early release and high pitches are common. Examination demonstrates tenderness over the top of the olecranon, a flexion contracture and discomfort with the Valgus Extension Overload Test. This test is performed by forcibly extending the elbow with valgus stress. It is also important in these patients to carefully examine for chronic medial collateral ligament instability. Radiographs often demonstrate an osteophyte or loose bodies over the tip of the olecranon.

Conservative treatment consists of rest, ice, anti-inflammatory medications, and rehabilitation involving an interval throwing programme. If conservative treatment fails, surgical treatment will relieve these symptoms.[28] Arthroscopy is utilised to remove loose bodies from the posterior compartment and to remove the posteromedial osteophyte from the tip of the olecranon[3,29] (Fig. 17.10). Return to pitching can be expected in 6–8 weeks.

OLECRANON APOPHYSITIS (STRESS FRACTURE)

Repetitive tensile stress of the triceps attachment to the olecranon, during the follow-through phase of throwing, can cause microfracture of the olecranon physis in the skeletally immature athlete.[22,30–32]

Subsequent delay in closure of the physis may occur or lead to a non-union.[33–35] The diagnosis is made by history and physical examination. Radiographs of both elbows may show the olecranon apophysis of the injured elbow to be separated or fragmented compared with the normal elbow. Initial treatment is conservative involving rest and ice, followed by a gradual return to sports activities once symptoms resolve. If conservative treatment fails to relieve symptoms or if significant displacement of the olecranon epiphysis occurs, open reduction and internal fixation is necessary.

INFLAMMATORY LESIONS

Triceps tendinitis is not uncommon, especially in the thrower, gymnast or weight lifter.[36] It is often associated with poor technique, improper training, or overuse. Repetitive locking of the elbow in hyperextension, especially during upper extremity weight bearing as in weight training and gymnastics, causes inflammation of the triceps tendon. Once other intra-articular pathology is eliminated, conservative treatment is initiated. Rest, ice, anti-inflammatories, physical therapy with emphasis on biceps strengthening usually leads to resolution of symptoms.

Olecranon bursitis results from direct trauma to the posterior aspect of the elbow, as occurs commonly in American football or rugby.[37] It is usually managed conservatively with anti-inflammatories, ice and a protective sports sleeve. If inflammatory bursitis persists, or if septic bursitis is suspected, aspiration should be performed. Recurrence of aseptic bursitis is decreased when aspiration is accompanied by corticosteroid injection. However, the patient should be advised that there is an increased chance of infection and subdermal atrophy with the use of steroids.[38] Chronic bursitis that has failed conservative treatment or infected olecranon bursitis should be surgically excised.

Anterior compartment disorders

ANTERIOR CAPSULITIS/BICEPS STRAIN

Acute hyperextension of the elbow, as is commonly seen with wrestling or American football injuries, leads to sprain of the anterior capsule as well as elbow flexor strain. This problem may also occur in baseball players. During the acceleration phase of throwing, the biceps is subjected to large eccentric loads. Poor preseason conditioning, hyperlaxity and improper mechanics can predispose the thrower to biceps overuse injury and tendinitis. Pain with passive elbow extension may be evident, as well as pain with resisted elbow flexion. Flexion contractures are common. Non-operative treatment involving rest, ice, stretching, and an eccentric biceps strengthening programme will usually improve the situation.

DISTAL BICEPS TENDON RUPTURE

Competitive weight lifters are predisposed to biceps tendon rupture due to degenerative changes in the tendon.[39] The rupture usually occurs with biceps eccentric contraction during curling exercises. The patient experiences acute pain in the anterior aspect of the flexed elbow. Weakness of elbow flexion and supination follows. Ecchymosis and swelling is present in the antecubital fossa. The biceps muscle appears deformed and the tendon is not palpable in the antecubital fossa. Treatment of complete rupture in athletes is surgical repair. A standard two incision technique directly reattaching the biceps tendon to the radial tuberosity (Boyd and Anderson) is preferred (Chapter 15).[40] Non-operative treatment usually leads to a 40% loss of flexion and supination strength.[41]

PRONATOR TERES SYNDROME

Median nerve entrapment at the elbow may occur in sports, but is very uncommon. Activities that involve repetitive gripping, or forearm pronation or wrist flexion such as racquetball, wrestling gymnastics and throwing sports cause flexor-pronator mass hypertrophy. This hypertrophic mass may compress the median nerve. Compression may also occur at several other locations such as the flexor sublimis arch and lacertus fibrosus.[42] The condition is more fully described in Chapter 21.

EXERTIONAL COMPARTMENT SYNDROME

There are no extensive studies of this condition in the literature as the condition is quite rare. In 1959, Bennett[30] described a syndrome of anteromedial elbow pain in baseball players. Muscle fatigue and oedema after exertion were though to result in increased pressure within the fascial compartment of the forearm producing chronic pain. Such a situation may disable a pitcher such that he is only able to pitch two to three innings. Conservative treatment involving rest, stretching and warm-up exercises and a 3- to 5-day rest period between pitching rotations usually resolves the problem. Bennett described surgery involving fascial division for pitchers failing conservative treatment.[30]

References

1. Schwab GH, Bennett JB, Woods GW *et al.* Biomechanics of elbow instability: The role of the medical collateral ligament. *Clin Orthop* 1980; **146:** 42–52.
2. Norwood LA, Snook JA, Andrews JR Acute medial elbow ruptures. *Am J Sports Med* 1981; **9:** 16–19.

3. Soffer SR, Andrews JR Arthroscopic surgical procedures of the elbow: common cases. In: *Elbow arthroscopy*. Andrews JR, Soffer SR (eds) St Louis: MOsby Inc. 1994.

4. Conway JE, Jobe FW, Glousman RE, Pin M Medial instability of the elbow in throwing athletes. *J Bone Joint Surg* 1992; **74A:** 67–83.

5. Jobe FW, Stark H, Lombardo SJ Reconstruction of the ulnar collateral ligament in athletes. *J Bone Joint Surg* 1986; **68A:** 1158–63.

6. Jobe FW, Nuber G Throwing injuries of the elbow. *Clin Sports Med* 1986; **5:** 621–36.

7. Del Pizzo W, Jobe FW, Norwood L Ulnar nerve entrapment syndrome in baseball players. *Am J Sports Med* 1977; **5:** 182–5.

8. Godshall RW, Hansen CA Traumatic ulnar neuropathy in adolescent baseball pitchers. *J Bone Joint Surg* 1971; **53A:** 359–61.

9. Rolfsen L Snapping triceps tendon with ulnar neuritis. *Act Orthop Scand* 1970; **41:** 74–6.

10. Spinner M *Injuries to the major branches of peripheral nerves of the forearm* (2nd edn). Philadelphia: WB Saunders Co, 1978.

11. Childress HM Recurrent ulnar nerve dislocation at the elbow. *J Bone Joint Surg* 1956; **38A:** 978–84.

12. Eaton RG, Crowe JF, Parkes JC Anterior transportation of the ulnar nerve using a non-compressing fasciodermal sling. *J Bone Joint Surg* 1980; **62A:** 820–5.

13. Ireland ML, Andrews JR Shoulder and elbow injuries in the young athlete. *Clin Sports Med* 1988; **7:** 473–94.

14. Leach RE, Miller JK Lateral and medial; epicondylitis of the elbow. *Clin Sports Med* 1987; **6:** 259–72.

15. Wares W Elbow injuries in javelin throwers. *Acta Chir Scand* 1946; **564:** 93.

16. Vangsness CT, Jobe FW Surgical treatment of medial epicondylitis. Results in 35 elbows. *J Bone Joint Surg* 1991; **73B:** 409–11.

17. Nestor BJ, O'Driscoll SW, Morrey BF Ligamentous reconstruction for posterolateral instability of the elbow. *J Bone Joint Surg* 1992; **74A:** 1235–41.

18. O'Driscoll SW, Bell DF, Morrey BF Posterolateral rotatory instability of the elbow. *J Bone Joint Surg* 1991; **73A:** 440–6.

19. Larson RL, Singer KM, Bergstrom R, Thomas S Little league survey: The Eugene study. *Am J Sports Med* 1976; **4:** 201–9.

20. Tullos HS, King JW Lesions of the pitching arm in adolescence. *J Am Med Assoc* 1972; **220:** 264–71.

21. McManama GB, Micheli LJ, Berry MV, Sohns RS The surgical treatment of osteochondritis of the capitellum. *Am J Sports Med* 1985; **13:** 11–21.

22. Pappas AM Elbow problems associated with baseball during childhood and adolescence. *Clin Orthop* 1982; **164:** 30–41.

23. Singer KM, Roy SP Osteochondritis of the humeral capitellum. *Am J Sports Med* 1984; **12:** 351–60.

24. Nirschl RP, Pettrone FA Tennis elbow: The surgical treatment of lateral epicondylitis. *J Bone Joint Surg* 1979; **61A:** 832–9.

25. Melholff TL, Bennett JB Elbow injuries. In: *The team physician's handbook*. Mellion MB, Walsh WM, Shelton GL (eds). Philadelphia: Hanley and Belfus Publishers, 1990.

26. Yocum LA The diagnosis and non-operative treatment of elbow problems in the athlete. *Clin Sports Med* 1989; **8:** 439–51.

27. Andrews JR, St Pierre RK, Carson WG Arthroscopy of the elbow. *Clin Sports Med* 1986; **5:** 653–62.

28. Wilson FD, Andrews JR, Blackburn TA, McCluskey G Valgus extension overload in the pitching elbow. *Am J Sports Med* 1983; **11:** 83–8.

29. Andrews JR, Carson WG Arthroscopy of the elbow. *Arthroscopy* 1985; **1:** 97–107.

30. Bennett GF Elbow and shoulder lesions ogf baseball players. *Am J Surg* 1959; **98:** 484–92.

31. Hunter LY, O'Connor GA Traction apophysitis of the olecranon. *Am J Sports Med* 1980; **8:** 51–2.

32. Torg JS, Moyer RA Nonunion of a stress fracture through the olecranon epiphysial plate observed in an adolescent baseball pitcher. *J Bone Joint Surg* 1977; **59A:** 264–5.

33. Kovach J, Baker BE, Mosher JF Fracture separation of the olecranon ossification center in adults. *Am J Sports Med* 1985; **13:** 105–11.

34. Micheli LJ The traction pophysitises. *Clin Sports Med* 1987; **6:** 389–404.

35. Pavlov H, Torg JS, Jacobs B, Vigorita V Nonunion of olecranon epiphysis: Two cases in adolescent baseball pitchers. *Am J Roentgenol* 1981; **136:** 819–20.

36. Aronen JG Problems of the upper extremity in gymnastics. *Clin Sports Med* 1985; **4:** 61–71.

37. Larson RL, Ostering LR Traumatic bursitis and artifactual turf. *J Sports Med* 1974; **2:** 183–8.

38. Weinstein PS, Canoso JJ, Wohlgethan JR Long-term follow-up of corticosteroid injections for traumatic olecranon bursitis. *Ann Rheum Dis* 1984; **43:** 44–6.

39. Davis WM, Yassine Z An etiology fractor in the tear of the distal tendon of the distal biceps brachialis. *J Bone Joint Surg* 1956; **38A:** 1368–70.

40. Boyd HB, Anderson LD A method for reinsertion of the distal biceps brachii tendon. *J Bone Joint Surg* 1961; **43A:** 1041–3.

41. Morrey BF, Askew LJ, An KH, Bobyns JH Rupture of the distal biceps tendon: Biomechanical assessment of different treatment options. *J Bone Joint Surg* 1985; **67A:** 418–21.

42. Hartz CR, Linscheid RL, Gramse RR, Daube JR The pronator teres syndrome: Compressive neuropathy of the median nerve. *J Bone Joint Surg* 1981; **63A:** 885–90.

CHAPTER 18

Elbow rehabilitation

GARY S FANTON, ALLAN MISHRA

Introduction

A careful clinical assessment of the elbow is necessary if the elbow is to be rehabilitated successfully. Realistic rehabilitation goals are needed in
order to maximise functional recovery and avoid
complications. The specific protocol to be followed, however, is highly dependent upon the
underlying disorder and its treatment. For example
a more aggressive rehabilitation programme can be
prescribed for a patient who has a loose body
removed arthroscopically than can be ordered for
an athlete who sustains a comminuted intra-articular distal humerus fracture. Clearly, the extent of
injury to the supporting skeletal, ligamentous and
muscular tissue about the elbow is predictive of the
eventual functional outcome. The degree of articular surface disruption, the motivation of the
patient and the potential for secondary gain are
also important parameters that can influence the
results.

Non-operative and postoperative rehabilitation

Elbow rehabilitation can be broadly divided into
treatment for soft tissue disorders and sports injuries,
and therapy to improve postoperative recovery.

Overuse injuries are the most common type of
disorder about the elbow and have been historically
treated with traditional physical therapy techniques. When elbow surgery has been performed
rehabilitation ideally should begin immediately.
The risks of wound breakdown, infection and loss
of soft tissue or bony fixation may, however,
require delaying the initiation of therapy.
Rehabilitation techniques must therefore be
designed according to the procedure performed.

In general, therapy can be started immediately
(on the day of surgery) early (within 3–4 days) or
in a delayed fashion (after 1–3 weeks). Immediate
therapy can be employed for arthroscopic procedures, manipulations, and superficial soft tissue

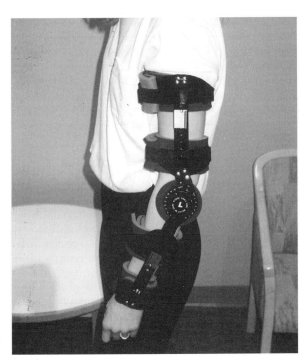

Fig. 18.1 Limited range of motion brace.

procedures. Early rehabilitation should be utilised for intermediate surgical cases such as ulnar nerve transpositions whilst delayed rehabilitation should only be considered in more complex situations i.e. posterolateral instability repairs.

In contrast to the prolonged immobilisation advised after posterolateral instability repairs (3–5 weeks)[1] medial ligament repairs and reconstruc-

Table 18.1 Postoperative elbow

Rehabilitation timing

Immediate (on the day of surgery)
Arthroscopic procedures
Manipulations
Superficial soft tissue procedures

Early (within 3–4 days)
Ulnar nerve transposition
Extensor tendon debridgement
Most radial head fractures
Stable elbow dislocation

Delayed (after 1–3 weeks)
Ligament repair/reconstruction
Biceps tendon reinsertion
Triceps repair
Comminuted articular fracture
Unstable elbow dislocation

tions are typically moved at about 10 days.[2] Both types of repair should be protected in a limited range of motion brace designed to prevent varus or valgus stress during the rehabilitation period (Fig. 18.1). Irrespective of which therapy regimen is used the patient must also be advised on shoulder and wrist exercises in order to prevent these joints from becoming stiff and painful.[3]

Overuse injuries

Repetitive type trauma to tendons, ligaments or even bone can produce significant pathology in and around the elbow. The most common forms include lateral and medial epicondylitis. Rehabilitation protocols (Table 18.2) for these overuse conditions focus on rest and activity modification. Specifically, the motion or sport that produces the pain is restricted while the patient participates in a programme designed not only to relieve the symptoms but also to prevent them from recurring. Proper equipment for racquet sports players such as low-vibrating frame materials, less tightly strung rackets, carefully sized grips and counterforce forearm bracing will help diminish the stress on the muscular origins at the epicondyles (Fig. 18.2). Pain and inflammation control with these conditions are typically achieved with oral non-steroidal anti-inflammatory medications and icing. A tapering dose of oral prednisone or methylprednisolone may on occasions be employed but never on a long-term basis. If the patient fails to respond to these measures, corticosteroid injection should be considered.

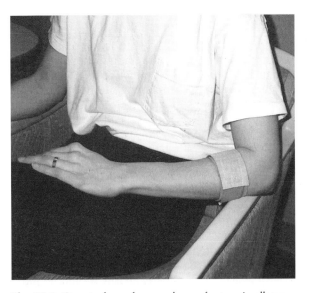

Fig. 18.2 Counterforce forearm brace for tennis elbow.

Table 18.2 Overuse rehabilitation

Protocol
Rest
Activity modification
Equipment modification
Pain and inflammation control
Flexibility programme
Strengthening programme
Sport- job-specific simulation
Return to activity

Table 18.3 Fracture rehabilitation

Protocol
Stabilise fracture
Short-term splinting
Start early motion progressive strengthening
(After osseous union)

Water based preparations such as dexamethasone sodium phosphate (Decadron) coupled with either lidocaine HCI or bupivacaine HCI should be used instead of crystalline corticosteroids such as methylprednisolone acetate because the crystals may cause an adverse flare reaction.[4] Most authors recommend no more than two or three of these injections.[5]

A comprehensive upper extremity stretching and strengthening protocol is then followed beginning with isometrics, ultrasound and electrical stimulation. Eccentric and concentric resistive exercises under supervision can typically be started after pain and tenderness subside. If the patient progresses, he or she is then advanced to a sport- or job-specific activity simulation. The patient is finally released to return only gradually to the duration and intensity or his or her previous exercise exposure. Failure of nonoperative treatment can be expected in 5–15% of cases. These patients will then either further modify their activity or undergo operative intervention.[4,5]

Trauma

Severe trauma about the elbow can result in irreparable damage. Restoring as much function as possible is the goal of treatment. For very difficult cases such as comminuted intra-articular fractures, early controlled movement following fracture fixation is crucial to achieving a functional arc of motion (Table 18.3). The type of fracture, ability to achieve anatomical congruity and the security of fixation often necessitates an individual rehabilitation programme. Jupiter[6] recommends a lightweight, removable thermoplastic resting splint for the early postoperative period. The splint can be discontinued at 10–14 days which will encourage elbow mobilisation and reincorporation of the limb into activities of daily living. Supine flexion and gravity assisted extension exercises should be initiated within the first week. For patients with an

olecranon osteotomy or a triceps tendon repair, active extension is avoided for the first 6 weeks postoperatively. Progressive muscle strengthening and endurance exercises are only instituted at 8–12 weeks after osseous union has been confirmed. If comminuted humeral shaft fractures require prolonged immobilisation elbow flexion contractures may result which will later require aggressive therapy in order to regain full elbow motion and strength. Indeed at times to improve the post-traumatic range of elbow movement an arthrolysis may be required (Chapter 16).

Pain and inflammation

A primary goal of all postoperative elbow therapy is limitation of pain and inflammation. This goal can be partially accomplished with cold therapy via an electronic cooling unit at the time of surgery over the dressing, by using crushed ice, or even by applying a bag of frozen vegetables. Intravenous or intramuscular narcotics occasionally are needed to control pain after complex procedures although oral pain medication, usually suffices. Pharmacologic inhibition of inflammation in the form of indomethacin can also be employed in those cases where extensive soft tissue damage (either from the initial injury or from the surgery) increases the risk of heterotopic ossification.

Restoration of full motion

After controlling pain and inflammation in the postoperative elbow patient, therapy should be directed toward restoring a full range of motion. Initially, elbow mobilisation exercises in the form of active assisted and gentle (not aggressive) passive assisted range of motion should be ordered. This early motion helps prevent the anterior capsule, brachialis and surrounding soft tissue from contracting. Wilk *et al.*[7] outlined a comprehensive programme for throwing athletes that is quite useful. They emphasised early active motion and passive stretching as well as isometric exercises. Specifically, passive elbow extension stretching using a lightweight handheld dumbbell and a rolled up towel under the distal humerus for a long duration in their programme was used to produce plastic elongation of the soft tissue. This exercise, however, must not be done if it produces excessive pain because it may lead to heterotopic ossification. Nirschl[8] improved flexibility with proprioceptive neuromuscular facilitation that he defined as active muscular contraction against resistance followed by static stretching. He found that an active biceps contraction for 2–3 seconds followed by a static extension stretch for 10–15 seconds significantly improved the progression of joint flexibility.

Contractures

If a flexion contracture persists postoperatively, serial casting, dynamic splinting, manipulation under anaesthesia (with or without continuous passive motion) or arthrolysis may be useful. Zander and Healy[9] improved extension 81% by applying serial casts over an 8-week period in patients with moderate flexion contractures. Static progressive stretching via a brace-like orthosis that takes advantage of the viscoelastic properties of soft tissue produced a 69% increase in mobility according to Bonutti et al.[10] The device used in their study was patient controlled and relied upon stress relaxation and creep to increase extension (Fig. 18.3).

Duke et al.,[11] however, reported an improved range of motion in only 55% of patients who underwent manipulation under anaesthesia.[11] Contracture release by arthrolysis[12] is discussed in Chapter 16. Finally, postoperative elbow continuous passive motion has been shown to produce satisfactory results but in some patients is not well tolerated.[13]

Strength and coordination

As the range of motion of the elbow is being restored, it is important to begin a strengthening and neuromuscular re-education programme (Table 18.4). The speed and intensity with which the therapy can advance are clearly related to the surgery performed. Initially, isometric exercises of the entire upper extremity are useful in limiting atrophy. Wilk et al.[7] then recommend free weight isotonic resistive exercises to improve muscular endurance. This is followed by neuromuscular control exercises both for the shoulder and elbow. Closed kinetic chain exercises are instituted as soon as possible. Therapy continues to progress to plyometric exercises, high speed strengthening and coordination drills if the patient demonstrates a full painfree range of motion with the initial programme (Fig. 18.4)

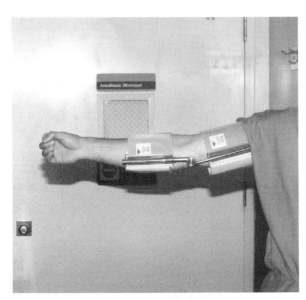

Fig. 18.3 Dyna elbow splint used to improve extension.

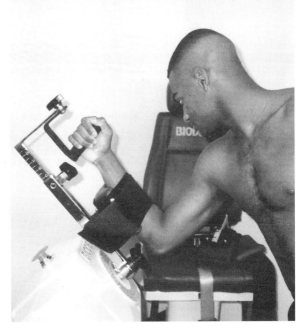

Fig. 18.4 Isokinetic strengthening.

Table 18.4 Postoperative rehabilitation

Protocol
Avoid wound complications
Pain and inflammation control
Active and gentle passive range of motion
Shoulder/wrist mobilisation
Early isometrics/electrical stimulation
Isotonics
Closed kinetic chain exercises
Plyometrics
Proprioceptive retraining
Activity specific therapy
Evaluate for secondary gain

Activity specific therapy

The concluding element of postoperative therapy is designing activity specific therapy. Most patients are not high performance athletes, but many engage in strenuous exercise either at work or home. It is therefore important to individualise a programme to help insure a successful surgical result. Often a customised brace is made to facilitate an earlier return to sports or work (Fig. 18.5). This brace typically serves as a protective device to help prevent reinjury. Paying particular attention to the motivational and emotional aspects of the patient can further improve the chances of a full recovery especially if litigation or workman's compensation is involved. Finally, Nirschl[8] recommends biofeedback, sympathetic blocks, or psychiatric counselling for those patients who are emotionally liable or have a low pain threshold.

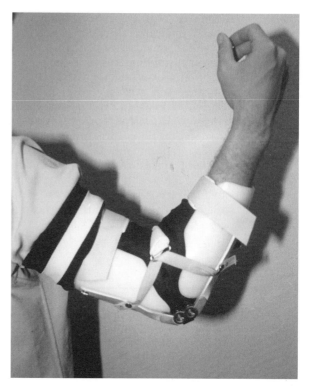

Fig. 18.5 Custom brace for throwing athlete after ligament reconstruction.

References

1. O'Driscoll SW, Bell DF, Morrey BF Posterolateral rotatory instability of the elbow. *J Bone Joint Surg (Am)* 1991; **73:** 440–6.
2. Conway JE, Jobe FW, Glousman RE, Pink M Medial instability of the elbow in throwing athlete. *J Bone Joint Surg (Am)* 1992; **1:** 67–83.
3. Bogard S, Fanton GS, Figgie MP *et al.* Elbow: Keep the whole arm in focus. *Patient Care* 29 February, 1992.
4. Kamien M A rational management of tennis elbow. *Sport Med* 1990; **9:** 173–91.
5. Jobe FW, Ciccotti MG Lateral and medial epicondylitis of the elbow. *J Am Acad Orthop Surg* 1994; **2:** 1–8.
6. Jupiter JB Complex fractures of the distal part of the Humerus and associated complications. *J Bone Joint Surg* 1994; **76A:** 1252–64.
7. Wilk KE, Arrigo C, Andrews JR Rehabilitation of the elbow in the throwing athlete. *J Orthop Sports Phys Ther* 1993; **17:** 305–17.
8. Nirschl RP Rehabilitation of the athlete's elbow. In: *The elbow and its disorders.* Morrey BF (ed) Philadelphia: WB Saunders Co, 1985: 599.
9. Zander CL, Healy NL Elbow flexion contractures treated with serial casts and conservative therapy. *J Hand Surg* 1992; **17A:** 694–7.
10. Bonutti PM, Windau JE, Ables BA, Miller BG Static progressive stretch to reestablish elbow range of motion. *Clin Orth Related Res* 1994; **303:** 128–34.
11. Duke JB, Tessler RH, Dell PC Manipulation of the stiff elbow with the patient under anaesthesia. *J Hand Surg* 1991; **16:** 19–24.
12. Breen TF, Gelberman RH, Ackerman GN Elbow flexion contractures: Treatment by anterior release and continuous passive motion. *J Hand Surg* 1988; **13:** 286–7.
13. Soffer SR, Yahiro MA Continuous passive motion after internal fixation of distal humerus fractures. *Orthop Rev* 1990; **19:** 88–93.

CHAPTER 19

Osteochondritis dissecans of the elbow

PER OLOF JOSEFSSON

Introduction

Osteochondritis dissecans is a crater-like lesion of a joint containing one or several osteochondral fragments. Often the osteochondral fragments will be detached to form loose bodies within the joint. The condition occurs at several locations but, after the knee the most frequent sites are the ankle and the elbow. In the reports by Green and Banks[1] and Lindholm *et al.*[2] osteochondritis dissecans of the elbow was second to that of the knee.

Removal of an intra-articular loose body was first described by Pare in 1558.[3] In 1870 Paget[4] described the process of 'quiet necrosis' of the femoral condyles in association with loose bodies within the knee joint. Konig[5] assumed the origin of the disease to be an inflammation and introduced the term osteochondritis dissecans. This name is still in use in spite of the fact that an inflammatory process as the cause of the disease has not been confirmed.

Osteochondritis dissecans of the humeral capitellum is a segmental disorder in contrast to osteochondrosis deformans juvenilis, also known as Panner's disease.[6] This latter condition is seen in children between the age of 4 and 10 years as an aseptic necrosis of the whole capitellar ossification nucleus similar to that of the femoral head in Legg-Calve-Perthes disease.[7] Loose bodies are not formed and the treatment is conservative.

Osteochondritis dissecans of the elbow usually involves the lateral or central portions of the capitellum humeri. Other locations include, the supratrochlear septum of the humerus,[8] the radial head[9,10] and the ulna.[2]

Aetiology

The aetiology of osteochondritis dissecans of the elbow is obscure. The time of onset of the disease is unknown although the diagnosis is often established in children and adolescents.[1] The diagnosis is for most patients established when the osteochondral lesion has become detached, probably a long time after the onset of the disease.[11,12] For some patients a relationship to trauma seems obvious.[13,14] In throwers osteochondritis dissecans of the elbow is a relatively common finding and is believed to be caused by valgus stress to the elbow.[15] For young baseball pitchers the term 'little leaguer's elbow' is used[15,16] to describe a series of pathologic conditions of the throwing elbow. This term includes osteochondritis dissecans of the capitellum and the radial head. The predominance of the right dominant elbow and the observation in several studies that it is more common in men supports a traumatic origin of osteochondritis dissecans of the elbow.

Another theory is that osteochondritis dissecans and Panner's disease represent different stages of the same disease, caused by avascular necrosis. The association with trauma might be that osteochondritis dissecans is caused by lateral overload with valgus stress at an age when the vascularity of the capitellum is fragile.[7]

A high incidence of bilateral disease and a common occurrence among relatives of affected patients also suggests the involvement of genetic factors in some patients.[17]

Clinical presentation

The most common clinical symptom in patients with osteochondritis dissecans of the elbow is pain. This is usually a dull ache which is poorly localised. It is made worse by activity, and is particularly troublesome if sports that involve throwing are undertaken.[12] Associated with the pain the patient may be aware of intermittent elbow swelling.

Another feature that is often present is reduced elbow movement. Extension is most commonly reduced but at times flexion, and forearm rotation may also be limited. The patient may complain of elbow stiffness particularly first thing in the morning.

Clicking, grinding and locking often follow fragment separation and are usually associated with acute elbow pain. If medical attention has not been sought previously, the acute pain of elbow locking will often lead to medical review.

Clinical examination of the elbow may reveal a reduced range of movement compared with the contralateral side. In addition, palpation may indicate the presence of a joint effusion. Frequently, however, the elbow appears normal.

Radiographic assessment

Although the diagnosis of osteochondritis dissecans is usually made on plain anteroposterior and lateral radiographs it is not unusual for radiographs taken in the early phase of the disease to appear normal. On the plain films the lateral and central portions of the capitellum should be carefully assessed followed by the supratrochlear septum of the humerus, radial head and ulna. If clinical symptoms persist despite normal radiographs further investigation is indicated. Standard tomography, computer tomography or magnetic resonance imaging should be performed since they may reveal evidence of osteochondritis dissecans not visible on plain radiographs (Fig. 19.1).

When osteochondritis dissecans is identified computed tomography can be valuable in assessing whether the cartilage overlying the damaged bone is intact, fissured, fractured, separated or detached. In addition, the size of the lesion can be more fully evaluated (Fig. 19.2) together with the number and size of any loose bodies.

The typical radiographic appearance consists of a crater in the capitellum with a sclerotic rim of subchondral bone (Fig. 19.2). If the central fragment separates, one or more loose bodies may be seen within the joint and it is these that give rise to the painful locking symptoms of which some patients complain. In late cases flattening of the capitellum is a common finding and at times the radial head appears larger compared with the opposite side. Finally with time degenerative changes occur within the elbow primarily affecting the radiocapitellar joint (Fig. 19.3).

Treatment

NON-OPERATIVE MANAGEMENT

The osteochondritis dissecans lesion may heal,[1] may remain unhealed *in situ* or become detached to form loose bodies. Healing of the lesion is thought to be related to the age of the patient, stage of the lesion, severity of the lesion, type and level of activities the patient has undertaken. The probability of healing is not known, but in children and adolescents with *in situ* lesions, recommendations against excessive use should be issued. In addition it is wise to consider above-elbow plaster cast immobilisation for 2 weeks. How long the elbow should be protected to facilitate healing is not know, although more than 6 months seems superfluous. Radiographic changes may persist for ever and therefore it is not reasonable to expect radiologic healing before full activity is permitted.

OPERATIVE MANAGEMENT

For adult patients with symptomatic osteochondritis dissecans *in situ* as well as all patients with

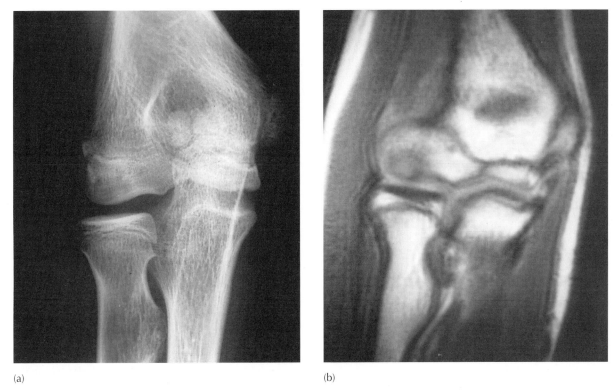

(a)   (b)

Fig. 19.1 A 14-year-old boy complained of pain and swelling in the right elbow for 3 years. The capitellum appeared normal on plain radiograms (a) but on magnetic resonance imaging the osteochondritis dissecans lesion in the capitellum was visualised (b).

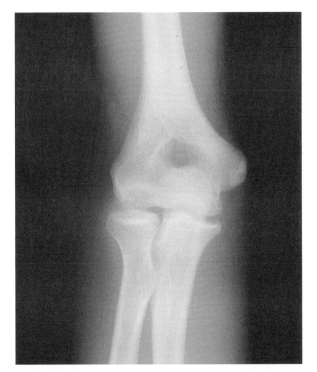

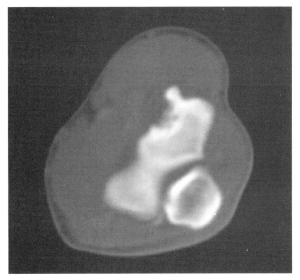

(b)

Fig. 19.2 Anteroposterior radiograph (a) and CT scan (b) of the elbow of a 15-year-old boy. The typical appearance and size of the osteochondritis dissecans lesion are clearly visualised.

(a)

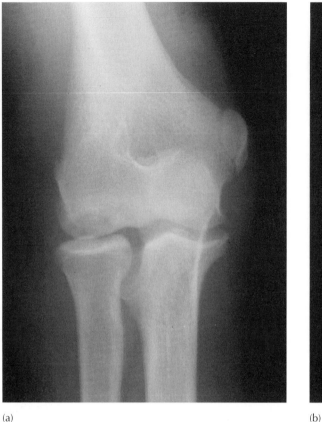

(a)

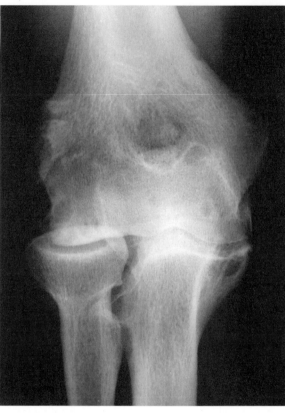

(b)

Fig. 19.3 Radiogram of the right elbow in a 16-year-old boy with pain and locking of the elbow for 3 months. Osteochondritis dissecans with loose bodies were found and removed (a). After 28 years when he was 44, osteoarthritis was present (b). Loss of extension was 25 degrees and loss of flexion 15 degrees. Pronation and supination were not reduced.

symptomatic loose bodies in the joint the treatment is surgical, with the removal of all loose osteochondral fragments. This can be undertaken either via a lateral arthrotomy or arthroscopically. Following surgery significant improvement can be expected in pain relief and increased range of motion.[12] When the crater is free from loose osteochondral fragments there is no evidence to support further procedures such as curetting or drilling, although I prefer to drill thin holes in the crater into bleeding bone according to Magnusson[18] and Pridie[19] in order to promote ingrowth of fibrous cartilage. Attempts to re-attach repelled lesions seem useless.[12,17] Excision of the radial head is without advantage and the results of procedures such as excision of the lateral condyle or bone grafting the defect are poor.[17]

Natural course and complications

In those patients whose osteochondral lesion has healed by joint protection residual symptoms are uncommon.

Unfortunately, however, in most patients the osteochondritis dissecans lesion does not heal and the lesion becomes detached. For these patients there is a high risk of developing degenerative joint disease. In a study of 31 patients, with an average time of follow-up of 23 years degenerative joint symptoms were noted in about half of the elbows and radiographic signs of degenerative joint disease in more than half of the patients.[11] Just as for osteochondritis dissecans of the knee,[20] patients who were children at the time of diagnosis seem to have a lower rate of degenerative joint disease. One-quarter of the children developed signs of degenerative disease compared with three-quarters of the adults.

Degenerative joint disease of the elbow results in a reduced range of motion and pain on effort. Although loss of flexion and pronation-supination were noted by Bauer *et al.*[11] loss of extension was the most common and for 7 of 23 adult patients was more than 10 degrees (15–60 degrees). Severe complaints were rare, unless the patient's occupation put great demand on the elbow.[11]

Lohr[21] found that all his patients showed premature epiphyseal closure and enlargement of the radial head. Bauer *et al.*[11] found enlargement of the radial head in two-thirds of the patients at follow-up examination and the diameter was increased by, on average, 4 mm (range 1–8 mm).

References

1. Green WT, Banks HH Osteochondritis dissecans in children. *Clin Orthop* 1990; **255:** 3–12.
2. Lindholm TS, Osterman K, Vankka E Osteochondritis dissecans of elbow, ankle and hip: A comparison survey. *Clin Orthop* 1980; **148:** 245–53.
3. Pare A *Oeuvres complètes* Vol III. Paris: JB Ballière, 1840–1: 32.
4. Paget J On the production of some of the loose bodies in joints. *St Bart Hosp Rep* 1870; **6:** 1–4.
5. Konig F Uber freie Korper in den Gelenken. *Deutsche Z Chir* 1888; **27:** 90–109.
6. Panner HJ A peculiar affection of the capitulum humeri resembling Calve-Perthes' disease of the hip. *Acta Radiol* 1929; **10:** 234.
7. Haraldsson S On osteochondrosis deformans juvenilis capituli humeri including investigation of intra-osseous vasculature in distal humerus. *Acta Orthop Scand* 1959; Suppl **38:** 1.
8. Hermans GP Osteochondrosis dissecans des Ellenbogengelenkes. *Orthopade* 1981; **10:** 335–7.
9. Gudmundsen TE Osteochondritis dissecans cubiti. *Tidsskriftfor Den Norsk Laegetidskrift* 1976; **96:** 355–7.
10. Nielsen NA Osteochondritis dissecans capituli humeri. *Acta Orthop Scand* 1933; **4:** 307–457.
11. Bauer M, Jonsson K, Josefsson PO, Linden B Osteochondritis dissecans ofthe elbow. A long-term follow-up study. *Clin Orthop* 1992; **284:** 156–60.
12. McManama GB Jr, Micheli LJ, Berry MV, Sohn RS The surgical treatment of osteochondritis of the capitellum. *Am J Sports Med* 1985; **13:** 11–21.
13. King JW, Brelsford HJ, Tullos HS Analysis of the pitching arm of the professional baseball pitcher. *Clin Orthop* 1969; **67:** 116–23.
14. Singer KM, Roy SP Osteochondrosis of the humeral capitellum. *Am J Sports Med* 1984; **12:** 351–60.
15. Tullos HS, King JW Lesions of the pitching arm in adolescents. *J Am Med Assoc* 1972; **220:** 264–71
16. Torg JS Little league. 'The theft of a carefree youth'. *Phys Sports Med* 1973; **1:** 72–41
17. Woodward AH, Bianco AJ Osteochondritis dissecans of the elbow. *Clin Orthop* 1975; **110:** 35–41.
18. Magnusson PB Technique of debridement of the knee joint for arthritis. *Surg Clin North Am* 1946; **26:** 249–66.
19. Pridie KH A method of resurfacing osteoarthritic knee joints. *J Bone Joint Surg (Br)* 1959; **41B:** 618.
20. Linden B Osteochondritis dissecans of the femoral condyles: A long-term follow-up study. *J Bone Joint Surg* 1977; **59A:** 769–76.
21. Lohr W Dauererfolge BEI Der Behandlung Der Osteochondritis Dissecans. *Arch F Klin Chir* 1929; **157:** 752–810.

CHAPTER 20

Inflammatory conditions of the elbow

NEVILLE RM KAY

Introduction

Pain primarily at the lateral aspect of the elbow (tennis elbow) is probably the most common reason for orthopaedic referral in patients with elbow disorders. Less frequently pain medially (golfer's elbow) posteriorly (triceps tendinitis) or anteriorly (biceps tendinitis) may also require assessment and treatment.

Morris[1] in 1882 noted that certain morbid changes were associated with many types of sports and amusements. His paper entitled 'the riders sprain' also included a discussion of the lawn tennis arm. He attributed pain along the region of the pronatus radii as being due to frequent backstroke. Rest and support were the treatment recommendations that Morris advised. Following this initial description the term tennis elbow rapidly became accepted[2] in the English literature though Wadsworth[3] notes that Runge[4] had previously described the condition in 1873. Cyriax[5] attributes the very first description of tennis elbow to Renton[6] in 1830 and interestingly this is perhaps the first description of acupuncture to cure the condition. In Europe, the condition is termed lateral epicondylitis.

By common consent medial epicondylitis is distinguished 'golfer's elbow' and in Coonrad and Hooper's[7] extensive series of tennis elbow patients 22 cases involved patients with golfer's elbow. Unlike tennis elbow there does not appear to be a single person to whom the description golfer's elbow can be attributed.

Posterior tennis elbow (triceps tendinitis) and tenderness at the insertion of the biceps tendon are uncommon conditions which have received little attention in the literature.

In this chapter tennis elbow, golfer's elbow, posterior (triceps) tendinitis and bicipital tendinitis will be discussed.

Tennis elbow

AETIOLOGY

It is difficult to describe the syndrome of tennis elbow until consideration has been given to its aetiology. If pain at the lateral aspect of the elbow in its widest sense is accepted as tennis elbow then the potential list of causes is endless. Cyriax's[8] classic paper lists 26 distinct causes of the condition each one supported by appropriate references. Priest[9] increases the list to 43 separate pathologies. Various attempts have been made to separate the clinical syndromes on the basis of the theoretical pathology and Cyriax[8] lists four principle groups on this basis, namely:

1. Acute – following indirect trauma
2. Sub-acute – following indirect trauma
3. Chronic – occupational
4. Following direct trauma

Similarly attempts have been made to identify the cause of tennis elbow by determining which is the most tender area on clinical examination.[10,11] This local assessment together with an appreciation of systemic factors is useful in the understanding of the various theories and pathologies that have been postulated as the cause of this condition.

Local causes
1. The epicondylar ridge
2. The musculotendinous junction
3. The elbow capsule
4. The articular surface
5. The synovium
6. The orbicular ligament
7. Nerve entrapment

Systemic causes
1. Age
2. Sex
3. 'Collagen' background
4. Hormones
5. Occupation/sports/litigation

Local causes

The epicondylar ridge

The epicondylar ridge has long been identified as a possible pathological site for the causative lesion of tennis elbow. Certainly in many patients, direct pressure over the epicondylar ridge causes pain and reproduces symptoms. Cyriax[5] believed that most cases resulted from a tear between the tendinous origin of the extensor carpi radialis brevis and the periostum of the lateral epicondyle. He relied heavily on continental literature for pathological support.

Garden[12] also accepts this theory and notes that the pain may be localised to the wrist extensors particularly during extension of the wrist in radial deviation. On this basis he proposed the operation of Z elongation of the tendon of the extensor carpi radialis brevis. However, although this was popular for

a time the operation has now largely been abandoned. Nonetheless Garden echoes the views of just about every writer on tennis elbow when he states 'with such a clearly defined clinical diagnostic feature the continued obscurity of the pathology of tennis elbow is surprising'.

Thermography[13] and ultrasound[14] have both been used to investigate the concept that tennis elbow results from a musculoperiosteal tear, but neither has convincingly demonstrated such a lesion. Thermography has shown hot spots over the lateral epicondyle whilst ultrasound has revealed thickening of the periosteal lining. Both these studies, however, were undertaken in patients who had already undergone treatment and thus interpretation of the results is difficult.

McKee[15] also believed that the pathology was at the musculoperiosteal level and suggested that a traumatic periostitis developed. This he felt should be regarded as synonymous with tennis elbow. Such a situation might be expected to result in calcification at the epicondylar ridges and although this has been variously reported,[16,17] in the author's experience it is unusual. In addition an inflammatory respose might also be expected. However, Verhaar et al.[17] in an extensive series of 63 surgical releases for tennis elbow found 'no evidence of an inflammatory reaction'. Essentially therefore although a lesion of the musculoperiosteal junction of the epicondylar ridge has for many years been considered a cause of tennis elbow there is little scientific evidence for its existence.

Tears of the musculotendinous junction

Tears of the extensor muscles at or near their musculotendinous origin is another theory that has been postulated as the pathological lesion in many cases of tennis elbow. Cyriax[5] quotes reference to 'tears of the extensor muscles, supinator muscles, extensor carpi radialis longus and brevis'. Coonrad and Hooper[7] in their extensive series of patients identified tears of the extensor tendon principally the superficial portion. Grey amorphous material was noted at surgery and histologically 'brown cell infiltrate, scattered foci of fine calcification and scar tissue with marginal areas of cystic degeneration' were noted. They further observed that in nine patients with no microscopic tear, biopsy of the 'abnormal tissue' yielded a similar microscopic picture.

Theoretically those studies investigating muscle tears reported before the advent of steroid injections are likely to be more reliable since, the average number of presurgical steroid injections, per patient in Coonrad's series[7] was six. The problems of preoperative treatment raises questions over the histology of biopsy specimens obtained surgically since no control tissue is available. Thus, the possibility of the biopsy lesion being produced by the steroid injection must be considered. As Wadsworth[3] elegantly illustrated in his review of tennis elbow the recommended site of the steroid injection is all too often the site of the abnormal tissue identified at surgery. More recently, Verhaar[17] has noted the presence of an amorpheous substance believed to be the residuum of local steroid injections in five of his 63 patients.

Reports of muscle tears seen at surgery prior to the introduction of steroid injections suffer from the disadvantage that, forced manipulation of the elbow was often recommended prior to surgery[18] and in these cases iatrogenic tears cannot be excluded.

Non-surgical attempts to demonstrate tears have not been universally successful although Maffulli *et al.*[14] using ultrasound showed that the tendon of extensor carpi radialis brevis was enlarged and areas of 'dyshomogeneous hypoechogenicity' were evident with loss of the normal microscopic wave form structure of the tendon collagen. Jobe and Ciccotti[19] accepted that a micro tear most often within the origin of extensor carpi radialis brevis was the pathological lesion. On that basis they recommended an operation which effectively strips the origin of extensor carpi radialis brevis from bone and decompresses the elbow joint.

Nirschl and Pettrone[20] in a large series of 1013 cases of which 88 were treated surgically, concluded, 'the basic underlying lesion is in the origin of the extensor carpi radialis brevis when overuse has resulted in a microscopic rupture and subsequent tendinous non-repair with immature reparative tissue'. Sadly this important paper has resulted in significant medico/legal litigation and the scientific validity of this concept must be questioned since all of their operative patients, had received several steroid injections prior to surgery. In addition the authors also noted a surprising and comprehensive range of musculoskeletal abnormalities in their patients. Thus, though a tear of the musculotendoneus junction principally of the extensor carpi radialis brevis is an undoubted pathological lesion seen in tennis elbow, it cannot be considered the 'single' clinical cause. Surgical and histological demonstration of such a lesion is of doubtful significance in the presence of preoperative treatment particularly forceful manipulation and repeated steroid injections.

The elbow capsule

The capsule of the elbow has been described in Chapter 2. Changes within the capsule do not appear to feature prominently in the pathology of tennis elbow although Boyd[21] noted that there are several pathological processes that can occur in the soft tissues of the lateral aspect of the elbow that may cause this syndrome.

Cyriax[8] cites a 'torn capsule' as a possible pathological cause and this is reiterated by Curwin and Standish.[22] Undoubtedly some capsular changes do occur in chronic tennis elbow but whether these are due to secondary scarring and contraction, due to a combination of treatment and painful full extension or whether, in some cases there is a primary pathological lesion within the capsule is speculative. Nonetheless, decompression of the elbow is achieved in many of the surgical procedures that are advocated and this capsular release may in part account for the operative success.

The articular surface

Bosworth[23] in a surgical series of 62 patients with chronic tennis elbow noted four cases of chondromalacia of the head of the radius. Later Goodfellow and Bullough[24] carefully documented the age related changes in the radial head. These authors drew attention to the particular mechanical environment of the radial head likening its movement on the capitellum to that of a 'pot scourer'. They concluded that in early adult life areas of articular cartilage of the radial head that do not normally articulate with opposed cartilage of the capitellum all show some degree of chondromalacia. In addition they stated that the subsequent 'almost inevitable' degeneration of the radio capitellum joint with age relates to the combination of rotation and hinge movements that occur at that joint.

In a subsequent clinical paper Newman and Goodfellow[25] identified a series of 25 patients with resistant tennis elbow who had abnormalities of the articular cartilage of the head of the radius. They documented that division of the orbicular ligament and excision of the abnormal cartilage gave good results. Clinically this group of patients had characteristic tenderness over the head of the radius as distinct from the lateral epicondyle. There was maximum tenderness on full pronation which was increased by palmar flexion of the wrist, thus compressing the head of the radius against the capitellum. Stanley[26] notes that osteoarthritis of the elbow may present with pain on the lateral side of the elbow as the initial symptom.

Synovium

Systemic synovial diseases, (rheumatoid arthritis and gout) are recognised causes of tennis elbow. However, localised changes within the synovium such as a small synovial bursa between the radio-humeral joint[27] the trapping of synovial fronds[18] have been described as localised synovial causes of tennis elbow. Surgery directed to the appropriate lesion is recorded as being successful.

The orbicular ligament

Bosworth[23] in a classic paper on tennis elbow drew attention to the anatomy of the radial head and noted:

1. The radial head is not quite circular when seen from above.
2. The radial head is not quite concentric with the radial shaft and is slightly offset.
3. One margin is considerably elevated above the opposite margin.
4. The peripheral border varies in width.
5. The lateral border is not smoothly moulded throughout its circumference but shows considerable irregularity.

He concluded that 'rotation of this distorted head in a changing plane on a changing stress axis, inside a sensitive membrane, compressed by powerful muscles and tendonous structures would be capable of producing the pain of tennis elbow'. On this basis Boswoth[23] recommended resection of the orbicular ligament. More recently this has been modified with only partial resection of the orbicular ligament.

In attempting to assess the success of surgery on the orbicular ligament in the relief of symptoms for tennis elbow it must be appreciated that of necessity, operations on the orbicular ligament demand an arthrotomy of the elbow joint. Whether it is the 'joint decompression' resulting from that arthrotomy, or the surgery to the orbicular ligament that produces the symptomatic relief is difficult to define.

Nerve entrapment

Roles and Maudsley[28] in their classic paper entitled 'Radial tunnel syndrome – resistant tennis elbow as nerve entrapment' presented a series of cases in which symptoms thought to be due to tennis elbow were relieved by radial nerve decompression. They described the salient anatomy of the radial tunnel (Fig. 20.1) drawing attention to the arcade of

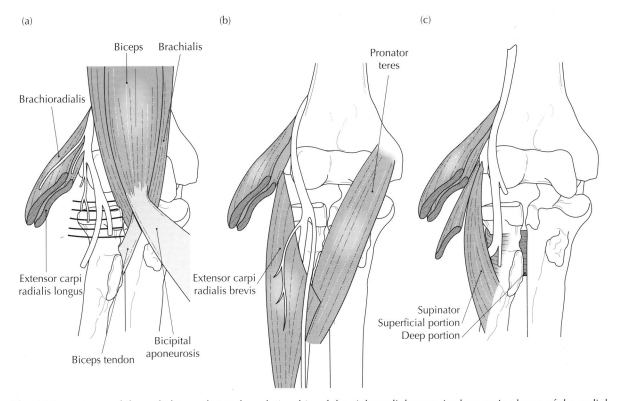

(a)   (b)   (c)

Biceps   Brachialis

Brachioradialis

Pronator teres

Extensor carpi radialis longus

Extensor carpi radialis brevis

Supinator
Superficial portion
Deep portion

Biceps tendon   Bicipital aponeurosis

Fig. 20.1 Anatomy of the radial tunnel. (a) The relationship of the right radial nerve in the proximal part of the radial tunnel. The transverse lines represent the fibrous bands tethering the radial nerve and its branches in front of the radial head. (b) The relationship of the extensor carpi radialis brevis to the right posterior interosseous nerve. The prolongation of the origin medially is variable. (c) The relationship of the superficial portion of the supinator to the right posterior interosseous nerve. Redrawn after Ref. 28.

Frosche and the close association of the radial nerve with the radial recurrent artery. They pointed out that the concept of radial nerve entrapment neuropathy had been previously described by Kaplan[29] Somerville[30] and Capner.[31]

Kaplan[29] reported a series of three patients treated by radial nerve denervation of the lateral aspect of the elbow. He stated that prior to surgery selective nerve blocks had been used to identify suitable cases.

The criteria Roles and Maudsley[28] used to select patients for surgery were: 1) failure of previous tennis elbow treatment; 2) tenderness along the course of the radial nerve; 3) pain on restricted extension of the middle finger. In addition a number of patients underwent radial nerve conduction studies and were noted to have delayed motor latency to the medius portion of extensor digitorum communis. Although in some patients nerve conduction improved postoperatively the precise value and reliability of such studies remains controversial.

Spinner and Linscheid[32] note 'Electro-myographic studies in cases of resistant tennis elbow due to the entrapment of the posterior interosseous nerves are often disappointing even if the condition has been present for some months' whilst Eversmann[33] has stated that the electro diagnostic studies of the radial nerve are helpful if signs of denervation are present on the electromyogram. Conduction velocity of the radial nerve across the radial tunnel has not been helpful in his experience. More recently Campion[34] has suggested that electrodiagnostic testing is the most appropriate test for possible radial tunnel syndrome.

Whilst radial tunnel syndrome must occupy a place in the differential diagnosis of tennis elbow these patients are best considered as a true nerve entrapment. Pathologically and surgically they are a different entity to tennis elbow and if accurately diagnosed surgical decompression should offer a very high level of symptomatic relief.

Systemic causes

Age

Tennis elbow can occur at any age but the two incidence peaks of presentation are in young sporting adults and in middle age. True sporting injuries (Chapter 17) require different evaluation and often a different management regime to the condition seen in middle age. Verhaar[35] estimates that the incidence of tennis elbow is between 1% and 2% whereas Allander[36] gives an annual incidence of less than 1%.

Goldie[37] noted that with increasing age degenerative changes were not found in the tendoneus attachment of the forearm extensors. This is somewhat surprising as age related changes in collagen tissue are increasingly well recognised, and documented.[38] Nonetheless, most authors accept that tennis elbow is most common in the 40–50 age group[19,20] and Dimberg[39] has stated that increasing age is the only positive factor associated with tennis elbow.

Sex

There does not appear to be a sex specific incidence for tennis elbow and the male/female prevalence rates appear to be approximately equal.[40]

Collagen background

It is a common clinical experience to note the comorbidity of tennis elbow, carpal tunnel syndrome, trigger digits and shoulder problems in the same patients. It is by no means unusual to treat a patient for all, or many of these conditions and Phalen[41] has stated that the co-existence of these various disorders (trigger finger, trigger thumb, carpal tunnel syndrome, De Quervain's tenovaginitus) as well as tennis elbow, peri-arthritis of the shoulder and calcific tendonitis is all too frequent to deny an aetiological relationship.

Certainly in any male patient a serum uric acid is a mandatory check since gout may present as an elbow problem. If there is a clinical suspicion of multiple joint disease then a collagen immune screen, especially in the female may be equally useful.

Hormones

The effect of hormones especially oestrogen on articular cartilage and joints in general is well documented and increasing attention is being focused on the effect of changes in female hormones on the presentation of musculoskeletal disease.[42] This may partly explain the development of bilateral tennis elbow in peri-menopausal women.

Occupation

The concept that work, especially repetitive work can cause tennis elbow has long been championed. Goldie[37] regarded tennis elbow as an overuse syndrome resulting in the deposition of hypervascular granulation tissue in the subtendoneous space at the site of the insertion of the forearm extensors of the epicondyle. Surgical removal of this tissue was stated to result in a cure and a return to work within 5 weeks. No explanation, however, was given as to why the granulation tissue did not recur when work was resumed.

Gellman[43] reiterated this view noting that such work-related overuse syndromes were difficult to treat and often required surgery. Workplace epidemiological studies, however, note no difference in the incidence between manual and non-manual workers[39] although some epidemiological studies have shown an increase in food factory workers over shop workers.[44]

Several factors limit the value of epidemiological studies. Kuppa *et al.*,[45] have noted 'increasing claims for compensation for tennis elbow with the implementation of more lenient insurance practices'. They also note the fact that the extent to which a person affected is occupationally disadvantaged depends upon the demands of the job; pointing out that a meat cutter may seek medical attention whilst a foreman may wait for the symptoms to disappear. These two factors significantly influence the incidence of tennis elbow in epidemiological studies and their apparent relationship to work.

Although there is as yet no scientific proof that movements such as repetitive dorsiflexion of the wrist and prosupination of the forearm are causative for tennis elbow syndrome[46] the view that occupation is the cause of tennis elbow appears to be having a significant effect on the morbidity of the condition.

It is interesting to compare the morbidity of tennis elbow before and after 'lenient insurance criteria'. Goldie[37] reported complete recovery and a return to work after 5 weeks following his operation and Cyriax[8] noted that the condition usually settled in 8–12 months without any treatment. He stated, however, that some longer lasting cases were encountered. This was also the experience of Roles and Maudsley[28] who referred to resistant tennis elbow.

The recent explosion of medico/legal claims relating to tennis elbow, especially within the UK and the significant sums awarded by the Courts (£50 000) does pose the question as to whether the perceived morbidity of tennis elbow has now been significantly altered by the existence of such compensation. Although there can be little doubt that such compensation claims crystallise medical views and expose woolly thinking and scientific inconsistency; it would apear that we are still some distance from the answers. This is recognised in the report of the Industrial Injuries Advisory Council[47] who note that the evidence from studies which have examined the relationships between occupational activity and medial and lateral epicondylitis is inconsistent. The data is difficult to interpret, largely because of small numbers, poor study design and difficulties in establishing reliable diagnostic criteria.

Author's view

The cause of tennis elbow is not known and is certainly multifactorial. The existence of intra-articular pathology is an undoubted cause of some tennis elbow conditions and the surprising silence of other investigators to confirm the findings of Nirschl and Pettrone[20] suggests[45] that the views expressed by the British Orthopaedic Association Working Party report[48] are correct. They state 'It is clear that the pathology of tennis elbow is still a subject for speculation, but that this common condition does not show a predilection for manual workers and is not clearly associated with working activity. However, when it does occur the symptoms are more likely to be troublesome in those doing manual work and re-occurrence which is quite common, is likely to occur when manual activities are resumed'.

Occasionally the author has been satisfied that tennis elbow has resulted from a single blow to the outside of the elbow. In tennis and squash players who develop the syndrome there appears little doubt that the game itself is a factor in the pathological development of the syndrome, either on the basis of a traumatic incident (hitting the wall with the squash racquet) or effective overuse in a degenerative elbow.

Though overuse either at work or on the tennis court can initiate symptoms in a degenerative elbow the fundamental problem is the degeneration of the joint and the surrounding tissues as distinct from the sport or work.

CLINICAL PRESENTATION

Pain localised to the lateral aspect of the elbow is consistent with a diagnosis of tennis elbow. The onset is usually gradual but occasionally a single traumatic episode may be identified. In racquet players an inadvertent stroke striking a fixed object with the racket can sometimes be recalled but usually tennis elbow presents as an increasing and progressive discomfort on active use of the elbow. Although the dominant arm is usually affected this is not invariable.

The pain over the lateral aspect of the elbow is frequently described as diffuse, toothache-like, or nagging. It often radiates up the arm and down the forearm and may occur on specific use of the index and long finger in activities such as writing. In addition activities such as gripping consistently produce pain.

It is important to differentiate pain at the elbow from pain referred from the neck. Clinically this can be assessed since if moving the neck against the examiner's resistance produces elbow pain, the neck is the likely source of the pain. A neurological diagnosis must also be considered if the patient complains of paraesthesia affecting the hand or fingers.

The signs

The 'signs' of tennis elbow are subjective and depend upon the examiner's assessment of the patient's pain. It is of practical importance to differentiate the most painful areas and care should be taken to try and determine whether the maximum site of tenderness is over the epicondylar ridge (indicating a teno/pathology) or over the radio-humeral articulation (indicating joint pathology).

The elbow should be examined in 90 degrees of flexion in order to enable accurate differentiation of the site of the pain (Fig. 20.2). If the tenderness is maximal over the extensor muscle mass especially if it is anterior and slightly medial to the lateral border of the forearm then, the possibility of radial – tunnel syndrome should be suspected. Mills manoeuvre and a finger/wrist extension test should be routinely performed.

Mills manoeuvre

The elbow is fully extended, fingers lightly clenched into a fist and the wrist flexed. The forearm is then

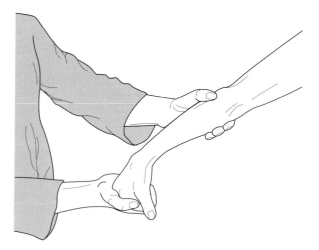

Fig. 20.3 Mills manoeuvre. Forced pronation of the extended forearm combined with wrist flexion produces pain over the common extensor origin.

fully pronated by the examiner and pain produced at the elbow is diagnostic of tennis elbow (Fig. 20.3).

Finger/wrist extension test

This is performed with the elbow in full extension, the wrist slightly extended 15–20 degrees and with the fingers in full extension. The patient attempts to extend his wrist and fingers against the examiner's resistance. Pain over the epicondylar ridge suggests a musculo/tendinous/periostal origin of the pain due to stretching of the extensors (Fig. 20.4). If the pain is most marked on resisted extension of the middle finger the site of pathology is considered to be the origin of the extensor carpi radialis brevis.

General examination

In any patient presenting with tennis elbow, a general examination to exclude polyjoint arthropathy, referred pain from the neck or shoulder and other systemic causes should be performed.

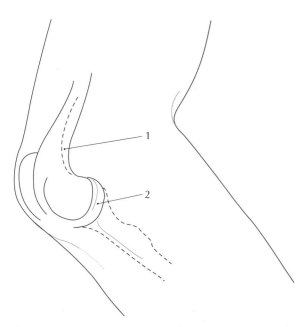

Fig. 20.2 Lateral aspect of the elbow joint. Note that the lateral supercondylar ridge (1) is easily palpated and that the head of the radius (2) can be felt to move under the examining finger as the forearm is rotated. Clinical identification of the most painful area is helpful in treatment.

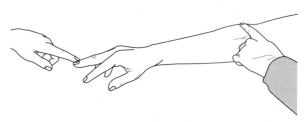

Fig. 20.4 The finger extension test relied on by Roles and Maudsley to identify 'resistant tennis elbow'.

INVESTIGATIONS

Radiographs

Anteroposterior and lateral x-rays of the elbow are useful to exclude arthritis, loose bodies or other joint pathologies. Particular care should be taken to look at the soft tissue shadow on the radiographs for a joint effusion and specks of calcification over the lateral epicondyle.

Magnetic resonance imaging of the elbow

This may be helpful in patients who present with elbow pain associated with sporting activities. The investigation may reveal osteochondritis of the capitellum or evidence of ligamentous injury as the underlying cause of the elbow pain. Treatment appropriate for the pathology can then be instituted.

Haematological investigations.

In middle aged males especially if hypertensive and on therapy, a serum uric acid should be performed. If systemic disease is suspected appropriate investigations are necessary.

TREATMENT

Conservative management

Rest and support

Stopping the provoking cause of the pain is the first line of treatment – and often the most difficult. Racquet players are reluctant to give up their sport and workers need to work.

In racquet players particular attention should be paid to the grip; the stroke and the pre-playing (warm up). Every sports physiotherapist has a specific view on the grip for racquet sports, but the author's own observations suggest a wide variety in the 'natural grip' and very careful thought is necessary before suggesting any serious alteration in the player's grip. In class racquet players, consultation with the coach on this matter is essential. Nirschl illustrates his method of assessing the racket handle diameter[49] but other workers[50] who have attempted to control forearm torque stresses have concluded that the grip size should be as large as is comfortable. In racquet players who insist on playing through an episode of tennis elbow the importance of pre-match and pre-training warm-ups cannot be overstated. The author's personal preference is to allow the patient to do the appropriate stretching exercises for 5 minutes then rub the affected elbow with liniment and keep the elbow warm with a light elastic support (tubigrip). In workers it is often possible to obtain a period of light duties and thus avoid the activity which initiated the symptoms.

Support for the elbow is not always easy or acceptable. A light-weight elasticised elbow support is helpful in mild cases and an epicondyler clamp is sometimes tolerated.

Physiotherapy

This has to be tailored to individual needs. A whole variety of agents are helpful. Icing the painful elbow; ultrasound for chronic periosteal/tendinitis lesions and stretching exercises are helpful in the prevention of contractures. The treatment of sports tennis elbow is fully discussed in Chapter 17 but a combination of treatments is useful both in the sporting elbow and the degenerative elbow. Prevention of contractures is important.

Drugs

These may be either systemic or local.

Systemic

The use of non-steriodal anti-inflammatory drugs in the treatment of an acute episode of tennis elbow is often beneficial. The side-effects particularly gastrointestinal irritation should not be underestimated and the long-term use of non-steroidal anti-inflammatory drugs for mild tennis elbow is questionable. Nonetheless a short 3-week course of non-steroidal anti-inflammatory drugs combined with physiotherapy is often all that is needed to settle many patients.

Local injection

The local injection of steroid to the tender area has been one of the principal mainstays of conservative treatment for some years. The choice of steriod preparation is a matter of individual preference but the author uses triamcinolone acetonide (Kenalog®) since there is some evidence that it is slightly longer lasting at its local site and less irritant. Routinely, this is mixed with 2 ml of 2% lignocaine without adrenalin prior to injection.

There is no precise agreement where best to inject the mixture though Wadsworth[3] suggests that it should be injected into the tendinous origin of the extensor carpi radialis brevis at the humeral lateral epicondyle.

The author prefers to be guided by clinical examination. If the maximum tenderness is over the lateral epicondyle then 75% of the mixture is injected at this site and 25% into the radiohumeral articulation. If the radiohumeral joint is the principal site of the tenderness then 75% of the mixture is injected into the joint and 25% injected at the lateral epicondyle. Many patients express concern at the possibility of injection having been advised by friends and colleagues that it is often particularly painful. Most of my personal patient population, however, express surprise and some delight that the injection is not painful and gives fairly instant relief.

The importance of a deep injection of steroid mixture cannot be overemphasised. Subcutaneous injection especially if the skin is pigmented will inevitably result in depigmentation and subcutaneous fat necrosis producing an ugly cosmetic deficit.

Author's injection technique

A suspension of 40 mg of triamcinoline acetonide in 1 ml fluid is mixed in the barrel of a syringe (5 ml syringe 21 g 1½ inch needle) with 2 ml of 2% plain lignocaine. With the patient standing and the elbow flexed at 90 degrees the most painful area is identified and 75% of the mixture is injected at that site. Although the point of the needle may be moved and re-inserted several times to cover the painful area it is seldom necessary to make another skin puncture with the needle. The remaining mixture should be delivered to the secondary site (see above).

After injection gentle pressure on the injection site with the thumb and a plug of cotton wool helps further distribute the mixture into the tissues whilst the elbow is gently passively flexed and extended. After a minute or so the treatment is completed by two or three Mills manoeuvres. By now the local anaesthetic solution will be acting on the local tissue and pain is rarely produced by this manoeuvre. The Mills manipulations are an essential part of the injection technique for they stretch out any contractures that may have developed from the patient protecting the painful elbow.

The frequency at which such injections can be repeated is by no means scientifically established. The author's preference is to limit the course to three injections with a minimum interval between each injection of 3 weeks.

Very occasionally, and usually in a 'class' sportsman, an injection of local anaesthetic may help in a critical match of a tournament. In these circumstances 0.5% Marcaine® is the local anaesthetic of choice. The volume of local anaesthetic used is critical – too much and muscle function is impaired and performance blunted. Usually 1 ml is adequate in these circumstances.

SURGICAL MANAGEMENT

The surgical operations offered in the treatment of tennis elbow are so many and as varied as the perceived surgical pathology. Mills offered manipulation under anaesthesia[51] Bosworth[23] recommended surgery to the orbicular ligament; and there are subsequent modifications to this procedure. Goldie[37] excised the subaponeurotic areolar tissue; Garden released the extensor radialis brevis at the wrist.[12]

Readers who have found a particular surgical technique effective are advised to continue using that procedure. For the last 20 years the author has adopted the view that if surgery is necessary for tennis elbow it should address as many of the potential causes as possible. For this reason a three-in-one procedure, which effectively slides the extensor origin by subperiosteal dissection decompresses the elbow joint by arthrotomy and divides the orbicular ligament, has been performed.

AUTHOR'S PREFERRED MANAGEMENT

Under general anaesthetic with a high tourniquet the patient is positioned on the operating table with the arm on an elbow table. The elbow is flexed to 90 degrees. The lateral epicondylar ridge is carefully palpated and the site of the radiohumeral joint is identified by rotation of the forearm. A curved incision along the epicondylar ridge is continued across the radiohumeral articulation and into the forearm (Fig. 20.5). The dissection is taken between the triceps muscle posteriorly and the brachioradialis and extensor carpi radialis longus muscles anteriorly. This enables exposure of the lateral condyle and the capsule over the lateral aspect of the joint. The joint capsule is incised and the elbow joint inspected. Particular attention is paid to the radiohumeral articulation and the synovium looking for any abnormality. The presence or absence of a joint effusion is noted. The orbicular ligament is then divided and the forearm rotated whilst observing the incision in the orbicular ligament. Occasionally as soon as the ligament is divided a gap of 2–3 mm appears suggesting that tension in this ligament was an important source of pain. More commonly there is no more than slight widening of the incision as the forearm rotates. Segments of the orbicular ligament are not routinely excised.

Finally, the epicondylar area is carefully assessed. Tears and granulation tissue are sought particularly in the extensor carpi radialis brevis and the extensor origin is slid off the epicondyle and front of the humerus by subperiosteal dissection.

(a)

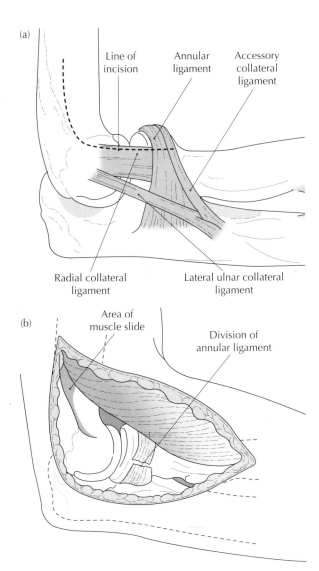

Line of incision

Annular ligament

Accessory collateral ligament

Radial collateral ligament

Lateral ulnar collateral ligament

(b)

Area of muscle slide

Division of annular ligament

Fig. 20.5 (a) Diagram of the ligaments of the lateral aspect of the elbow with the line of the incision for release of tennis elbow identified. (b) Indication of area of the muscle slide from the epicondylar ridge and also the division of the orbicular ligament.

This subperiosteal dissection should begin at the distal end of the epicondylar ridge and extend proximally to that part of the humerus where the epicondylar ridge merges with the shaft of the humerus.

The capsule of the elbow is closed with continuous absorbable sutures, and haemostasis secured prior to wound closure. Early mobilisation of the elbow is encouraged and the patient warned that in the early postoperative phase a mild self correcting extensor lag of the index and long finger may be present for 2–3 weeks.

Golfer's elbow

This occurs less commonly than tennis elbow. However, in a study of human epicondylitis associated with carpal tunnel compression and cervical spondylosis, Murray-Leslie and Wright[52] noted the association of medial and lateral epicondylitis in the same patients.

CLINICAL PRESENTATION

Patients with golfer's elbow frequently present with pain well localised to the medial side of the elbow and accurately pin-pointed to the medial epicondyle. If the pain is diffuse, paraesthesia in the forearm is a dominant feature or if pressure over the ulnar nerve reproduces the symptoms then nerve conduction studies should be undertaken. These are helpful in differentiating medial epicondylitis, ulnar neuritis and referred pain from cervical spondylosis. The co-existence of these three pathologies is not unusual, nor is it uncommon for the patient to have associated tennis elbow symptoms.

CLINICAL SIGNS

The classic clinical sign is tenderness accurately located over the medial epicondyle which is consistently reproduced. A reverse Mills manoeuvre producing pain (supination of the extended forearm with the wrist extended), and pain on resisted flexion of the wrist are both useful confirmatory signs. Particular care must always be taken to exclude ulnar nerve lesions and a careful neurological examination to exclude ulna neuritis is essential. In addition the elbow should be assessed for evidence of medial collateral ligament pathology since this also may mimic medial epicondylitis.

TREATMENT

Conservative management

The same basic principles are used as in the management of tennis elbow. Thus, initially rest, avoidance of the provoking activity, support (an epicondylar clamp can be useful) together with analgesics, liniments and a 3-week course of non-steroidal anti-inflammatory drugs should always be tried. Physiotherapy may also be helpful with specific emphasis on re-training in sporting/occupational activities. Although steroid injections are useful, special care must be taken to avoid inadvertant injury to the ulnar nerve, and damage to the medial collateral ligament.

Technique of injection

The same mixture as is used for tennis elbow is recommended (40 mg of triamcinolone acetonide in 1 ml fluid mixed with 2 cc of 2% plain lignocaine). With the patient standing and the elbow flexed at 90 degrees the ulnar groove is carefully palpated posterior to the medial epicondyle. Two fingers of the left hand keep the ulnar nerve in its gutter and the thumb of the left hand stretches the skin and subcutaneous tissue over the anterior surface of the medial epicondyle. This provides a safe area for needle insertion (Fig. 20.6). The steroid is then injected into the maximally tender area of the medial epicondyle.

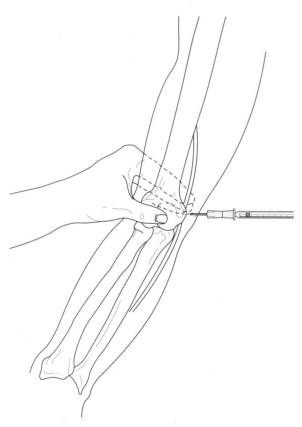

Fig. 20.6 Technique of injecting medial epicondyle and note that the thumb of the left hand stretches the skin over the volar aspect of the forearm whilst the index and long fingers do the same at the posterior aspect, but primarily stabilise the ulnar nerve. This exposes the medial epicondyle which can then be safely injected.

Surgical management

Few authorities precisely detail the surgery for golfer's elbow and many standard textbooks of operative surgery give no details. Vangsness and Jobe,[53] however, have described their technique of detachment of the flexors, removal of degenerative granulation tissue, and re-attachment of the forearm flexors to the roughened and drilled bone. They reported good results using this technique.

Author's preferred management

My own preference is to excise the medial epicondyle and perform a subperiosteal slide of the forearm flexors without resuturing them. When excising the medial epicondyle, care must be taken to protect the ulnar nerve and create a soft tissue sleeve of periosteum and loose areolar tissue to cover the bleeding osteotomy site and so prevent the ulnar nerve adhering to the bone.

TECHNIQUE

Under general anaesthesia and with a high tourniquet the elbow is flexed and placed on a hand table. The medial epicondyle, ulnar groove and ulnar nerve are carefully identified. A curved incision over the medial epicondyle is deepened and the ulnar nerve identified and protected. A subperiosteal dissection of the medial epicondyle is performed with preservation of the medial collateral ligament. As this is performed the common flexor origin is released from the medial epicondyle allowing the flexor muscles to slide. The medial epicondyle is osteotomised and a triangle of bone removed. The bleeding base of the bone is covered by periosteum but no attempt is made to relocate the forearm flexors (Fig. 20.7).

The wound is closed in layers and early mobilisation of the elbow instituted.

Triceps tendinitis

Triceps tendinitis is not an infrequent cause of elbow pain (Chapter 17). The pain is accurately located to the point of the olecranon and is not usually confused with either tennis or golfer's elbow.

Conservative treatment with rest, ice, non-steroidal anti-inflammatory drugs and physiotherapy is usually all that is required. Occasionally, a local steroid injection may be appropriate if symptoms are persistent.

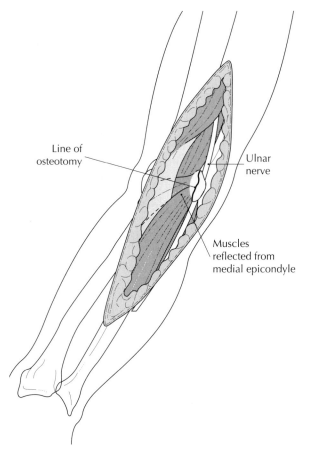

Line of osteotomy

Ulnar nerve

Muscles reflected from medial epicondyle

Fig. 20.7 Medial release for golfer's elbow showing line of osteotomy of medial epicondyle and slide of flexor muscles.

Biceps tendinitis

Tendinitis of the biceps insertion is uncommon. The patient presents with anterior elbow pain which is accurately located to the insertion of the biceps tendon at the radial tuberosity. The diagnosis can be tested by asking the patient to supinate the flexed forearm against the examiner's resistance and the reproduction of pain at the site of the insertion of the biceps tendon is good confirmatory evidence.

Very occasionally the symptoms may be related to a partial rupture of the biceps insertion (Chapter 15) or may result from inflammation of the bursa that separates the tuberosity of the radius from the biceps tendon. To fully assess these patients magnetic resonance imaging scanning is recommended.

Treatment is conservative and includes rest, ice, non-steroidal anti-inflammatory drugs, and physiotherapy.

References

1. Morris H The riders sprain. *Lancet* 1882; **ii:** 557.
2. Major HP Lawn tennis elbow. *Brit Med J* 1883; **2:** 557.
3. Wadsworth TH Tennis elbow. Conservative and manipulative treatment. *Brit Med J* 1987; **294:** 631–3.
4. Runge F Zur Genese Und Behandlung Des Schreibekrampfes. *Berl Klin Wschr* 1873; **1:** 245.
5. Cyriax J The elbow. In: *Textbook of orthopaedic medicine.* London: Baillière Tindall, 1978: 268–77.
6. Renton J Observations on acupuncturation. *Edinb Med J* 1830; **34:** 100.
7. Coonrad RW, Hooper WR Tennis elbow: Its course, natural history, conservative and surgical management. *J Bone Joint Surg* 1973; **55A:** 1177–82.
8. Cyriax J The pathology and treatment of tennis elbow. *J Bone Joint Surg* 1936; **18:** 921–40.
9. Priest JD Tennis elbow – the syndrome and a study of average players. *Minn Med* 1976; **59:** 367–71.
10. Fisher AGT *Treatment by manipulation.* London: HK Lewis and Co, 1928: 171.
11. Trethowen WH Diseases and minor injuries of the elbow. *Joint Proc Roy Soc Med* 1929; **23:** 319.
12. Garden RS Tennis elbow. *J Bone Joint Surg* 1961; **43B:** 100–6.
13. Binder A, Parr G, Thomas PP, Hazleman B A Clinical and thermographic study of lateral epicondylitis. *Brit J Rheum* 1983; **22:** 77–81.
14. Maffulli N, Regine R, Carrillo F *et al.* Tennis elbow. an ultrasound study in tennis players. *Brit J Sports Med* 1990; **24:** 151–5.
15. McKee GK Tennis elbow. *Brit Med J* 1937; **2:** 434.
16. Brailsford JF *The radiology of bone and joints.* London: JA Churchill, 1935: 73.
17. Verhaar J, Walenkamp G, Kester A *et al.* Lateral extensor release for tennis elbow. *J Bone Joint Surg* 1993; **75:** 1034–43.
18. Moore M Jr Symposium on ambulant surgery: Radiohumeral synovitis, cause of persistent elbow pain.
19. Jobe FW, Ciccotti MG Lateral and medial epicondylitis of the elbow. *J Am Acad Orthop Surg* 1994; **2:** 1–8.
20. Nirschl RP, Pettrone FA Tennis elbow. The surgical treatment of lateral epicondylitis. *J Bone Joint Surg* 1979; **61A:** 832–9.
21. Boyd HB, McLeod AC Jr Tennis elbow. *J Bone Joint Surg* 1973; **55A:** 1183–7.
22. Curwin S, Standish WD *Tendinitis its etiology and treatment.* Lexington Mass: Collamore Press, 1984.
23. Bosworth DM The role of the orbicular ligament in tennis elbow. *J Bone Joint Surg* 1955; **37A:** 527–33.
24. Goodfellow JW, Bullough DG The pattern and aging of articular cartilage in the elbow. *J Bone Joint Surg* 1967; **49B:** 175–81.
25. Newman JH, Goodfellow JW Fibrillation of the head of the radius as one cause of tennis elbow. *Brit Med J* 1975; **2:** 328–30.
26. Stanley D Primary osteoarthritis of the elbow In: *Surgery of the elbow: Practical and scientific aspects.* Stanley D, Kay NRM (eds) London: Arnold, 1998: 354–64.

27. Osgood RB Radiohumeral bursitis, epicondylitis, epicondylalgia (tennis elbow). *Arch Surg* 1922; **4:** 420

28. Roles NC, Maudsley RH Radial tunnel syndrome. Resistant tennis elbow as a nerve entrapment. *J Bone Joint Surg* 1972; **54B:** 499–508.

29. Kaplan EB Treatment of tennis elbow (epicondylitis) by denervation. *J Bone Joint Surg* 1959; **41A:** 147–51.

30. Somerville EW Pain in the upper limb. *J Bone Joint Surg* 1963; **45B:** 62D–1.

31. Capner N The vulnerability of the posterior interosseous nerve of the forearm: A case report and an anatomical study. *J Bone Joint Surg* 1966; **48B:** 770–3.

32. Spinner M, Linscheid RL Nerve entrapment syndromes. In: *The elbow and its disorders.* Morrey BF (ed) Philadelphia: WB Saunders Co, 1993: 813–32.

33. Eversmann WW Entrapment and compression neuropathies. In: *Operative hand surgery* (3rd edn). Green DP (ed) New York: Churchill Livingstone, 1993: 1341–86.

34. Campion D Electrodiagnostic testing in hand surgery. *J Hand Surg* 1996; **21A:** 947–56.

35. Verhaar J Tennis elbow. Anatomical, epidemiological and therapeutic aspects. *Int Orthop* 1994; **18:** 263–7.

36. Allander E Prevalence, incidence and remission rate of some common rheumatic disorders and syndromes. *Scand J Rheum* 1974; **3:** 145–53.

37. Goldie I Epicondylitis lateralis humeri (epicondylalgia or tennis elbow). A pathogenetical study. *Acta Chir Scand Suppl* 1964; 339.

38. Buckwalter JA, Woo SL, Goldberg UM *et al.* Current concepts review – soft tissue aging and musculoskeletal function. *J Bone Joint Surg* 1993; **75A:** 1533–48.

39. Dimberg L The prevalence and causation of tennis elbow in a population of workers in an engineering industry. *Ergonomics* 1987; **30:** 573–9.

40. Greuchlow HW, Pelletier D An epidemiological study of tennis elbow – incidence recurrence and effective prevention strategies. *Am J Sports Med* 1979; **7:** 234–8.

41. Flynn GS Stenosing tenosynovitis: Trigger fingers and trigger thumb, De Quervain's disease, acute calcification in wrist and hand. In: *Hand surgery* (3rd edn). Flynn JE (ed) Baltimore: Williams and Wilkins, 1982: 489–99.

42. McGuire JL, Lambert RE Arthropathies associated with endoczine disorders In: *Textbook of rheumatology* (4th edn). Kelly WN, Harris ED, Ruddy S, Sledge CB (eds) Philadelphia: WB Saunders Co, 1993: 1527–44.

43. Gellman H Tennis elbow – epicondylitis. *Orthop Clin North Am* 1992; **23:** 75–82.

44. Luopajar VI, Kivi P, Kuorinkal I *et al.* Prevalence of tenosynovitis and other injuries of the upper extremities in repetitive work. *Scand J Work Envir Health* 1979; Supp 3: 48–55.

45 Kuppa K, Viikari-Juntura E, Kuosma E, Huuskonen M Incidence of tenosynovitis or peritendinitis and epicondylitis in a meat-processing factory. *Scand J Work Envir Health* 1991; **17:** 32–7.

46. Viikarri-Juntura E Tenosynovitis, peritendinitis, tennis elbow syndrome. *Scand J Work Envir Health* 1984; **10:** 443–9.

47. Harrington JR *Report on work related upper limb disorders.* London: HMSO, 1992.

48. Barton NJ, Hooper G, Noble J, Steel WM Report of the British Orthopaedic Association Working Party on occupational causes of upper limb disorders. London: Royal College of Surgeons, 1992.

49. Nirschl RP Muscle and tendon trauma: tennis elbow. In: *The elbow and its disorders.* Morrey BF (ed) Philadelphia: WB Saunders Co, 1993: 537–52.

50. Bernhang AM, Dehner W, Fogarty C Tennis elbow – A biomechanical approach. *J Sports Med* 1974; **2:** 235–60.

51. Mills GP Treatment of tennis elbow. *Brit Med J* 1928; **1:** 12.

52. Murray-Leslie CF, Wright V Carpal tunnel syndrome, humeral epicondylitis and the cervical spine. A study of clinical and dimensional relationships. *Brit Med J* 1976; **1:** 1439–42.

53. Vangsness CT, Jobe FW Surgical treatment of medial epicondylitis. *J Bone Joint Surg* 1991; **73B:** 409–11.

CHAPTER 21

Neurological injury and entrapment at the elbow

FRANK D BURKE, DAVID STANLEY

Introduction

The three major nerves of the forearm and hand are intimately related to the elbow joint and are frequently affected by injury or disease processes in this area. Neurological damage resulting in loss of function of the elbow affects the patient's ability not only to position the hand in space but also affects manipulative dexterity. It is essential therefore that patients presenting with injuries around the elbow are fully clinically assessed with regard to sensory and motor function distal to the site of injury.

In a similar way patients with suspected nerve entrapment syndromes also require careful clinical assessment before being considered for special investigations. In this chapter the assessment and management of nerve injuries and entrapment syndromes will be considered.

Lacerations to nerves around the elbow

Although the site of a laceration at the elbow will give some guide as to the major nerves at risk, oblique penetrating injuries can cause remote nerve damage. For this reason a comprehensive clinical examination is essential.

Testing for sensory loss is a crucial part of the initial assessment and should be undertaken by lightly touching an area of the injured limb and comparing it with the equivalent area on the uninjured limb. Care should be taken during this process to avoid joint movement since innervated capsular receptors may be stimulated giving the impression that sensation is intact even though the nerve being assessed is divided. The distal sensory supply of the three major nerves crossing the elbow is shown in Fig. 21.1, whilst Fig. 21. 2 outlines the motor supply.

Distribution of cutaneous nerves to the palm and
to the dorsum of the hand

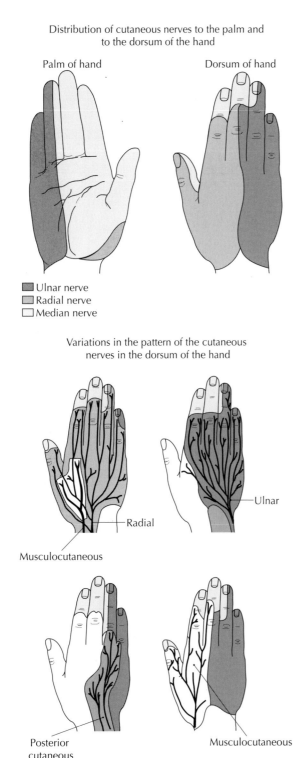

Fig. 21.1 The distal cutaneous supply of the three major
nerves which cross the elbow.

Nerve exploration

Probing oozing wounds in accident and emergency
departments with inadequate equipment, poor
lighting and no tourniquet is a recipe for disaster. If
there is concern over the integrity of the major
nerves, exploration is required in a satisfactory
operating theatre environment under tourniquet
control with appropriate delicate instruments.

The wound should be extended proximally to
enable identification of the major vessels and
nerves. The dissection should then be extended distally into the lacerated area in order to assess
whether there is neurological damage.

The ulnar nerve lies superficially on the medial
border of the upper arm and can most easily be
located by palpation behind the medial epicondyle.
It may then be followed distally between the heads
of flexor carpi ulnaris. The radial nerve should be
identified by exploration of the space between brachioradialis and brachialis on the proximal lateral
aspect of the antecubital fossa. It can be followed
distally to its division into the radial sensory branch
and the posterior interosseous nerve. The latter
then enters the supinator tunnel at the arcade of
Frohse. The median nerve is located in the lower
part of the upper arm on the medial border of
biceps and brachialis in the upper part of the antecubital fossa. It can be traced distally with the
brachial artery in the antecubital fossa where the
anterior interosseous nerve arises from the main
trunk.

Investigation of nerve injury

Smith and Mott[1] and Lynch and Quinlan[2] working
on distal nerve injuries have both observed the
short-term conductance of transected nerve if the
ends are in contact. This phenomenon is only temporary and rapidly disappears as distal Wallerian
degeneration occurs. Some appreciation of sensibility may occur for 24–36 hours in these cases. In
addition the distal segment of the transected nerve
may exhibit some ability to conduct for 2–3 weeks
after transection. For this reason, nerve conduction
studies are rarely used for the acute assessment of
nerve injuries.

If doubt exists as to whether a nerve has been
transected, the ninhydrin[3,4] or O'Riain[5] tests may
clarify the situation. Both tests assess the sympathetic function in the hand. Nerve injury gives rise
to an absence of sweating in the area denervated.
The ninhydrin test, using hydrophylic dyes

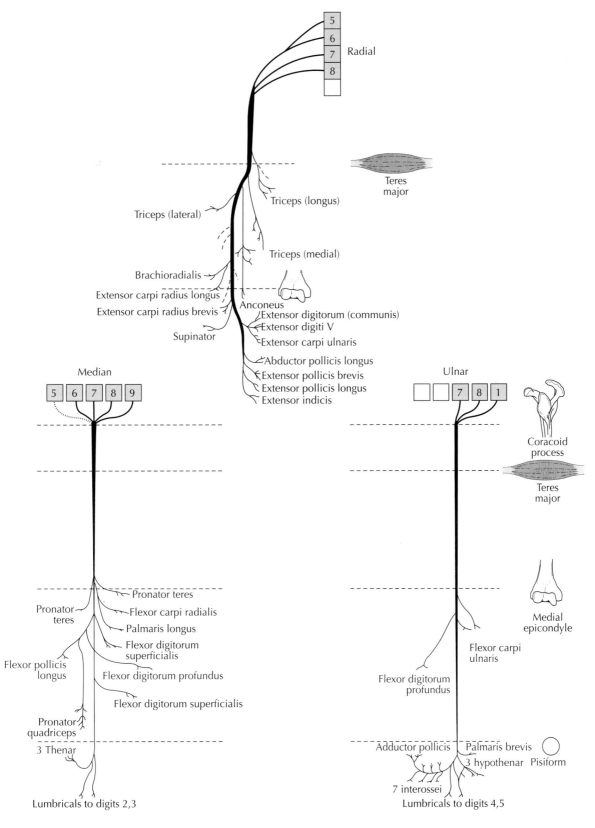

Fig. 21.2 The motor supply of the three major nerves crossing the elbow.

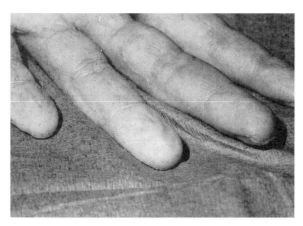

Fig. 21.3 O'Riain's test in a median nerve laceration. Wrinkling is limited to the ulnar innervated pulps.

demonstrates absent sweating by colour changes in the denervated non-sweating area.

O'Riain demonstrated that denervated skin exhibited a loss of wrinkling following immersion of the area in water for 30 minutes (Fig. 21.3).

Nerve repair

Although the specific techniques of nerve repair are beyond the remit of this chapter the following principles are important:

1. The nerve ends should be trimmed if there is a significant crush element to the transection.
2. Repair should be performed with magnification using fine interrupted monofilament nylon sutures (not thicker than 8/0).
3. The repair should be by epineural sutures.
4. The repair should not be under undue tension.

THE RESULTS OF NERVE REPAIR

Reinnervation following nerve repair is always partial and patients should be advised of the limitations of surgical intervention. Patients need to be told that from the moment of injury a subnormal outcome is inevitable. Failure to impart this information to patients leads to misplaced optimism, then disappointment and often disgruntlement. Children under the age of 12 years do best with a gradual deterioration in potential outcome, even if repair is optimal.

Over and above this general prognosis for nerve recovery lies a varying prognosis related specifically to each nerve which is dependent upon the particular functions the nerve provides.

The radial nerve

The radial nerve supplies a relatively unimportant contact area of the limb but a very large number of muscles on the extensor surface of the forearm. Despite this, repair of the nerve will often give gratifying results with functional return of wrist and finger extension. However, should nerve repair fail, tendon transfers provide a valuable and predictable secondary surgical option (Fig. 21.4).

The classical transfers are pronator teres to extensor carpi radialis brevis (Fig. 21.5), flexor carpi ulnaris or flexor carpi radialis to extensor digitorum communis (Fig. 21.6) and, if available palmaris longus to extensor pollicis longus.[6,7]

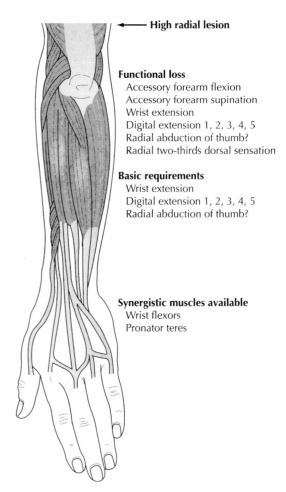

◀━━ High radial lesion

Functional loss
Accessory forearm flexion
Accessory forearm supination
Wrist extension
Digital extension 1, 2, 3, 4, 5
Radial abduction of thumb?
Radial two-thirds dorsal sensation

Basic requirements
Wrist extension
Digital extension 1, 2, 3, 4, 5
Radial abduction of thumb?

Synergistic muscles available
Wrist flexors
Pronator teres

Fig. 21.4 High radial nerve palsy. Refrawn after Ref. 65.

Some surgeons couple radial nerve repair or graft with the single transfer of pronator teres to extensor carpi radialis brevis. This gives the patient immediate control of the most disabling part of the motor loss. If subsequently reinnervation produces overly strong wrist extension forces the tendon transfer can be reversed.

The median nerve

The median nerve provides an important sensory supply for precision skills and is also primarily responsible for power grasp and power pinch. As such although reinnervation may occur following nerve repair the sophisticated requirements of the nerve undermine results in all but the young. For this reason tendon transfers are often necessary[8,9] (Fig. 21.7).

Residual weakness or paralysis of individual digital flexors may be balanced by buddying the affected tendon to a powerful neighbour in the

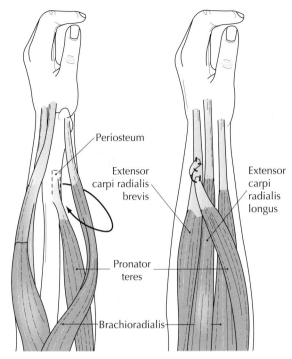

Fig. 21.5 Radial nerve palsy: Pronator teres transfer to extensor carpi radialis brevis. Redrawn after Ref. 69 with permission from Churchill Livingstone, Edinburgh.

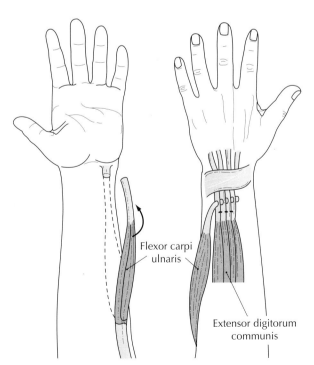

Fig. 21.6 Radial nerve palsy: Flexor carpi ulnaris transfer to extensor digitorum communis. Redrawn after Ref. 69 with permission from Churchill Livingstone, Edinburgh.

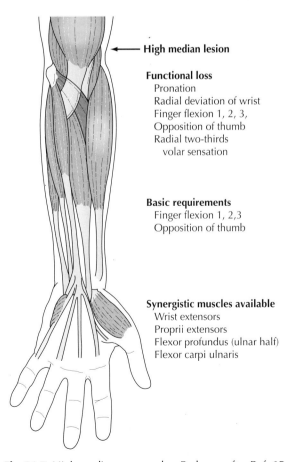

Fig. 21.7 High median nerve palsy. Redrawn after Ref. 65.

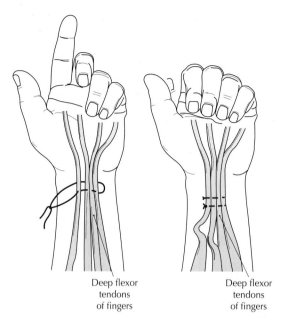

Fig. 21.8 In high median nerve palsy the profundus tendons of the index and middle fingers are tightened and sutured to the profundus tendons of the ring and little fingers. Redrawn after Ref. 10.

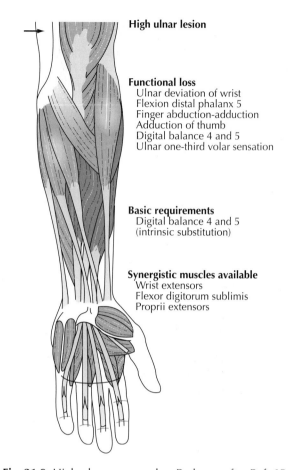

Fig. 21.9 High ulnar nerve palsy. Redrawn after Ref. 65.

forearm[10] (Fig. 21.8). Brachioradialis can be mobilised and joined end-to-side to power flexor pollicis longus.[11] Opposition can be corrected by an extensor indicis proprius transfer. The tendon is taken long at the level of the metacarpal phalangeal joint and mobilised extensively proximally. It is then re-routed around the ulnar border of the wrist and sutured to the abductor brevis insertion.[12]

The ulnar nerve

Of the three major nerves, the ulnar is the most exposed and easily transected. The characteristics of the nerve reduce the prospects of a satisfactory result from surgical repair. The sensory component is similar to the median in terms of distance the axons are required to grow to reinnervate the distal end organs. The contact area is less critical to precision skills and it is the motor component that creates the greatest difficulty. If the branches to flexor carpi ulnaris and the ulnar digital long flexors are involved in lacerations above the elbow, satisfactory reinnervation may follow accurate repair since the distance from the repair to the motor ends plates is short. However, the remaining motor fascicles are required to supply the majority of the intrinsic muscles much more distally in the hand.

Motor end plates in the intrinsic muscles deteriorate during the prolonged phase of axon regeneration in the forearm and hand. The reinnervated nerve is less well myelinated and conducts more slowly. Intrinsic function is a sophisticated activity requiring rapidly adjusting co-ordinated multiple muscle movements. Partial reinnervation with slowly conducting fibres with multiple crossovers fundamentally prejudices intrinsic recovery even if repair has been meticulous. Satisfactory intrinsic function after high ulnar nerve transection is therefore rare in adults. To improve upper limb function, tendon transfers are frequently required (Fig. 21.9).

Residual weakness or paralysis of ulnar innervated digital long flexors may be corrected by side-to-side suture to median innervated digital flexors in the forearm. Clawing can be corrected by a variety of techniques: volar plate reefing, tenodesis or tendon transfer.[13–17] Clawing limited to the ring and little fingers can be controlled by the use of the extensor indicis proprius taken long at the metacarpophalangeal joint level and realigned proximally.[14] The tendon is split distally and passed through the intrinsic muscles volar to the intermetacarpal ligament. It is then passed along the lumbrical canal and the distal slips are sutured to the ring and little finger central extensor tendons at their insertion at the base of the middle phalanges. The transfer strengthens metacarpophalangeal joint flexion and proximal interphalangeal joint extension thereby correcting the claw deformity. Extensor indicis proprius can be readily spared without loss and has the benefit of being a synchronous musculotendinous unit.

An additional transfer is available for patients with ulnar intrinsic dysfunction. A tendon transfer can be performed to recreate adductor function to the thumb. Brachioradialis[15] or extensor carpi radialis brevis[16] may be advanced with a tendon graft between the third and fourth metacarpals and across the palm to the adductor or abductor insertion on the thumb. The transfer recreates adductor power to the thumb improving stability of the thumb in power pinch.

Thumb-index pinch may occasionally be improved by using abductor pollicis longus.[17] A slip of the tendon is raised distally and swung ulnarly. It is advanced with a graft and sutured to the insertion of the first dorsal interosseous on the index finger at metacarpal–phalangeal joint level. The transfer is designed to recreate the action of the first dorsal interosseous by strengthening the index component of thumb-index pinch.

Entrapment syndromes

Nerve compression around the elbow gives rise to the various nerve entrapment syndromes. Classically these are associated with local pain and nerve discomfort together with altered sensation distal to the site of compression and in severe cases muscle wasting. The diagnosis will usually be apparent if these features are present but often the overlap in clinical features with conditions such as medial or lateral epicondylitis, early degenerative arthritis or more distal nerve compression such as carpal tunnel syndrome may make accurate appreciation of the underlying pathology difficult.

ULNAR NERVE ENTRAPMENT

Aetiology

The ulnar nerve may be compressed by a variety of fibrous bands; the arcade of Struthers proximal to the elbow,[18] the medial intermuscular septum more distally,[19] Osbourne's band at the level of the flexor carpi ulnaris aponeurosis[20,21] or, rarely, more distally within flexor carpi ulnaris muscle.[22] Compression can also be caused by rheumatoid synovium arising from within the elbow joint or bony exostoses associated with an arthritic joint.

Sleep patterns can also give rise to local compression and need to be considered in this section. The effect is partly local pressure but there is also a traction element to the problem. A minority of patients sleep prone with their hands under the pillow. This is a particularly unsuitable posture for the ulnar nerve and results in local pressure over the nerve at the elbow. The shoulder is abducted and the elbow flexed which additionally provides longitudinal traction to the nerve and may restrict the blood supply to the nerve at the elbow.

Clinical features

The initial clinical features of ulnar nerve entrapment are tingling and numbness affecting the little and ring fingers. These symptoms are often more pronounced at night particularly in prone sleepers. Motor symptoms most frequently appear later and since there is usually paralysis of flexor digitorum profundus to the little and ring fingers, clawing of the hand is not a conspicuous feature. Since, however, the ulnar nerve supplies most of the small muscles of the hand wasting of the interosseous particularly the first dorsal interosseous and of the hypothenar muscles occur in advanced entrapment.

Examination reveals diminished sensation over the little and ring fingers although often it is only the medial half of the ring finger which is affected. Sensory loss in the dorsoulnar aspect of the hand is a classic feature. Motor weakness of flexor carpi ulnaris (supplied by the ulnar nerve at the level of the elbow) can be appreciated by asking the patient to actively flex the wrist whilst the tension of the tendon at lower forearm level is assessed. Weakness of flexor digitorum profundus to the little and ring fingers can be tested by assessing the power of active flexion across the distal interphalangeal joints of the involved fingers. Active abduction of the little finger (abductor digiti minimi) or the index finger (first dorsal interosseous) will test the function of the individual ulnar innervated intrinsic muscles.

In normal use, firm pinch between the thumb and the side of the index finger is performed with the interphalangeal joint of the thumb in full extension. Loss of the ulnar innervated adductor pollicis function destabilises the thumb during firm pinch which is only controlled by an increased flexor pollicis longus action. Firm pinch in these cases can only be performed in a position of interphalangeal joint flexion (Froment's sign).

Investigations

Following clinical assessment, anteroposterior, lateral and cubital tunnel radiographs should be performed. Whilst these are often normal they may reveal osteophytic narrowing of the cubital tunnel.

Electromyographic and nerve conduction studies are helpful if positive but frequently, particularly in early entrapment, they fail to show any abnormality. Comparison of postoperative nerve conduction studies with preoperative values is, however, a reliable indicator of nerve recovery.[23]

Treatment

Conservative

Altered sensibility to ring and little fingers without subluxation of the ulnar nerve at the elbow in flexion and extension should first be treated in a night splint, holding the elbow semi-extended. This is particularly worthwhile if the history suggests that the patient is a prone sleeper. The elbow is held in a position of 40 degrees from full extension in a well moulded and cushioned splint. A trial of several weeks is required and in many early cases lasting relief of symptoms will be obtained. Failure to respond to conservative treatment necessitates consideration of surgery.

Surgical

A range of surgical procedures has been advocated for the treatment of ulnar nerve entrapment[24–33] but until recently there have been no prospective randomised clinical studies.[34]

SUPERFICIAL TRANSPOSITION OF THE ULNAR NERVE

Under tourniquet control with the arm abducted and externally rotated the skin incision begins approximately 8 cm proximal to the medial epicondyle and extends in the line of the ulnar nerve for a similar distance beyond this landmark. The anterior and posterior skin flaps are raised taking care to avoid damage to the medial antebrachial cutaneous nerve. The ulnar nerve is identified and carefully mobilised with its blood supply and with preservation of its branches to flexor carpi ulnaris and flexor digitorum profundus. To enable adequate mobilisation of the nerve the arcade of Struthers is released and the medial intermuscular septum is excised. The nerve is then transposed anterior to the medial epicondyle and allowed to rest on the fascia of the flexor–pronator group of

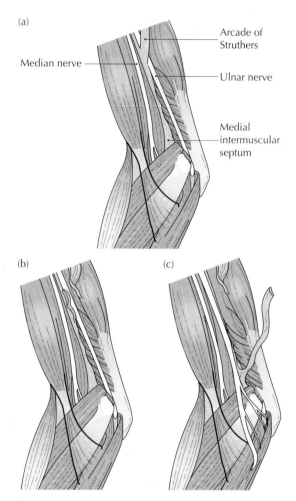

Fig. 21.10 Anterior transposition of the ulnar nerve. (a) The normal position of the ulnar nerve. (b) After division of the arcade of Struthers. (c) After excision of the medial intermuscular septum, the ulnar nerve can be transposed anteriorly. Redrawn after Ref. 66.

muscles beneath the thick fat of this region (Fig. 21.10). Passive flexion and extension of the elbow is then undertaken in order to be certain that the nerve is not compressed or kinked during elbow movement. Providing the nerve lies freely, two interrupted absorbable sutures are placed through the fascia and subcutaneous fat medial to the nerve in order to prevent the nerve returning to its anatomical position posterior to the epicondyle.

The tourniquet is deflated and haemostasis achieved. The wound is closed over a suction drain which is removed at 24 hours. It is important when undertaking any of these procedures on the ulnar nerve to prevent haematoma formation since this may result in further nerve compression postoperatively.

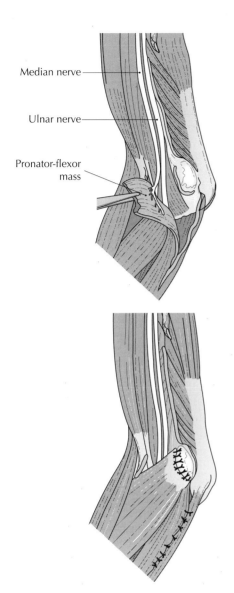

Median nerve

Ulnar nerve

Pronator-flexor mass

Fig. 21.11 Submuscular anterior transposition of the ulnar nerve. The flexor–pronator group of muscles are released in order to allow transposition of the ulnar nerve such that it can lie adjacent to the median nerve. The muscles are then reattached to the medial epicondyle. Redrawn after Ref. 66.

SUBMUSCULAR TRANSPOSITION OF THE ULNAR NERVE

If a submuscular transposition of the ulnar nerve is to be undertaken the initial stages of ulnar nerve mobilisation are as described above. The median nerve is then identified medial to the brachial artery and the lacertus fibrosus is incised longitudinally. A haemostat is placed beneath the flexor–pronator group of muscles which are then released from their attachment to the medial epicondyle and reflected distally. The ulnar nerve is transposed to lie beside the median nerve. The tourniquet is deflated and haemostasis achieved. The flexor pronator muscles are reattached to the medial epicondyle and the wound closed as for a superficial transposition of the nerve (Fig. 21.11).

MEDIAL EPICONDYLECTOMY

Under tourniquet control with the arm abducted and externally rotated, a 10-cm skin incision centred on the medial epicondyle is made in the line of the ulnar nerve. The medial brachial and antebrachial cutaneous nerves are identified and protected. The medial epicondyle is exposed and the flexor pronator origin is reflected distally from the bone by subperiosteal dissection. As this is done, care must be taken to protect the ulnar collateral ligament. The ulnar nerve is then retracted posteriorly and protected whilst the medial epicondyle is excised using an osteotome. A bone rasp and nibblers are used to remove any residual sharp edges in the region of the epicondylectomy. The medial intermuscular septum is excised and the arcade of Struthers is released. The flexor pronator origin is reattached to the humeral condyle. The ulnar nerve is allowed to seek its own position adjacent to the medial humeral condyle and the elbow is passively flexed and extended to be sure the nerve is not kinked or compressed during this movement (Fig. 21.12).

The tourniquet is deflated and the wound closed over a single suction drain which is left *in situ* for 24 hours.

Decompression of the ulnar nerve

A decompression of the ulnar nerve without anterior transposition or medial epicondylectomy requires the division of fascial or muscular bands overlying the nerve from the arcade or Struthers to where the nerve passes between the two heads of flexor carpi ulnaris. The procedure is most useful for patients with altered sensibility but without intrinsic muscle wasting.

Postoperative management

For each of the described surgical procedures a soft bulky dressing should be applied with the elbow at 90 degrees and the forearm in neutral rotation. The arm should be supported in a sling for 10 days at which stage the dressing should be reduced and sutures removed. The patient is then allowed to begin gentle active elbow mobilisation.

(a)

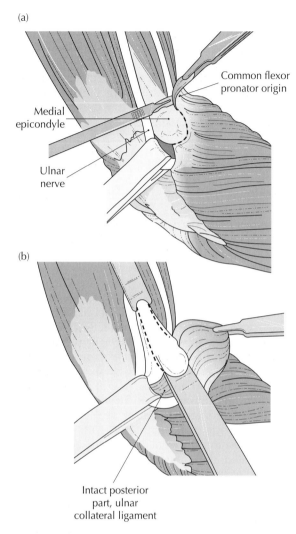

Common flexor pronator origin

Medial epicondyle

Ulnar nerve

(b)

Intact posterior part, ulnar collateral ligament

Fig. 21.12 Medial epicondylectomy. (a) The ulnar nerve is protected and the common flexor pronator origin is elevated from the medial epicondyle. (b) Technique for osteotomy. Redrawn after Ref. 67.

Surgical results for ulnar nerve entrapment

Varying results have been reported following surgery for ulnar nerve entrapment. Adelaar *et al.*[26] prospectively compared release of the cubital tunnel, subcutaneous anterior transposition and submuscular anterior transposition in 32 patients. They found no significant differences in the results of the three procedures. Craven and Green[31] investigating the outcome of medial epicondylectomy found relief of pain and improvement in

nerve conduction velocities in 93% of patients. Less satisfactory results for medial epicondylectomy were, however, noted by Jones and Gauntt.[35] They reported only 48% good with 17% fair and 35% poor.

In 1989 Dellon[36] reviewed the world literature on ulnar nerve compression and found that excellent results could be achieved in half of the patients treated conservatively and in almost all those undergoing any of the surgical procedures. He found that for moderate compression the largest number of excellent results with fewest recurrences were obtained by anterior submuscular transposition of the nerve. He noted that an essential part of the surgical procedure was excision of the medial intermuscular septum.

Most recently, Geutjens *et al.*[34] have undertaken a randomised prospective study comparing medial epicondylectomy with anterior transposition of the ulnar nerve. They found that neither procedure had a significant effect on elbow function. They noted, however, that after anterior transposition of the nerve significantly more patients complained of mild pain in the hand whilst after epicondylectomy significantly more patients were satisfied and would have the operation again. It was suggested that the symptoms in those undergoing anterior transposition of the nerve might relate to damage to the vascular supply during nerve mobilisation.

Authors' preferred management

For patients with sensory symptoms which have failed or only partially responded to conservative treatment we perform electromyographic and nerve conduction studies. If these are negative but the patient has persisting symptoms the ulnar nerve is explored and a decompression without anterior transposition is undertaken.

For patients with both sensory and motor signs and slowed nerve conductance we prefer at present a superficial transposition of the ulnar nerve. We accept that some studies have shown good results with medial epicondylectomy and in particular note the prospective randomised study by Geutjens *et al.*[34] which showed somewhat better results for this technique than anterior transposition of the ulnar nerve.

RADIAL NERVE ENTRAPMENT

Aetiology

Entrapment syndromes of the radial nerve occur when the nerve is compressed at any point along its course. Proximal to the elbow this may be caused by the fibrous arch of the long head of the triceps[37] or the lateral head of the triceps.[38]

More commonly, however, it is the posterior interosseous nerve which is most at risk of compression, and this may be caused by the fibrous arcade of Frohse,[39] the exit from supinator[40] fracture dislocations around the elbow,[41,42] tumours[43] ganglia,[44] and rheumatoid synovitis of the elbow.[45–47]

Occasionally an isolated superficial radial nerve entrapment may occur.

Clinical features

Patients who present with sensory disturbance of the dorsal and radial aspects of the wrist will have involvement of the superficial branch of the radial nerve. Since this nerve always passes superficial to the arcade of Frohse the level of compression must be proximal to the arcade.

Motor weakness can be of two types with some patients presenting with paralysis of all the muscles supplied by the nerve (extensor digitorum communis, extensor indicis proprius, extensor digiti quinti, extensor carpi ulnaris, abductor pollicis longus and extensor pollicis brevis). In others only one or two muscles may be paralysed. Compression of the entire nerve results in an inability to extend the metacarpophalangeal joints of the thumb and fingers together with radial deviation of the wrist on wrist extension. With partial compression the patient retains the ability to extend some of the fingers at the metacarpophalangeal joints.

Roles and Maudsley[48] and more recently Lawrence et al.[49] have emphasised that entrapment of the posterior interosseous nerve may resemble resistant tennis elbow. With posterior interosseous nerve entrapment, however, tenderness is localised over the radial nerve as distinct from the lateral epicondyle. In addition a constant aching pain is most commonly localised to the region of the arcade of Frohse and patients often complain of discomfort when writing.

The differentation between entrapment neuropathy and neuralgic amyotrophy can also be difficult. Hashizume et al.[50] from their own studies and the studies of others[51–56] identified a number of distinguishing features:

1. Severe pain usually precedes paralysis in neuralgic amyotrophy but is usually absent or slight in entrapment neuropathy.
2. Neuralgic amyotrophy is often preceded by other features including a common cold, influenza, minor trauma, vaccination, the recovery period from major surgery, acute hepatism or toxic exposure.
3. The degree of paralysis in neuralgic amyotrophy varies from mild to severe. It is changeable and sometimes reversible. Paralysis due to entrapment is progressive and becomes complete.
4. Full examination sometimes reveals additional paralysis and possible sensory disturbance around the shoulder girdle and upper arm in neuralgic amyotrophy. The sensory distribution of the radial nerve is often involved but sensory change is not seen in nerve entrapment unless it is proximal to the arcade of Frohse.
5. Evidence of denervation of the brachioradialis or more proximal muscles may be seen in neuralgic amyotrphy but never in entrapment neuropathy.

Investigations

Nerve conduction studies may offer evidence of a local conduction delay but the reliability of investigations discriminating accurately between nerve and tendon pathology in lateral elbow pain is limited. Ultasonography and magnetic resonance imaging are useful for identifying space-occupying lesions.

Treatment

Surgical

In order to release entrapment of the radial nerve surgical decompression is required. The skin incision is shown in Fig 21.13. Dissection begins proximally allowing identification of the radial nerve in the interval between brachioradialis and brachialis. The nerve is then traced distally to where it passes below the arcade of Frohse between the two heads of supinator. As this is performed vessels or fibrous bands crossing the nerve are released, and the arcade of Frohse if tight is divided.

In order to free the nerve within the supinator tunnel it is then necessary to develop the plane between extensor digitorum communis and extensor carpi radialis longus and brevis. This provides an excellent view of supinator which can then be carefully incised from proximal to distal. Particular care must be taken distally where the posterior interosseous nerve gives off several small branches innervating the adjacent muscles. Meticulous haemostasis reduces the risk of subsequent haematoma and adhesions. Early active mobilisation of the elbow postoperatively is advised and may be important in reducing the risk of nerve adhesions with a consequent traction neuritis.

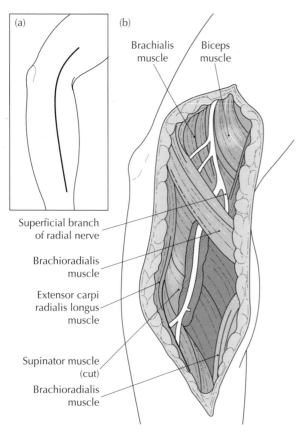

Fig. 21.13 Exposure of the posterior interosseous branch of the radial nerve. (a) Incision. (b) Surgical anatomy Redrawn after Ref. 68.

MEDIAN NERVE ENTRAPMENT

Aetiology

The median nerve may be compressed at several sites around the elbow. These include the supracondylar process and its extension to the medial epicondyle the ligament of Struthers,[18,57,58] muscular anomalies (Gantzer muscle), and fractures or fracture dislocations.[59]

Important types of compression that are recognised are the pronator syndrome[60,61] and the anterior interosseous syndrome.[62,63]

With pronator syndrome compression may occur at the lacertus fibrosus, between the superficial and deep heads of pronator teres, or occasionally more distally within the flexor digitorum superficialis arch. Although the clinical features for the anterior interosseous syndrome differ from those of the pronator syndrome the aetiological factors are similar.

Clinical features

The pronator syndrome

The clinical features of pronator syndrome are often rather vague. They consist primarily of diffuse proximal forearm discomfort and weakness. In addition there may be associated distal sensory changes in the distribution of the median nerve. This can give rise to an erroneous diagnosis of carpal tunnel syndrome. However, Phalen's test and Tinel's sign are negative at the wrist whilst percussion over the median nerve at the elbow results in tingling distally. Provocation tests when positive are helpful to confirm the diagnosis (Fig. 21.14). These tests consist of 1) resisted pronation for 60 seconds; 2) resisted elbow flexion and forearm supination; and 3) resisted middle finger flexion at the proximal interphalengeal joint.

The anterior interosseous syndrome

Patients with this syndrome usually present with an abrupt weakness or total paralysis of flexor pollicis longus and usually the profundus flexor tendon of the index finger (Fig. 21.15). Occasionally, the flexor digitorum profundus tendon to the middle finger is also affected.

The superficial flexors to the index and middle fingers are not involved. There is often diffuse forearm discomfort in the flexor compartment around the time of onset of the nerve palsy. The anterior interosseous nerve does not contain sensory fibres from the skin but does contain many proprioceptive fibres from the flexor muscles and it is these fibres which are responsible for the appreciation of forearm discomfort.

Abrupt loss of function of flexor pollicis longus in association with flexor forearm pain readily suggests a diagnosis of tendon rupture to the unwary clinician. There are, however, several clinical checks which can be applied to avoid the not uncommon error of misplaced surgery to a tendon when nerve decompression is indicated more proximally. An apparent rupture of the flexor pollicis longus tendon should immediately provoke close assessment of the index profundus tendon function. Any weakness suggests that it is likely there is anterior interosseous nerve dysfunction. Weakness of pronator quadratus (the only other muscle supplied by the nerve) may be checked by assessing power of pronation with the elbow in maximal flexion to diminish the effect of pronator teres. On occasions quite a marked disparity in power between the limbs is apparent although the value of this test is variable. It is usually possible to make an assessment of flexor pollicis longus

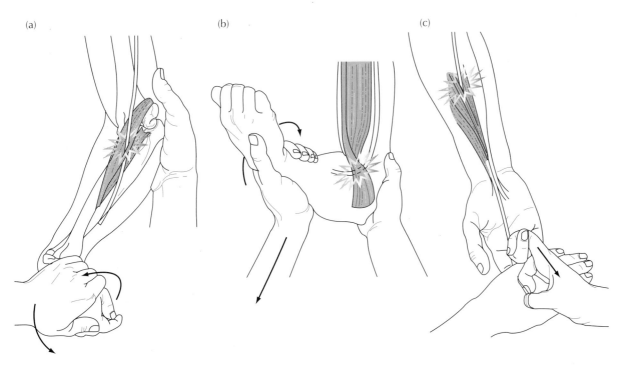

(a)   (b)   (c)

Fig. 21.14 Provocation tests for the assessment of pronator syndrome. (a) Resisted pronation. (b) Resisted elbow flexion and forearm supination. (c) Resisted middle finger flexion at the proximal interphalangeal joint. Redrawn after Ref. 66.

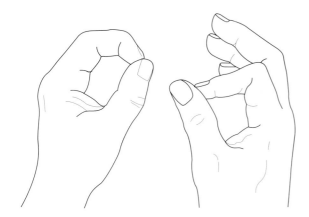

Fig. 21.15 Clinical appearance of anterior interosseous nerve palsy.

integrity by clinical examination. With the patient's wrist and thumb relaxed in full extension, press deeply to the extreme radial border of the flexor compartment while observing the interphalangeal joint of the thumb. Firm pressure to the flexor pollicis longus muscle or tendon will usually produce some active flexion of the interphalangeal joint of the thumb, indicating integrity of the musculotendinous unit.

Investigations

Plain radiographs of the elbow may show a supracondylar process as the cause of median nerve compression.

Pronator syndrome

Electromyography is not usually sufficiently sensitive to detect the pronator syndrome. The diagnosis is dependant on clinical awareness and the findings on clinical examination.

Anterior interosseous syndrome

Electromyographic studies of flexor pollicis longus or pronator quadratus should be undertaken in order to confirm the diagnosis of anterior interosseous syndrome.

Treatment

Conservative

Anterior interosseous nerve palsy has been treated by two contrasting methods in the last few years. Surgeons have considered release of nerve compression to be required. Physicians have considered many such cases to be an amyotrophy without a requirement for decompression. Review of a 16-case series by Sood and Burke[64] justifies the physicians view that many patients do not require decompression and will do as well treated conservatively. Surgery is indicated in complete lesions with no evidence of recovery at 6 months. Incomplete lesions or those with additional loss outwith the territory of the nerve merit conservative management in the first instance.

Surgical

If surgery is indicated an approach to the anterior aspect of the elbow is required. This involves a longitudinal incision curved at the antecubital skin crease. The medial antebrachial cutaneous nerve is identified and protected. The medial and lateral skin flaps are raised. The lower humerus is then palpated in order to exclude a supracondylar process and examination made for a ligament of Struthers.

In the arm the brachial artery and vein are retracted to expose the median nerve (Fig. 21.16). The nerve enters the forearm beneath the lacertus fibrosus and then passes between the two heads of pronator teres. It continues distally beneath flexor digitorum superficialis lying on flexor digitorum profundus.

At the elbow the nerve is exposed by reflection of the brachial fascia and release of the lacertus fibrosus. The forearm is then pronated and the humeral head of pronator teres retracted. The ulnar head of pronator teres is released and if the flexor digitorum superficialis arch is tight this is divided.

Careful haemostasis is required at all stages in the decompression in order to avoid the risk of haematoma formation and subsequent further nerve compression.

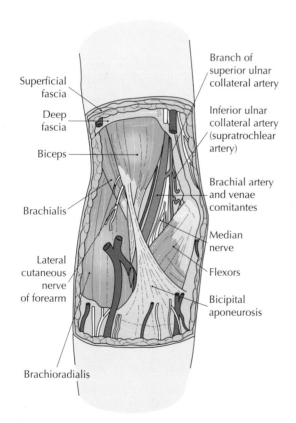

Fig. 21.16 Surgical anatomy for exposure of the median nerve.

Superficial fascia

Deep fascia

Biceps

Brachialis

Lateral cutaneous nerve of forearm

Brachioradialis

Branch of superior ulnar collateral artery

Inferior ulnar collateral artery (supratrochlear artery)

Brachial artery and venae comitantes

Median nerve

Flexors

Bicipital aponeurosis

References

1. Smith PJ, Mott G Sensory threshold and conductance testing in nerve injuries. *J Hand Surg* 1986; **11B:** 157–61.
2. Lynch G, Quinlan D Jump function following nerve division. *Brit J Plast Surg* 1986; **39:** 364–6.
3. Aschan W, Moberg E The ninhydrin finger printing test used to map out partial lesions to hand nerves. *Acta Chir Scand* 1962; **123:** 365–40.
4. Stromberg WB, McFarlane RM, Bell JL *et al.* Injury to the median and ulnar nerves: One hundred and fifty cases with an evaluation of Moberg's ninhydrin test. *J Bone Joint Surg* 1961; **43A:** 717–30.
5. O'Riain S New and simple test of nerve function in the hand. *Brit Med J* 1973; **3:** 615–6.
6. Riordan DC Radial nerve paralysis. *Orthop Clin North Am* 1974; **2:** 283–7.
7. Boyes JH Tendon transfers for radial palsy. *Bull Hosp Joint Dis* 1960; **21:** 97–105.
8. Spinner M Reconstruction of the hand in high median nerve injuries. *Bull Hosp Joint Dis* 1965; **26:** 191–7.
9. Burkhalter WE Tendon transfers in median nerve palsy. *Orthop Clin North Am* 1974; **2:** 271–81.
10. Omer GE Jr Evaluation and reconstruction of the forearm and hand after acute traumatic peripheral nerve injuries. *J Bone Joint Surg* 1968; **50A:** 1454–78.
11. Waters R, Moore KR, Graboff SR, Paris K Brachioradialis to flexor pollicis longus tendon transfer for active lateral pinch in the tetraplegic. *J Hand Surg* 1985; **10A:** 385–91.
12. Burkhalter W, Christensen RC, Brown P Extensor indicis proprius opponensplasty. *J Bone Joint Surg* 1973; **55A:** 725–32.
13. Zancolli EA Claw-hand caused by paralysis of the intrinsic muscles: A simple surgical procedure for its correction. *J Bone Joint Surg* 1957; **39A:** 1076–80.
14. Riordan DC Tendon transplantations in median-nerve and ulnar-nerve paralysis. *J Bone Joint Surg* 1953; **35A:** 312–20.
15. Boyes JH Selection of a donar muscle for tendon transfer. *J Hosp Joint Dis* 1962; **23:** 1–4.
16. Smith RJ Extensor carpi radialis brevis tendon transfer for thumb abduction: A study of power pinch. *J Hand Surg* 1983; **8:** 4–15.

17. Neviaser RJ, Wilson JN, Gardner MM Abductor pollicis longus transfer for replacement of first dorsal interosseus. *J Hand Surg* 1980; **5A:** 53–7.
18. Fragiadakis EG, Lamb DW An unusual cause of ulnar nerve compression. *Hand* 1970; **2:** 14–6.
19. Spinner M, Kaplan EP The relationship of the ulnar nerve to the medial intermuscular septum in the arm and its clinical significance. *Hand* 1976; **8:** 239–242.
20. Osborne G The surgical treatment of tardy ulnar neuritis. *J Bone Joint Surg* 1957; **39B:** 782.
21. Osborne G Compression neuritis of the ulnar nerve at the elbow. *Hand* 1970; **2:** 10–13.
22. Harrelson JM, Newman M Hypertrophy of the flexor carpi ulnaris as a cause of ulnar-nerve compression in the distal part of the forearm. Case report. *J Bone Joint Surg* 1975; **57A:** 554–5.
23. Friedman RJ, Cochran TP A clinical and electro physiological investigation of anterior transposition for ulnar neuropathy at the elbow. *Arch Orthop Trauma Surg* 1987; **106:** 375–80.
24. Clark CB Cubital tunnel syndrome *J Am Med Assoc* 1979; **241:** 801–2.
25. MacNicol MF The results of operation for ulnar neuritis. *J Bone Joint Surg* 1979; **61B:** 159–64.
26. Adelaar RS, Foster WC, McDowell C The treatment of the cubital tunnel syndrome. *J Hand Surg* 1984; **9A:** 90–5.
27. Lundborg G, Surgical treatment for ulnar nerve entrapment at the elbow (Editorial). *J Hand Surg* 1992; **17B:** 251–4.
28. Learmonth JR Technique for transplanting the ulnar nerve. *Surg Gynecol Obstet* 1942; **75:** 792–3.
29. Leffert RD Anterior submuscular transposition of the ulnar nerve by the Learmonth technique. *J Hand Surg* 1982; **7:** 147–55.
30. King T, Morgan FP Late results of removing the medial humeral epicondyle for traumatic ulnar neuritis. *J Bone Joint Surg* 1959; **41B:** 51–5.
31. Craven PR, Green DP Cubital tunnel syndrome: Treatment by medial epicondylectomy. *J Bone Joint Surg* 1980; **62A:** 986–9.
32. Froimson AI, Zahrawi F Treatment of compression neuropathy of the ulnar nerve at the elbow by epicondylectomy and neurolysis. *J Hand Surg* 1980; **5A:** 391–5.
33. Robinson D, Aghasi MK, Halperin N Medial epicondylectomy in cubital tunnel syndrome: An electrodiagnostic study. *J Hand Surg* 1992; **17B:** 255–6.
34. Geutjens GG, Langstaff RJ, Smith NJ *et al.* Medial epicondylectomy or ulnar-nerve transposition for ulnar neuropathy at the elbow? *J Bone Joint Surg* 1996; **78B:** 777–9.
35. Jones RE, Gauntt C Medial epicondylectomy for ulnar nerve compression syndrome at the elbow. *Clin Orthop* 1979; **139:** 174–8.
36. Dellon AL Review of treatment results for ulnar nerve entrapment at the elbow. *J Hand Surg* 1989; **14A:** 688–700.
37. Lotem M, Fried A, Levy M *et al.* Radial palsy following muscular effort. A nerve compression syndrome possibly related to a fibrous arch of the lateral head of the triceps. *J Bone Joint Surg* 1971; **53B:** 500–6.

38. Nakamichi K, Tachibana S Radial nerve entrapment by the lateral head of the triceps. *J Hand Surg* 1991; **16A:** 748–50.
39. Spinner M The arcade of Frohse and its relationship to posterior interosseous nerve paralysis. *J Bone Joint Surg* 1968; **50B:** 809–12.
40. Derkash RS, Niebauer JJ Entrapment of the posterior interosseous nerve by a fibrous band in the dorsal edge of the supinator muscle and erosion of a groove in the proximal radius. *J Hand Surg* 1981; **6A:** 524–6.
41. Spinner M, Freundlich BD, Teicher J Posterior interosseous nerve palsy as a complication of Monteggia fracture in children. *Clin Orthop* 1968; **58:** 141–5.
42. Lichter RL, Jacobsen T Tardy Palsy of the posterior interosseous nerve with a Monteggia fracture. *J Bone Joint Surg* 1975; **57A:** 124–5.
43. Richmond DA Lipoma causing posterior interosseous nerve lesion. *J Bone Joint Surg* 1953; **35B:** 83.
44. Bowen T.L, Stone K.H Posterior interosseous nerve paralysis caused by a ganglion at the elbow. *J Bone Joint Surg* 1966; **48B:** 774–6.
45. Millender LH, Nalebuff EA, Holdsworth DE Posterior interosseous nerve syndrome secondary to rheumatoid synovitis. *J Bone Joint Surg* 1973; **55A:** 375–7.
46. Marshall SC, Murray WR Deep radial nerve palsy associated with rheumatoid arthritis. *Clin Orthop* 1974; **103:** 157–62.
47. Popelka S, Vainio K Entrapment of the posterior interosseous branch of the radial nerve in rheumatoid arthritis. *Acta Orthop Scand* 1974; **45:** 370–2.
48. Roles NC, Maudsley RH Radial tunnel syndrome: Resistant tennis elbow as a nerve entrapment *J Bone Joint Surg* 1972; **54B:** 499–508.
49. Lawrence T, Mobbs P, Fortems Y, Stanley JK Radial tunnel syndrome: A retrospective review of 30 decompressions of the radial nerve. *J Hand Surg* 1995; **20B:** 454–9
50. Hashizume H, Nishida K, Nanba Y *et al.* Non-traumatic paralysis of the posterior interosseous nerve. *J Bone Joint Surg* 1996; **78B:** 771–6.
51. Turner JWA, Parsonage MJ Neuralgic amyotrophy (paralytic brachial neuritis) with special reference to prognosis. *Lancet* 1957; **ii:** 209–12.
52. Magee KR, Dejong RN Paralytic brachial neuritis. discussions of clinical features with review of 23 cases. *J Am Med Assoc* 1960; **174:** 1258–62.
53. Furusawa S, Hara T, Maehiro S *et al.* Neuralogic amyotrophy. *Seikeigeka* 1969; **20:** 1286–90.
54. Tsairis P, Dyck PJ, Mulder DW Natural history of brachial plexus neuropathy – report on 99 patients. *Arch Neurol* 1972; **27:** 109–17.
55. Torikata Y, Hozumi Y, Hiyama T *et al.* On the neuralgic amyotrophy with chief symptom of anterior and/or posterior interosseous nerve paralysis. *Saigaiigaku* 1976; **14:** 885–91.
56. Futami T Clinical investigations on anterior or posterior interosseous nerve palsy: From the etiological view point. *J Jpn Sol Surg Hand* 1987; **4:** 86–90.

57. Gessini L, Jandolo B, Pietrangeli A Entrapment neuropathies of the median nerve at and above the elbow. *Surg Neurol* 1983; **19:** 112–6.

58. Braun RM, Spinner RJ Spontaneous bilateral median nerve compressions in the distal arm. *J Hand Surg* 1991; **16A:** 244–7.

59. Pritchard JD, Linscheid RL, Svien HJ Intra articular median nerve entrapment with dislocation of the elbow. *Clin Orthop* 1973; **90:** 100–3.

60. Johnson RK, Spinner M, Shrewsbury MM Median nerve entrapment syndrome in the proximal forearm. *J Hand Surg* 1979; **4:** 48–51.

61. Hartz CR, Linscheid RL, Gramse RR., Daube JR The pronator teres syndrome: Compressive neuropathy of the median nerve. *J Bone Joint Surg* 1981; **63A:** 885–90.

62. Farber JS, Bryan RS The anterior interosseous nerve syndrome. *J Bone Joint Surg* 1968; **50A:** 521–3.

63. Spinner M The anterior interosseous nerve syndrome with special attention to its variations. *J Bone Joint Surg* 1970; **52A:** 84–94.

64. Sood MK, Burke FD Anterior interosseous nerve palsy. *J Hand Surg* 1997; **22B:** 64–8.

65. White WL Restoration of function and balance of the wrist and hand by tendon transfers. *Surg Clin North Am* 1960; **40:** 427.

66. Spinner M *Injuries to the major branches of peripheral nerves of the forearm* (2nd edn). Philadelphia: WB Saunders Co, 1978.

67. Eversmann WW Entrapment and compression neuropathies. In: *Operative hand surgery* (2nd edn). Green DR (ed) New York: Churchill Livingstone, 1968.

68. Mayor JH Jr, Mayfield FH Surgery of the posterior interosseous branch of the radial nerve – Analysis of 58 cases. *Surg Gynecol Obstet* 1947; **84:** 979.

69. Burke FD, McGrouther DA, Smith PJ *Principles of hand surgery*. Edinburgh: Churchill Livingstone, 1990.

CHAPTER 22

The neurological elbow

WJW SHARRARD

Introduction

Neurological lesions may affect elbow function in a number of ways. They may cause:

1. paralysis of paresis of elbow flexion, with or without concomitant extension contracture;
2. paralysis or paresis of elbow extension, with or without concomitant flexion contracture;
3. complete paralysis of the elbow – a flail elbow;
4. spasticity in the elbow flexor muscles, possibly in association with contracture.

The first three conditions arise as a result of a lower motor neuron lesion which, in children, may be due to poliomyelitis, obstetrical palsy or neurological arthrogryposis and, in adults, to poliomyelitis, a lesion of the brachial plexus or post-traumatic quadriplegia. The fourth condition arises as the results of an upper motor neuron lesion due, in children, to palsy or in adults to a cerebral vascular accident.

Paralysis of elbow flexion

Complete paralysis of elbow flexion is disabling. The arms hangs down by the side and the hand cannot be lifted up to place it on a surface nor can objects be lifted up. Bilateral complete paralysis is severely disabling. Paresis such that the elbow cannot be flexed against gravity is also disabling and many need to be strengthened by a tendon transfer.

CAUSATION

Poliomyelitis

In the first half of the twentieth century, the most common cause of elbow flexor paralysis in children or adults was poliomyelitis. Caused by one of three varieties of poliovirus, poliomyelitis develops as an acute infection of the spinal cord and brain. It results in meningitic symptoms followed by the sudden development of paralysis due to destruction of anterior horn motor cells. With the development of vaccination against the poliovirus, poliomyelitis has disappeared in Europe and North America but it is still prevalent in India, the Middle East and South America.

The extent of the paralysis is extremely variable. It may affect one or both lower limbs and one or both upper limbs. A variable number of muscles may be affected any of which may be completely paralysed or paretic. The elbow flexors are more often paretic than paralysed. During the acute stage, which usually lasts for 1–2 weeks, the affected muscles must be rested and the joints positioned to avoid contracture. The elbow needs to be splinted during the first 3 weeks in semiflexion because of the liability for it to develop an extension deformity. Daily passive elbow movements are given to maintain elbow mobility. After this, active exercises are given to strengthen any remaining active motor fibres. The aim of this treatment is to make each affected muscle act against the force of gravity but not beyond the maximum power of the muscle. At the end of a year following the onset of paralysis, the muscles will have reached their maximum recovery. If the power of elbow flexion is of grade 2, such that the elbow can be flexed only if gravity is eliminated, or there is total loss of elbow flexor power, tendon transfer to enhance or restore flexion should be considered. However, surgical restoration of elbow flexion is only indicated if there is sufficient power in the finger flexors to provide a reasonable grip. An important feature of paralysis in poliomyelitis is that there is no sensory deficit.

Neurogenic arthrogryposis

This rare paralysis develops *in utero* and is due to congenital absence of anterior horn motor cells. In the upper limb, a frequent pattern of involvement affects the 5th and 6th cervical spine cord segments, which results in paralysis of all the flexors of the elbow and of the deltoid, supraspinatus, infraspinatus and teres muscles. Activity in the triceps muscles is preserved and, as a result of active elbow extension *in utero* and complete loss of flexion, the elbow joint becomes fixed in extension, which is present at birth. Since the condition is usually bilateral, function is greatly disturbed and the infant, who cannot reach his or her mouth to feed, is very frustrated. As in poliomyelitis, sensory function is preserved. Before undertaking tendon transfer to restore elbow flexion, the triceps usually needs to be lengthened.

Obstetrical paralysis

Paralysis due to injury to the 5th and 6th cervical nerve roots during childbirth is known as Erb's palsy. There is usually a history of a difficult delivery. The newborn infant does not abduct his shoulder or flex his elbow but does show activity in the triceps and in the wrist and hand muscles. The condition differs from neurogenic arthrogryposis in that there is no fixed extension deformity of the elbow provided that early passive elbow movements are maintained. In addition the condition is almost always unilateral. Spontaneous recovery occurs in 75% of cases. In more than one-third, the lesion is a neurapraxia and recovery starts within 6 weeks. If no recovery is seen after 3 months, surgical exploration of the brachial plexus and possibly nerve suture may be possible. It is therefore appropriate to wait for at least 6 months before considering tendon transfer. In the meantime, daily passive movements are needed to prevent shoulder adduction and medial rotation contracture or extension contracture of the elbow.

Brachial plexus injury

In adults, injury to the brachial plexus with a traction lesion of the 5th and 6th cervical nerve roots results in the same distribution of paralysis as in Erb's obstetrical paralysis. Some partial spontaneous recovery or recovery following operative repair of the plexus may take place during the first 6 months following injury but if the elbow flexors have not shown any recovery at all, or elbow flexion power does not recover to grade 3 (elbow flexion against gravity) or better, tendon transfers may be required.

The management of paralytic lesions of the elbow

The first, and most important step in the management of any paralysis is the assessment by muscle testing of the extent of the paralysis both in the affected limb and in the other limbs. At the same time, the presence of any limitation of elbow flexion or extension due to muscle and tendon contracture should be recorded.

In the acute stage of a paralysis, treatment should consist of exercises to encourage activity in the weaker muscles together with daily passive movements to stretch any contracted muscles and tendons. In paralysis due to poliomyelitis, some recovery may take place for up to a year after the acute stage. For this reason no final decisions as to the need for reconstructive procedures should be made until the end of this period when the final distribution and extent of the paralysis can be determined. Similarly, in acute lesions of the brachial plexus, recovery can occur, either spontaneously or following operative repair of the plexus lesion for as long as 2 years. By contrast in cases of neurological arthrogryposis, the paralysis commences when the child is *in utero* and the paralysis that is present at birth is unlikely to change. The contracture, however, may respond to passive movements.

When the state of the paralysis and contracture has become static, the possibility of reconstructive surgery can be considered. The main function of elbow movements is to allow the hand to be placed in a position to perform manipulative activities and to provide power for lifting, pushing or carrying. It is seldom appropriate to perform operations to regain elbow function unless the hand has sufficient power to grip. In cases of poliomyelitis, the state of paralysis in the remainder of the limb and in the lower limbs may be taken into consideration. In this situation if walking requires the use of elbow crutches, the power of elbow extension is important. In traumatic quadriplegia, elbow extension may be needed bilaterally to propel a wheelchair.

Before any tendon transfer is made to regain or improve the power of elbow flexion or extension, any significant residual contracture due to tight and short muscles and tendons must be corrected by tendon lengthening and release of the joint capsule. This is particularly required in neurogenic arthrogryposis in which paralysis of elbow flexion is associated with an extension contracture which is present at birth and is due to a short triceps.

The choice of muscles for transfer depends on the availability of a strong active muscle which can be spared from its normal function without unduly disturbing function in the limb as a whole.

Surgical restoration of elbow flexion

There are several methods of restoring or improving active elbow flexion. The three best methods available are as follows: 1) proximal transfer of the common flexor and extensor origins; 2) transfer of the pectoralis major muscle; 3) anterior transfer of the triceps brachii tendon. The choice of transfer depends on whether the flexor paralysis is complete or partial; whether there is adequate power and range of action in the muscle chosen for transfer and whether the transferred tendon or muscle can be spared from its previous function.

As mentioned earlier the patient must have satisfactory hand function prior to undergoing elbow surgery. Appropriate reconstructive hand surgery may be necessary before performing a transfer to restore elbow flexion. It may also be necessary to undertake a triceps lengthening before attempting to restore elbow flexion if the patient has any fixed extension (a loss of more than 30 degrees range of flexion). This particularly applies in cases of neurogenic arthrogryposis in which fixed extension of the elbow with a short triceps is almost always present at birth.

TRICEPS LENGTHENING

The operation is performed under general anaesthetic with the patient prone. In a child aged 3–4 years a pneumatic tourniquet is not easy to apply without limiting the exposure. It must be applied as high as possible just below the axilla. A long skin incision is made posteromedially from the middle of the upper arm passing distally to the medial side of the olecranon and then curving laterally across the olecranon (Fig. 22.1). The triceps brachii tendon is exposed and cleared on its medial, lateral and anterior aspects. The ulnar nerve is identified medially and the radial nerve laterally. Both are retracted and protected from injury. The medial head of the triceps is mobilised with a rugine from the posterior aspect of the lower third of the humerus.

The triangular tendon of the triceps is elongated using a reversed V–Y plasty (Fig. 22.2). It is important to make as long an incision as possible because the tendon may need to double its length. The elbow is flexed, keeping the ulnar nerve under view to ensure that it is not stretched. If necessary, the posterior capsule of the elbow joint is divided by a

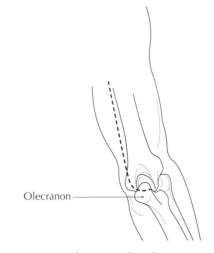

Olecranon

Fig. 22.1 Incision for triceps lengthening.

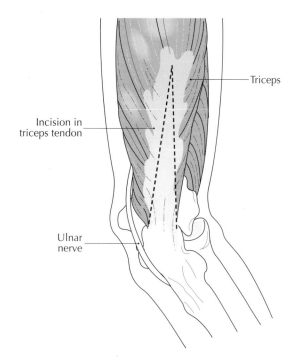

Fig. 22.2 Inverted V-incision in the triceps tendon.

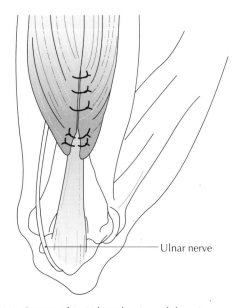

Fig. 22.3 Suture of V–Y lengthening of the triceps.

transverse incision. The elbow can usually be flexed fully and the triceps tendon reconstituted by suturing the tip of the distal portion of the tendon to the proximal portions of the muscle (Fig. 22.3). Closure is performed in two layers with suction drainage. The elbow is kept in as much flexion as possible. A collar-and-cuff sling and posterior plaster back slab are applied for 3 weeks.

PROXIMAL TRANSFER OF THE COMMON FLEXOR AND EXTENSOR ORIGINS (STEINDLER FLEXORPLASTY)

In this operation, the common flexor origin of the pronator teres, the flexor carpi radialis and ulnaris, the palmaris longus and the flexor digitorum superficialis are detached from the medial epicondyle and transferred proximally by about 5 cm so that these muscles 'bowstring' across the anterior aspect of the medial side of the elbow.[1-4] The operation is only appropriate if the muscles are strong (grade 4) or normal in power. Mayer and Green[3] described a preoperative test which they used to assess the common flexor origin muscles in order to decide whether it was appropriate to undertake the transfer. Gravity was eliminated by abducting the arm to 90 degrees. If in this position elbow flexion was possible using the common flexor origin muscles then surgery was indicated. In a similar way, the extensor carpi radialis brevis, the extensor digitorum communis, the extensor pollicis longus and the extensor indices arising from the common extensor origin attached to the lateral epicondyle and the extensor carpi radialis longus and the brachioradialis muscles attached to the lateral intermuscular septum above the lateral epicondyle can be transferred proximally by about 5 cm.[1] Although Steindler initially reported this extensor origin transfer[1] in later publications it was the flexor transfer that was stressed.

The major advantage of this transfer is that it does not prevent any of the transferred muscles from performing their normal function and its does not involve any alteration in the direction of action of the muscles. Its only disadvantage is that it produces limitation of extension by 30 or 40 degrees. Its ideal indication is when the elbow flexors are not completely paralysed in poliomyelitis or there has been some partial recovery in cases of brachial plexus injury.

The operation is performed under general anaesthesia with a pneumatic tourniquet applied to the upper arm. The patient lies supine with the arm on a hand table. Through a 16 cm L-shaped incision on the medial side of the elbow (Fig. 22.4), the common flexor origin and the muscles attached to it are exposed. Care is taken to identify and protect the ulnar nerve. The median nerve and brachial vessels which pass beneath the pronator teres muscle on the anteromedial surface of the elbow, are identified and retracted. The muscles attached to the medial epicondyle are mobilised from the brachialis and the common flexor origin is detached from the medial epicondyle with a small flake of bone. The muscles are mobilised distally for 4 or

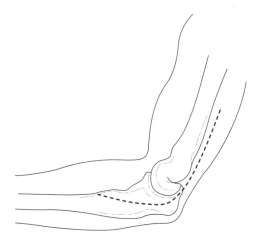

Fig. 22.4 Medial incision for proximal transfer of the common flexor origin.

5 cm and then with the elbow flexed to a right angle the block of muscle is moved proximally for 5 cm. It is attached under tension to the intermuscular septum between the triceps and brachialis by strong non-absorbable sutures (Fig. 22.5). Although less frequently undertaken a similar operation may be performed on the lateral side of the elbow with transfer of the common extensor origin and origins of the extensor carpi radialis longus brachioradialis. The muscles are attached 5 cm proximally to the lateral intermuscular septum. On the lateral side the radial nerve should be identified and retracted, making sure that the nerve branches supplying the extensor carpi radialis longus and the muscles arising from the common extensor origin are preserved. After closure of the incisons, the elbow is

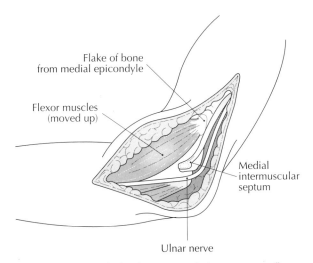

Flake of bone
from medial epicondyle

Flexor muscles
(moved up)

Medial
intermuscular
septum

Ulnar nerve

Fig. 22.5 Proximal displacement of the common flexor origin.

immobilised in 110 degrees of flexion for 3 weeks using a collar-and-cuff sling and a plaster back slab. This is followed by the application of a removable splint to allow active flexion mobilisation during the next 6 weeks. A fixed flexion of 30–40 degrees can be expected and is desirable for the best result.

If the residual elbow flexion following the paralysis is of grade 2 or 3 and the forearm muscles are acting to power grade 4 or more, elbow flexion can be expected to be improved to grade 3 or 4+. This will enable the patient to lift light objects with their hand.

TRANSFER OF THE PECTORALIS MAJOR MUSCLE

Clark in 1946[5] was the first to report the successful transfer of the pectoralis major muscle for paralysis of the elbow flexors in brachial plexus injury. The muscle of the distal part of the pectoralis major was detached from the ribs and mobilised into the upper arm. It was attached to the tendon of the biceps in the distal third of the upper arm. The technique left intact the insertion of the pectoralis major to form the origin of the reconstituted elbow flexor. Although the procedure works well, it is a major procedure requiring an extensive exposure of the thorax. In addition the preoperative power of the transferred pectoralis major muscle must be normal since only the distal part of the muscle is transferred. After this transfer there is a tendency for elbow flexion to be accompanied by medial rotation of the shoulder due to activity in the remaining clavicular portion of the pectoralis major muscle. This may require tendon transfers to enhance lateral rotation of the shoulder or arthrodesis of the shoulder joint to prevent medial rotation. In poliomyelitis or brachial plexus injury, the pectoralis major may remain partially paralysed and a transfer of the whole muscle is needed. Atkins and co-workers[6] have shown that, by detaching the clavicular origin of the muscle it is possible to mobilise the muscle and its tendon of insertion downwards to reach the biceps tendon close to the elbow. The operation is indicated whenever the pectoralis major muscle is strong (grade 4) or normal in power and the elbow flexors are completely paralysed or very weak. Such a situation may exist in poliomyelitis, neurogenic arthrogryposis or brachial plexus injury.

The operation is performed under general anaesthesia with the patient supine. The upper limb is draped to allow free movement of the joints of the upper limb. A curved incision (Fig. 22.6) is made from 4 cm below the middle third of the clavicle, along the deltopectoral groove and the lateral side

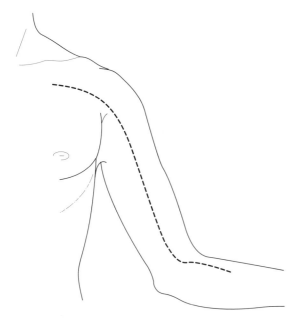

Fig. 22.6 Incision for transfer of pectoralis major to biceps.

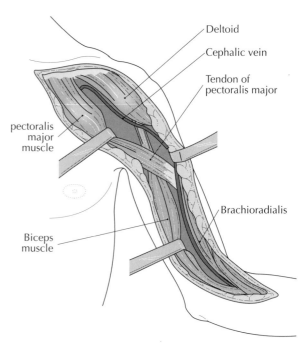

Fig. 22.7 Exposure and definition of the pectoralis major.

of the biceps tendon into the upper forearm. The upper part of the pectoralis major is exposed along its outer side down to its tendon of insertion and the shaft of the humerus is exposed for 2 cm below the tendon (Fig. 22.7). The clavicular head is detached from the clavicle and the upper part of the sternum and mobilised downwards. As this is undertaken care is necessary to protect its neurovascular supply which passes to the deep surface of the muscle. The tendon of insertion of the muscle is detached from the humerus as far distally as possible together with a strip of fascia and periosteum (Fig. 22.8). This enables the muscle and its tendon of insertion to be mobilised distally to reach the lower third of the upper arm.

The tendon of the biceps is exposed on the anterior aspect of the lower third of the upper arm. The median nerve and brachial vessels are retracted and the biceps tendon is traced distally. The lacertus fibrosus is divided at the elbow and the pronator teres is retracted medially and the brachioradialis laterally. This allows the biceps tendon to be followed to the bicipital tubercle.

The biceps tendon is mobilised from the anterior aspect of the capsule of the elbow joint allowing it to bowstring forwards so that tension on it causes the elbow to flex. The tendon of insertion of pectoralis major is then passed subcutaneously to be attached to the biceps tendon by weaving it through the biceps tendon and suturing it with nonabsorbable sutures with the elbow flexed as fully as

possible (Fig. 22.9). The incisions are closed over suction drains and the limb is immobilised with the elbow flexed fully and held by elastic strapping to the chest for 3 weeks. The elbow is then allowed to gradually extend over the course of the next 6 weeks. The technique enables good power of elbow flexion to be restored up to power grade 3 or 4.

If the pectoralis major transfer proves to give insufficient elbow flexor power, it may be strengthened further by transfer of the pectoralis minor.

TRANSFER OF THE BICEPS BRACHII

Transfer of the triceps brachii to the biceps[7–9] has limited indications in paralysis of elbow flexion. Although extension of the elbow results from the simple action of gravity, the total loss of active extension which the transfer causes has important consequences. Crutches or sticks cannot be used when there is concomitant paralysis in the lower limbs and in addition triceps action is essential when transferring from a bed to a wheelchair. In poliomyelitis, and neurogenic arthrogryposis in the upper limbs there is frequently paralysis in the lower limbs. If there is significant weakness in one or both lower limbs, triceps transfer is contraindicated. Triceps transfer is acceptable in Erb's palsy or in adult lesions of the 5th and 6th cervical nerve roots. To be effective, the triceps must be strong or normal in power. The triceps tendon will not reach

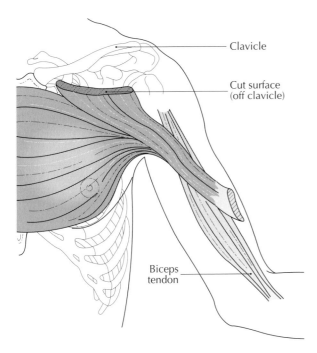

Fig. 22.8 Detachment of pectoralis major from the clavicle and downward mobilization.

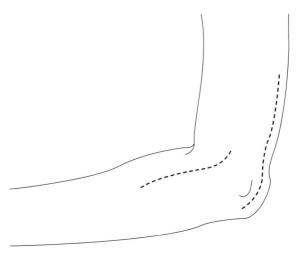

Fig. 22.10 Incisions for transfer of the triceps tendon to the biceps tendon.

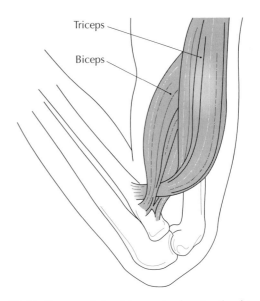

Fig. 22.11 Suture of the triceps tendon to the biceps tendon with the elbow fully flexed.

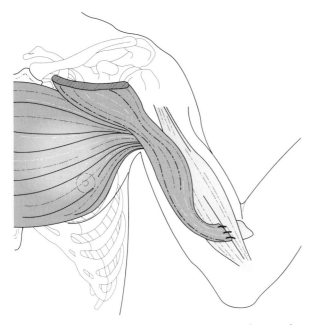

Fig. 22.9 Suture of the pectoralis major tendon to the biceps tendon.

the tuberosity of the radius but it can be attached to the distal tendon of the biceps provided that the biceps is mobilised from the anterior capsule of the elbow joint.

The triceps tendon is exposed through a posterolateral incision (Fig. 22.10) and the tendon is divided as far distally as possible from the olecranon and mobilised proximally for 5–6 cm so that it can be rerouted round the lateral aspect of the lower end of the humerus. Through an anterior incision over the elbow, the brachioradialis and pronator teres muscles are retracted to expose the biceps tendon which is mobilised from the capsule of the elbow as described above. The triceps tendon is interwoven into the biceps tendon with the elbow in over 90 degrees of flexion (Fig. 22.11). An alternative method is to prolong the triceps tendon by means of a tube of fascia lata so that the tendon can be attached to the bicipital tuberosity. The incisions are closed and the elbow is immobilised in flexion by a collar-and-cuff sling and a plaster back slab for 3 weeks.

It is important to transfer the whole of the triceps tendon and not part of it because the triceps cannot act as both an extensor and a flexor of the elbow at the same time.

Whatever transfer technique is used to restore elbow flexion, the postoperative management must include a period of 2–3 months of re-education of the transferred tendon. In small children play activities are usually sufficient but in older children and adults, formal training using springs and slings is usually necessary. The results of all types of tendon transfer, if performed for appropriate indications, are good. Segal *et al.*[10] in a comparative review of Steindler flexorplasty, pectoralis major transfer and triceps transfer in poliomyelitis found the best results with Steindler flexorplasty, followed by pectoralis major transfer.

The management of paralysis of elbow extension

Weakness or paralysis of elbow extension is sometimes thought to be of little importance since gravity can extend the elbow passively. However, in addition to the problems described above with the use of crutches and transfer activities in patients with lower limb paralysis, triceps paralysis also affects activities such as cutting bread or meat. It is particularly disabling if the paralysis is bilateral. In poliomyelitis, the triceps (sometimes bilaterally) is one of the more frequently paralysed muscles, and in cervical quadriplegia at C6/7 level, bilateral triceps paralysis is a serious disability.

Surgical restoration of elbow extension

Several methods of tendon transfer have been described using the brachioradialis,[11] the latissimus dorsi,[12–14] and the posterior part of the deltoid muscle or biceps.[15–19] The author only has experience of the use of the posterior part of the deltoid muscle, as described by Moberg.[15] In traumatic quadriplegia the transfer must be combined with tendon transfers to restore pinch grip in the hand. Before performing a transfer, any flexion deformity

needs to be corrected. This can often be achieved by a course of passive movements but if this is not successful surgery with lengthening of the biceps tendon and fractional lengthening of the brachialis is required.

TRANSFER OF THE POSTERIOR DELTOID MUSCLE TO THE TRICEPS

The posterior part of the deltoid muscle, is separately innervated from the remainder of the muscle. It is sufficiently powerful if its innervation is normal and has a suitable range for transfer to the triceps aponeurosis in order to restore elbow extension. The transfer does, however, also require the use of free tendon grafts taken from the toe extensors.

The operation is performed with the patient prone through two incisions (Fig. 22.12). Proximally, an incision is made along the posterior border of the deltiod muscle. Distally, an incision 7.5 cm long is made over the triceps tendon above the olecranon. The deltoid is exposed in the proximal incision and the posterior third of the muscle is defined and detached from its insertion. The aponeurosis of the

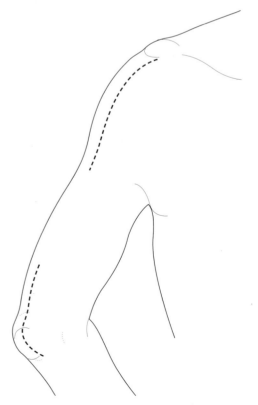

Fig. 22.12 Incisions for transfer of the posterior deltoid to the triceps.

triceps is exposed through the lower incision. The distance between the deltoid and the triceps is estimated to indicate the length of tendon grafts needed to span the gap by two strands of tendon. The knee on the same side is flexed to allow the dorsum of the foot to be approached. The extensor tendons to the third and fourth toes are removed through four short transverse incisions on the dorsum of the foot taking the tendons from the base of the toes to just above the extensor retinaculum. The triceps is then pulled proximally and the deltoid distally with Kocher forceps putting both under tension. One end of each tendon graft is sutured to the triceps aponeurosis distally. Each graft is passed subcutaneously to the distal end of the deltoid interlacing it through four small incisions (Fig. 22.13). If possible the graft is then returned back to the triceps. The elbow, which is in full extension, is flexed slightly to confirm the adequacy of the sutures and grafts. The skin and subcutaneous tissues are closed with suction drains and a plaster cast applied from the axilla to the wrist with the elbow in 10 degrees of flexion. Moberg[15] advises infiltration of local anaesthetic into the deltiod before closure to avoid detachment of the transfer whilst the patient is recovering from anaesthesia.

The plaster cast is retained for 6 weeks and then replaced by serial plaster back slabs flexing the elbow by 10 degree increments weekly until elbow flexion to a right angle has been obtained. At that stage exercises are recommended.

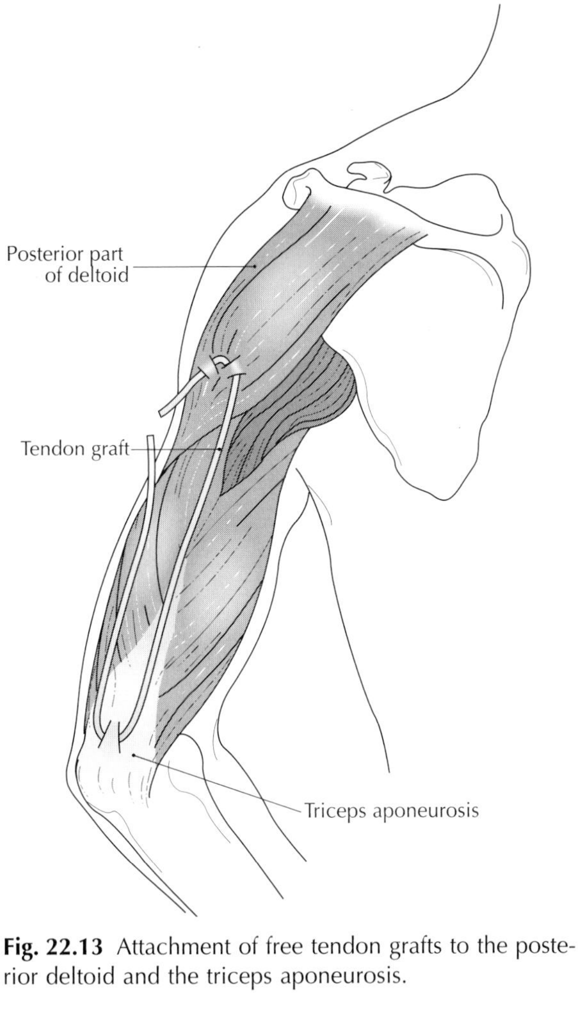

The management of the flail elbow

Complete paralysis of all muscles acting on the elbow can occur in poliomyelitis. This is most likely in children, in whom inoculations or injections were made into the limb during the initial stages of the acute poliomyelitic illness. The limb is effectively useless and the arm hangs down by the side of the trunk. Rarely, severe paralysis may occur bilaterally and very rarely bilateral upper limb paralysis may be present at birth as the result of neurogenic arthrogryposis.

There is limited scope for surgical treatment. If the sternomastoid muscle is active and strong, its sternoclavicular attachment can be mobilised and prolonged by a long fascial graft to reach the bicipital tubercle[7,20] (Fig. 22.14). The operation is an

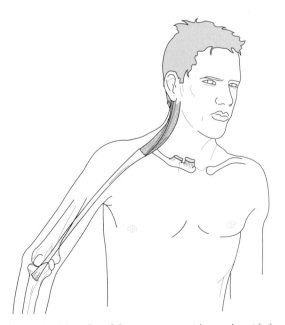

Fig. 22.13 Attachment of free tendon grafts to the posterior deltoid and the triceps aponeurosis.

Fig. 22.14 Transfer of the sternomastoid muscle with free fascial graft for flail elbow.

extensive one and gives only a limited degree of flexion. A posterior bone block at the elbow formed by elevating the posterior cortex of the humerus just above the olecranon and packing bone chips beneath it to abut against the olecranon and thus limit extension to a right angle can be tried. With time, however, this is likely to fail because of stretching of the anterior joint capsule.

Flexion has been successfully provided in some patients by using free muscle transplants.[21-23] This technique involves nerve grafting which at times may be unsuccessful.[24]

Whichever method is used, it is only appropriate if there is some function in the hand. In cases with total paralysis of the wrist and hand, limited function can be achieved by arthrodesis of the wrist and tenodesis of the finger flexors to provide a passive grip.

Spastic flexion deformity of the elbow

Spastic hemiplegia and quadriplegia in children and spastic hemiplegia following a cerebral vascular accident in adults is associated with spasticity in the flexors of the elbow. In most cases, passive extension of the elbow can be maintained by regular passive movements.

In adolescence, flexion deformity of the wrist and fingers may be associated with some flexion deformity of the elbow. If the deformity becomes sufficiently severe as to warrant surgical release, partial correction of the elbow flexion deformity may be achieved in the course of correction of the wrist and hand deformities by release of the muscles from the common flexor origin, lengthening of the biceps tendon and fractional lengthening of the brachialis muscle.

References

1. Steindler A Operative treatment of paralytic conditions of the upper extremity. *J Orthop Surg* 1919; **1:** 608.
2. Steindler A Tendon transplantation in the upper extremity. *Am J Surg* 1939; **44:** 260–71.
3. Mayer L, Green W Experiences with Steindler flexorplasty of the elbow. *J Bone Joint Surg* 1954; **36A:** 775–89.
4. Lindholm TS, Einola S Flexorplasty of paralytic elbow: Analysis of late functional results. *Acta Orthop Scand* 1973; **44:** 1–11.
5. Clark JMP Reconstruction of the biceps brachis by pectoral muscle transplantation. *Brit J Surg* 1946; **34:** 180–1.
6. Atkins RM, Bell MJ, Sharrard WJW Pectoralis major transfer for paralysis of elbow flexion in children. *J Bone Joint Surg* 1985; **67B:** 640–4.
7. Bunnell S Restoring flexion to the paralytic elbow. *J Bone Joint Surg* 1951; **33A:** 566–71.
8. Carroll RE Restoration of flexor power to the flail elbow by transplantation of the triceps tendon. *Surg Gynecol Obstet* 1952; **95:** 685–8.
9. Carroll RE, Hill NA Triceps transfer to restore elbow flexion. A study of fifteen patients with paralytic lesions and arthrogryposis. *J Bone Joint Surg* 1970; **52A:** 239–44.
10. Segal A, Seddon HJ, Brooks DM Treatment of paralysis of the flexors of the elbow. *J Bone Joint Surg* 1959; **41B:** 44–50.
11. Ober FR, Barr JS Brachioradialis muscle transposition for triceps weakness. *Surg Gynecol Obstet* 1938; **67:** 105–7.
12. Harmon PH Muscle transplantation for triceps palsy: The technique of utilising the latissimus dorsi. *J Bone Joint Surg* 1949; **31A:** 409–12.
13. Hovnanian AP Latissimus dorsi transplantation for loss of flexion or extension at the elbow. *Ann Surg* 1956; **143:** 493–9.
14. Landra AP The latissimus dorsi musculo cutaneous flap used to resurface defects on the upper arm and restore extension to the elbow. *Brit J Plast Surg* 1979; **32:** 275–7.
15. Moberg E Surgical treatment for absent single-hand grip and elbow extension in quadriplegia. *J Bone Joint Surg* 1975; **57A:** 196–206.
16. Bryan RS The Moberg deltoid-triceps replacement and key pinch operations in quadriplegia: Preliminary experiences. *Hand* 1977; **9:** 207–14.
17. Hentz VR, Brown M, Keoshain LA Upper limb reconstruction in quadriplegia: Functional assessment and proposed treatment modifications. *J Hand Surg* 1983; **8:** 119–31.
18. Freehafer AA, Kelly CM, Peckham PH Tendon transfer for the restoration of upper limb function after a cervical spinal cord injury. *J Hand Surg* 1984; **9A:** 887–93.
19. Friedenberg ZB Transposition of the biceps brachii for triceps weakness. *J Bone Joint Surg* 1954; **36A:** 656–61.
20. Carroll RE Restoration of elbow flexion by transplantation of sternocleidomastoid muscle. *J Bone Joint Surg* 1962; **44A:** 1039.
21. Hirayama T, Takemitsu Y, Atsuta Y, Ozawa K Restoration of elbow flexion by complete latissimus dorsi muscle transposition. *J Hand Surg* 1987; **12B:** 194–8.
22. Dumontier C, Gilbert A Traumatic brachial plexus palsy in children. *Ann Hand Surg* 1990; **9:** 351–7.
23. Akasaka Y, Hara T, Takahashi M Restoration of elbow flexion and wrist extension in brachial plexus paralyses by means of free muscle transplantation innervated by intercostal nerve. *Ann Hand Surg* 1990; **9:** 341–50.
24. Botte MJ, Wood MB Flexor plasty of the elbow. *Clin Orthop* 1989; **245:** 110–6.

CHAPTER 23

The medical management of rheumatoid arthritis

DAVID PROPPER, VERNA WRIGHT

Introduction

In order to adopt a rational approach to the treatment of rheumatoid arthritis, it is necessary to know the natural history of the disease. In the past, rheumatoid arthritis was viewed as a relatively benign disorder. This view arose because of data derived from population based studies. These showed that a high proportion of patients fulfilling American Rheumatism Association (ARA) criteria for probable or possible rheumatoid arthritis had no evidence of the disorder 3–5 years later.[1] In distinct contrast, clinic based studies now show that in the majority of patients, rheumatoid arthritis is a progressive, lifelong disorder associated, in time, with radiographic damage, significant disability, loss of earnings and increased mortality. For instance, 50% of patients with rheumatoid arthritis

are work disabled by 10 years.[2] After 20 years, 50% are disabled or dead,[3] by then most will have some degree of functional impairment, and only 20% will be in remission.

Rheumatoid arthritis, however, is a heterogeneous disease. Identifying, at the onset, those patients who will progress rapidly, those who will progress slowly and those who will remit is difficult, but important. This is because the aggressiveness and speed of inception of potentially toxic treatments will depend on the perceived eventual outcome. Speed of onset, high titre rheumatoid factor, extra-articular features, female gender, early onset of disease, persistently raised acute phase reactants, polyarticular disease and early disability have some correlation with eventual poor outcomes. In the future, genetic markers may allow disease severity to be predicted more accurately.

Management of rheumatoid arthritis

The principle aims of treatment in rheumatoid arthritis are to prevent disability, to relieve pain and, where disability has occurred, to maximise function. The non-surgical treatment of rheumatoid arthritis is therefore complex. The various modalities available include drugs, physical therapies, orthotics, appliances (such as those to ease activities of daily living), patient education, and psychological therapies (Table 23.1). Due to the complexity of therapy, and the heterogeneity of the disorder, attempting to show whether these modalities alter the long-term impact of rheumatoid arthritis has been difficult.

Management also depends on the stage of the disease. Arbitrarily, rheumatoid arthritis can be divided into early, established, or end-stage disease. In early disease, the focus is primarily on suppressing inflammation and preventing disability, predominantly by drugs. In late disease, the focus is on reducing pain and disability. However, different joints in an individual may be at different stages of the disease.

Drug management, in particular, depends on the clinical and laboratory assessment of whether the disease is active and progressing or, in contrast, whether the disease is inactive. It is important to realise that pain may be due to ongoing immune attack, existing damage, psychological factors, or a combination of these.

Table 23.1 Non-surgical modalities involved in the management of rheumatoid arthritis

Drugs
    analgesics
    non-steroidal anti-inflammatory agents (NSAIDs)
    disease modifying anti-rheumatic drugs (DMARDs)
Physiotherapy
    active/passive
Education
    on rest and joint protection
    about the disease
    about drugs
    on pain and stress management
Vocational assessment and training
Orthoses
Appliances and aids to daily living
Psychotherapy and counselling
Footwear
Chiropody
Social service support

Assessment of disease activity is often difficult. If joint damage occurs and is due to immune attack, then patients need to have their disease modifying therapy changed. Ongoing joint damage and pain may, however, simply reflect a cycle initiated by synovitis, but then perpetuated, in the absence of immune mediated synovitis, by mechanical forces subsequent on this damage. Changing or instituting second-line agents in such instances will be ineffective, and exposes patients to the potential toxicity of alternative drugs which may be less effective than existing therapy.

Assessment of disease activity is often done intuitively by the treating physician. Factors that should be included in assessing disease activity are pain level, stiffness and its duration, the number of affected joints, systemic symptoms, disability and laboratory parameters of inflammation. These last include erythrocyte sedimentation rate, plasma viscosity and C-reactive protein (CRP). Radiological investigations may help in that they provide an indication of disease progression. Changes in these factors over time are of more importance than single-time point assessments. Clearly the benefits of long-term follow-up by a single physician help in the detection of such changes.

Clinical parameters of disease can be formally quantified, for instance by health assessment questionnaires, by measurements of an articular index, (such as the Ritchie articular index), and the measurement of grip strength. Nevertheless, all assessments of disease activity in rheumatoid arthritis are imperfect. Not least because psychological factors contribute considerably to pain perception and levels of disability. The ability to detect ongoing immune mediated joint damage in the midst of these factors is often difficult and is dependent on the cognitive skills of therapists and their relationship with patients. In this review, we first concentrate on drug treatment and then on non-pharmacological treatments.

PHARMACOLOGICAL MANAGEMENT OF RHEUMATOID ARTHRITIS

The principle drugs used in rheumatoid arthritis are analgesics, non-steroidal anti-inflammatory drugs (NSAIDs), corticosteroids and the so-called disease modifying anti-rheumatic drugs (DMARDs; Table 23.2). The last comprise the traditional second-line agents, established immunosuppressive drugs, and recently introduced but still experimental therapies, which target more specific points of immune function. Disease modifying anti-rheumatic drugs differ from NSAIDs in that they alter disease progression, at least in the short term. Unlike NSAIDs,

Table 23.2 Disease modifying drugs used in rheumatoid arthritis

Gold (oral or intramuscular)	
Hydroxychloroquine	
(Chloroquine)	
Sulphasalazine	Traditional second line agents. No
Penicillamine	immunosuppressive properties, with
Methotrexate	the possible exception of methotrexate
Corticosteroids	
Azathioprine	
Cyclosporin A	Established immunosuppressive agents
Chlorambucil	
Cyclophosphamide	
Monoclonal antibodies	Experimental therapies
to T cell determinants	
Specific cytokine inhibitors	

DMARDs suppress laboratory markers of inflammation, such as ESR and CRP. Unlike NSAIDs, most DMARDs take some weeks to months to show an effect.

THE PROBLEM WITH THE CONCEPT OF DISEASE MODIFYING ANTI-RHEUMATIC TREATMENT

Although it is clear that DMARDs are effective in the short term there are two important points. First, traditional second-line agents usually do not fully control rheumatoid arthritis. In fact, it is not known how effective second-line drugs are in the long-term. Most published clinical trials have been conducted over 2–12 months. There are few published trials of treatment longer than 3 years.

Second, favourable short-term responses on second-line agents are not strongly associated with favourable long-term responses.[4] For instance, fewer than 10% of patients maintained on an individual second-line agent will be taking that drug 3 years later, because of withdrawal for inefficacy or toxicity. Methotrexate and prednisolone are, however, exceptions to this.[5]

Last, obtaining clear cut answers about the efficacy of DMARDs is complex and difficult. It is complex for several reasons, either to do with the methodology of the trials or because of the nature of the disease. Maintaining patients in trials on a single second-line agent for several years is difficult because these agents do not fully control the disease, and as discussed, the efficacy of a second-line agent appears to decrease with time.

Rheumatoid arthritis is also a hetergenous disorder, and has both intra- and inter-patient intrinsic variability. Individual trials, however, have often included patients at different stages of the disease. Many trials include patients with treatment-resistant late-stage disease. The effects of a second-line agent given to patients with early rheumatoid arthritis may differ from those in patients with established disease.

Comparing the results of various trials is difficult because of considerable variation in the outcomes measured. Trials need to include measurements of articular activity, health status and clinical, laboratory and radiological measurements. Consensus on what measurements to include had not, until recently, been reached. Moreover, the outcomes assessed are, to some extent, arbitrary, and there is a need to decide what emphasis should be placed on parameters such as symptoms, signs, disability, joint destruction, employability and survival when assessing the effects of a drug. In addition, trials which compare one second-line agent with another may not use 'equivalent' suppressive doses of the drugs. Furthermore, to discern significant differences between the effects of specific second-line agents requires a much larger trial population than where comparisons are made with placebo. Thus trials showing that one drug is as effective as another are open to type II statistical errors.

It is difficult, and probably unethical, to recruit patients with early rheumatoid arthritis into trials comparing drug treatment with placebo treatment. Hence trials have often compared effects of a test drug with an established second-line agent, such as gold. Although this overstates the case, much of the evidence that such established second-line drugs are effective comes from studies which could be construed as having methodological problems. Nevertheless, empirically, it seems likely that suppression of clinical and laboratory parameters of disease activity by DMARDs correlates to some extent with a retardation of joint damage in the long term.

Despite the above, it is justified to say that second-line drugs slow the progression of rheumatoid arthritis in the short term, and this is important. Any slowing of the disease reduces the amount of time that a patient is disabled. It is important that both therapist and patient are aware of the fact that the disease is only likely to be partially controlled, rather than cured, by DMARDs.

INCEPTION OF TREATMENT

Until recently, rheumatoid arthritis was treated by a step-up approach. Initial treatment was rest, patient education, physical therapy and NSAIDs. If, after 6–12 weeks, the response was inadequate, or if erosions developed, then second-line agents were started. There are, problems with waiting several months, and then starting a single second-line agent. First, many patients do not respond to an individual second-line drug. Second, most second-line agents take at least 2–3 months for the full efficacy to develop, and it may take up to 6 months to decide that a drug is ineffective.

Hence, in a significant proportion of patients, many months elapse during which the disease is not controlled. It is now known that most patients develop erosions within 2 years of onset.[6] If a patient is refractory to most drugs, this is the period required to have tried the range of standard second-line agents. Hence a policy based on the expectation that a second-line agent will suppress disease is clearly not an effective approach in a significant proportion of patients.

In addition, in the past there was considerable bias against corticosteroid therapy. Many only used corticosteroids once the range of second-line agents had been exhausted. This attitude to corticosteroid treatment stemmed from experience of the side-effects when corticosteroids were first introduced and used at considerably higher doses than is the norm today. The benefit of corticosteroids is that they suppress disease activity within days.

As it is now known that joint damage occurs early in rheumatoid arthritis, the trend in recent years has been to start second-line agents earlier than used to be the practice, before any irreversible damage has occurred. This approach has to be balanced with the fact that, in some patients, polyarthritis is self-limiting and may not justify the use of potentially toxic treatments. However, modern approaches to drug dosage and monitoring probably minimise this problem.

The effects of early and aggressive use of disease modifying agents, at least in the short term, appear favourable. Nevertheless, any long-term effects on disease outcome are unknown.[7,8] We favour the use of corticosteroids at diagnosis to bring the disease under control and if, after withdrawal, the disease becomes active, to institute a second-line agent. The early use of steroids provides time for any instituted second-line agent to become effective. We use intramuscular long-acting corticosteroids, such as triamcinolone or Depo-Medrone, rather than oral corticosteroids. This reduces the possibility of patients becoming accustomed to taking oral corticosteroids and consequent abuse. An alternative approach, advocated by others, is to use methotrexate early, rather than corticosteroids, in conjunction with a more traditional second-line agent. This is because the suppressive effects of methotrexate develop within a few weeks, unlike other traditional second-line agents. Once the second-line agent has brought the disease under control, then methotrexate is withdrawn. Despite the above it is important to realise that rheumatoid arthritis is a heterogenous disorder. Management will vary considerably from patient to patient.

Analgesia

Patients often require analgesics in addition to NSAIDs, or are unable to take NSAIDs because of side-effects. Simple analgesics such as paracetamol may be as effective as NSAIDs in a significant proportion of patients.[9] Paracetamol is much safer than NSAIDs. Preparations of paracetamol combined with codeine or other analgesics, such as dextropropoxyphene, have a large place in the treatment of rheumatoid arthritis. Other drugs such as nefopam and buprenorphine are also sometimes useful, although many patients cannot take these drugs because of side-effects. Low-dose tricyclic antidepressants are useful pain modifying drugs. It is important that patients are aware that such drugs can be taken in combination with NSAIDs.

Non-steroidal anti-inflammatory drugs

The inflammatory process in rheumatoid arthritis is complex. Although NSAIDs inhibit prostaglandin

Table 23.3 Principle classes of non-steroidal anti-inflammatory drugs

Salicylic acids and esters	Phenylacetic acids	Carbo- and heterocyclic acids	Propionic acids	Fenamic acids	Pyrazolones	Oxicams	Non-acidic drugs
Aspirin Benorylate Diflunisal	Diclofenac	Etodolac Indomethacin Sulindac Tolmetin	Fenbufen Fenoprofen Fluiprofen Ibuprofen Ketoprofen Naproxen Tiaprofenic acid	Mefanamic acid	Phenylbutazone	Piroxicam Tenoxicam	Nabumetone

synthesis, it is now thought that this property does not entirely account for their therapeutic effects in rheumatoid arthritis.

It is known that NSAIDs are well absorbed. They are predominantly metabolised in the liver and cleared by the kidney. They are highly protein bound, but the active moiety is the non-protein bound component. Since protein binding is reduced in certain disease states, including hypoalbuminaemia, hepatic disease and renal impairment, NSAIDs must be used with caution in patients with these disorders.

On the basis of plasma clearance times, NSAIDs fall into two groups – those with short and those with long clearance times. These differences are not of such relevance in rheumatoid arthritis because NSAIDs diffuse slowly into joints, resulting in the synovial fluid half-life being considerably longer than the plasma half-life.

There are several classes of NSAIDs (Table 23.3). Differences in physiochemical properties between these classes lead to differences in efficacy and side-effects. For instance, the more lipid soluble propionic acid derivatives, such as ketoprofen, ibuprofen and naproxen, penetrate the central nervous system readily, and are associated with side-effects, such as mood alterations, dizziness and cognitive changes. There is also considerable interindividual variation in responses to individual NSAIDs. Hence, if one NSAID is ineffective, or is associated with unacceptable side-effects, it is important to prescribe alternative NSAIDs, preferably of different chemical classes, before concluding that NSAID therapy is ineffective or causes unacceptable side-effects in a specific patient.

SIDE-EFFECTS OF NSAIDS

The side-effects of NSAIDs are listed in Table 23.4. The incidence of these effects increase with age.

Hence it is important that elderly patients receive low doses when initiating treatment. The most prominent side-effects of NSAIDs are on the gastrointestinal tract. The risk of patients developing an endoscopy-proven gastric or duodenal ulcer with NSAIDs is 15–20%, 3% of whom develop a major haemorrhage or perforation.[10] Also NSAIDs frequently caused oesophageal and small and large bowel ulceration. A point to note is that the correlation between gastrointestinal symptoms and ulceration is poor. Patients with gastrointestinal symptoms may not have ulcers and those without

Table 23.4 Principle side-effects of NSAIDs

Gastrointestinal	Dyspepsia Gastrointestinal ulceration
Renal	Interstitial nephritis Papillary necrosis Decreased glomerular filtration rate Transient creatinine rise Salt retention Hyperkalaemia
Liver	Hepatocellular injury Cholestasis
Haematological	Inhibition of platelet aggregation Thrombocytopenia Aplastic anaemia Haemolytic anaemia Neutropenia
Cutaneous	Photosensitivity Urticaria Erythema multiforme
Pulmonary	Bronchospasm
Central nervous system	Headache Dizziness Cognitive dysfunction

may.[11,12] Individual case control studies suggest that major gastrointestinal bleeding or perforation in patients receiving NSAIDs will occur once every 300–1500 patient years, and death once every 3000 to 10 000 patients years.[13]

The risks of NSAID-induced gastrointestinal disease are increased in the elderly, in patients with previous gastrointestinal side-effects or ulceration, and in patients with rheumatoid disease who are physically disabled, or receiving concomitant anticoagulant or corticosteroids. They are also much higher in the first few months of therapy.[14] Hence, if a patient has managed to take a drug for some weeks, the risks of gastrointestinal complications fall.

The relative risk of bleeding or gut perforation from individual NSAIDs varies from study to study, and is correlated with the daily drug dose.[15] The Committee on Safety of Medicines (CSM) ranks ibuprofen as having the lowest risk, diclofenac, indomethacin and naproxen as intermediate, and azapropazone as high risk.

There has been considerable recent interest in reducing NSAID-induced gastrointestinal damage. Since NSAIDs inhibit prostaglandin synthesis, it has been postulated that prostaglandin replacement might protect the gastrointestinal tract from NSAID-induced ulceration. Misoprostol is a prostaglandin analogue specifically developed for this purpose. In patients taking NSAIDs, a 12-week course of misoprostol 200 µg four times daily reduced the incidence of gastric ulcers from 7.7% to 1.9%, and of duodenal ulcers from 4.6% to 0.6%.[16] Ranitidine has also been shown to reduce the frequency of endoscopically-proven duodenal ulcers, but it has no effect on the frequency of gastric ulcers.[17] Omeprazole also reduces the incidence of NSAID-induced ulceration.[18]

Whether any of these agents reduce the rate of more serious complications of NSAIDs, such as major haemorrhage or perforation, is not yet known, but seems likely. The council of perfection is to stop NSAIDs in patients with gastrointestinal ulceration. Nevertheless, either omeprazole or ranitidine or misoprostol will heal a proportion of such ulcers.[18]

Skin reactions to NSAIDs are usually mild and respond to changing the drug class. It is known that NSAIDs can cause bronchospasm and should be used with extreme caution in patients with a previous allergic reaction. Rarely, blood dyscrasias have been reported during NSAID treatment. Nonsteroidal anti-inflammatory drugs, particularly diclofenac and sulindac, may cause transient elevations in liver enzymes. These abnormalities are usually mild and transient. Changing to another NSAID will often resolve this problem.

Although NSAIDs can also increase serum creatinine levels, this usually resolves despite continued therapy. However, NSAIDs occasionally cause renal failure, and because many NSAIDs are excreted by the kidneys, it is important to reduce or avoid their use in more than mild renal failure, particularly because they can cause hyperkalaemia. Also NSAIDs may reduce renal sodium excretion, which can exacerbate heart failure.

Ibuprofen, fenbufen, diflunisal and phenylbutazone interact with warfarin to increase the prothrombin index.[18] Although several studies have shown that other NSAIDs do not affect the prothrombin index there are occasional reports to the contrary.[19] Such effects may be idiosyncratic. It is therefore important to monitor the prothrombin index more frequently when starting or withdrawing an NSAID, and to avoid the drugs listed above.

Indomethacin significantly inhibits gentamicin clearance and caution is advocated for use of all NSAIDs in patients receiving aminoglycosides. Since NSAIDs may also precipitate lithium toxicity by reducing its renal clearance, lithium levels should be monitored more frequently when commencing NSAIDs. Other drug interactions are listed in Table 23.5. In practice, many of these drug interactions do not occur, and if it is necessary to prescribe drugs which potentially interact with NSAIDs, then an awareness of the possible problems is usually sufficient.

Table 23.5 Principle drug interactions with NSAIDs

Warfarin	Increase in prothrombin time
Lithium	Increase in lithium levels by effects on tubular excretion
Phenytoin	May increase or decrease phenytoin levels
Oral hypoglycaemics	Increased risk of hypoglycaemia by prolonging half-life
Digoxin	Reduction in digoxin clearance increasing risk of toxicity
Aminoglycosides	Reduction in drug clearance, increasing risk of toxicity
Antihypertensives	Reduction in antihypertensive effects
Cholestyramine	Reduction in NSAID absorption

Disease modifying anti-rheumatic drugs

CHOICE OF DRUG

Meta-analysis of 66 placebo controlled studies indicates that intramuscular gold, methotrexate, penicillamine and sulphasalazine are equally effective in suppressing ongoing rheumatoid arthritis, at least in the short term.[20] Oral gold is less effective than most of these drugs. The anti-malarials (hydroxychloroquine and chloroquine) are probably also less effective.[20] Azathioprine, cyclophosphamide and chlorambucil appear to have an efficacy similar to intramuscular gold.[21]

The caveats already discussed about such efficacy ranking need to be remembered. Moreover, it is important to note that there is considerable inter-individual variation in responses to DMARDs, and so this efficacy ranking does not necessarily hold true at the level of the individual patient.

Although second-line agents, when effective, will suppress clinical and laboratory parameters of disease activity this does not necessarily mean that the underlying progression in joint destruction has been retarded. In fact the relevance of short-term improvements to long-term outcome has become controversial.[1] Nonetheless, many believe, empirically, that suppressing laboratory parameters of disease activity, particularly when taken in conjunction with clinical response, has some correlation with slowing the progression of the disease, and there is some evidence to support this contention.[5]

The choice of which second-line drug agent to use varies and is often a combination of physician and patient preference. For most, it is dependent on the clinical features of the disease. Patients with mild rheumatoid arthritis might be commenced on hydroxychloroquine or oral gold, because these drugs have a low incidence of serious toxicity. If the disease is more aggressive, falls into a prognostic category signifying an aggressive arthritis, or is refractory to these agents, then one of the other traditional second-line agents is chosen. If the disease is still refractory, then consideration must be given to treatment with either corticosteroids or other immunosuppressive drugs.

Potential toxicity is a factor that influences the choice of DMARD. Meta-analysis has shown that intramuscular gold has the greatest toxicity whilst antimalarial drugs, oral gold and methotrexate have the least.[22] The toxicities of penicillamine, sulphasalazine and azathioprine are intermediate.

Gold

MECHANISM OF ACTION

Gold was first used in arthritis because it was postulated that it had anti-microbial effects. This was at a time when it was believed that rheumatoid arthritis had an infective aetiology. Gold is concentrated in macrophages and inhibits many *in vitro* immune responses. These include neutrophil chemotaxis, phagocytosis, and the neutrophil oxidative burst. Gold also inhibits mitogen-induced proliferation and immunoglobulin synthesis in T and B cells, respectively. These latter effects are probably secondary to the effects of gold on macrophage activation. However, gold does not inhibit disease progression in animal models of autoimmune arthritis. It is therefore not clear just how gold modifies rheumatoid arthritis in man, although this is likely to be related to effects on macrophage function.

EFFICACY

Gold is effective in about 20–35% of patients after 6–12 months of treatment, but sustained responses beyond 1 year are only seen in about 50% of these responders.[23] Almost complete remission is rare and may simply reflect a group of patients who would have entered remission spontaneously. Nevertheless, about 20% of patients are able to take gold for more than 4 years.[23]

TOXICITY

The adverse effects of gold treatment are shown in Table 23.6. These effects are much more common in patients treated with intramuscular gold than in those receiving oral gold, although the latter is less effective. Toxicity does not correlate well with the length of time of treatment. In fact, if patients are able to take gold for a year or more the incidence of toxicity falls.[23] The commonest side-effects of gold are mucocutaneous, particularly pruritus. Rashes are common and, if not exfoliative, gold can be withdrawn and restarted under careful supervision at a lower dose. If there are any signs of exfoliative dermatitis then gold should be permanently withdrawn. This is because exfoliative dermatitis, although rare, is a potentially fatal complication of therapy.

Proteinuria is a common side-effect of gold. If present at low levels, (2 g per day) there is no absolute indication for withdrawal but if the proteinuria increases, or miscroscopic haematuria

Table 23.6 Adverse effects of gold treatment

	Prevalence (%)		Management
	Intramuscular	Oral	
Very common			
Pruritus and rashes (other than exfoliative dermatitis)	>35	30	Temporary withdrawal
Mouth ulcers	13	15	Temporary withdrawal
Eosinophilia	<50		Increased vigilance
Gastrointestinal	<1	40	Often causes withdrawal
Common			
Thrombocytopenia	1–3	2	Permanent withdrawal
Proteinuria	0.7–8	<1	Temporary withdrawal if more than 1–2 g/24 h; permanent withdrawal if heavy proteinuria or if haematuria supervenes
Rare			
Neutropenia	<1	<1	Permanent withdrawal
Marrow aplasia	Very rare		Permanent withdrawal
Hepatic necrosis	Very rare		Permanent withdrawal
Enterocolitis	Very rare		Permanent withdrawal
Pneumonitis	Very rare		Permanent withdrawal
Exfoliative dermatitis	Very rare		Permanent withdrawal

supervenes, then gold should be withdrawn. It is possible to restart gold once the proteinuria has resolved. The renal lesions of gold-induced nephritis are reversible, but in occasional instances may take some years to do so.

Apart from eosinophilia, the most common haematological side-effects of gold are reductions in one or more of the blood cell lines, particularly platelets. These reductions usually occur as a trend, and indicate that gold should be withdrawn permanently. Gold rarely causes marrow aplasia of sudden onset, for which there are no warning signs. This occurrence may be fatal. Gold commonly induces an eosinophilia. This is not an indication for cessation of therapy, but should prompt particular vigilance and perhaps dose reduction, because it may herald more serious haematological side-effects. Serious marrow toxicity, if these guidelines are followed, is uncommon.

DOSAGE AND ADMINISTRATION

Intramuscular gold is first given as a test injection of 10 mg, provided a preceding platelet count is normal. Rare side-effects at this stage are hyper-sensitivity or a severe skin rash. One week later, after a further check of the platelet count, a second test injection of 20 mg is given and the platelet count rechecked afterwards. If this is still normal, patients proceed to regular therapy.

Each week, patients receive intramuscular gold 50 mg, preceded by a full blood count check and a urine dipstick text for albumin. The results of these tests must be known before giving the gold. Injections should be withheld if more than a trace of albuminuria is present but can be reinstated if this has gone on retesting. If albuminuria (more than a trace) persists, then the amount should be quantified by 24-hour urine collection. Patients continue with weekly 50 mg injections to a total cumulative loading dose of between 700 and 1000 mg, according to their response. Patients are normally reviewed in clinic at this stage to determine whether response has occurred. Once the loading dose has resulted in response, the drug is gradually reduced to a lower maintenance level, usually 50 mg per month but sometimes higher or lower according to the need and size of the patient. During long-term treatment, the frequency or amount of the monthly injection can be altered slightly to cope with natural variation in the severity of the arthritis. Patients may remain on gold for many years and it should not be stopped if the arthritis is in remission. This is because there is evidence to suggest that if patients relapse after gold withdrawal, they are refractory to further courses of the drug.

D-Penicillamine

Penicillamine has been used for treating rheumatoid arthritis for 25 years. Its mode of action in rheumatoid arthritis, however, is unknown. It may exert its effect by reducing sulphydryl exchange reactions on or in immunoreactive cells. At a dose of 500 mg/day, it is effective in approximately 60–70% of patients by 6 months,[24] yet the evidence that it retards the progression of erosions is poor. Moreover, there have been no trials of the drug lasting more than 1 year.

The rate of drug withdrawal amongst penicillamine treated patients, due to inefficacy or side-effects, is high and similar to that of gold. About 50% of patients experience some form of toxicity within 6 months of starting treatment, half of whom have to stop the drug.[24]

The side-effects of penicillamine are similar to those of gold. They are shown in Table 23.7. The development of gold toxicity does not indicate that patients should not be commenced on penicillamine, and vice versa. The principle side-effects of penicillamine are mucocutaneous, renal, gastrointestinal and haematological. The most common mucocutaneous problems are taste disturbances, urticaria and macular or papular rashes. These side-effects resolve rapidly on drug withdrawal. Pemphigus, although rare, is the most serious dermatological side-effect of the drug and is potentially fatal.

A significant number of penicillamine-treated patients develop proteinuria. As with gold, this almost always resolves within 1 year of stopping the drug. Haematuria, however, is a serious but very rare problem, which may indicate a progressive glomerulonephritis, necessitating renal biopsy and systemic immunosuppression.

Table 23.7 Adverse effects of penicillamine

Reaction	Prevalence (%)	Management
Gastrointestinal		
Taste disturbances	25	
Nausea/vomiting		
Stomatitis		
Renal		
Proteinuria	9–15	If significant(>2 g/24h) necessitates withdrawal, reversible on withdrawal.
Glomerulonephritis	Rare	Withdraw, monitor renal function
Haematological		
Thrombocytopenia	10	Withdraw. May be possible to restart
Neutropenia	5	Withdraw permanently
Marrow plasia	Rare	Withdraw
Dermatological		
Pruritis	8	May need withdrawal, may be possible to restart
Alopecia	Rare	May reverse on stopping
Pemphigus	Rare	Withdraw, immunosuppression
Autoimmune disorders		
Myasthenia gravis	Rare	Withdraw, immunosuppression
Polymyositis	Rare	
Goodpasture's syndrome	Rare	
Systematic lupus erythematosus	Rare	
Others		
Hepatotoxicity	Rare	
Neuropathy	Rare	
Pulmonary fibrosis	Rare	

The main haematological complications of penicillamine are thrombocytopenia and, less commonly, leukopenia and marrow aplasia. These can occur at any time during treatment. Penicillamine should be withdrawn if these effects occur.

DOSAGE AND ADMINISTRATION

The standard dose regime of penicillamine is 125 mg/day for 2 weeks, then 250 mg/day for 2 weeks, then 375 mg/day for 2 weeks, and 550 mg/day thereafter. The dose may be further increased if the patient fails to respond. The drug takes some months to exert its full action. A weekly full blood count is advisable as patients build up the dose, and fortnightly or monthly platelet counts should be checked thereafter. Early toxicity is indicated by a fall in platelet count. Patients should be taught to check their urine each week with dipsticks. They should be warned about the symptoms of the possible side-effects, such as bruising, rashes, taste disturbance and infections.

Sulphasalazine

Sulphasalazine is a conjugate of the salicylate 5-aminosalicylic acid and the sulphonamide sulfapyridine. Its mode of action is unknown. Its efficacy appears to be equivalent to gold or penicillamine, but with a lower incidence of serious side-effects.[25] Hence the drug is fairly safe. The withdrawal rate of side-effects of sulphasalazine is similar or slightly lower than traditional second-line agents with equivalent efficacy (with the exception of methotrexate).

SIDE-EFFECTS

The principle side-effect of sulphasalazine is gastrointestinal intolerance, often in association with headache and dizziness. Although sulphasalazine may cause dyspepsia it does not predispose to gastrointestinal ulceration. Less commonly, the drug has haematological side-effects. The most common of these is neutropenia, which has a frequency of between 1 and 5%.[25] This usually develops early during treatment. Agranulocytosis is rare, but usually occurs within the first 2 months of treatment, hence the necessity to monitor the full blood count fortnightly during the first months of treatment. Thrombocytopenia is a rare side-effect.[25] The drug can also cause a reversible hepatitis, mani-

fested by a rise in liver transaminases. Reversible male infertility may occur, but there is little evidence for a teratogenic effect. Nevertheless, the drug should be avoided during pregnancy. Occasionally patients develop a late folate sensitive macrocytic anaemia after 1 or 2 years therapy.

DOSAGE AND ADMINISTRATION

The normal dose regime (enteric-coated formulation) is 0.5 g/day for 1 week, then 1.0 g/day for a further week, then 1.5 g/day for a further week and 2.0 g/day thereafter. The main side-effect at this stage is dyspepsia, necessitating discontinuation in up to 30% of patients. Should this occur, the drug should be omitted for a period of 3–4 days, then reintroduced at a dose lower than that which caused the side-effects. If a therapeutic response fails to occur after 8–12 weeks at 2.0 g/day, patients may proceed up to 3.0 g/day in stepwise fashion, provided there are no side-effects. A 2-weekly full blood and platelet count is recommended during the first 3 months of treatment, and 3-monthly when patients are established on treatment. Like most other second-line agents the drug takes some weeks to exert its full clinical action.

Anti-malarials: hydroxy-chloroquine and chloroquine

The anti-malarials hydroxychloroquine and chloroquine have been used for many years to treat rheumatoid arthritis. Their mode of action is unknown. Almost all of the drug becomes tissue bound and with both it takes several months to reach a steady plasma level. Plasma levels also take several months to fall following drug withdrawal. The anti-malarials are less effective than other traditional second-line drugs (with the exception of oral gold).[20] They are, however, significantly less toxic than most other second-line agents.[20,22]

SIDE-EFFECTS

The principle side-effect of either hydroxychloroquine or chloroquine is retinopathy. Other side-effects include gastrointestinal intolerance and mild skin rashes, both of which are uncommon. The retinopathy is generally irreversible and, if associated with high dose therapy, is sometimes progressive, despite drug withdrawal. In the past, the reported frequency of retinal toxicity was 10% for chloroquine and 3–4% for hydroxychloroquine.[26] Hence there was considerable concern over the use of the two drugs in rheumatology. However, in large series of patients, retinopathy was not observed in those taking doses of less than chloroquine 3.5 mg/kg/day, or hydroxychloroquine 6.5 mg/kg/day.[27] These studies did not, however, take into account lean body mass, which is important because both drugs are fat insoluble. Furthermore, Easterbrook described retinopathy in patients taking 250 mg chloroquine/day.[28] Since retinopathy has not been described in patients taking less than 600 mg/day hydroxychloroquine,[29] this drug is preferable to chloroquine.

DOSAGE AND MONITORING

The normal maintenance therapy for hydroxychloroquine is 200–400 mg/day. Usually patients commence on hydroxychloroquine 400 mg/day and after 3 months reduce to 200 mg/day. Occasionally the drug is given at a higher dose of 600 mg for a short period. The drug takes some weeks or months to exert its activity.

Provided patients keep below a total cumulative dose amounting to approximately 20 months therapy at 400 mg/day, it is exceptional for retinopathy to occur. Hepatic and renal impairment may predispose to retinal toxicity, and should be checked before commencing treatment. After 12 months, regular ophthalmological examination is recommended, including visual acuity, ophthalmoscopy and central visual field testing (usually with Ishihara colour charts or Amsler red charts) at 6-monthly intervals. In an effort to limit the cumulative dose, and because the drug is highly tissue bound, patients whose disease is well controlled should try to reduce to alternate day dosing at 200 mg, or to omit the drug for a period of weeks at regular intervals.

Methotrexate

Methotrexate has been used for many years in the treatment of cancer and for psoriasis. In patients with malignancy treated with methotrexate, side-effects, most particularly hepatic cirrhosis, pulmonary fibrosis and myelosuppression are well documented. Concerns over these adverse effects retarded the widespread acceptance of the drug for treating rheumatoid arthritis. Due to the lower doses used in rheumatoid arthritis these side-effects are uncommon in rheumatological practice. Thus,

over the last decade, methotrexate has gained widespread acceptance as one of the treatments of choice for rheumatoid arthritis.

At high doses methotrexate is a folate antagonist, inhibiting thymidylate synthetase, thereby blocking DNA synthesis. In rheumatoid arthritis, however, the drug is used at low doses, at which there is no conclusive evidence that it is immunosuppressive. Hence it is not clear how the drug modifies rheumatoid arthritis.

EFFICACY

There are contrasting clinical data on the efficacy of methotrexate. On one hand, a body of evidence suggests that about 80% of methotrexate-treated rheumatoid arthritis patients respond. In about half of these, the improvement is maintained for up to 2 years.[30] Certain trials indicate that methotrexate will slow the appearance of erosions, at least in the first 3 years.[31,32] Analysis of the length of time patients with rheumatoid arthritis are able to continue on methotrexate shows that this drug is prescribed for longer periods than other second-line agents. This indicates a toxicity-efficacy weighting which is superior to other second-line drugs.

On the other hand, there has been considerable debate about the efficacy of methotrexate and possible flaws in some of the methotrexate studies have been considered.[33,34] Other clinical trials have indicated that although the drug is at least as effective as gold, it is not significantly better.[35,36] In these trials, although more patients were able to continue on methotrexate compared with intramuscular gold, because of a lower incidence of side-effects, these differences were not statistically significant. In addition, despite the fact that methotrexate may improve symptoms, signs and laboratory parameters of disease activity, this does not necessarily mean that it stops the progression of erosions.[37] There is also a view that patients taking methotrexate do not enter remission. Nonetheless, most rheumatologists view the drug as effective.

SIDE-EFFECTS

The incidence of withdrawal due to side-effects from methotrexate is low, occurring in only about 20% of patients in trials of drug efficacy.[20] The most common side-effects are gastrointestinal, particularly nausea, as well as dyspepsia and stomatitis. The stomatitis may be responsive to folate therapy.

The side-effects of particular concern are hepatic, haematological and pulmonary. Concerns over hepatic toxicity arose because cirrhosis occurs in patients treated at higher doses than are used in rheumatoid arthritis. In rheumatoid arthritis, however, the results of several long-term follow-up studies show that the risk of cirrhosis, when recommended doses are not exceeded, is very low but not unreported.[38,39] It is important to note that there may be little correlation between abnormalities in hepatic transaminases and underlying liver damage.

Pneumonitis secondary to methotrexate is uncommon (less than 5%). Its appearance does not correlate with the dose of methotrexate, and it may be a hypersensitivity reaction. It can be very serious, but is usually reversible on drug withdrawal. There is controversy, but little evidence whether methotrexate causes pulmonary fibrosis during long-term treatment.[21] Whether methotrexate is oncogenic is unresolved. In patients treated for psoriasis, who generally receive higher methotrexate doses than those with rheumatoid arthritis, there is no evidence for such an effect. Nevertheless, there have been reports of lymphoma in patients with rheumatoid arthritis treated with methotrexate.[21]

Whether methotrexate is associated with an increase in infections following orthopaedic surgery is also controversial. Several small studies described an increased infection rate in methotrexate-treated patients. In the largest series, however, Perhala *et al.*[40] reported on 60 methotrexate-treated patients who underwent 92 arthroplasties. The infection rate in these patients was similar to that in 61 non-methotrexate treated patients receiving 110 arthroplasties. This issue therefore requires further investigation.

The frequency of haematological side-effects in methotrexate-treated patients with rheumatoid arthritis varies from 1% to 24%.[38,39] However, permanent discontinuation for leukopenia or thrombocytopenia is uncommon.[38] These side-effects may be linked to impaired renal function, folate deficiency and co-trimoxazole therapy. Methotrexate is teratogenic, and should not be given in pregnancy or to patients wishing to conceive.[39,41] As methotrexate is excreted by the kidneys it should not be given to patients with significantly impaired renal function.

DOSAGE AND ADMINISTRATION

Methotrexate is usually given as a weekly oral dose, although it can be given intramuscularly or subcutaneously. In some patients, in order to overcome nausea, it is given as a divided dose. The usual dose is 7.5–15 mg per week. The recommended maintenance dose in rheumatoid arthritis, 10 mg a week,

has been reached as a result of a series of controlled clinical trials. It is reached over 4 weeks by 2.5 mg incremental increases in doses, starting at 2.5 mg/week. Since the most common mistake is for patients to take methotrexate daily, patients should be advised to choose a particular day each week for their methotrexate treatment and adhere to this.

Patients should have fortnightly full blood and platelet count checked during the first 6 weeks of therapy, reducing to monthly thereafter once the patient is on a constant dosage. Liver function tests should be performed monthly as monitoring for hepatoxicity. This is first manifested by a rise in transaminases.

INTERACTIONS

In practice the interaction of methotrexate with NSAIDs is of little consequence, although aspirin should probably be avoided. Patients should be instructed not to take probenecid, trimethoprim or sulphonomides while on methotrexate. Live vaccines should not be given whilst patients are taking methotrexate, although influenza vaccines are safe.

Azathioprine

Azathioprine is an oral purine analogue which suppresses DNA synthesis in lymphocytes and other dividing cells. It is therefore a non-specific immunosuppressive agent. The usual dose is 1.5–2.5 mg/kg/day and it is often combined with corticosteroid therapy. The efficacy of azathioprine appears greatest at a dose of 2.5 mg/kg/day, and it is probably ineffective at a dose of 1 mg/kg/day or less.[42] There is little evidence that doses higher than 2.5 mg/kg/day are any more effective than standard doses.[43]

Most studies show that the efficacy of azathioprine in rheumatoid arthritis is comparable with gold, penicillamine, sulphasalazine or methotrexate.[21,43] Due to concerns over side-effects many physicians only use the drug in refractory rheumatoid arthritis, after more conventional agents have failed. Traditionally azathioprine has also been used as a corticosteroid sparing agent.

The most important side-effects of azathioprine are marrow suppression (infrequent) and oncogenesis. However, although the incidence of tumours in organ allograft recipients receiving azathioprine, as part of a cocktail of immunosuppressive agents, is increased above normal, the incidence of tumours in azathioprine-treated rheumatoid arthritis patients is not high. Silman's data suggest that the risk of lymphoma is increased in patients with rheumatoid arthritis treated with azathioprine, but the incidence of solid tumours is not.[44]

Other side-effects of azathioprine are gastrointestinal upsets and hepatoxicity. Patients taking the drug require full blood and liver function testing over the first few months, and thereafter, monthly or 2-monthly tests. Once patients are established on azathioprine, it is usually well tolerated. It is essential that patients are not treated with concomitant allopurinol, because this drug inhibits the excretion of azathioprine metabolites, and therefore can induce serious toxicity. It is recommended that pregnant females should discontinue azathioprine. Nevertheless, there are many reports of transplant recipients conceiving and giving birth to healthy infants whilst taking azathioprine.

Alkylating agents

The use of the alkylating agents chlorambucil and cyclophosphamide in rheumatoid arthritis is restricted either to disease complicated by vasculitis, or to refractory disease. For both these indications, however, the evidence for efficacy is at best partial. Both drugs significantly increase the risks of serious infections and malignancy and hence they are used only as a last resort.

Cyclosporin A

Cyclosporin A has been used, mainly on a experimental basis, in rheumatoid arthritis for over 10 years. It is likely that it exerts its effects in rheumatoid arthritis via its well described inhibitory effects on the transcription of T cell cytokines necessary for T helper cell activation. The efficacy of cyclosporin A is similar to that of azathioprine. It is not generally possible to use the drug in particularly high doses because of complicating nephrotoxicity and hypertension. Despite these problems, when used with caution and within the prescribing guidelines it is a useful adjunct, particularly in patients unable to tolerate more conventional second-line agents.

Combination therapy

Since the results of single second-line agent treatment for rheumatoid arthritis are often poor, there have been attempts to determine whether combination therapy is of value.[45] Another rationale for the combination approach is that it takes several months to determine whether a second-line agent is effective. If the drug is ineffective then during this time joint destruction will continue unchecked. Moreover, although the short-term effects of individual second-line agents are often good, (with the exception of methotrexate) fewer than 10% of patients continue on an individual drug for more than 3 years.[5] Whether combination therapy is more effective than single second-line therapy is, however, controversial.[5]

Credible results have been obtained with the combination of methotrexate, azathioprine and hydroxychloroquine in patients who had failed on individual drug treatment – including methotrexate and azathioprine.[5] Likewise, impressive results have been obtained with the combination of prednisolone 10 mg, methotrexate 15 mg, oral gold 6 mg and hydroxychloroquine.[5]

The results of other trials of combination treatment have been equivocal.[5] This may be partly because combination therapy has often been used as a last attempt to treat late-stage refractory rheumatoid arthritis. This may not be representative of possible effects on early disease. Moreover, although the guiding principle for combination therapy is to ensure that the clinical and laboratory features of active rheumatoid arthritis are suppressed, whether this actually correlates particularly well with an endpoint of preserved joint function is not clear.

Corticosteroids

Corticosteroids were first used to treat rheumatoid arthritis more than 40 years ago. Initially they were used at high dose, with resulting side-effects, and because of this physicians, until recently, overcompensated by not using them enough, and thus their benefits may have been underestimated. Corticosteroids are useful for gaining control of rheumatoid synovitis before the slower acting second-line agents have effect. They are also useful for rapidly rescuing patients from rheumatoid flares.

There are some data suggesting that low dose corticosteroids may retard the development of osteoporosis, at least in early rheumatoid arthritis.[46] This may be because any effects on bone loss are outweighed by reducing the osteoporosis that occurs secondary to synovitis. Whether early corticosteroid use retards the progression and the development of erosions is unknown. The place of low-dose steroids in treating rheumatoid arthritis is therefore unresolved.[8]

At doses of below 10 mg in males, and 7.5 mg in females, there is evidence that prednisolone has little effect on bone stock. If higher doses are required, it seems prudent, although not yet substantiated that measures are taken to retard steroid induced bone loss. Hence post-menopausal females should take at least 1 g of calcium per day, and consideration should be given to biphosphonate therapy. Preliminary data suggest that these drugs in combination with vitamin D (1000 international units/day), will retard steroid-induced bone loss.[47] Hormone replacement therapy for post-menopausal females is also of potential benefit. Another method of reducing potential side-effects is to concomitantly prescribe a steroid sparing drug to reduce corticosteroid doses. Traditionally azathioprine has been used, but there is evidence that methotrexate is an effective steroid sparing agent.

INTRA-ARTICULAR STEROIDS

Intra-articular corticosteroids are indicated for patients with rheumatoid arthritis where one or a few joints are active. Moreover, there is evidence that intra-articular corticosteroids will significantly retard the progression of erosions.[48]

The effects of intra-articular corticosteroid injections are dependent on the anti-inflammatory strength of the compound, its solubility, and the joint injected. The more inflamed a joint, the faster the dispersal of the compound out of the joint. Also, the larger the surface area of the joint then the greater the potential for drug dispersal. Indeed, many patients with rheumatoid arthritis report an overall amelioration of joint symptoms following intra-articular corticosteroid injections indicating systemic anti-inflammatory effects. In fact intra-articular injections can suppress the hypothalamic-pituitary axis.

Hydrocortisone acetate and methylprednisolone acetate are more soluble than triamcinolone hexacetonide, despite the latter two drugs having similar anti-inflammatory potency. This suggests that triamcinolone hexacetonide is the drug of choice for intra-articular injections when the physician is confident that the drug will be administered into the joint. This is born out by clinical data on the duration of pain relief.[49] In small joints, where the volume injected is limited, such as the interphalangeal joints, a dose of triamcinolone hexacetonide 5–10 mg is usually sufficient. In larger joints, such as the knee and elbow, triamcinolone hexacetonide 20–40 mg may be necessary,

With care, serious complications, such as infection, are rare following intra-articular corticosteroid injections. The benefit of resting a joint after joint injection is controversial. Some patients experience a post-injection flare following joint injection, which may represent a crystal synovitis. This needs to be distinguished from infection. Leakage of corticosteroids from the joint or incorrect instillation may cause skin discolouration or atrophy.

Future pharmacological treatment of rheumatoid arthritis

Treatment designed to inactivate or modulate the immune system at specific points, compared with the more global inhibition caused by standard immunosuppressive drugs is being evaluated in rheumatoid arthritis. Encouraging results have been observed with monoclonal antibodies directed to the CD-4 molecule or other T cell antigens, although there are problems with such antibody therapy. The antibodies have to be given intravenously; they make patients more susceptible to infections, and it is not yet known whether anti-T cell therapy is oncogenic. In transplantation, the monoclonal antibody OKT3, which is directed to the pan-T cell antigen CD-3, is strongly associated with the development of subsequent malignancies. A further problem is that after repeated courses, patients synthesise antibodies against the therapeutic antibody, so reducing their efficacy. Other drugs, which inactivate or block the activity of certain specific cytokines are also undergoing evaluation.[50]

Non-pharmacological management of rheumatoid arthritis

The non-pharmacological, non-surgical management of rheumatoid arthritis involves a host of disciplines. These include physiotherapy, occupational therapy, orthotics, chiropody, psychology, vocational assessment and social services. Many of these disciplines will provide education for the patients, both about the disease, and about facilities and opportunities available to them.

Education and psychobehavioural therapies are a neglected area of treatment in rheumatoid arthritis, but are particularly important. Data support the view that patients experience improvements in global function when they are active rather than passive participants in the management of their arthritis.[51] Measures which promote active participation, knowledge and reduction of stress have economic impact because they reduce the number of visits to physicians and have been shown to reduce physical disability, psychosocial problems and pain, and increase compliance and surveillance for drug side-effects.[51]

Education of patients about a complex disease is necessarily involved. Patients need to be advised about the clinical course of the disease, exercise, joint protection, and drug treatment. It is useful for patients to know about stress management, and to have knowledge of the community resources available to them.

Physical therapy

Physical therapies for rheumatoid arthritis have been extensively used for many years.[52] Unfortunately, scientific data on their mode of action and efficacy are often lacking. The various physical modalities available include rest, heat, cold, electrical stimulation, hydrotherapy, and other forms of active muscle exercise. Many of these modalities ease pain and allow the institution of a programme of active physiotherapy. Active physiotherapy decreases disability, and may increase psychological health.[53]

References

1. Pincus T, Callahan LF What is the natural history of rheumatoid arthritis? *Rheum Dis Clin North Am* 1993; **19:** 123–51.
2. Yelin E, Henke C, Epstein W The work dynamics of the person with rheumatoid arthritis. *Arth Rheum* 1987; **30:** 507–12.
3. Scott DL, Symmons DPM, Coulton BL, Popert AJ Long-term outcome of treating rheumatoid arthritis: results after 20 years. *Lancet* 1987; **i:** 1108–11.
4. Pincus T The paradox of effective therapies but poor long-term outcomes in rheumatoid arthritis. *Semin Arth Rheum* 1992; **9**(Suppl 3): 2–15.
5. Wilske KR, Healey LA The need for aggressive therapy of rheumatoid arthritis. *Rheum Dis Clin North Am* 1993; **19:** 153–61.
6. Fuchs HA, Kaye JJ, Callahan LF *et al.* Evidence of significant radiographic damage in rheumatoid arthritis within the first 2 years of disease. *J Rheumatol* 1989; **16:** 585–91.
7. Kushner I, Dawson NV Aggressive therapy does not substantially alter the long-term course of rheumatoid arthritis. *Rheum Dis Clin North Am* 1993; **19:** 163–72.
8. Weisman MH Should steroids be used in the management of rheumatoid arthritis? *Rheum Dis Clin North Am* 1993; **19:** 189–99.
9. March L, Irwig L, Schwartz J *et al.* Trials comparing a non-steroidal anti-inflammatory drug with paracetamol in osteoarthritis. *Brit J Med* 1994; **309:** 1041–5.
10. Lanza FL Gastrointestinal toxicity of newer NSAIDs. *Am J Gastroenterol* 1993; **88:** 1318–23.
11. Skander MP, Ryan FP Non-steroidal anti-inflammatory and pain free peptic ulceration in the elderly. *Brit J Med* 1988; **297:** 833–4.
12. Jorde R, Burhol PG Asymptomatic peptic ulcer disease. *Scand J Gastroenterol* 1987; **22:** 129–34.
13. Bossingham D, Hawkey CJ Gastroenterology in the rheumatoid diseases. In: *Oxford textbook of rheumatology* Vol 1. Madison PJ, Isenberg DA, Woo P, Glass DN (eds) Oxford: Oxford University Press, 1993: 138–45.
14. Carson JL, Strom BL, Soper KA *et al.* The association of nonsteroidal anti-inflammatory drugs with upper gastrointestinal tract bleeding. *Arch Intern Med* 1987; **147:** 85–8.
15. Bateman DN, NSAIDs: time to re-evaluate gut toxicity. *Lancet* 1994; **343:** 1051–2.
16. Graham DY, White RH, Moreland LW *et al.* Duodenal and gastric ulcer prevention with misoprostol in arthritis patients taking NSAIDs. *Ann Intern Med* 1993; **119:** 257–62.
17. Ehsanullah RS, Page MC, Tildesley G, Wood JR Prevention of gastroduodenal mucosal damage induced by non-steroidal anti-inflammatory drugs; controlled trial of ranitidine. *Brit J Med* 1988; **297:** 1017–21.
18. Walan A, Bader JP, Classen M *et al.* Effect of omeprazole and ranitidine on ulcer healing and relapse rates in patients with benign gastric ulcer. *New Engl J Med* 1989; **320:** 69–75.
19. Furst DE, Paulus HE Aspirin and other nonsteroidal anti-inflammatory drugs. In: *Arthritis and allied conditions.* McCarty DJ, Koopman WJ (eds) Philadelphia: Lea and Febiger, 1993: 567–602.
20. Felson DT, Anderson JJ, Meenan RF The comparative efficacy and toxicity of second line drugs in rheumatoid arthritis – results of two metaanalyses. *Arth Rheum* 1990; **33:** 1449–61.
21. Cash JM, Klippel JH Second-line drug therapy in rheumatoid arthritis. *New Engl J Med* 1994; **330:** 1368–75.
22. Felson DT, Anderson JJ, Meenan RF The use of short term efficacy/toxicity trade offs to select second line drugs in rheumatoid arthritis: a metaanalysis of published clinical trials. *Arth Rheum* 1992; **35:** 1117–25.
23. Champion G, Graham G, Zeigler J The gold complex. *Ballière's Clin Rheumatol* 1990; **4:** 491–534.
24. Joyce DA D-Penicillamine. *Ballière's Clin Rheumatol* 1990; **4:** 553–74.
25. Porter DR, Capell HA The use of sulphasalazine as a disease modifying antirheumatic drug. *Ballière's Clin Rheumatol* 1990; **4:** 535–51.
26. Bernstein HN Ophthalmological considerations and testing in patients receiving long term antimalarial therapy. *Am J Med* 1983; **75:** 25–34.

27. Mackenzie AH Dose refinements in long-term therapy of rheumatoid arthritis with antimalarials. *Am J Med* 1983; **75:** 40–5.

28. Easterbrook M Dose relationships in patients with early cloroquine retinopathy. *J Rheumatol* 1987; **14:** 472–5.

29. Urowitz MB, Lee P The risks of antimalarial retinopathy, azathioprine lymphoma and methotrexate hepatoxicity during the treatment of rheumatoid arthritis. *Ballière's Clin Rheumatol* 1990; **4:** 193–206.

30. Denman AM, Brooks PM, Antirheumatic drugs. In: *Oxford textbook of rheumatology* Vol. 1. Madison PJ, Isenberg DA, Woo P, Glass DN (eds) Oxford: Oxford University Press, 1993: 329–9.

31. Reykdal S, Steinsson K, Sigurjonsson K, Brekkan A Methotrexate treatment of rheumatoid arthritis: effects on radiological progression. *Scand J Rheum* 1989; **18:** 221–6.

32. Jeurissen MEC, Boerbooms AMT, van de Putte LB *et al.* Influence of methotrexate and azathioprine on radiological progression in rheumatoid arthritis: a randomized double-blind study. *Ann Intern Med* 1991; **114:** 999–1004.

33. Porter DR, Capell HA Methotrexate and rheumatoid arthritis. *Ann Intern Med* 1991; **115:** 745–6.

34. Epstein WV Methotrexate and rheumatoid arthritis. *Ann Intern Med* 1991; **115:** 746.

35. Suarez-Almozor M, Fitzgerald A, Grace M, Russell AS A randomized controlled trial of parenteral methotrexate compared to sodium aurothiomalate (myochrysine) in the treatment of rheumatoid arthritis. *J Rheumatol* 1988; **15:** 753–6.

36. Morassut P, Goldstein R, Cyr M *et al.* Gold sodium thiomalate compared with low dose methotrexate in the treatment of rheumatoid arthritis: a randomized, double blind, 26-week trial. *J Rheumatol* 1989; **16:** 302–6.

37. Nordstrom DM, West SG, Anderson PA, Sharp JT Pulse methotrexate therapy in rheumatoid arthritis. A controlled prospective roentogengraphic study. *Ann Intern Med* 1987; **107:** 797–801.

38. Furst DE Methotrexate. In: *Arthritis and allied conditions.* McCarty DJ, Koopman WJ (eds) Philadelphia: Lea and Febiger, 1993: 621–36.

39. Goodman TA, Polisson RP Methotrexate: Adverse reactions and major toxicities. *Rheum Dis Clin North Am* 1994; **20:** 513–28.

40. Perhala RS, Wlke WS, Clough JD, Segal AM Local infectious complications following large joint replacements in rheumatoid arthritis patients treated with methotrexate versus those not treated with methotrexate. *Arth Rheum* 1991; **34:** 146–52.

41. Songsiridej N, Furst DE Methotrexate – the rapidly acting drug. *Ballière's Clin Rheumatol* 1990; **4:** 575–93.

42. Woodland J, Chaput de Saintonge DM, Evans SJW *et al.* Azathioprine in rheumatoid arthritis: double blind study of full versus half dose placebo. *Ann Rheum Dis* 1981; **40:** 355–9.

43. Luqmani RA, Palmer RG, Bacon PA Azathioprine, cyclophosphamide and chlorambucil. *Ballière's Clin Rheumatol* 1990; **4:** 595–619.

44. Silman AJ, Petrie J, Hazleman B, Evans SJ Lymphoproliferative cancer and other malignancies in patients with rheumatoid arthritis treated with azathioprine: a 20 year follow up study. *Ann Rheum Dis* 1988; **47:** 988–92.

45. Cannon GW, Ward JR Cytotoxic drug and combination drug therapy. In: *Arthritis and allied conditions.* McCarty DJ, Koopman WJ (eds) Philadelphia: Lea and Febiger, 1993: 645–63.

46. Harris EB Treatment of rheumatoid arthritis. In: *Textbook of rheumatology.* Kelley WN, Harris E, Ruddy S, Slidge CB (eds) Philadelphia: WB Saunders Co, 1993: 912–23.

47. Worth H, Stammen D, Keck E Therapy of steroid-induced bone loss in adult asthmatics with calcium, vitamin D and a biphosphonate. *Am J Resp Crit Care Med* 1994; **150:** 394–7.

48. McCarthy DJ Treatment of rheumatoid joint inflammation with triamcinolone hexacetonide. *Arth Rheum* 1972; **15:** 157–73.

49. Bird HA Intra-articular and intralesional therapy. In: *Rheumatology.* Klippel JH, Dieppe PA (eds) St Louis: CV Mosby, 1994; 8.16.1–8.16.6.

50. Elliott MJ, Maini RN, Feldmann M *et al.* Treatment of rheumatoid arthritis with chimeric monoclonal antibodies to tumour necrosis factor. *Arth Rheum* 1993; **36:** 1681–90.

51. Lorig K, Chastain RL, Ung E *et al.* Development and evaluation of a scale to measure perceived self-efficacy in people with arthritis. *Arth Rheum* 1989; **32:** 37–44.

52. Gerber LH Nonpharmacologic modalities in the treatment of rheumatoid diseases. In: *Rheumatology.* Klippel JH, Dieppe PA (eds) St Louis: CV Mosby, 1994: 8.4.1–8.4.4.

53. Maehlum S Strategies to improve strength and stamina. In: *Rheumatology.* Klippel JH, Dieppe PA (eds) St Louis: CV Mosby, 1994: 8.51–5.8.

CHAPTER 24

The surgical management of rheumatoid arthritis: synovectomy

FRANK W HAGENA

Introduction

The importance of the elbow joint to the complex function of the upper limb is perhaps best seen in patients with rheumatoid arthritis. Inflammatory destruction of the joint limits elbow extension and flexion as well as forearm pronation and supination. This restriction of movement can significantly reduce the patient's ability to perform activities of daily living; in particular patients may be unable to dress without help, or reach their mouth, hair or perineum. In addition, since rheumatoid arthritis frequently also involves the patient's lower limb joints those with elbow disease find it increasingly difficult to use walking aids.

The first report on synovectomy of a chronic infectious elbow was published in 1923.[1] This was followed in 1924 by a second publication on three elbow synovectomies in rheumatoid arthritis.[2]

The procedure was extended in 1943 by Smith-Petersen et al. to include resection of the radial head.[3] This improved elbow movement and enabled a more radical synovectomy to be performed.

The first systematic follow-up of 92 elbow synovectomies, performed between 1965 and 1967 was reported by Laine and Vainio 1969,[4] with good results in 80% of the patients.[5] This positive outcome has been reproduced in other series with up to 87% of patients having complete pain free elbow function.[6-15] The European, multinational, multicentre study supported by ERASS (European Rheumatoid Arthritis Surgical Society) demonstrated pain relief in 82% of elbows that had undergone synovectomy.[16] In this study 265 elbow synovectomies were reassessed in 11 international rheumatoid centres at an average follow-up time of 4.1 years (min 2.5 years; max 14 years). Significant joint swelling was reduced in 90% of the cases. At the time of follow-up 57.6% of the elbows did not show any sign of synovitis. The range of motion was increased in terms of flexion/extension by 14.3 degrees and pronation/supination by 19.8 degrees. Within the observation time radiographic deterioration was noted from an average (Larsen, Dale, Eek: LDE) of 2.6 + 1.5 (see classification below). The conclusive statement was that radical synovectomy produces good long-term results. This was supported by the patients, 83.5% of whom would have undergone the procedure a second time.

Epidemiology

The elbow is the first joint to be affected by rheumatoid arthritis in only 2.1–3.0%.[17,18] In long-standing rheumatoid disease, however, the elbow joint is involved in 41–68% of patients.[4,18] In a retrospective study of seropositive rheumatoid patients 33% of the elbows showed clinical symptoms after an observation period of 17 years with 20% of the joints having significant radiographic changes.[19]

Elbow synovectomies account for 2.3–5.5% of all operations performed for rheumatoid arthritis.[2,20,21]

Clinical examination

Clinical examination will detect early signs of synovitis at the 'soft spot' between the lateral epicondyle and the radial head. Crepitus and pain may be produced by compression of the examiner's thumb over the patients radial head whilst turning the patient's forearm in pronation and supination. In addition it is also important to record the active and passive range of elbow movement together with the range of pronation and supination. The ulnar nerve must be assessed for signs of entrapment.

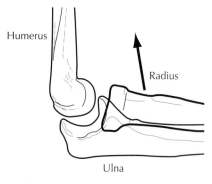

Fig. 24.1 The anterior drawer sign for instability of the radial head.

Instability of the radial head should be documented. This can be demonstrated by fluoroscopic radiography. The technique involves an 'anterior drawer' test with the elbow flexed at 90 degrees. The patient is requested to contract their biceps muscle whilst the examiner holds the hand resisting the movement. The biceps tendon subluxes the radial head. This is associated with crepitus and in most cases subjective pain provocation (Fig. 24.1).

Classification

The patient's history including medication, detailed physical and neurological examination and radiographic classification are essential in the assessment of surgical management. Increasing knowledge and experience with magnetic resonance imaging may enable the differentation of synovectomy into those cases that are best managed arthroscopically and those in which open synovectomy is to be preferred.

The standard radiographic assessment of rheumatoid arthritis was proposed by Larsen, Dale Eek in 1975.[22] It grades the disease into six (LDE) stages (Fig. 24.2) and enables the results from one centre to be compared with those from another.[16,23]

Grade 0: Normal.
Grade I: Slight abnormality. One or more of the following changes are present: periarticular soft tissue swelling, periarticular osteoporosis and slight joint space narrowing. When possible it is wise to use a normal contralateral or a previous normal radiograph of the same joint (Grade 0). Soft tissue swelling and osteoporosis are sometimes reversible changes. This is an early, uncertain phase of arthritis. Compatible changes may occur without arthritis in old age, in traumatic conditions or in Sudeck's atrophy.
Grade II: Definite early abnormality. Erosions (an obligatory sign) and joint space narrowing is noted.
Grade III: Medium destructive abnormality. Erosions and joint space narrowing are more marked.
Grade IV: Severe destructive abnormality. Marked erosion and joint space narrowing. Bone deformation is also present.
Grade V: Mutilating abnormality. The original articular surfaces have disappeared. Gross bone deformation is present.

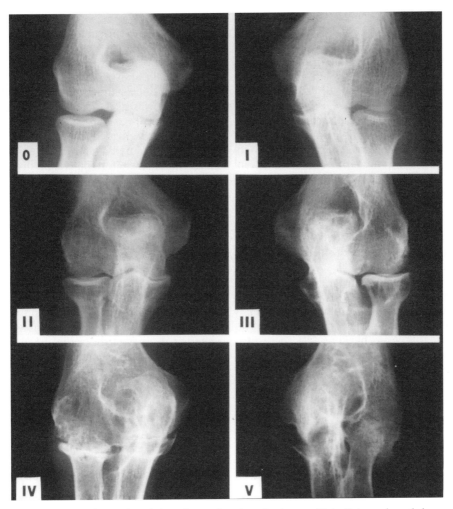

Fig. 24.2 Standard radiographs of the elbow showing the Larsen Dale Eek grades of rheumatoid elbow disease.

For prospective studies on the natural history of rheumatoid elbow disease and postoperative evaluation of outcome this standardised method of radiographic analysis is a prerequisite.

MANAGEMENT OPTIONS

Indication for conservative surgical treatment

There is overall agreement that synovectomy and debridement is indicated when swelling and/or pain persists for 3–6 months despite medical treatment and physiotherapy.

Early synovectomy is justified in LDE Grade 0–I [2,10,16,24,25] with the highest rate of pain relief being achieved in LDE Grades II and III. Synovectomy together with radial head excision can be used in LDE Grades III and IV. It offers considerable pain relief in up to 80% but the patient may have reduced function postoperatively.[26]

Early versus late synovectomy

The largest single study on synovectomy was published 20 years ago by Vainio.[6] Of 262 elbow synovectomies, 154 cases were available for follow-up. True early synovectomies, which by definition must be performed before radiographic or morphologic changes occur within the joint, were not reported. A total of 60% of Grade 2 cases had satisfactory results whilst only 50% were satisfactory in Grade 3. The radiographic Grade 4 cases had 57% satisfied patients. Although this study showed different outcomes depending on the severity of the disease when the synovectomy was performed, this is not true in other studies. Eichenblat *et al.*[24] and Linclau *et al.*[27] have shown no significant difference between early and late synovectomy. The improvement obtained, however, following synovectomy has been shown to be maintained for up to 10 years.[28]

Resection of the radial head

Just as the problem of the best surgical approach remains unsolved, the value of resection of the radial head remains controversial. Some authors generally combine synovectomy with radial head resection[9,29–31] while others view it as a 'vital part' of the procedure.[32] Still others see no significant benefit from removal of the radial head.[15,28] The negative effect of resection of the radial head has been documented in biomechanical studies. These have revealed increased loading of the ulnar compartment of the elbow joint. In addition resection of the radial head has been shown to result in deterioration of postoperative results from 70% to 45% during a 6-year follow-up period.[33] These results were confirmed by Summers *et al.*[34] in 1987. Gschwend[9] pointed out in 1977 that resection of the radial head leads to an increased rate of symptoms at the caput ulnae, which in turn may also have to be resected. The results of a multicentre study of German speaking orthopaedic rheumatologists, suggests that in cases of early synovectomy without cartilage destruction, the radial head should be preserved, but for late synovectomy radial head resection should routinely be included in the procedure.[25]

Surgical approaches

Rather than performing a medial approach to the elbow, many surgeons prefer a lateral approach to reduce the risk of ulnar nerve irritation.[13,32,35–38] A medial and lateral approach is stated to give improved postoperative results[7] but is more likely to be associated with postoperative ulnar nerve symptoms. Gschwend and Steiger[11,21] have shown that such neurological complications can be avoided by taking advantage of the dorsoradial approach and it is this which is the authors' preferred option.

Author's preferred procedure

The operative technique has been described by Gschwend.[10,20,39]

The patient is positioned supine with the arm flexed on an arm table over a small cushion to prevent ulnar nerve compression. A high tourniquet is applied. The incision is marked with a marker pen and begins 4.5 cm distal to the radial head. It follows the proximal radial shaft before curving towards the lateral epicondyle and then ending 3 cm proximal to the tip of the olecranon. The fascia is divided between the extensor carpi ulnaris and extensor digitorum muscles. The anconeus muscle tendon is then divided at its insertion on the lateral epicondyle, and the triceps is released from the distal humerus and lateral intermuscular septum.

With the elbow extended and the anconeus retracted, the olecranon fossa and synovial pouch are identified. The synovium is carefully resected.

With the elbow flexed, the flexor carpi radialis brevis and the lateral border of flexor carpi radialis longus are dissected from the distal humerus. An anterior compartment synovectomy is performed (Fig. 24.3). If the cartilage of the radial head is destroyed the radial head is resected at a distance of 1.5 cm from the joint surface. The elbow joint is once more inspected and the synovectomy completed. Only if preoperatively there are signs of ulnar nerve compression is it necessary to perform a medial incision with decompression and anterior subcutaneous transposition of the nerve (Chapter 7).

After completing the synovectomy the tourniquet is released and haemostasis performed. The annular ligament is tightened. A suction drain is inserted, the muscles repaired and the wound closed.

Postoperatively the arm is rested in a plaster slab for 5 days after which the patient has intensive physiotherapy.

Complications

Sensory dysfunction of the ulnar nerve has been reported in up to 17% when a medial approach and transposition of the ulnar nerve has been performed.[4,7,15,40] The dorsoradial approach potentially enables a radical synovectomy to be undertaken without the risk of neurological damage.[39,41]

Rarely is wound healing or infection a problem.[12,34]

Revision surgery for incomplete synovectomy or recurrent synovitis has been reported in up to 23.8% of cases.[7,12,35] The ERASS study and ARO study showed revision rates of 5.8% and 6.7% respectively.[23,25]

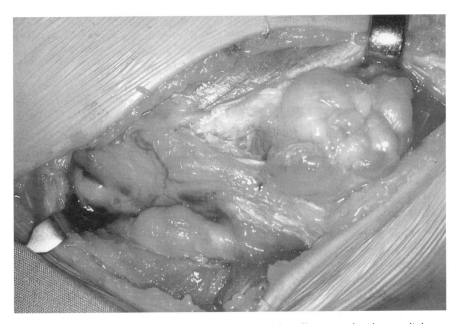

Fig. 24.3 An open anterior compartment synovectomy of the elbow via the dorsoradial approach. This figure is reproduced in colour in the colour plate section.

References

1. Swett PP Synovectomy in chronic infectious arthritis. *J Bone Joint Surg* 1923; **5:** 110–20.
2. Raunio, P Synovectomy of the elbow in rheumatoid arthritis. *Reconstr Surg Traumat* 1981; **18:** 63–9.
3. Smith-Petersen, MN, Aufanc OE, Larson CB Useful surgical procedures for rheumatoid arthritis involving joints of the upper extremity. *Archs Surg* 1943; **46:** 770.
4. Laine V, Vainio K Elbow. In: *Rheumatoid arthritis: synovectomy of the elbow*. Symposium on early synovectomy in rheumatoid arthritis. Amsterdam, 1967.
5. Laine V, Vainio K Synovectomy of the elbow. In: *Early synovectomy in rheumatoid arthritis*. Hijmans W, Paul WD, Herschel H (eds) Amsterdam: Excerpta Medica Foundation, 1969: 117–8.
6. Vainio K Eingriffe am rheumatischem Schulter – und Ellenbogengelenk. *Therapiewoche* 1970, **20:** 727.
7. Porter BB, Richardson BA, Vainio K Rheumatoid arthritis of the elbow: The results of synovectomy. *J Bone Joint Surg* 1974; **56B:** 427–37.
8. Brattstrom H, AL-Khudairy HA Synovectomy of the elbow in rheumatoid arthritis. *Acta Orthop Scand* 1975; **46:**744–50.
9. Gschwend N *Die operative Behandlung der chronischen Polyarthritis.* Stuttgart: Thieme, 1977: 63–8.
10. Gschwend N Die Ellenbogensynovektomie: Operationstechnik und Ergebnisse. *Akt Rheumatol* 1981, **6:**49–53.
11. Gschwend N, Steiger JU Elbow synovectomy. *Ann Chir Gynaecol* 1985, **74:** Suppl 198: 31–6.
12. Brumfield RH, Resnick RT Synovectomy of the elbow in rheumatoid arthritis. *J Bone Joint Surg* 1985; **67A:** 16–20.
13. Ferlic DC, Patchett CE, Clayton ML, Freeman AC Elbow synovectomy in rheumatoid arthritis. Long-term results. *Clin Orthop* 1987, **220:** 119–25.
14. Grimm J Spatsynovektomie des Ellenbogens und Resektion des Radiuskopfchens bei chronischer Polyarthritis. *Acta Orthop* 1989; **127:** 77–81.
15. Copeland SA, Taylor JG, Synovectomy of the elbow in rheumatoid arthritis: the place of excision of the head of the radius. *J Bone Joint Surg* 1997; **61B:** 69–73.
16. Hagena FW Synovectomy of the elbow. A review of the literature and results of an ERASS multicenter study. *Rheumatology* 1991; **15:** 6–21.
17. Boni A Die progrediente chronische Polyarthritis. In: *Klinik der rheumatischen Erkrankungen*, Berlin: Springer, 1970.
18. Fleming A, Cronen JM, Corbett M Early rheumatoid disease: I Onset; II Pattern of joint involvement. *Ann Rheum Dis* 1976; **35:** 357–64.
19. Hamalainen M, Ikavalko M Epidemiology of the elbow joint involvement in rheumatoid arthritis. *Rheumatology* 1991; **15:** 1–5.
20. Gschwend N Our operative approach to the elbow joint. *Arch Orthop Traumat Surg* 1981; **98:** 143–6.
21. Gschwend N, Steiger JU Ellbogengelenk. *Orthopade* 1986, **15:** 304–12
22. Larsen A, Dale K, Eek M Radiographic evaluation of rheumatoid arthritis and related conditions by standard reference films. *Acta Radiologica Diagnosis* 1977; **18:** 481–91.
23. Hagena F-W, Zwingers Th, Schattenkirchner M, Bracker W Die ARO-Dokumentation am Beispiel der Ellbogen-Synovektomien. In: *Aktuelle Probmleme in Chirurgie und Orthopadie*. Wessinghage D, Zacher J, Weseloh G (eds) Bern, Stuttgart, Toronto: Hans Huber, 1989.

24. Eichenblat M, Hass A, Kessler I Synovectomy of the elbow in rheumatoid arthritis. *J Bone Joint Surg* 1982; **64A:** 1074–8.

25. Siekmann W, Beyer W, Hagena FW, Weseloh G, Refior HJ Einfluß der Radiuskopfchenresektion auf das Ergebnis der Synovektomie des Ellbogengelenks bei chronischer Polyarthritis. In: *Aktuelle Probleme in Chirurgie und Orthopadie.* Wessinghage D, Zacher J, Weseloh G (eds) Bern, Stuttgart, Toronto: Hans Huber, 1989, 67.

26. Zena PW, Schwagerl W, Wanivenhaus A Expanded elbow synovectomy – An alternative to total arthrosplasty? *Rheumatology* 1991; **15:** 27–36.

27. Linclau LA, Winiawe CA, Korst JK Synovectomy of the elbow in rheumatoid arthritis. *Acta Orthop Scand* 1983; **54:** 935–7.

28. Tulp NJ, Winia WPCA Synovectomy of the elbow in rheumatoid arthritis. *J Bone Joint Surg* 1989; **71B:** 664–6.

29. Wilson BW, Arden GP, Ansell BM Synovectomy of the elbow in rheumatoid arthritis. *J Bone Joint Surg* 1973; **55B:** 106–11.

30. Goldie IF Synovectomy in rheumatoid arthritis: Theoretical aspects and a 14–year follow-up in the knee joint. *Reconstr Surg Traumat* 1981; **18:** 2–7.

31. Inglis AI Correction of arthritic deformities. In: *Arthritis and allied conditions. A textbook of rheumatology.* McCarty DJ (ed) Philadelphia: Lea and Febiger, 1985: 742–750.

32. Taylor AR, Mukerjea SK, Rana NA Excision of the head of the radius in rheumatoid arthritis. *J Bone Joint Surg* 1976; **58B:** 485–7.

33. Rymaszewski LA, Mackay I, Amis AA, Miller JH Long-term effects of excision of the radial head in rheumatoid arthritis. *J Bone Joint Surg* 1984; **66B:** 109–13.

34. Summers GD, Webley M, Taylor ARA Reappraisal of synovectomy and radial head excision in rheumatoid arthritis. *Brit J Rheum* 1987; **26:** 59–61.

35. Torgerson WR, Leach RE Synovectomy of the elbow in rheumatoid arthritis. *J Bone Joint Surg* 1970; **52A:** 371–5.

36. Marmor L Surgery of the rheumatoid elbow. *J Bone Joint Surg* 1972; **54A:** 173–8.

37. Low WG, Evans JP Synovectomy of the elbow and excision of the radial head in rheumatoid arthritis. *South Med J* 1980, **73:**707–9.

38. Ferlic D Management of the rheumatoid elbow. In: *Surgery for rheumatoid arthritis.* Clayton ML, Schmith CJ (eds) New York: Churchill Livingstone, 1992: 133–54.

39. Gschwend N Die Ellbogensynovektomie. *Operat Orthop Traumatol* 1989; **1:** 1–7.

40. Tillmann K Synovektomie und Arthroplastiken des Ellenbogengelenkes BEI Chronischer Polyarthritis. *Orthop Prax* 1975; **11:** 895–9.

41. Hagena, F W: Die Ellenbogensynovektomie bei chronischer Polyarthritis. *Akt Rheumatologie* 1994; **19:** 38–43.

CHAPTER 25

The surgical management of rheumatoid arthritis: interpositional arthroplasty

KARL TILLMANN, WOLFGANG RUTHER

Introduction

Arthroplasty in the original and pure sense can be defined as any mobile reconstruction of a functionally and anatomically damaged joint.

In contrast to an arthrolysis the joint surfaces require reshaping with or without endoprosthetic replacement.

Technically there are several options: a resection arthroplasty (RAP) involves either excising the whole joint or remodelling more or less congruent joint surfaces. This also applies to the resection and interposition arthroplasty (RIAP) but in this procedure homologeous or autologeous material, is interposed between the joint surfaces. A variation on this is the resection interposition and suspension arthroplasty (RISAP). In contrast to these procedures, distraction arthroplasty has become more of an adjunct rather than an autonomous surgical procedure in the management of post-traumatic conditions.

This chapter is confined to the management of rheumatoid elbow arthritis using the resection and interposition arthroplasty. In addition, the new technique of resection interposition and suspension arthroplasty is described. This is felt to be a suitable alternative for some rheumatoid patients.

Historical perspective

The underlying principles and ideas for resection arthroplasties go back to the last century. Ollier[1] in France is regarded as the first person to try and mobilise stiff elbow joints. In 1882 he reported on 106 resection arthroplasties. Helferich[2] (1894) introduced interposition of muscle flaps to prevent reankylosis. In the following 30 years, important contributions were made by McAusland[3] (1921) and Campbell[4] (1922) from the USA, by Putti[5] (1913) from Italy and by Payr[6] (1910) and Lexer[7] (1910) from Germany. Payr

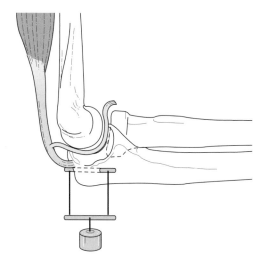

Fig. 25.1 Resection interposition arthroplasty of the elbow with distraction device Redrawn from Ref. 6.

Indications for resection arthroplasty

In the authors' experience resection interposition arthroplasty fills a gap between late synovectomy and total joint replacement in younger co-operative patients with a high need for function. An important pre-condition for the procedure is that the patient must have sufficient bone stock with reconstructable collateral ligament stability. Late synovectomy can be performed providing the joint is stable and mobile enough and has sufficient cartilage left to make its preservation worthwhile. Persisting pain after late synovectomy can also be an indication for an interpositional arthroplasty as a second step. Mutilating types of rheumatoid arthritis are a contraindication for this procedure.

Surgical technique

For reconstructive surgery in rheumatoid elbow arthritis a dorsal approach with a long V-shaped dissection of the triceps-tendon is preferred (Chapter 7). The distal flap remains based on the olecranon. Usually the ulnar nerve is translocated anteriorly.

A radical synovectomy and capsulectomy is always performed with the synoveum first being excised from the dorsal side and below the collateral ligaments. Following the bone resections the synovectomy is completed with removal of the synovium from the cubital and radial part of the joint.

In cases of marked joint stiffness it is advisable to mobilise the collateral ligaments up to their proximal origin at the epicondyles. In addition the distal insertion of the anconaeus muscle should be stripped with the medial head of triceps from the radial margin of the ulna. This preserves the nerve supply to anconeus.

The tips of the olecranon and the coronoid processes are both resected together with the frequently found large and shallow osteophyte on the medial side of the ulna. During this part of the procedure the ulnar nerve is at risk of damage and must therefore be protected. The joint surfaces of the ulna and humerus are then reshaped as congruently as possible. It is important, however, for mobility that the radius of the humerus should generally be somewhat smaller compared with the concave surface of the ulna. This reshaping is critical since a marked disparity between the surfaces of the humerus and ulna will result in joint instability postoperatively. The radial head is resected and the annular ligament which can be very slack after synovectomy is tightened and stabilised.

proposed resection arthoplasties for many joints.[6] He even recommended resection arthroplasty of the elbow with a distraction device (Fig. 25.1), which in principle is now being recommended again by Morrey[8] (1994). The aim of resection arthroplasties at that time was to remobilise stiff joints. The interposed material was therefore essential to prevent reankylosis. It was Herbert[9] (1958) in France and Vainio[10] (1967) in Finland who recommended resection arthroplasty not only for post-traumatic stiff joints but also for destroyed painful elbow joints in rheumatoid arthritis. Nowadays resection arthroplasties are mainly confined to rheumatoid patients, and it is not only stiffness of the joint that is the main indication for surgery, but pain. This is very important in terms of the interposed material.

In general the classical surgical methods, such as osteotomies and arthrodeses have gradually been forced aside with the introduction of modern artificial joints. However, resection arthroplasty still plays an important role in the modern management of rheumatoid elbow disease.

It is generally accepted that in early stage rheumatoid elbow arthritis synovectomy gives good results, particularly as regards pain relief. Even in advanced destruction of the elbow late synovectomies have been recommended. However, if the articular surface is destroyed and deformed and prevents congruous motion either a resurfacing by endoprosthetic replacement or a remodelling and reshaping by resection arthroplasty is required.[11–19]

The need for an interponant remains controversial. If early mobilisation is anticipated most patients feel more comfortable if an interponant is used. The authors recommend using lyophilised dura mater allograft and advise that only the humeral surface is covered by this material. The edges of the interponant are fixed by resorbable sutures to the adjacent soft tissues. The procedure is facilitated by transosseous fixation of the cubital and dorsal tip of the flap by two small drill holes through the fossa olecrani.

If detached, the anconeus-insertion is repaired by drill holes in the bone of the ulna. The triceps tendon is then reconstructed using resorbable sutures and the wound closed over suction drainage. An elastic compressive dressing is applied and the patient provided with three dorsal splints. These support the elbow in flexion, extension, and at 90 degrees respectively. The splints are exchanged at least four times per day. The forearm is kept in neutral rotation with the wrist in the position of function.

The drain is removed at 48 hours and physiotherapy commenced. Due to the repair of the triceps muscle active elbow extension is avoided for 3 weeks.

In rare cases gentle manipulation under anaesthesia may become necessary if the patient has poor elbow mobility. If required it should be performed within the first 3 weeks following surgery.

For the past 5 years the senior author has preferred a new technique of resection interposition and suspension arthroplasty for rheumatoid elbows (Fig. 25.2). Instead of a V-shaped division of the triceps tendon a 12–15 mm long and 15–20 mm wide distally based central tendon loop is formed. The dorsal capsule is approached between the long and the medial head of the triceps muscle for capsulectomy and synovectomy. The reshaping of the articular surfaces and the resection of the radial head is performed as described above. After this, in the thinnest region of the olecranon fossa a drill hole of approximately 10 mm diameter is made between the posterior and anterior elbow compartments. The completion of the cubital compartments synovectomy is made easier by this drill hole.

The triceps tendon loop is then pulled from the dorsal surface to the cubital surface through the reshaped joint space and back from there to the dorsal surface through the drill hole (Fig. 25.2a,b). Its proximal part and tip is fixed to the dorsal surface of the distal humeral metaphysis by transverse drill holes in the bone. This provides interposition and suspension of the ulna against the humerus and minimises the risk and disadvantage of dorsal tilting of the olecranon – a frequent and functionally impairing sequel of resection interposition arthroplasty at the elbow. Closing the gap in the triceps tendon by transverse sutures (Fig. 25.2c) improves the collateral stability of the joint in an

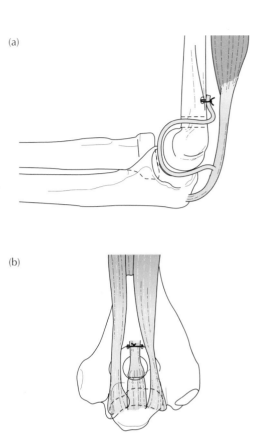

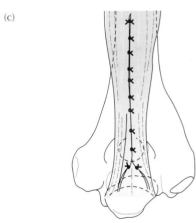

Fig. 25.2 Resection interposition suspension arthroplasty (RISAP) of the elbow: course of the central triceps tendon loop through joint and humerus: (a) lateral view; (b) posterior view; (c) narrowing of the triceps tendon by closing sutures.

often surprising way. Stability of the margins of the triceps tendon is enhanced by a boot lace suture (1 mm PDS) which is fixed distally to the reduced tip of the olecranon through a transverse drill hole. Passive motion and full active flexion is permitted after removal of the suction drain. Active extension begins 3 weeks after surgery and is slowly increased.

Postoperative results

There are very few publications reporting the results of interposition arthroplasty in rheumatoid patients.[12–14,20–23] Most have described reshaping of the joint surfaces[12,13,20–22,24]although complete joint excision has been occasionally reported.[1,9,21,23]

The published results indicate that postoperatively two-thirds of patients become completely pain free. The remainder suffer generally tolerable pain such that revision surgery is rare.[12,13,20,22,23] The reported gain in mobility averages 40 degrees (20–60 degrees) for flexion and extension and 40 degrees (35–50 degrees) for forearm rotation.[12–14,20,21] The Ollier–Herbert technique has been shown to give better pain relief and mobility but less stability and strength.[21]

Our own work has involved the study of 61 interpositional arthroplasties of the elbow which have been followed for 7.1 (1–19) years.[22] Twenty were followed to 5 years, 28 for 5–10 years and 12 for more than 10 years.

With regard to pain, 57% of our patients were completely pain free; 22% experienced mild, 15% moderate and 4% severe pain. The pain score did not deteriorate during the observation period (Table 25.1).

Joint mobility improved by an average of 26 degrees (71 degrees to 97 degrees) for flexion and extension (Fig. 25.3) and by 15 degrees (76 degrees to 91 degrees) for forearm rotation. Pronation remained unchanged. These results are inferior to other studies[12–14,20] and the reason for this may be because our indications for surgery were somewhat wider than those of other studies. In our study the gain in extension and supination returned to the preoperative values after 10 years. The gain in flexion, however, was fully maintained. This we believe is due to the patients' functional requirements during activities of daily living.

Table 25.1 Evaluation of pain after resection – interposition arthroplasty

Pain (postop)	Joints		Follow-up (years)		
	No	%[a]	<5	5–10	>10
Severe	4	(7)	3	1	–
Moderate	9	(15)	2	6	1
Mild	13	(22)	6	2	5
None	34	(57)	9	19	6
Total	60		20	28	11

[a] % approximated to nearest 'whole patient'.

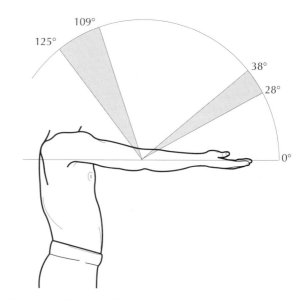

Fig. 25.3 Flexion and extension in resection interposition arthroplasty preoperatively 38 degrees to 109 degrees and postoperatively 28 degrees to 125 degrees.

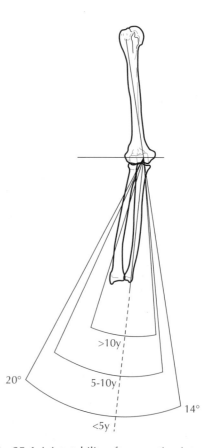

Fig. 25.4 Joint stability after resection interposition arthroplasty. Diagram to show improvement in stability with progression of time.

Collateral ligament stability in the extended position of the elbow was impaired after the operation by an average of 30 degrees (10 degrees in varus and 20 degrees in valgus). However, some improvement was noted with time. Instability of 35 degrees during the first 5 years reduced to 30 degrees after 5–10 years and 15 degrees after more than 10 years (Fig. 25.4). The dorsocubital stability measured in centimetres at 90 degrees of flexion improved in a similar way during the same period. This went from an average of 1.5 cm in the first 5 years to 1 cm after 5–10 years and 0.5 cm after more than 10 years.

A correlation was found between mobility and instability. Eight joints with 125 degrees or more of flexion and extension had varus–valgus instability of about 45 degrees whilst eight joints with 60 degrees or less flexion and extension had only approximately 20 degrees of varus–valgus instability.

Bone resorption is the main long-term concern after resection interposition arthroplasty. In our study there was no proven correlation between the extent of bone resorption and joint stability. Radiographic analysis of the humeral side of the elbow joint revealed no evidence of bone resorption

in 22% of cases, little bone resorption (confined to the intercondylar joint surfaces) in 29%, moderate bone resorption (approaching the fossa olecrani) in 18% and severe bone resorption (including the fossa) in 31% of our cases.

Severe bone resorption implies the risk of a condylar fracture but usually does not jeopardise joint stability (Fig. 25.5). Usually the progress of bone resorption stops spontaneously after some months or years, but it can continue for more than 10 years.

Complications

The most frequent complication that we have seen is ulnar neuritis. In four patients symptoms existed prior to surgery but in 12 they developed postoperatively. These were successfully treated by extensive neurolysis. Fractures occurred in five patients, two of whom involved the olecranon and three the ulnar epicondyle. Three fractures were caused by trauma and two occurred spontaneously (one 11 years postoperatively). Two of the fractures were treated by osteosynthesis and two were left

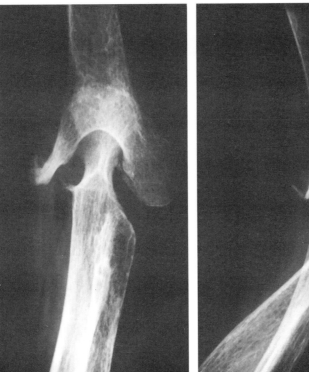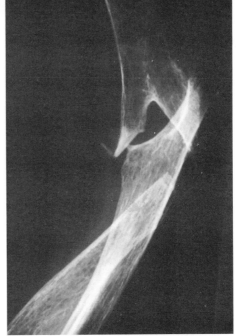

Fig. 25.5 Massive bone resorption in the intercondylar area including the olecranon fossa, 12 years after resection interposition arthroplasty in a patient with rheumatoid arthritis.

untreated as the patients were asymptomatic. In one patient the bony fragment was excised.

Two superficial wound breakdowns healed with conservative treatment. There were no deep infections.

Revision and endoprosthetic replacement was necessary in three cases (5%) due to painful stiffness.

The patients assessment of their surgery was generally less enthusiastic than after endoprothetic replacement; 69% of our patients were fully satisfied, 11% had some reservation and 20% were dissatisfied due to pain, instability and/or insufficient mobility.

A detailed assessment of our new resection, interposition and suspension arthroplasty has not as

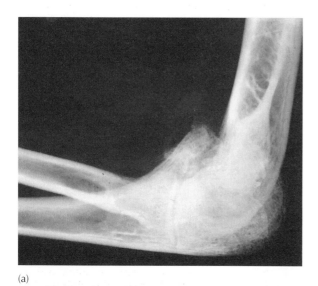

(a)

Fig. 25.6 x-Rays of a 26-year-old rheumatoid female patient with ankylosis of the right elbow – lateral view (a) preoperatively; (b) postoperatively active flexion; (c) postoperatively, active extension.

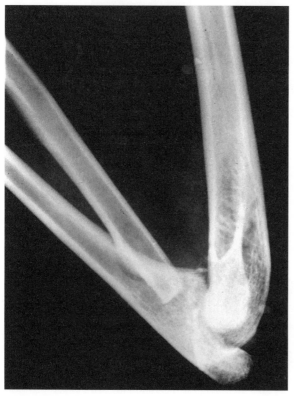

(b)

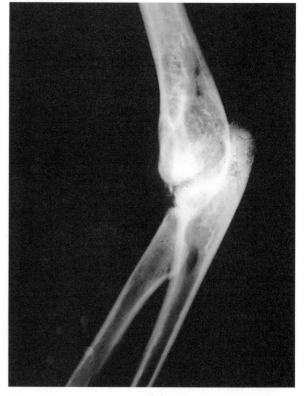

(c)

yet been undertaken since to date we have only treated 10 patients with a maximum follow-up of 5 years. However, our initial impression is that the gain in mobility and the postoperative stability are both superior to what has been achieved by the interposition arthroplasty (Fig. 25.6a-c). In addition the postoperative treatment is less demanding for the patients.

References

1. Ollier L Demonstration anatomique de la reconstitution du coude après la resection sousperiostée. Examen d'une serie de 106 cas des cette operation. *Zentralbl Chir* 1982; **9:** 548–9.
2. Helferich H Ein Neues Operationsverfahren zur Heilung der knochernen Kiefergelenksankylose. *Verh Dtsch Ges Chir* 1984; **23:** 504–10.
3. McAusland WR Arthroplasty of the elbow. *New Engl J Med* 1947; **236:** 97–9.
4. Campbell WC Arthroplasty of the elbow. *Ann Surg* 1992; **76:** 615.
5. Putti V Arthroplasty. *Am J Orthop Surg* 1921; **3:** 421.
6. Payr E Uber die operative Mobilisierung ankylosierter. *Gelenke Munch Med Wochenschr* 1910; **57:** 1921–7.
7. Lexer E Uber Gelenktransplantationen. *Arch Klin Chir* 1909; **90:** 263.
8. Morrey BF Distration arthroplasty. In: *The elbow.* Morrey B (ed) New York: Raven Press, 1994: 307–28.
9. Herbert JJ Traitement des ankyloses du coude dans le rhematisme. *Rev Chir Orthop* 1958; **44:** 87–90.
10. Vainio K Arthroplasty of the elbow and hand in rheumatoid arthritis. In: *Synovectomy and arthroplasty in rheumatoid arthritis.* Chapehal G (ed). Stuttgart: George Thieme, 1967: 66–70.
11. Porter BB, Richardson C, Vainio K Rheumatoid arthritis of the elbow: The results of synovectomy. *J Bone Joint Surg* 1974; **56B:** 427–37.
12. Bontemps G. Meyer G. Tillmann K Synovektomie und Arthroplastiken des Ellenbogengelenkes beichronischer Polyarthritis arthritis. *Orthop Praxis* 1975; **11:** 895–9.
13. Gschwend N *Die operative Behandlung der chronischen Polyarthritis.* Stuttgart:Thieme, 1977; 63–8.
14. Thabe H, Tillmann K Spatergebnisse von Resektions-Arthroplastiken der oberen Extremitaten bei chronischer Polyarthritis im Bergleich zur Alloarthroplastik. *Orthop. Praxis* 1983; **19:** 662–70.
15. Linclau LA, Winiawe CA, Korst JK Synovectomy of the elbow in rheumatoid arthritis. *Acta Orthop Scand* 1983; **54:** 935–7.
16. Brumfield RH, Resnick CT Synovectomy of the elbow in Rheumatoid Arthritis. *J Bone Joint Surg* 1985; **67A:** 16–20.
17. Inglis AE, Figgie MP Rheumatoid arthritis. In: *The elbow and its disorders.* Morrey BF (ed) Philadelphia: WB Saunders Co, 1993: 751–66.
18. Ferlic DC, Patchett CE, Clayton ML, Freeman AC Elbow synovectomy in rheumatoid arthritis. *Clin Orthop* 1987; **220:** 119–25.
19. Tillmann K Recent advances in the surgical treatment of rheumatoid arthritis. *Clin Orthop* 1990; **258:** 62–72.
20. Dickson RA, Stein H, Bentley G Excision arthroplasty of the elbow in rheumatoid disease. *J Bone Joint Surg* 1976; **58B:** 227–9.
21. Raunio P, Jakob R Die Ellenbogenarthroplastik in der rheumatoiden Arthritis. *Orthopade* 1973; **2:** 102–4.
22. Ruther W, Tillmann K Resection interposition arthroplasty of the elbow in rheumatoid arthritis. In: *Replacement and non-endoprosthetic procedures.* Ruther W (ed) Berlin: Springer Verlag, 1996; 57–67.
23. Uupaa V Anatomical interposition arthroplasty with dermal graft A study of 51 elbow arthroplasties on 48 rheumatoid patients. *Z Rheumatol* 1987; **46:** 132–5.
24. Hass J Die Mobilisierung ankylotischer Ellenbogen – und Kniegelenke mittels Arthroplastik. *Arch Klin Chir* 1930; **160:** 693–715.

CHAPTER 26

Total elbow arthroplasty

HIROSHI KUDO, ALAN LETTIN, DAVID STANLEY

Introduction

The development of elbow arthroplasties has significantly improved the quality of life for many patients suffering with disabling elbow disorders. The ability to successfully replace a severely damaged elbow joint results not only in that joint frequently becoming pain free but also often results in an improvement in the range of movement. In addition because of the reduction in elbow pain the function of the whole ipsilateral limb may often benefit markedly.

Historical review

Robineau in 1927[1] was the first to describe an artificial replacement for the elbow. The design was a hemiarthroplasty for the distal humerus comprising a metal implant covered with rubber. More recent distal humeral designs have been made with acrylic,[2,3] nylon,[4] Teflon[5] and Vitallium.[6–8] The implants have usually incorporated loops for muscle

attachment to the condyles and intramedullary stems with holes in order to enable screw fixation to the humerus (Fig. 26.1). In addition to humeral hemiarthroplasties ulnar[9] and radial head replacements have also been designed.[10,11] With a few exceptions,[9,12] however, the long-term results of these implants have not been satisfactory and interest has now focused on total joint replacement.

Total elbow replacement began in the early 1940s when Boerema and de Waard[13] reported their experience of using a single-axis metallic hinge arthroplasty for elbow reconstruction. This was followed by other hinge designs[14–16] all of which gave encouraging early results but were noted quite quickly to be associated with loosening predominantly on the humeral side of the joint.[17] Souter[18] suggested that loosening had several causes including the cyclical loading of the distal humerus, posterior pull of the elbow flexors on the forearm with the elbow at 90 degrees, lateral rotational stresses during supination and pronation, and distraction forces during full elbow flexion. However, it was his opinion that the primary cause of loosening was the transfer of rotational forces across the elbow to the humeral cement/bone interface rather than via the collateral ligaments which had been resected with the epicondyles in order to allow insertion of these early implants.[17]

Further development aimed at reducing the frequency of loosening and improving elbow function led to three different groups of elbow arthroplasty being designed.

1. Constrained hinge arthroplasties
   Early second-phase development rarely used nowadays
2. Semi-constrained arthroplasties
   Linked implants with valgus/varus laxity at the articulation
3. Unlinked or resurfacing arthroplasties
   Depend for stability on implant orientation and soft tissue tensioning.

CONSTRAINED HINGE ARTHROPLASTIES

To overcome humeral loosening Nederpelt[19] supplemented his humeral component with a posteriorly positioned metal plate which was fixed with screws to the intramedullary humeral implant (Fig. 26.2). Later a further modification involved the use of an anterior high density polyethylene plate. This

was added in order to resist rotational and posteriorly displacing forces.

An alternative hinge prosthesis, the Stanmore elbow developed in England by Lettin and Scales[20] enabled preservation of the collateral ligaments. The implant, a slim metal design with long humeral and ulnar stems had a high density polyethylene bushing between the two components (Fig. 26.3).

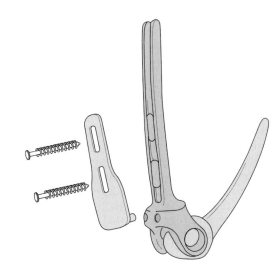

Fig. 26.2 Nederpelt's prosthesis. This was a fully constrained hinge implant which was supplemented by a posteriorly positioned metal plate. Later an anterior high density polyethylene plate was also added. Despite these modifications loosening remained a problem.

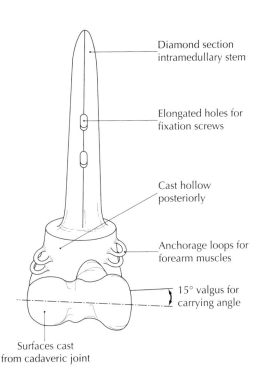

Diamond section intramedullary stem

Elongated holes for fixation screws

Cast hollow posteriorly

Anchorage loops for forearm muscles

15° valgus for carrying angle

Surfaces cast from cadaveric joint

Fig. 26.1 The distal humeral implant of Mellen and Phalan (1947),[2] which was hand-carved acrylic and used as an alternative to excision arthroplasty.

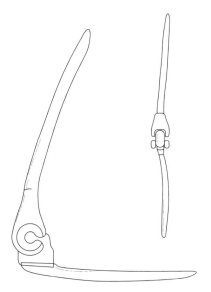

Fig. 26.3 The Stanmore elbow replacement. This implant had long humeral and ulnar stems with a high-density polyethylene bushing between the components.

Although the overall results of this implant were much better than the original hinge designs, radiological loosening remained a problem and has been reported at 20%.[21] In addition 9% have required revision.[21]

SEMI-CONSTRAINED ARTHROPLASTIES

Semi-constrained implants differ significantly from constrained hinge prostheses since although the humeral and ulnar components are linked the design permits valgus and varus laxity. The articulation between the components is able, at least in part, to accommodate the valgus and varus changes of normal elbow movement. This is of importance since theoretically it reduces the stress forces at the bone/cement interface[22] and should therefore in practice reduce implant loosening. Elbows incorporating this principle include the Schlein,[23] Pritchard-Walker,[24] and Triaxial.[25] All of these arthroplasties have been shown to give improved results over the original constrained hinge prostheses although the incidence of loosening still remains a problem.[23,25,26]

More encouraging results have been obtained with the Gschwend–Scheier–Bahler (GSB) and the Coonrad–Morrey arthroplasties. These devices whilst being semi-constrained also have additional features which provide improved humeral fixation.

The GSB implant (Fig. 26.4) has a humeral component that is fan-shaped distally and has flanges that are impacted over the humeral condyles. In addition the link axle between the humeral and ulnar components is surrounded by high density polyethylene and allows 4 degrees of valgus and varus angulation during elbow movement.[27,28]

The Coonrad–Morrey prosthesis has a triangular humeral stem with a link articulation to the ulna which permits 7–10 degrees of hinge laxity. The distal humerus and proximal ulnar stems are porous coated and there is an anterior flange at the distal humerus (Fig. 26.5). Bone graft is inserted between the flange and anterior distal humeral cortex enhancing fixation of the humeral component.[29] The implant is designed for fixation with methylmethacrylate cement and has been used for a wide variety of indications including the treatment of rheumatoid arthritis, post-traumatic arthritis and revision surgery.[30–32]

UNLINKED OR RESURFACING ARTHROPLASTIES

The early resurfacing arthroplasties required minimal bone resection and were designed as shell fit replacements to the distal humerus and proximal ulna. The components were unlinked and depended for their stability on accurate implant orientation and appropriate soft tissue tensioning. They included the Wadsworth,[33] Lowe–Miller[34] and original Kudo implant (Fig. 26.6).

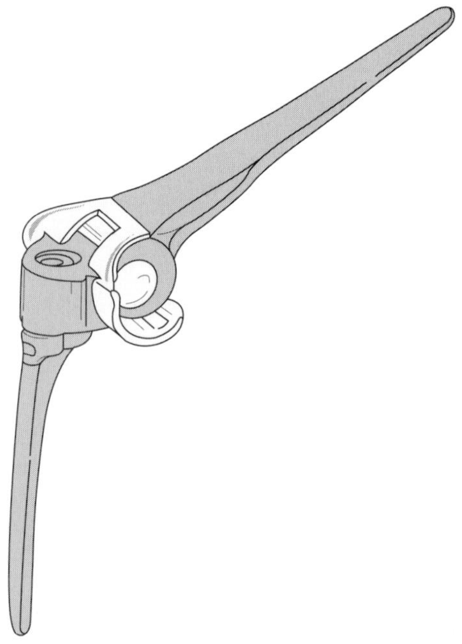

Fig. 26.4 The GSB III prosthesis. A semi-constrained implant with 4 degrees of valgus and varus angulation. The metal flanges are impacted over the humeral condyles.

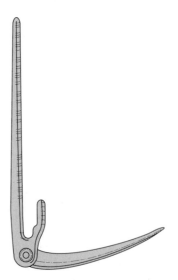

Fig. 26.5 The Coonrad–Morrey prosthesis. A semi-constrained implant. The anterior humeral flange provided improved fixation of the humeral component.

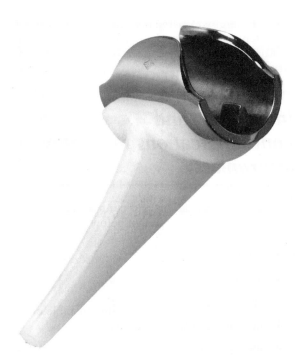

Fig. 26.6 The original Kudo implant. The shape of the humeral component was basically similar to a cylinder.

Unfortunately although these prostheses were unlinked, loosening remained a problem.[34,35] To overcome this complication the Kudo elbow underwent several modifications. The initial cylindrical humeral implant was changed to a saddle shape whilst the opposing articular surface of the ulnar component underwent reciprocal change. The new design appeared successful and interim results published in 1980[36] were very encouraging. However, with longer follow-up it became apparent that loosening of the humeral component was more frequent than previously realised and thus in 1983 the humeral component was modified by adding an intramedullary stem in order to achieve more secure fixation. The stem was set at 5 degrees valgus and 20 degrees anterior flexion to the articular portion of the component. In 1988 a cementless prosthesis was introduced and in 1991 the base of the humeral stem was reinforced in order to resist the high stresses experienced at this site (Fig. 26.7).

In addition to the Kudo arthroplasty two other unlinked prostheses are currently widely used. These are the capitello–condylar implant designed by Ewald, and the Souter–Strathclyde replacement developed in Edinburgh.

The capitellar–condylar implant is a shell fit prosthesis with an intramedullary stem (Fig. 26.8). It

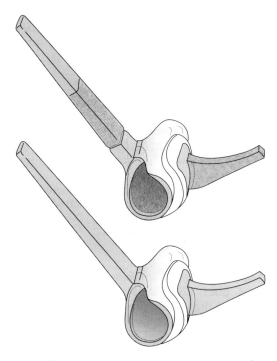

Fig. 26.7 The Kudo type-5 implant (current prosthesis). The humeral component is made of cobalt-chromium alloy, and the base of the stem is mechanically reinforced to prevent breakage. Only one-third of the surface area of the stem is porous coated. The ulnar has an option without metal back support.

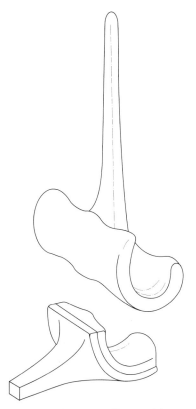

Fig. 26.8 The capitello–condylar implant designed by Ewald. It is an unlinked resurfacing prosthesis.

OPERATIVE TECHNIQUE FOR THE KUDO ARTHROPLASTY

The patient is placed in the semi-lateral position with the arm across the chest and with the posterior aspect of the elbow facing superiorly. A high tourniquet is applied. A straight midline skin incision is made with its centre at the tip of the olecranon. The ulnar nerve is extensively released and protected before exposure of the joint space. The nerve is dissected free as far distally as possible beyond the cubital tunnel. This is done by splitting the muscle of the flexor carpi ulnaris and also by releasing the nerve from the deep pronator–flexor aponeurosis. Occasionally in rheumatoid arthritis the ulnar nerve is constricted or kinked at this site.[56]

To expose the joint Campbell's posterior approach is used[57] (Chapter 7). This provides an excellent exposure even in elbows with severe deformity. In addition, if necessary, it permits lengthening of the triceps tendon. The radial head is always excised, and the ulnar collateral ligament, including the tight anterior band is usually cut in order to allow dislocation and adequate access to the interior of the joint. Distal humeral preparation (Fig. 26.10) followed by preparation of the ulna (Fig. 26.11) is then undertaken. It should be noted that secure fixation of the ulnar component depends not only on the presence of good bone stock in the coronoid process but also on adequate bony support in the olecranon.

After placement of the trial components and reduction of the dislocation a check is made for

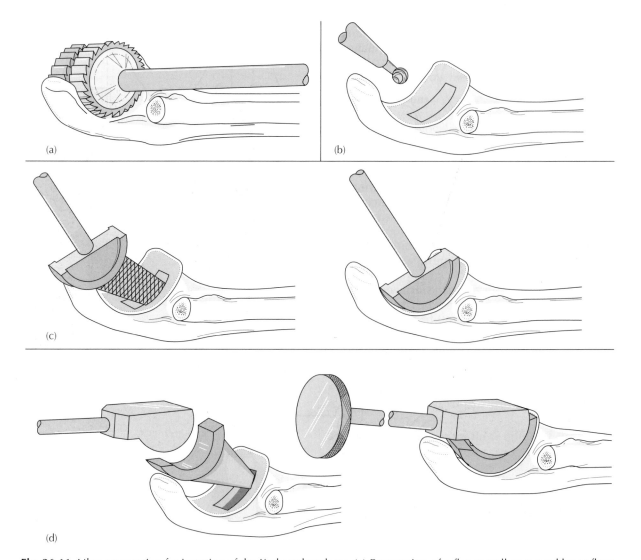

Fig. 26.11 Ulna preparation for insertion of the Kudo arthroplasty. (a) Preparation of a flat as well as curved bone floor using a barrel trimmer. (b) A rectangular hole is made to open the medullary canal. (c) Rasping of the medullary canal of the ulna. (d) Final insertion of the ulna component.

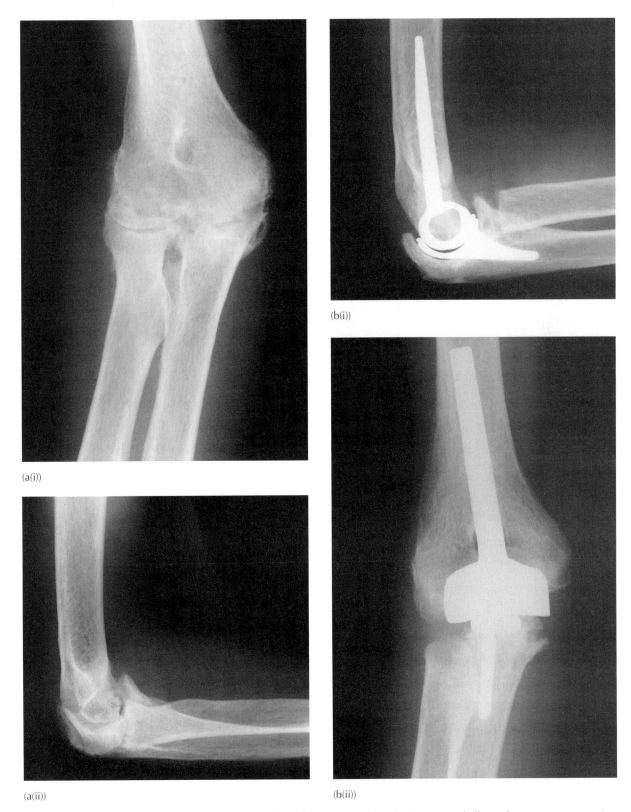

(a(i))

(a(ii))

(b(i))

(b(ii))

Fig. 26.12 (a) Preoperative anteroposterior (i) and lateral (ii) radiographs of a rheumatoid elbow showing severe erosion of the joint. (b) Postoperative radiographs of the same patient. Both the humeral and ulnar components were inserted without cement.

impingement of bone on the prosthesis. If present the bone is trimmed. The range of motion is then examined. Usually it will be possible to obtain more than 120 degrees of flexion although full extension is rare.

Acrylic cement fixation is necessary in 70% of the ulnar components whilst the other 30% are inserted as a press fit. In contrast the humeral component can be inserted as a press fit in almost 95% of cases (Fig. 26.12).

In order to prevent postoperative dislocation or residual instability, the incised ends of the triceps tendon and the incised margins of the dorsal fascial layer of the radial side of the olecranon are meticulously sutured. This is a key factor in preventing dislocation. In some instances the triceps tendon may need to be lengthened in a V-Y fashion to achieve a good arc of flexion.

Kudo transposes the ulnar nerve anteriorly and subcutaneously before closing the wound over a suction drain. The elbow is then immobilised in 60 degrees of flexion in a posterior splint for 1 week before mobilisation is permitted.

RESULTS OF UNLINKED RESURFACING ARTHROPLASTIES

Resurfacing arthroplasties can give good or excellent results in up to 90% of patients providing the indications for surgery have been appropriate.[36,38,48,47] Pain relief is frequently significantly improved[47,54] (Table 26.1) as is the patient's ability to undertake activities of daily living[47] (Table 26.2). Range of elbow motion is also generally better postoperatively. Kudo noted that the average preoperative flexion increased from 106 degrees to 131 degrees postoperatively whilst there was no significant improvement in extension.[54] The average range of pronation increased from 39 degrees to 46 degrees whilst average supination increased from 40 degrees to 61 degrees postoperatively.[54] All of these improvements were statistically significant.

Table 26.1 Pre- and postoperative pain levels in 26 elbows of 25 patients (Souter–Strathclyde implant)

Pain	Preoperative	Postoperative
None	0	14
Occasional twinges usually at night	0	8
Mild	4	2
Substantial	10	2
Severe	12	0

Adapted from Ref. 47.

Table 26.2 Daily living activities pre- and postoperatively in 26 elbows of 25 patients (semi-Strathclyde implant)

Activity	Preoperative	Postoperative
Hand to mouth	20	26
Can lift teacup	13	24
Can lift kettle	7	22
Hand to perineum	12	22
Light household tasks	17	23
Most household tasks	4	10

Adapted from Ref. 47.

Management of rheumatoid elbow disease using semi-constrained arthroplasties

The rationale for using semi-constrained arthroplasties for the treatment of rheumatoid elbow disease lies in the fact that although the humeral and ulna components are linked the angular laxity at the articulation reduces the stresses on the bone/cement interface.[22,29] In addition, this type of implant can be used in patients with more extensive bone loss, where ligament and soft tissue stability is poor, and in patients who require revision surgery.

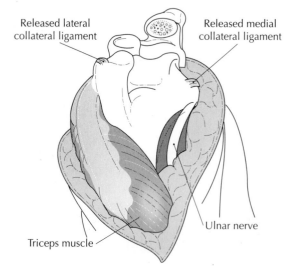

Fig. 26.13 The Bryan–Morrey approach to the elbow. The tip of the olecranon is excised. The ulnar nerve is transposed anteriorly. The medial and lateral collateral ligaments are released and the radial head debrided or excised.

OPERATIVE TECHNIQUE FOR THE COONRAD–MORREY ARTHROPLASTY

Although various posterior approaches to the elbow have been reported[57–59] the approach that will be outlined here is that described by Bryan and Morrey[60] (Chapter 7). The operative technique is as described by Morrey and Adam[29]

The patient is placed in the supine position with a sandbag under the shoulder and with the arm across the chest. A high tourniquet is applied and the arm is prepared and draped. A straight skin incision approximately 15 cm in length is made just medial and centred on the tip of the olecranon. The ulnar nerve is identified freed and transposed anteriorly.

By sharp dissection the triceps extensor mechanism together with the periosteum on the proximal ulna and forearm fascia are reflected laterally. This allows exposure of the distal humerus, proximal ulna and radial head. The medial and lateral collateral ligaments are released and the tip of the olecranon is excised (Fig. 26.13). The elbow is dislocated. Preparation of the humerus and ulna are undertaken using the Coonrad–Morrey guides and rasps (Fig. 26.14). The excised trochlea, removed at the time of humeral preparation is made into an appropriate shape and used as bone graft. The humeral and ulnar meduallary canals are then cleaned and the prosthesis is cemented in place with the trochlea bone graft being inserted between the distal anterior humeral surface and the anterior flange of the humeral component (Fig. 26.15).

The triceps is reattached to the ulna with sutures that pass through the tip of the olecranon and the

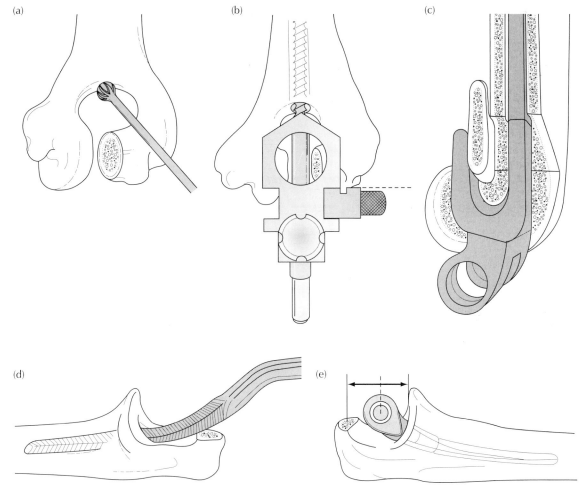

(a)　　　(b)　　　(c)

(d)　　　(e)

Fig. 26.14 Preparation of the humerus and ulna for insertion of the Coonrad–Morrey prosthesis. (a) Opening of the humeral medullary canal. (b) Use of the Coonrad–Morrey instruments to accurately prepare the humerus. (c) Insertion of the humeral component with anterior bone graft. (d) Preparation of the ulna. (e) Insertion of the ulnar component. The centre of the ulnar component should align with the projected centre of the greater sigmoid fossa.

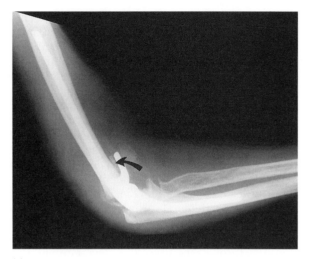

(a)

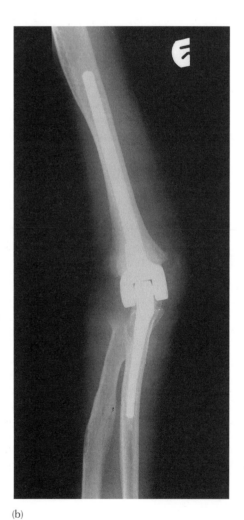

(b)

Fig. 26.15 Radiographs showing a total elbow replacement using the Coonrad–Morrey prosthesis. The bone graft between the anterior humeral cortex and flange of the humeral component is clearly seen.

proximal ulna. The tourniquet is deflated, haemostasis achieved and the wound closed over two suction drains. A compressive dressing is applied with the elbow splinted in full extension by an anteriorly placed plaster slab. Mobilisation of the elbow is permitted after 3–5 days.

RESULTS OF SEMI-CONSTRAINED ARTHROPLASTIES

Semi-constrained arthroplasties can be used for all patients who meet the criteria for total elbow replacement.[28,51,52,61–63] The results obtained by using these prostheses in rheumatoid patients are comparable with the results of unlinked surface replacement.

Gschwend *et al.* found a significant reduction in elbow pain postoperatively in patients undergoing elbow replacement with the GSB III prosthesis[28] (Table 26.3). In addition he noted that most of the patients had satisfactory flexion power of 4+ to 5 (5 being normal) although extension power was often weaker. Despite this, 70% of the patients with extension power of 4 to 4+ were able to extend their arms against resistance even through the last 30 degrees of extension.[28] The improvement in range of motion is shown in Table 26.4.

The Mayo clinic experience of semi-constrained prostheses has been primarily with the Pritchard Mark II implant[26] and more recently with the Mayo modified Coonrad (Coonrad–Morrey) implant.[29] Using the Pritchard Mark II implant, pain relief was obtained in 90% of patients. The mean arc of flexion and extension was from 30 degrees – 135 degrees with 60 degrees of pronation and 65 degrees of supination.[29]

Since 1981 over 250 Mayo modified Coonrad implants have been inserted at the Mayo clinic; 45% have been for rheumatoid arthritis with the

Table 26.3 Pre- and postoperative pain levels in 57 patients undergoing total elbow replacement using the GSB III prosthesis

Pain	Preoperative		Postoperative	
	No	%	No	%
None	0		41	(72)
Mild	2	(3.5)	12	(21)
Moderate	10	(17.5)	3	(5.5)
Severe	45	(79)	1	(1.5)

Adapted from Ref. 28.

Table 26.4 Pre- and postoperative range of motion in patients undergoing total elbow replacement using the GSB III prosthesis

	Preoperative	Postoperative
Fixed flexion	37.9 degrees + 19.8 degrees	29.2 degrees + 15.5 degrees
Flexion	119.5 degrees + 23.5 degrees	140 degrees + 9.1 degrees
Pronation	59.7 degrees + 23.9 degrees	68.6 degrees + 17.4 degrees
Supination	43.3 degrees + 29.3 degrees	64.2 degrees + 24.8 degrees

Adapted from Ref. 28.

remainder being inserted for post-traumatic arthritis and revision procedures.[29] Within the rheumatoid arthritis group of patients Morrey and Adams have reported 91% to have little or no pain when followed for a mean of 3.8 years.[30] In addition they reported that flexion improved by an average of 11 degrees and extension by an average of 12 degrees (average arc 20 degrees – 129 degrees). The average arc of pronation was 78 degrees, an increase of 14 degrees and the average arc of supination was 77 degrees, an increase of 18 degrees.[30]

Complications

Gschwend in a review of the literature 1986–92 identified a high complication rate following total elbow arthroplasty[64] (Table 26.5). This Morrey feels is related to the elbow, being:

1. an anatomically and biomechanical complex joint;
2. poorly covered with soft tissue;
3. intimately related to the ulnar nerve.[65]

The complications that are associated with total elbow replacement may be grouped into those

Table 26.5 Literature 1986–92 (total of 828 elbow arthroplasties)

	No of arthroplasties	%
All complications	357	43.1
Revision rate	151	18
Permanent complications	124	15

Adapted from Ref. 64.

occurring at the time of surgery (intraoperative) and those occurring following surgery (postoperative).

INTRAOPERATIVE COMPLICATIONS

Bone fractures

Intraoperative fractures occur in less than 3% of total elbow replacements.[65] If this happens during bone preparation for an unlinked resurfacing implant it may be necessary to consider inserting a semi-constrained prosthesis in order to obtain a sufficiently sound prosthetic fixation. The fracture itself should be fixed with either Kirschner wires[65] or screws.

Ulnar neuritis

The incidence of ulnar neuritis following total elbow replacement has been reported from 1.7%[64] to 26%.[41] The majority of cases are neuropraxias which fully recover and persisting sensory and motor deficits occur in less than 5%.[35,66,67] The cause of this complication is probably multifactorial but undoubtedly the nerve will be damaged if its blood supply is compromised during mobilisation, if traction is applied to the nerve or if the nerve is incompletely released. It is to prevent this complication that Kudo releases the nerve to the level of the deep pronator–flexor aponeurosis. Other factors that may damage the nerve include direct surgical trauma, haematoma formation, and thermal injury from methylmethacrylate cement. It has also been suggested that minor lengthening of the limb can be produced by inserting an elbow arthroplasty and that this can stretch and damage the ulnar nerve.[64]

Patients who develop this complication require careful assessment. Further surgery is usually not indicated unless there is concern that the nerve may have been injured by direct surgical trauma or by haematoma formation.

POSTOPERATIVE COMPLICATIONS

Wound problems

Although occasionally wound healing problems may occur they can be minimised by careful attention to detail. The skin incision should be straight, and large skin flaps should be avoided. The tourniquet should be deflated prior to closure and haemostasis achieved. The wound should then be closed over two suction drains. Immediate postoperative splinting should either be in extension or slight flexion in order to reduce the pressure on the skin incision.

Infection

Gschwend in his review of late complications of elbow arthroplasty identified an infection rate of 8.1%.[64] This is similar to Morrey's literature review figure of 7.0% for unlinked resurfacing arthroplasties and 6% for semi-constrained implants.[65] However, both Gschwend *et al.*[64] and Morrey[65] state that their own infection rates are less than 3%.

The treatment options for an infected total elbow replacement are either removal of the prosthesis with conversion to a resection arthroplasty or a revision joint replacement.[63,64] Occasionally if infection is diagnosed early, debridement and antibiotic therapy may be successful and avoid the need to remove the prosthesis.[63] If reimplantation surgery is considered Gschwend advises a one-stage revision in the presence of a Gram-positive bacteria but a two-stage procedure if the infecting organism is Gram-negative. The first operation involves removal of the implant and bone cement together with a thorough debridement of the soft tissues. The second operation to reinsert an elbow arthroplasty is usually undertaken after 6–8 weeks.[64]

Extensor mechanism insufficiency

Morrey has stated that triceps insufficiency probably occurs more frequently than is reported.[65] It may result from stretching or dehiscence of the suture line when the Campbell approach to the elbow is used[57] or it may be secondary to pull-off of the triceps from the ulna when the Bryan–Morrey approach is used.[60]

To reduce the incidence of this complication the extensor mechanism should be carefully repaired after insertion of the elbow prosthesis.

Instability

Instability is a complication of unlinked resurfacing implants. Gschwend in an analysis of the world's literature between 1986 and 1992 found an average rate of 6.5% dislocations and subluxations.[64] The direction of the instability may be laterally, anteriorly or dorsally and it results from ligamentous insufficiency, inadequate soft tissue tensioning or inaccurate implant alignment[68–70] (Fig. 26.16).

If the soft tissues are incompetent, reconstruction with particular attention to the ulnar collateral ligament or revision to a semi-constrained implant is usually required. Occasionally immobilisation with the elbow in flexion for 3–6 weeks may be of benefit. When soft tissue reconstruction is undertaken the patient should be advised that the price for improved stability may well be increased elbow stiffness.[68] Despite this, soft tissue reconstruction is usually preferable to revision of a well fixed resurfacing prosthesis to a semi-constrained implant since such a procedure has a high complication rate.

Ectopic bone

Although ectopic bone formation has been reported after total elbow arthroplasty[50] it appears to be an uncommon complication which is rarely seen.

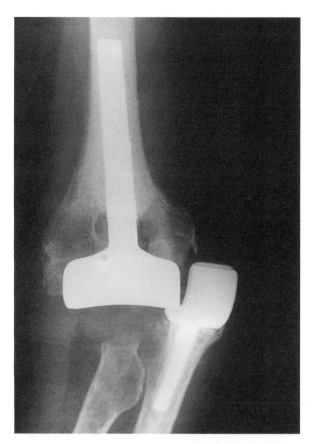

Fig. 26.16 Instability in the form of subluxation of a Kudo total elbow arthroplasty.

Aseptic loosening

Aspectic loosening of elbow arthroplasties is a well recognised complication which first became apparent with the follow-up of the original hinge arthroplasties.[14–17,19,21,71] The Mayo experience is that approximately 25% of constrained hinge elbow arthroplasties loosen within 5 years.[72] Loosening in this group of implants has several causes of which transfer of rotational forces across the elbow to the humeral cement/bone interface is probably the most important.[17] Loosening of unconstrained resurfacing implants without humeral stems[73,74] is thought to be related to insufficient bone stock preventing solid primary stability (despite cement fixation) and also inadequate ligament support to transmit the rotational forces across the elbow.[64] These problems at least in part have been overcome by the development of semi-constrained implants and resurfacing arthroplasties with improved humeral fixation usually in the form of an intramedullary stem. In a review of the recent literature on total elbow replacements in rheumatoid patients, Morrey found a loosening rate of approximately 2% in patients treated with unconstrained resurfacing implants and a rate of less than 2% for those having semi-constrained prostheses.[65]

Another important factor as a cause of aseptic loosening is surgical technique. An inaccurately inserted poorly cemented prosthesis will have an increased risk of loosening compared with an appropriately positioned and well cemented implant.

When loosening occurs it usually affects the humeral side of the arthroplasty[72,75] and results in the proximal tip of the implant displacing anteriorly (Fig. 26.17). Loosening of the ulnar component is less frequent.[21]

The treatment options for aseptic loosening are either to remove the implant leaving a resection arthroplasty or to undertake a revision arthroplasty. Both these techniques have been discussed earlier in this chapter and are dealt with in greater detail in Chapters 25 and 27.

Implant failure

In Gschwend's review of elbow arthroplasty complications an incidence of 0.6% prosthetic fractures was noted.[64] This complication, usually associated with implant loosening, occurs most often at the junction between the stable and loosened parts of the prosthesis.

Kudo also noticed this problem with breakage of the stem of the humeral component (Fig. 26.18). To

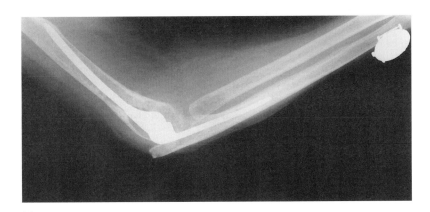

(a)

Fig. 26.17 Aseptic loosening of a Stanmore total elbow replacement. The tip of the humeral component has displaced anteriorly.

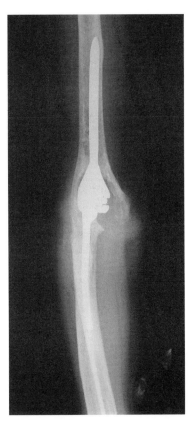

(b)

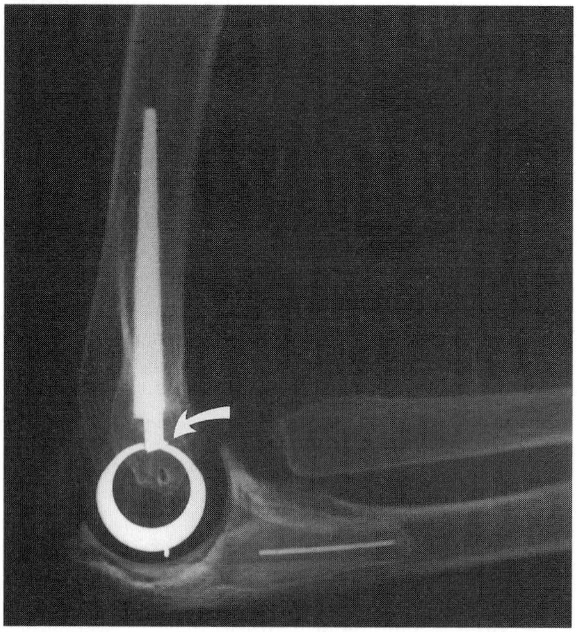

Fig. 26.18 Lateral radiograph of the type-4 Kudo prosthesis. It had been *in situ* 2½ years. A fracture at the base of the stem humeral component can be clearly seen.

overcome this complication strengthening of the humeral stem was introduced in 1991.

Disassembly or uncoupling is another important problem that may occur with semi-constrained prostheses. Gschwend had an incidence of 3.5% in his series using the GSB prosthesis.[64] He suggested that it occurred if the soft tissue release was too extensive or if the centre of rotation was incorrectly located.[76]

Wear of both unlinked resurfacing implants and semi-constrained prostheses produces high-density polyethylene debris which damages the bone cement interface and ultimately results in implant loosening. With semi-constrained prostheses the small articular bushings are perhaps more prone to wear because of the local force concentration.

Although it may be possible to treat some of these implant failures by replacement of the articular bushings or reassembly of an uncoupled implant, revision joint replacement is often necessary. This topic is dealt with fully in the following chapter (Chapter 27).

References

1. Robineau R Contribution à l'etude des prosthèses osseuses. *Bull Mim Soc Nat Chir* 1927; **53:** 886.
2. Mellen RH, Phalen GS Arthroplasty of the elbow by replacement of the distal portion of the humerus with an acrylic prosthesis. *J Bone Joint Surg* 1947; **29:** 348–53.
3. Silva JF Arthroplasty of the elbow-acrylic prosthesis for the distal humerus. *Singapore Med J* 1967; **8:** 222–9.
4. MacAusland WR Replacement of the lower end of the humerus with a prosthesis. *J Surg Gyn Obst* 1954; **62:** 557–66.
5. Silva JF The problems relating to old dislocations and the restriction on elbow movement. *Acta Orthop Belg* 1975; **41:** 399–411.
6. Venable CS Elbow and elbow prosthesis – case of complete loss of the lower third of the humerus. *Am J Surg* 1952; **83:** 271–5.
7. Barr JS, Eaton RG Elbow reconstruction with a new prosthesis to replace the distal end of the humerus. *J Bone Joint Surg* 1965; **47A:** 1408–13.
8. Kestler OC Replacement of the distal humerus for reconstruction of the elbow joint. *Bull Hosp Joint Dis* 1970; **31:** 85–90.
9. Johnson EW, Schlein AP Vitallium prosthesis for the olecranon and proximal part of the ulna. *J Bone Joint Surg* 1970; **52A:** 721–4.
10. Cherry JC Use of acrylic prosthesis in the treatment of fracture of the head of the radius. *J Bone Joint Surg* 1953; **35B:** 70–1.
11. Knight DJ, Rymaszewski LA, Miller JH, Amis AA Primary replacement of the fractured radial head with a metal prosthesis. *J Bone Joint Surg* 1993; **75B:** 572–6.
12. Shifrin PG, Johnson DP Elbow Hemiarthroplasty with 20 year follow-up study. A case report and literature review. *Clin Orthop* 1990; **254:** 128–33.
13. Boerema I, de Waard DJ Osteoplastische Verakening von Metall prosthesen bei Pseudarthrose and bei Orthoplastik. *Acta Chir Scand* 1942; **86:** 511–24.
14. Dee R, Sweetnam DR Total replacement arthroplasty of the elbow joint for rheumatoid arthritis: two cases. *Proc Royal Soc Med* 1969; **63:** 653–5.
15. McKee GK Total replacement of the elbow joint. *Proceedings of 12th Sicot Congress*. Amsterdam: Excerpta Medica, 1973: 891–3.
16. Shiers LGP Replacing the shot-out joint. *Roy Naval Med Serv* 1976; **62:** 149–51.
17. Souter WA The evolution of total replacement arthroplasty of the elbow. In: *Elbow joint*. Kashiwagi D (ed) Amsterdam: Elsevier Science Publishers (Biomedical Division), 1985: 255–26.
18. Souter WA Total replacement arthroplasty of the elbow. In: *Joint replacement in the upper limb*. London: Institute of Mechanical Engineers Conference Publications, 1977: 99–106.
19. Nederpelt KJ Eight years of experience with endoprostheses for the elbow joint. *Acta Orthopaedica Belgica* 1975; **41:** 499–504.
20. Scales JT, Lettin AWF, Bayley I The evolution of the Stanmore hinged total elbow replacement 1967–1976. In: *Joint replacement in the upper limb*. London: Institute of Mechanical Engineers Conference Publications, 1977: 53–62.

21. Johnson JR, Getty CJM, Lettin AWF, Glasgow MMS The Stanmore total elbow replacement for rheumatoid arthritis. *J Bone Joint Surg* 1984; **66B:** 732–6.

22. O'Driscoll SW, An KN, Korinek S, Morrey BF Kinematics of semi-constrained total elbow arthroplasty. *J Bone Joint Surg* 1992; **74B:** 297–9.

23. Schlein AP Semi-constrained total elbow arthroplasty. *Clin Orthop* 1976; **121:** 222–9

24. Pritchard RW Flexible elbow joint replacement. In: *Joint replacement in the upper limb.* London: Institute of Mechanical Engineers Conference Publications, 1977: 63–8.

25. Inglis AE, Pellicci PM Total elbow replacement. *J Bone Joint Surg* 1980; **62A:** 1252–8.

26. Pritchard RW Long-term follow-up study: Semi-constrained elbow prosthesis. *Orthopaedics* 1981; **4:** 151–5.

27. Steigher JU, Gschwend N, Bell S GSB elbow arthroplasty: A new concept, and six years experience. In: *Elbow joint.* Kiashiwagi D (ed) Amsterdam: Elsevier Science Publishers (Biomedical Division), 1985: 285–94.

28. Gschwend N, Loehr J, Ivosevic-Radovanovic D *et al.* Semi-constrained elbow prosthesis with special reference to the GSB III prosthesis. *Clin Orthop* 1988; **232:** 104–11.

29. Morrey BF, Adam RA Semi-constrained elbow replacement arthroplasty: Rationale technique and results. In: *The elbow and its disorders.* Morrey BF (ed) Philadelphia: WB Saunders Co, 1993: 648–64.

30. Morrey BF, Adams RA Semi-constrained elbow replacement for rheumatoid arthritis of the elbow. *J Bone joint Surg* 1992; **74A:** 479–90.

31. Morrey BF, Adams RA, Bryan RS Total replacement for post-traumatic arthritis of the elbow. *J Bone Joint Surg* 1991; **73B:** 607–12.

32. Morrey BF Revision of failed total elbow arthroplasty. In: *The elbow and its disorders.* Morrey BF (ed) Philadelphia: WB Saunders Co, 1993: 676–89.

33. Wadsworth TG A new technique of total elbow replacement. *Engineering Med* 1981; **10:** 69–74.

34. Lowe LW, Miller AJ, Allum RL, Higginson DW The development of an unconstrained elbow arthroplasty: A clinical review. *J Bone Joint Surg* 1984; **66B:** 243–7.

35. Rydholm U, Tjornstrand B, Pettersson H, Lidgren I Surface replacement of the elbow in rheumatoid arthritis. Early results with the Wadsworth prosthesis. *J Bone Joint Surg* 1984; **66B:** 737–41.

36. Kudo H, Iwano K, Watanabe S Total replacement of the rheumatoid elbow with a hingeless prosthesis. *J Bone Joint Surg* 1980; **62A:** 277–85.

37. Ewald FC Total elbow replacement. *Orthop Clin North Am* 1975; **6:** 685–96.

38. Ewald FC, Scheinberg RD, Poss R *et al.* Capitello–condylar total elbow arthroplasty two to five year follow-up in rheumatoid arthritis. *J Bone Joint Surg* 1980; **62A:** 1259–63.

39. Ewald FC, Jacobs MA Total elbow arthroplasty. *Clin Orthop* 1984; **182:** 137–42.

40. Davis RF, Weiland AJ, Hungerford DS *et al.* Non-constrained total elbow arthroplasty. *Clin Orthop* 1982; **171:** 156–60.

41. Tranick T, Wilde AH, Borden LS Capitello-condylar total elbow arthroplasty: two to eight year experience. *Clin Orthop* 1987; **223:** 175–80.

42. Dennis DA, Clayton ML, Ferlic DC *et al.* Capitello–condylar total elbow arthroplasty for rheumatoid arthritis. *J Arthroplasty* 1990; **5:** S83–8.

43. Ruth JT, Wilde AH Capitello–condylar total elbow replacement: A long term follow-up study. *J Bone Joint Surg* 1992; **74A:** 95–100.

44. Nicol AC Elbow joint prosthesis design: Biomechanical aspects. PhD thesis University of Strathclyde, Glasgow, 1977.

45. Souter WA A new approach to elbow arthroplasty. *Engineering Med* 1981; **10:** 59–64.

46. Jonsson B, Larsson SE Elbow arthroplasty in rheumatoid arthritis. *Acta Orthop Scand* 1990; **61:** 1344–7.

47. Poll RG, Rozing PM Use of the Souter-Strathclyde total elbow prosthesis in patients who have rheumatoid arthritis. *J Bone Joint Surg* 1991; **73A:** 1227–33.

48. Lyall HA, Cohen B, Clatworthy M, Constant CR Results of the Souter–Strathclyde total elbow arthroplasty in patients with rheumatoid arthritis. *J Arthroplasty* 1994; **9:** 279–84.

49. Street DM, Stevens PS A humeral replacement prosthesis for the elbow: Results in ten elbows. *J Bone Joint Surg* 1974; **56A:** 1147–58.

50. Figgie MP, Inglis AE, Mow CS, Figgie HE Salvage of non-union of supracondylar fracture of the humerus by total elbow arthroplasty. *J Bone Joint Surg* 1989; **71A:** 1058–65.

51. Figgie HE, Inglis AE, Mow CS Total elbow arthroplasty in the face of significant bone stock and soft tissue losses. *J Arthroplasty* 1986; **1:** 71–81.

52. Figgie MP, Inglis AE, Mow CS, Figgie HE Total elbow arthroplasty for complete ankylosis of the elbow. *J Bone Joint Surg* 1989; **71A:** 513–20.

53. Kudo H, Iwano K Total elbow arthroplasty with a non-constrained surface-replacement prosthesis in patients who have rheumatoid arthritis, a long-term follow-up study. *J Bone Joint Surg* 1990; **72A:** 355–62.

54. Kudo H, Iwano K, Nishino J Cementless or hybrid total elbow arthroplasty with titanium-alloy implants. A study of interim clinical results and specific complications. *J Arthroplasty* 1994; **9:** 269–78.

55. Larsen A, Dale K, Eek M Radiographic evaluation of rheumatoid arthritis and related conditions by standard reference films. *Acta Radiologica Diagnosis* 1977; **18:** 481–91.

56. Gabel GT, Amadio PC Reoperation for failed decompression of the ulnar nerve in the region of the elbow. *J Bone Joint Surg* 1990; **72A:** 213–9.

57. Campbell WC Incision for exposure of the elbow joint. *Am J Surg* 1932; **15:** 65–7.

58. Gschwend N Our operative approach to the elbow joint. *Arch Orthop Trauma Surg* 1981; **98:** 143–6.

59. Wolfe SW, Ranawat CS The osteo-anconeus flap. *J Bone Joint Surg* 1990; **72A:** 684–8.

60. Bryan RS, Morrey BF Extensive posterior exposure of the elbow. A triceps-sparing approach. *Clin Orthop* 1982; **166:** 188–92.

61. Goldberg VM, Figgie HE, Inglis AE, Figgie MP Current concepts review – total elbow arthroplasty. *J Bone Joint Surg* 1988; **70A:** 778–83.
62. Inglis AE, Pellicci PM Total elbow replacement. *J Bone Joint Surg* 1980; **62A:** 1252–8.
63. Morrey BF, Bryan RS Infection after total elbow arthroplasty. *J Bone Joint Surg* 1983; **65A:** 330–8.
64. Gschwend N, Simmen BR, Matejovsky Z Late complications in elbow arthroplasty. *J Shoulder Elbow Surg* 1996; **5:** 86–96.
65. Morrey BF Complications of elbow replacement surgery. In: *The elbow and its disorders.* Morrey BF (ed) Philadelphia: WB Saunders Co, 1993: 665–75.
66. Soni RK, Cavendish ME A review of the Liverpool elbow prosthesis from 1974 to 1982. *J Bone Joint Surg* 1984; **66B:** 248–53.
67. Sourmelis SG, Burke FD, Varian JPW A review of total elbow arthroplasty and an early assessment of the Liverpool elbow prosthesis. *J Hand Surg* 1986; **11B:** 407–13.
68. Rosenberg GM, Turner RH Non-constrained total elbow arthroplasty. *Clin Orthop* 1984; **187:** 154–62.
69. Evans BG, Serbousek JC, Mann RJ *et al.* Comparison of mechanical design parameters in current total elbow prostheses. *Trans Orthop Res Soc* 1985; **10:** 100.
70. Figgie HE, Inglis AE Current concepts in total elbow arthroplasty. *Adv Orthop* 1986; **9:** 195–212.
71. Dee R Total replacement arthroplasty of the elbow for rheumatoid arthritis. *J Bone Joint Surg* 1972; **54B:** 88–95.
72. Morrey BF, Bryan RS, Dobyns JH, Linscheid RL Total elbow arthroplasty: A five year experience at the Mayo Clinic. *J Bone Joint Surg* 1981; **63A:** 1050–63.
73. Roper BA, Tuke M, O'Riordan SM, Bulstrode CJ A new unconstrained elbow. A prospective review of 60 replacements. *J Bone Joint Surg* 1986; **68B:** 566–9.
74. Lowe LW The development of an elbow prosthesis at Northwick Park Hospital. *J Roy Soc Med* 1978; **72:** 117–20.
75. Ross AC, Sneath RS, Scales JT Endoprosthetic replacement of the humerus and elbow joint. *J Bone Joint Surg* 1987; **69B:** 652–5.
76. London JT Kinematics of the elbow. *J Bone Joint Surg* 1981; **63A:** 529–35.

CHAPTER 27

Revision total elbow arthroplasty

MARK P FIGGIE

Introduction

Advances in surgical technique and implant design combined with the recognition of the importance of restoring the anatomic relationships of the elbow have led to a decreased complication rate associated with total elbow arthroplasty. However, when failures do occur it may lead to a very complex situation. The surgical solutions for the failed total elbow replacement are usually extremely challenging with high complication rates. The options range from implant removal with resection arthroplasty to revision total elbow arthroplasy and even amputation in severe cases. When faced with a failed total elbow replacement, the surgeon must understand the failure mode, evaluate the remaining soft tissues, bone and neurovascular status and then individualise the treatment option for the patient.

Failure modes

The most common methods of failure necessitating revision elbow replacement include:

1. Loosening
2. Infection
3. Instability
4. Implant failure involving either polyethylene wear or implant fracture.

Periprosthetic fractures which require revision may also occur but are usually associated with loosening. Other causes for poor results include nerve dysfunction, triceps insufficiency, and stiffness. However, these usually do not require revision of the prosthesis.

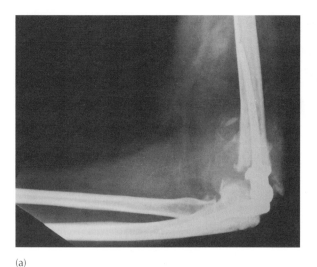

(a)

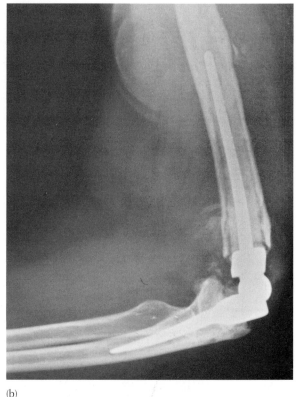

(b)

Fig. 27.1 (a) Total elbow replacement showing characteristic features of loosening with anterior migration of the tip of the humeral component and posterior migration of the distal part of the humeral implant. (b) Revision with centralisation of the humeral stem.

LOOSENING

Aseptic loosening is usually felt to be an implant specific complication with non-constrained implants having lower loosening rates than semi-constrained and constrained devices. Theoretically, non-constrained implants rely on soft tissue stability secondary to ligament support. Thus, loosening rates should be lower because stresses are absorbed by the ligaments and are not transferred directly to the bone–cement interface. However, when used in patients with rheumatoid arthritis, marked osteopenia secondary to steroid use can result in implant loosening.

Most authors have noted low revision rates for humeral loosening with the capitello–condylar prosthesis with rates ranging between 0 and 2%.[1–7] The rates of ulnar component loosening have been higher but the revision rates have been similar.[1–7] Other non-constrained type devices have had higher rates of loosening especially those without humeral stems. The rates of revision for loosening have ranged up to 36%.[8–17] In addition, Kudo documented a 70% humeral subsidence rate with humeral components without stems.[8]

Semi-constrained implants have been associated with higher rates of revision for loosening (Fig. 27.1) ranging between 0 and 14%.[18–29] The early

Coonrad and Mayo devices had revision rates reported at 14% and were later modified to provide more laxity at the articulation.[20,25] With this modification, there have been no revisions for loosening in the latest study with follow-up ranging from 2 to 8 years.[24] In addition, Figgie and associates reported no revisions for loosening among 137 semi-constrained implants using both the Triaxial and Osteonics devices at up to 13-year follow-up.[21]

The fully constrained devices provided excellent initial results but had high failure rates as a result of loosening.[30] This was due to the high stresses at the bone–cement interface due to implant constraint combined with particulate debris from the metal-on-metal articulation. In addition, several of the designs required complete resection of the distal humerus including the origins of flexor and extensor muscles. The loss of the soft tissue supporting sleeve created further stress on the bone–cement interface and resulted in failure due to rotational stresses and torsional loads.

INFECTION

Deep infection is one of the most devastating complications of total elbow replacement (Fig. 27.2). The rates of infection have ranged from 0 to 11%

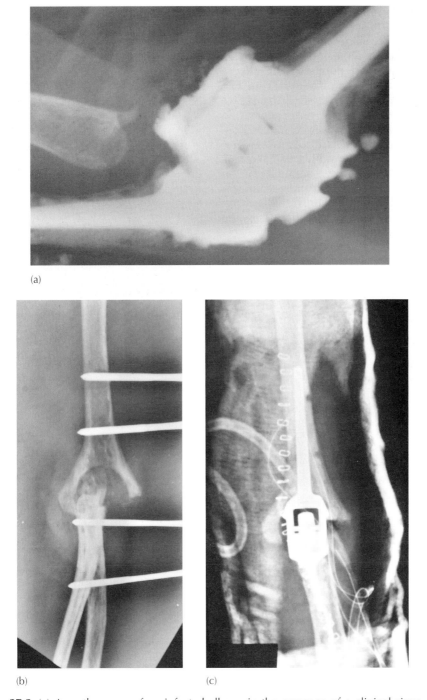

(a)

(b)   (c)

Fig. 27.2 (a) An arthrogram of an infected elbow, in the presence of a clinical sinus. (b) The elbow arthroplasty was removed, cement was debrided and an external fixator applied. (c) After 6 weeks of antibiotic treatment a revision elbow arthroplasty was performed.

but in the larger series, Morrey and Bryan reported a 9% infection rate[31] and Wolfe and associates reported a rate of 7.3%.[32] However, the risk of infection has decreased due to improvements in surgical technique and the use of antibiotic-impreg-

nated cement in some series. Kraay and associates have reported no deep infections in primary total elbow replacements for rheumatoid arthritis since the introduction of antibiotic impregnated cement in 1986.[23] In spite of these improvements, however, the risk of infection still exists due to several reasons. First, the lack of subcutaneous tissue about the elbow makes it more vulnerable to pressure and skin necrosis. In addition, total elbow replacements are usually performed on patients with severe rheumatoid arthritis or post-traumatic arthritis. The patients with end-state rheumatoid arthritis are often taking disease modifying anti-rheumatoid drugs including methotrexate as well as corticosteroids. These patients also place a great deal of pressure on the elbow as they often use them as weight bearing joints during ambulation on platform crutches. Patients with post-traumatic arthritis have often undergone previous surgery, compromising skin vascularity and increasing the risk of wound breakdown.

In the series by Morrey and Bryan,[31] and Wolfe and associates,[32] several risk factors for infection were evaluated. Patients undergoing primary total elbow replacement have a higher risk for infection if they have had any previous elbow surgery. This increase was 12% in Morrey's study[31] and 19% in Wolfe's study.[32] In addition, any subsequent surgery placed the elbow at a 20% risk of infection. Other risk factors for infection included previous infection of the elbow, psychiatric illness, class IV rheumatoid arthritis, postoperative wound drainage, spontaneous drainage after 10 days and ipsilateral shoulder arthritis.[32] The patients with class IV rheumatoid arthritis and ipsilateral shoulder arthritis tend to place greater demands upon the elbow. Morrey and Bryan[31] showed a significantly increased risk of infection in patients taking steroids while Wolfe and colleagues[32] had a 7% risk of infection with those patients undergoing steroid therapy as opposed to 6.6% of those not taking steroids. Combining the two series, the responsible bacteria was *Staphylococcus aureus* in 18 elbows, *Staphylococcus epidermidis* in five and a different organism in each of the five remaining elbows. Nine of these infections occurred between 3 months and 1 year postoperatively while ten occurred after 1 year. The clinical presentation of these patients was extremely varied. In Wolfe's series, 12 of 14 patients had severe pain and 12 had drainage. However, only seven had increased temperature whereas five had erythema and four had swelling. Radiolucency was detected in 10 of the 14 elbows but only four had the scalloping that is typical of infected joint replacements.

INSTABILITY

Non-constrained prostheses

Instability may occur in non-constrained implants if soft tissue balance is not present (Fig. 27.3).

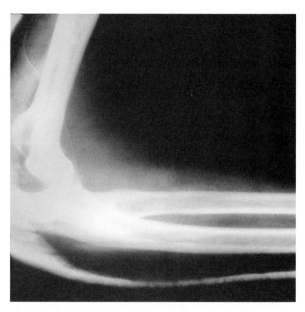

Fig. 27.3 This demonstrates an unstable capitello–condylar replacement. Options for treatment include casting, revision of the humeral component, exploration of the medial side or revision to a semi-constrained device.

Instability may range from subluxation or translocation to frank dislocation. Usually those patients with translocation, where the ulnar component articulates with the capitellum, are functioning well and do not require revision surgery. Frank dislocation has occurred between 3 and 15% in series of capitello–condylar implants.[1–7] In the majority of these series, the dislocations were initially treated by closed reduction and casting for a 4-week period, after which the elbows were gradually mobilised. This form of treatment was successful in more than 50% of the reported cases. In other cases, the medial side of the elbow was explored and attempts were made to reconstruct the medial collateral ligament. The results of this procedure have been inconsistent.[1–3,8,9] Other options for unstable non-constrained implants include revision of the humeral component to increase the carrying angle which tightens the medial soft tissue tension. This has been described in one case each by Ewald and colleagues,[3] Tuke,[16] and Rydholm *et al*.[13] It was successful in two of the three reported cases. A final option for patients with recurrent instability is revision to a semi-constrained implant.

Semi-constrained prostheses

Instability among semi-constrained prostheses has been rare, except with the Pritchard–Walker and

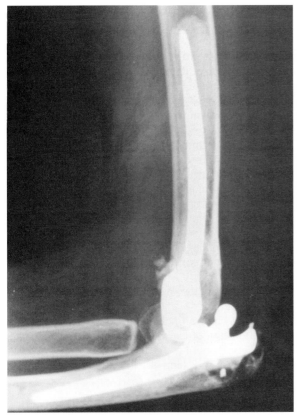

Fig. 27.4 Radiograph showing dislocation of Triaxial component 4½ years postoperatively, secondary to polyethylene wear.

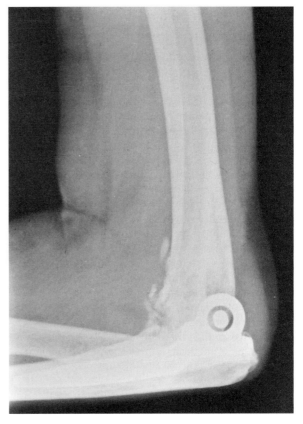

Fig. 27.5 Radiograph of failed Pritchard–Walker implant. Note the humeral component is made of polyethylene which fractured.

Triaxial components. The other semi-constrained devices are usually linked and dislocation only occurs when the locking mechanism has failed. In a study on the original Pritchard–Walker implant, 10 of 269 cases had instability due to faulty locking of the axial pin.[26] Instability in the Triaxial implant is secondary to polyethylene failure (Fig. 27.4). Figgie and associates reported eight late dislocations[27] after 4 years. This led to the redesign of the Triaxial implant to change the load-bearing surface from the condyles to the central region to improve stress distribution and decrease polyethylene wear. In addition, a non-load bearing restraining axle was added to prevent dislocation.

IMPLANT FAILURE

Non-constrained prostheses

There have been few reported fractures in non-constrained prostheses. Two have occurred in capitello–condylar devices with polyethylene ulnar components. One fracture, reported by Rosenberg and Turner, occurred 36 months after surgery as a result of a traumatic incident.[33] The second fracture, reported by Ruth and Wilde, was noted on a 12-year follow-up radiograph.[4] Neither of the patients with fractured prostheses have undergone revision surgery.

Semi-constrained prostheses

The original Pritchard–Walker implant had a high failure rate due to fracture of its all-polyethylene humeral component (Fig. 27.5). Pritchard reported eight humeral component fractures among 269 implants for a rate of 3%.[26]

There has been only one reported fracture of a metal total elbow component and this was reported by Morrey and Adams who had a patient fracture the ulnar component of a Coonrad elbow replacement 27 months after surgery.[24] This patient had resumed heavy manual work which may have contributed to the fracture. Revision of the ulnar component was undertaken.

Initial evaluation

Evaluation of the failed total elbow replacement may be extremely complex. As reported by Wolfe *et al.*[32] the initial presentation of an infected elbow replacement may be varied. Thus, any patient who presents with a painful elbow arthroplasty should be evaluated for possible infection. The same is true for any patient who presents with a loose elbow replacement. In evaluating the failed total elbow replacement, a careful physical examination must be performed. Blood tests are often not helpful as patients with rheumatoid arthritis frequently have elevated sedimentation rates. However, a high white cell count may be suggestive of infection.

During clinical examination a careful assessment of the range of movement and comparison with the previously recorded range of movement is essential. The elbow should be evaluated for stability and swelling. Assessment of ulnar nerve function is critical, but the radial and median nerves should not be ignored. Skin incisions must be carefully reviewed and the patient's biceps and triceps power must be determined.

High quality x-rays are important in evaluating the failed total elbow replacement. These are essential for the assessment of radiolucencies and for comparison with previous x-rays. Loosening may present with minimal changes, but in other cases there can be gross bone destruction due to particulate debris. Cortical thinning may occur with 'ballooning' of the humerus or ulna. Bone resorption can also occur. In a frequent pattern of loosening, the distal part of the humeral implant migrates posteriorly with the tip migrating anteriorly (Fig. 27.1). Fractures, especially at the level of the epicondyles, should be sought and if there is any question as to the quality of the remaining bone stock, computed tomography (CT) scans should be performed in order to determine bone geometry. In the loose total elbow replacement, or if infection is suspected, aspiration should be performed and the sample sent for microscopy, culture and sensitivity. Bone scans may be helpful in the work-up of a potentially infected elbow but we find no use for magnetic resonance imaging in a failed total elbow replacement. An electromyogram is often an excellent preoperative study in patients who present with any neurologic dysfunction.

In cases where there may be elbow instability that is not demonstrable on plain x-rays, fluoroscopy is useful. This can evaluate potential subluxations in patients with non-constrained implants.

Treatment options

The treatment options for the failed total elbow replacement are determined by the underlying cause for failure:

1. Aseptic loosening
   implant removal with arthrodesis
   implant removal with resection type
      arthroplasty
   revision arthroplasty
2. Septic loosening
   debridement with antibiotic suppression
   implant removal with arthrodesis
   implant removal with resection type
      arthroplasty
   two-stage reimplantation
3. Instability
   reconstruction of the medial collateral
      ligament
   addition of a thicker polyethylene component
   alteration of the valgus angle of the humeral
      component
   revision to a semi-constrained implant

ARTHRODESIS

Arthrodesis of the elbow is an operation to be avoided whenever possible. Loss of motion at the elbow is extremely disabling and patients find that they are unable to perform most activities of daily living. Arthrodesis is only considered for the failed total elbow if there is loss of the humeral epicondyles such that the elbow would be flail (Fig. 27.6) In this instance, an arthrodesis would be deemed preferable to a flail elbow or an amputation. Arthrodesis after a failed elbow replacement, however, is extremely difficult to achieve due to marked bone loss.

RESECTION ARTHROPLASTY

The preferred treatment for an infected total elbow replacement where reimplantation is not considered appropriate is a resection type arthroplasty. This is a modified resection of the original resection arthroplasty first described by Verneuil in 1860,[34] included removing the distal humerus above the epicondyles along with resection of a portion of the olecranon and excision of the radial head. This leaves the elbow as a flail, useless joint. Currently, with an infected elbow, we will remove the implant and all cement and place the patient in an external hinged device. This provides for soft

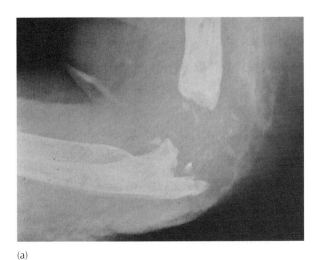

(a)

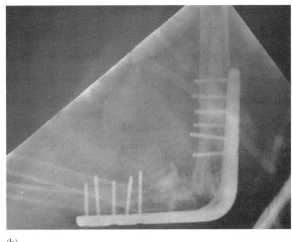

(b)

Fig. 27.6 (a) Radiograph showing loss of bone stock following failure and removal of a total elbow arthroplasty. (b) Arthrodesis with contoured internal fixation device.

tissue healing while maintaining stability of the elbow. The goal is to achieve an anatomic reduction of the olecranon within the humeral epicondyles (Fig. 27.7).

The hinged device will allow for early range of motion and provide alignment of soft tissues and healing in the plane of motion.[35] The fixator is usually used for a 6–8 week period and the pins are placed under direct vision to prevent injury to the radial nerve on the lateral side and the ulnar nerve on the medial side. In a series of patients undergoing removal of failed total elbow replacements, Figgie and associates[35] reported that seven of eight patients who achieved an anatomic alignment had satisfactory results. All eight elbows were pain free with an average arc of motion of 85 degrees. Flexion was usually excellent but triceps strength was often compromised. No excellent results were obtained but there was only one failure secondary to a radial nerve palsy. Of the three patients in whom an anatomic reduction could not be achieved, all experienced failure and two required arthrodesis.

ANTIBIOTIC SUPPRESSION

Antibiotic suppression alone is not recommended. It should be combined with debridement and a 6-week course of intravenous antibiotics followed by oral antibiotic suppression. This should only be considered for sensitive bacteria and well fixed components. There is an extremely high failure rate. In the series by Morrey and

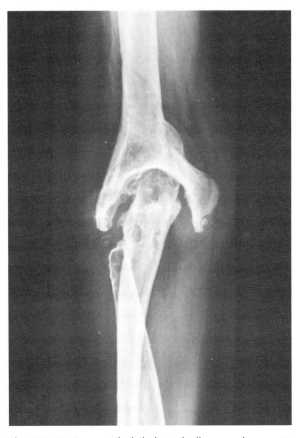

Fig. 27.7 Patients with failed total elbow replacements may do well with a resection type arthroplasty if an anatomic reconstruction can be obtained with containment of the olecranon within the epicondyles.

Bryan[31] only one of 14 elbows was salvaged by suppression and in Wolfe and associates' series[32] only three of 13 elbows were successfully treated by suppression.

REIMPLANTATION

Reimplantation after infection is performed rarely and only in carefully selected patients. Primary selection criteria includes the ability to eradicate the infection adequately as determined by minimum inhibitory concentration levels and the presence of adequate bone stock with sufficient soft tissues. We recommend the removal of the original infected elbow replacement and all the cement and the placement of an external fixator for 3–4 weeks. This should then be removed and the patient placed in a removable splint while intravenous antibiotics are continued. The proper antibiotic levels must be obtained according to the minimum inhibitory concentration levels. Reimplantation can be considered after 6 weeks of antibiotic treatment. In general, reimplantation is recommended only when resection arthroplasty has failed as a result of pain or instability.

SURGERY FOR INSTABILITY

Non-constrained total elbow replacements that are unstable (in the early perioperative period) and have had a frank dislocation are usually treated by a 4-week period of cast immobilisation. However, for patients who fail that treatment or have late dislocations, then one option is exploration of the medial aspect of the elbow with reefing of the capsule, reconstruction of the medial collateral ligament and postoperative immobilisation. However, the results are unpredictable especially in patients with rheumatoid arthritis where soft tissues may be marginal.

HUMERAL COMPONENT REVISION

Another option that exists for the unstable non-constrained elbow is to revise the humeral component to one that has an increased valgus angulation. This will tighten the medial structures and may improve the stability. However, one must be aware of the increased angulation of the humerus which changes the carrying angle and kinematics of the elbow. Motion may be altered if significant changes occur. In addition, the ulnar nerve may be subject to tension which might result in an ulnar neuropathy. The other option is to place a new ulnar component with a thicker component which would serve to tighten the joint and the existing soft tissues. However, if this fails then revision to a semi-constrained implant would be the procedure of choice.

POLYETHYLENE REVISION

In the unstable semi-constrained devices, the source of instability must be identified. If there is failure of the locking mechanism this may be able to be revised, although sometimes the locking mechanism has been deformed and the humeral component would require revision. With the Triaxial total elbow arthroplasty, failure occurs secondary to polyethylene wear and revision of the polyethylene bushing provides stability. In many instances, a yoke is also applied in order to provide increased compression and reduce instability. However, this technique was successful in only 50% of the cases as reported by Gerwin and associates.[36] In patients whose components are malpositioned, revision of the polyethylene bushing alone will most likely not provide satisfactory results and revision of the components will be required.[37]

REVISION SURGERY

Implant revision is the procedure of choice in patients with loose components who have adequate bone stock for reconstruction. Patients with fractured components may also successfully undergo revision of the fractured component.

Author's preferred management

For the septic elbow, we prefer to perform a debridement with antibiotic suppression only in those cases where the infection is determined early on, the bacteria is extremely susceptible, the components are well fixed and removing them might cause significant damage. In addition, the patient should have good skin coverage without any draining sinus and must be able to take oral antibiotics for the rest of their life. If any of these conditions are not met or if adequate suppression cannot be obtained then we prefer to remove the implant, place the patient in an external fixator preferably with a hinge and treat the patient for 6 weeks with intravenous antibiotics. Creation of an anatomic arthroplasty with the olecranon reduced between the epicondylar pillars must be obtained in order to provide a good functional result. With this type of reconstruction, patients usually do well enough that they do not need further revision surgery. We would only consider reimplantation for a septic elbow if either excision arthroplasty left them with pain or dysfunction or if they had marked instability. Reimplantation would only be performed if a stable reconstruction seemed possible and adequate bacteriocidal levels of antibiotic could be obtained.

For the loose total elbow replacement reimplantation is the procedure of choice. Often, additional bone grafting will also be required. Again, salvage of the epicondyles is key and we prefer revision to a semi-constrained device. In patients with marked bone loss an anterior flange and longer stem may be appropriate.

For the unstable non-constrained implant the initial treatment should be closed reduction and casting but if this fails the option of reconstruction of the medial collateral ligament is often prone to failure. Revision of the component to increase the valgus alignment has been described but a more predictable option is revision to a linked semi-constrained implant. Although this is a more involved procedure, it has a greater chance of providing a stable elbow.

Preoperative planning for revision surgery

In addition to a thorough clinical and radiological evaluation there are several factors that must be considered prior to revision surgery. The soft tissues must be adequately evaluated including muscle strength. Neurological examination is also critical as is bone quality. In patients with questionable bone defects a CT scan is often helpful in order to evaluate this further.

The choice of revision implant is critical. Often a standard type of device may be utilised for revision if the bone structure is maintained. However, in those cases where there is loss of humeral bone then a long-stemmed version may be required. In cases where there is loss of one or both epicondyles we recommend the use of an anterior flanged device to help decrease rotational stress. Customised devices may be required to maintain the centre of rotation. With standard long-stemmed devices, the canal will determine the centre of rotation. In addition, humeral canal diameters vary markedly and components may need to be altered to fit. Longer stemmed devices are recommended when there are perforations or fractures and these devices should bypass defects by two bone diameters. However, one must be aware of interference with the humeral stems of shoulder replacements especially in patients with multiple joint arthritis. Usually ulnar components only need to vary based upon stem length and diameter. In cases where only the humeral component of a non-constrained device is being revised, the appropriate humeral components must be available at different valgus angulations.

As well as having the appropriate implant available, it is also important to consider non-prosthetic options including an external fixator as a temporising measure if revision cannot be performed. Proper revision tools and equipment are mandatory prior to any revision procedure. In addition the surgeon must be familiar with bone grafting techniques and should have taken advice from a plastic and reconstructive surgeon if the preoperative assessment indicates that the soft tissue and skin coverage may be problematic.

Implant selection

In general, we find that non-constrained components are difficult to utilise as revision prostheses. They are dependent upon soft tissue support and after failure of a prosthesis, the ligamentous stability is suspect. Thus, in almost all instances, revision surgery should be done with a semi-constrained type component. The decision to use a standard or customised component is based upon available bone quality. If there is a bony defect, a long-stem device should be utilised. However, too long a stem should be avoided as it can interfere with the humeral component of a shoulder replacement, create a large stress riser, and may alter the accurate positioning of the centre of rotation since the stem length and size will determine where the centre of rotation is placed. In addition, anterior flanges may be useful to help with rotational stresses but again may force the centre of rotation into a particular position if the flange ends up determining the rotation of the component (Fig. 27.8). Customised implants may be required in order to accurately place the centre of rotation within the available bone stock. The use of such implants is associated with a learning curve with regard to design, proper fit and implantation. The use of cementless components for revision surgery is still considered experimental.

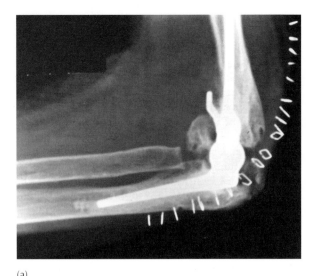

(a)

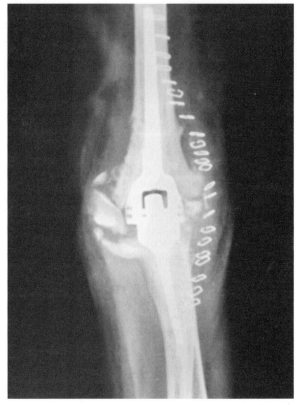

(b)

Fig. 27.8 (a) Patients with loss of the distal humerus may require an anterior flange to help with rotational control. (b) Note the suture holes within the component for attachment and stabilisation of the soft tissue sleeves.

Surgical technique

The usual surgical approach that we employ for revision operations is the Bryan–Morrey posteromedial reflection of the triceps.[38] However, in many instances, the implant can be disarticulated without reflecting the triceps, thus preserving the triceps attachment. If at all possible the approach should be made through a previous skin incision. If the previous incision was on the lateral side of the elbow then a new posteromedial approach should be used. If there is concern regarding skin viability then a preoperative assessment by a plastic and reconstructive surgeon is indicated.

With the posteromedial approach, the patient is placed in a supine position with the arm across the chest. The skin incision is made over the medial border of the triceps and extended to the level of the cubital tunnel. The incision then curves to the proximal third of the ulna. The subcutaneous tissues are divided and subcutaneous flaps are avoided. The ulnar nerve is identified at the cubital tunnel and is dissected free along its course proximally and distally. With revision surgery, the surgeon must be aware if the ulnar nerve was trans-

posed with the original operation. This should be reviewed from the previous operative note. When the nerve has been operated on previously and there is scar tissue, the proximal incision may need to be extended and the nerve found at the medial border of the triceps and carefully followed distally. The ulnar nerve must be identified, freed and protected in any revision operation. A Penrose drain is placed around the nerve and sutured instead of using a clamp to avoid undue tension. The nerve is dissected free and a passage is created between the two heads of the flexor carpi ulnaris to allow the nerve to be translocated anteriorly. The fascia of the flexor carpi ulnaris is then divided to the proximal third of the ulna from where the ulnar nerve enters beneath the fascia. The triceps muscle is dissected free medially and elevated laterally with care taken to avoid injuring the ulnar nerve that lies within the fibres of the proximal triceps muscle. If an extensile exposure is required then the triceps attachment is elevated at the tip of the olecranon along with the periosteum. A Beaver blade is helpful in this dissection. The sleeve of the triceps and the forearm fascia remain in continuity and are elevated across the capitellum to the lateral epicondyle, exposing the radial head. The anconeus muscle is also reflected. The capsule and scar tissue are excised and the medial aspect of the olecranon is exposed. The flexor carpi ulnaris is reflected to the sublime tubercle and the medial collateral ligament is subperiosteally elevated. The ulnar nerve is carefully protected as it lies in close proximity to the sublime tubercle. At this point the locking mechanism of the component can be removed and the elbow can be dislocated.

Another approach for revision surgery is via a posteromedial incision. The ulnar nerve is located, freed and protected. The triceps is then elevated both medially and laterally from the humerus and the locking mechanism of the elbow replacement is identified, the coupling mechanism is removed and the humerus and ulna are disassociated. The medial collateral ligament is reflected and the olecranon can be exposed leaving the triceps mechanism intact. The ulnar nerve must be carefully protected to ensure that it is not under tension. Once the ulna and humerus are exposed, an anterior capsulectomy is performed by placing a haemostat anterior to the capsule and excising it down to the brachialis muscle. At this point the original prosthesis can be removed. If it is loose it may be easy to remove.

Care must be exercised if the cement is well fixed to the component, since fractures may occur when trying to remove large pieces of cement. If the implant is well fixed it is often helpful to remove it before the cement is addressed. In cases of infection all cement must be removed whereas in cases of revision for dislocation or aseptic loosening, well fixed cement does not need to be removed if it does not interfere with the new implant. Removal of cement from the ulna and humerus is extremely difficult due to the small calibre of these bones. Most hand tools are still too large to remove the cement. We avoid using the Midas instruments except where excellent visualisation and control can be obtained since the Midas may chatter enough to cause perforations or fractures of the humerus or ulna. This creates great difficulty with the revision operation. In addition, perforations of the proximal humerus place the radial nerve at risk. If there is any question, the mid-shaft of the humerus must be well exposed and, in some cases, the radial nerve identified and protected. If the Midas equipment is to be used then the small diameter barrels must be obtained in order to be effective.

We currently prefer using the small tips on the ultrasonic devices which allow for safer cement removal within the shaft. However, even this can cause perforations in soft rheumatoid bone. If there is much difficulty removing the cement or there is an inaccessible area then a cortical window or posterior trough may be required. However, creating a posterior trough in the humerus will reduce the support for the revision prosthesis. The posterior cortex is extremely important since the vector force from the joint reaction force causes posterior loading. Most humeral components loosen by migrating posteriorly with the tip perforating anteriorly. During cement removal cultures should be taken and frozen sections identified in order to rule out a subclinical infectious process in the case of loose components.

When removing fractured implants, appropriate preparations for removing the distal stem must be made. This may involve the use of a special Midas device to drill the stem and remove it. However, this can be extremely difficult due to the small diameter of the component. A cortical window is an alternative approach.

With the ulna, a large subperiosteal reflection might be necessary in order to avoid perforation. Due to the angulation of the shaft of the ulna, cement removal with straight instruments is difficult. The small tip ultrasonic devices are again extremely helpful and, as in the humerus, well fixed cement does not need to be removed for non-infectious revision surgery.

Once sufficient cement has been removed, bone defects must be identified. Perforations should be grafted. If defects are significant in important areas, such as the posterior aspect of the humerus, then cortical strut grafts may be used along with morselized graft. The stems of the components should bypass any cortical defects by at least two bone diameters. If one or both of the humeral epicondyles has been fractured then these should be fixed to the humerus with pins or screws if feasible. The screws must be of the same type metal as the humeral component in order to avoid a 'battery' reaction due to dissimilar metals. If the epicondyles are not repairable then we often will place large Tevdek sutures through them and tie this behind the humeral component in order to preserve the soft tissue sleeve. In some instances we have created a custom implant with attachments on the humeral component to allow repair of the soft tissue sleeve or an epicondyle to the component.

Once the trial components have been placed, the range of motion should be tested. The component must track appropriately and the rotation must be judged. This is sometimes difficult due to the loss of normal structures but the humeral component should be internally rotated approximately 5 degrees with respect to the epicondyles. It is also important to be certain that the humerus is not lengthened as this may cause undue stress and loss of motion. It can cause greater problems with the polyethylene bushing due to the increase in the joint reaction force. The centre of rotation should be maintained and can be moved slightly proximally but should not be moved distally in the humerus. Once the components have been tested, the canals can be irrigated and dried. We recommend the use of antibiotic impregnated cement with all revisions. In addition, we use methylene blue in the polymethylmethacrylate in case another revision is required. Often, an intramedullary plug cannot be utilised with long-stem components. The humeral and ulnar components can be cemented with the same batch of cement, but with difficult situations, such as a humeral non-union or fracture, then the implants should be cemented separately. During the cementing procedure, any perforations are exposed in order to prevent cement extrusion and possible damage to the radial nerve behind the distal humerus. Cement is trimmed, the tourniquet released, bone grafts placed, including strut grafts, and haemostasis obtained. The elbow is reduced, the components articulated and the locking mechanism placed. The wound is closed over drains and the triceps is restored by repairing the fascial sleeve. Sutures placed through drill holes in the olecranon help reinforce the repair. The ulnar nerve is evaluated and transposed with a fascial sling if necessary. The soft tissues are closed and the elbow is placed in a bulky dressing with a plaster splint which is split posteriorly to avoid pressure on the olecranon.

Postoperative management

The splint is left in place and the wound inspected after 3 days. If the wound is intact then early range of motion can be started. An orthoplast splint is made in order to protect the arm and is utilised with straps to alternate extension and flexion when the arm is at rest. The splint is usually discontinued after 6 weeks. A therapist guides the patient through the early rehabilitation stage, but the patient is encouraged to use the arm as much as possible for all activities of daily living except lifting. Flexion is usually regained more easily than extension as most activities of daily living require flexion. Pronation and supination are also encouraged during rehabilitation.

Revision of polyethylene bushing for a Triaxial component

The surgical approach is similar, using either a triceps flap elevation or dislocation of the component by elevating the triceps medially and laterally after identifying the ulnar nerve. There is often a metal synovitis which must be thoroughly debrided. The bushing may be fragmented and should be removed in its entirety. Exposure of the distal humerus must include removal of a portion of the epicondyle in order to have adequate access to the distal humerus. In some cases, the small bearings are difficult to remove from the sides of the humerus. The new high density polyethylene bushing should be tested to ensure it fits appropriately. Two small O-rings should be embedded in the polyethylene with the chamfer facing inward. The polyethylene is then fitted to the humerus and the ulnar component is reduced. This requires considerable force. The yoke, if it is to be used, can be placed posteriorly. Formerly, we placed it anteriorly but since its purpose is to squeeze the polyethylene and not block flexion, we find it works equally well when placed posteriorly. The small screws are then placed through the yoke and humeral component until they are just inside the edge of the yoke. The range of motion should be tested to make sure that there is no restriction. If there is, the screws are loosened slightly. Then, a small osteotome is used to score the threads, preventing the screws from backing out. The wound can then be closed in the previously described manner.

Results of revision surgery

The largest series of revision total elbow replacement was reported by Morrey and Bryan with 33 revisions performed over a 10-year period with an average 5-year follow up.[39] The cause of failure leading to revision varied in these patients, but pain was a common symptom. Loosening of the component was the most common factor leading to revision with 17 elbows having loose humeral components, three elbows having loose ulnar components, and eight elbows having both components loose. Of these, six elbows had fractures of the humerus or ulna due to bony resorption around the loose prosthesis. Three implants had material failure, and two implants were unstable. In all, 88% of elbows had moderate or severe bone loss, with loss of the trochlea or humeral condyles. Two-thirds of the patients had rheumatoid arthritis.

Reimplantation was performed with six different commercial prostheses and four custom prostheses, making comparison survival analysis difficult. Half of the implants had a long-stemmed humeral component. Three of the 33 revision prostheses became infected (9%), which is similar to the incidence of 7–9% found in the literature for primary elbow arthroplasties.[31,32] No mention was made of whether antibiotic impregnated cement was used, and perhaps this could account for the relatively lower than expected incidence of infection after revision surgery. Rheumatoid patients faired better after revision elbow surgery with 64% having a good result compared with 40% of those with traumatic arthritis. Rating was based on a scale previously described by Morrey and Bryan for evaluating pain, function, and stability.[31] The success of the re-implantation was correlated to the adequacy of the cementing technique. Neither the number of prior procedures nor the amount of bone loss at the time of revision was correlated with subsequent failure of the revision prosthesis. Cementation technique was considered inadequate if the cement did not extend beyond the tip of the prosthesis and there was greater than a 1-mm gap over more than half of the cement–prosthesis interface on the postoperative anteroposterior or lateral radiograph. Of those humeral components judged to have adequate cementation on postoperative radiographs, none became loose. Of those humeral components having inadequate cementation, five of 13 (38%) loosened. All of the ulnar components were judged to have adequate cementation techniques postoperatively, and 10% loosened. A total of 60% of patients had an intraoperative or postoperative complication. In all, one-third (11 of 33) of revision prostheses required a second operation to remove or revise the prosthesis for infection, loosening, implant failure or instability. Of the eight revised prostheses (second revision), five had a good result. At recent follow-up, 55% of these elbow replacements were still in place with satisfactory results.[40] Eleven elbows had an additional procedure performed.

A recent preliminary study reviewed the results of 47 patients who underwent revision total elbow replacement using a cemented modified Coonrad implant (Morrey and King, personal communications). All procedures were performed for pain, instability or loosening. Revisions for septic failure were excluded. Twenty patients had revision of a constrained elbow replacement, 16 had resurfacing devices, 10 patients had semi constrained implants and one had a silicone spacer; 41 of the 47 patients had more than 2 years follow-up and 36 of these (88%) had a satisfactory result at a mean of 5 years after their revision. Four patients underwent re-operation of their revision procedure; one patient had a fracture of the ulna and was revised to a long-stem ulnar component; two patients developed instability due to polyethylene wear of the bearing axle; and one patient had revision for titanium synovitis from the plasma spray on the humeral component. Overall, eleven patients (27%) sustained a significant complication which either influenced the end result or required further surgery.

Results of revision of semi-constrained Triaxial total elbow replacements for failure of the polyethylene articulation and resultant dislocation have been fair.[36] The mean time from elbow implantation to initial dislocation was 30 months. In all, 50% of elbows required more than one revision for polyethylene failure and dislocation. All elbows that dislocated within the first year of implantation redislocated. Radiographic evaluation revealed all implants outside the acceptable alignment criteria for good outcome of elbow arthroplasty.[37]

Complications

Complications after revision total elbow arthroplasty are similar to those after primary replacements, only the rates are significantly increased. These complications include the risk of infection, loosening, ulnar nerve palsy, and wound problems. In addition, the risk of implant fracture, instability, triceps rupture, heterotopic ossification and fracture are also increased with revision operations. The risk of wound problems is increased largely due to previous incisions which compromise the vascularity of the skin. In addition, the surgery required for revision procedures usually requires greater exposure with a greater likelihood that haematomas may develop resulting in wound necrosis or drainage. Thus, previous surgical incisions should be utilised whenever possible. Flaps should not be raised and careful haemostasis with the use of postoperative drains is advised. If there is any question as to the viability of the skin then early range of motion should not be initiated.

With regard to deep infection, the risk with revision surgery is greater, again due to the length of surgery and surgical exposure. In addition, there is more likelihood that there is a subclinical infection especially if there is gross loosening of the prosthesis. Thus, we recommend aspiration of loose total elbow arthroplasties before revision surgery together with intraoperative Gram stains, frozen sections and a culture. If there is any question of infection then we would not reimplant at that time but wait until final cultures are negative. In addition, we routinely use antibiotic impregnated cement in order to help reduce the risk of early infection. Late infection is more common in the immunosuppressed patient with multiple joint replacements. To reduce the risks of failure we advise that patients who develop chest infections or other bacterial conditions are aggressively treated. In addition, we advise that they avoid undue pressure on the elbows to prevent skin breakdown and possible late infection.

The incidence of ulnar nerve palsy is higher with revision surgery. Scar formation around the nerve together with vascular compromise render the nerve more vulnerable. The nerve should be isolated and freed whenever revision surgery is undertaken. It must also be carefully protected. Whether or not the nerve is transposed anteriorly as part of the procedure is determined at the time of surgery. With the extensive exposure that is usually required for revision procedures other nerves may also be at risk of injury. These include the radial nerve on the humeral side, the posterior interosseous nerve at the radial neck and the median nerve anteriorly. The radial nerve is especially at risk if extensive proximal exposure of the humerus is undertaken in order to remove the implant or if there is any bone defect.

Care of the triceps mechanism is extremely important in revision operations. We prefer to use an extensile triceps sparing approach such as that described by Bryan and Morrey.[38] This allows adequate exposure of the ulnar nerve and elevation of the triceps mechanism. However, in many instances, especially in revision procedures, the triceps mechanism may be extremely thin. In these instances a fleck of cortical bone may be elevated with part of the flap. We do not recommend detaching the triceps in any exposure. If the triceps mechanism is at risk then reinforcement is indicated and a longer period of postoperative immobilisation is recommended.

The risk of intraoperative or postoperative fracture is extremely high in revision operations due to the difficulty in removing the existing implant and the small diameter of the bone in the humeral and ulnar canals. The epicondyles are especially at risk with removal of a humeral component. In cases where there has been gross loosening with a balloon type radiolucency and thinning of the cortex, fractures often occur. The epicondyles must be carefully protected as they can provide support for the humeral components against rotational stress. An adequate soft tissue release must be performed when exposing the elbow with marked bone loss as the pull from the soft tissues may actually cause fractures to occur. If cortical perforations occur when removing cement these must be bypassed by two bone diameters when the new implant is inserted in order to provide adequate fixation and to avoid the stress rise where it has occurred. If postoperative fractures occur they are often at the epicondyles. These can be splinted and treated non-operatively. However, if fractures occur at the tip of the stem these are extremely difficult to treat as usually marked deformity will result and a non-union can occur.

The risk of loosening is higher after a revision operation because the bone stock is less optimal. Soft tissue deformities and muscle imbalance may also increase this risk. In order to gain adequate fixation, longer stemmed devices must be utilised. These, however, do not necessarily provide rotational stability but this may be improved by using an implant with an anterior flange.

Instability may occur after revision operations due to the higher demands placed upon the polyethylene as the result of muscle imbalance and loss of ligamentous support. Even the linked semi-constrained components may develop instability or problems due to wear of their polyethylene axles because of the soft tissue imbalance and increased stress. In the cases where there is marked instability at the time of surgery attempts at ligament balancing should be made with postoperative bracing to help with soft tissue healing.

The incidence of heterotopic ossification after revision surgery is extremely low. In our experience it is usually only Grade I or II and this does not interfere with the functional result. There is little need for postoperative prophylaxis for heterotopic ossification even in cases of ankylosis. The only exception might be a patient who had previously heterotopic bone formation due to a post-traumatic condition. In this instance we would recommend the use of Indocin to prevent this complication.

References

1. Davis RF, Weiland AJ, Hungerford DS, Moore JR, Volenec-Dowling S Non-constrained total elbow arthroplasty. *Clin Orthop* 1982; **171:**156–60.
2. Dennis DA, Clayton ML, Ferlic DC, Stringer EA, Bramlett KW Capitello–condylar total elbow arthroplasty for rhuematoid arthritis. *J Arthroplasty* 1990; **5**(Suppl): S83–8.
3. Ewald FC, Scheinberg RD, Poss R *et al.* Capitello–condylar total elbow arthroplasty: Two-to-five year follow-up in rheumatoid arthritis. *J Bone Joint Surg* 1980; **62A:** 1259–63.
4. Ruth JT, Wilde AH Capitello–condylar total elbow replacement. *J Bone Joint Surg* 1992; **74A:** 95–100.
5. Simmons ED, Sullivan JA, Ewald FC Long-term review of the capitello–condylar total elbow replacement. *Orthop Trans* 1990; **14:** 642.
6. Trancik T, Wilde AH, Borden LS Capitello–condylar total elbow arthroplasty. *Clin Orthop* 1987; **223:** 175–80.
7. Weiland AJ, Weiss A, Wills RP, Moore JR Capitello–condylar total elbow replacement. A Long-term follow-up study. *J Bone Joint Surg* 1989; **71A:** 217–22.
8. Kudo H, Iwano K Total elbow arthroplasty with a non-constrained surface replacement prosthesis in

patients who have rheumatoid arthritis: A long-term follow-up study. *J Bone Joint Surg* 1990; **72A:** 355–62.

9. Kudo H, Iwano K, Watanabe S Total replacement of the rheumatoid elbow with a hingeless prosthesis. *J Bone Joint Surg* 1980; **62A:** 277–85.

10. Lowe LW, Miller AJ, Allum RK, Higginson DW The development of an unconstrained elbow arthroplasty: A clinical review. *J Bone Joint Surg* 1984; **66B:** 243–7.

11. Pritchard RW Anatomic surface elbow arthroplasty: A preliminary report. *Clin Orthop* 1983; **179:** 223–30.

12. Roper BA, Tuke M, O'Riordan SM, Bulstrode CJ A new unconstrained elbow. *J Bone Joint Surg* 1986; **68B:** 566–9.

13. Rydholm U, Tjornstrand B, Pettersson H, Lidgren L Surface replacement of the elbow in rheumatoid arthritis: Early results with the Wadsworth prosthesis. *J Bone Joint Surg* 1984; **66B:** 737–41.

14. Soni RK, Cavendish ME, A review of the Liverpool elbow prosthesis from 1974 to 1982. *J Bone Joint Surg* 1984; **66B:** 248–53.

15. Souter WA A new approach to elbow arthroplasty. 1981; **10:** 269.

16. Tuke MA The ICLH elbow. 1981; **10:** 75.

17. Wadsworth TG A new technique of total elbow replacement. 1981; **10:** 69.

18. Brumfield RH Jr, Volz RG Total elbow arthroplasty: A clinical review of 30 cases employing the Mayo and AHSC prostheses. *Clin Orthop* 1981; **158:** 137–41.

19. Bryan RS Total replacement of the elbow joint. *Arch Surg* 1977; **112:**1092–3.

20. Coonrad RW Seven-year follow-up of Coonrad total elbow replacement. In: *Upper extremity joint replacement.* Inglis AE (ed) St Louis: CV Mosby, 1982.

21. Figgie MP, Inglis A.E, Figgie HE III, Mow CS Semi-constrained total elbow replacement in rheumatoid arthritis. *Orthop Trans* 1990; **14:** 104.

22. Inglis A.E, Pellicci PM Total elbow replacement. *J Bone Joint Surg* 1980; **62A:** 1252–8.

23. Kraay MJ, Figgie MP, Inglis AE Survivorship analysis of primary total elbow arthroplasty with a semi-contrained prosthesis. Presented at the 59th Annual Meeting of the American Academy of Orthopedic Surgeons, Washington DC, 1992.

24. Morrey BF, Adams RA Semi-constrained arthroplasty for the treatment of rheumatoid arthritis of the elbow. *J Bone Joint Surg* 1992; **74A:** 479–90.

25. Morrey BF, Bryan RS, Dobyns JH, Linscheid RL Total elbow arthroplasty: A five-year experience at the Mayo Clinc. *J Bone Joint Surg* 1981; **63A:** 1050–63.

26. Pritchard RW Long-term follow-up study: Semi-constrained elbow prosthesis. *Orthopedics* 1981; **4:** 151–5.

27. Rosenberg G, Figgie HE III, Ranawat CS *et al.* Total elbow replacement for rheumatoid arthritis. Long-term results with a semi-constrained prosthesis. *Orthop Trans* 1989; **12:** 732.

28. Rozenfeld SR, Anzel SH Evaluation of the Pritchard total elbow arthroplasty. *Orthopedics* 1982; **5:** 713.

29. Volz RG Development and clinical analysis of a new semi-constrained total elbow prosthesis. In: *Upper extremity joint replacement.* Inglis A (ed) St Louis: CV Mosby, 1982.

30. Garrett JC, Ewald FC, Thomas WH, Sledge CB Loosening associated with GSB hinge total elbow replacement in patients with rheumatoid arthritis. *Clin Orthop* 1977; **127:** 170–4.

31. Morrey BF, Bryan RS Infection after total elbow arthroplasty. *J Bone Joint Surg* 1983; **65A:** 330–8.

32. Wolfe SL, Figgie MP, Ingis AE *et al.* Management of infection about total elbow prosthesis. *J Bone Joint Surg* 1990; **72A:** 198–212.

33. Rosenberg GM, Turner RN Non-constrained elbow arthroplasty. *Clin Orthop* 1984; **187:**154–62.

34. Verneuil A De la Creation d'une fausse articulation par section ou resection partielle de l'os maxillaire inferieur, comme moyen de rededier l'anklylose orale de fausse de la machoire inferieur. *Arch Gen Med* **15:**284, 1860.

35. Figgie MP, Inglis AE, Mow CS *et al.* Results of reconstruction for failed total elbow arthroplasty. *Clin Orthop* 1990; **253:** 123–32.

36. Gerwin M, Figgie MP, Mabrey JD, Inglis AE Results of revision of semi-constrained total elbow replacement for dislocation. Presented at the 60th Annual American Academy of Orthopedic Surgeons, San Francisco, 1993.

37. Figgie HE, Inglis AE, Mow CS A critical analysis of alignment factors affecting functional outcome in total elbow arthroplasty. *J Arthroplasty* 1986; **1:** 169–73.

38. Bryan RS, Morrey BF Extensive posterior exposure of the elbow: A triceps-sparing approach. *Clin Orthop* 1982; **166:** 188–92.

39. Morrey BF, Bryan RS Revision total elbow arthroplasty. *J Bone Joint Surg* 1987; **69A:** 523–32.

40. Morrey BF Revision of failed total elbow arthroplasty. In: *The elbow and its disorders* (2nd edn). Philadelphia: WB Saunders Co, 1993: 676.

CHAPTER 28

Primary osteoarthritis of the elbow

DAVID STANLEY

Introduction

Osteoarthritis has been defined as a 'non-inflammatory disorder of moveable joints characterised by deterioration and abrasion of articular cartilage together with the formation of new bone at the joint surfaces'.[1] The condition has been studied in great detail in many joints of the body[2-4] although involvement of the elbow has received relatively little attention. In this chapter aetiology, pathology, clinical presentations and investigations will be described and treatment options discussed.

Aetiology

Artiological factors in the development of osteoarthritis of the elbow have been debated for many years with interest focusing particularly on the relative importance of heavy manual work and the use of pneumatic tools.

Holtzmann[5] in a study of heavy manual workers was the first to suggest that the use of pneumatic tools might be an important predisposing factor. This view was further substantiated by the work of Rostock[6] who investigated 744 miners using pneumatic boring tools and found 32.8% (244) had degenerative arthritis of the elbow, whilst only 6% (45) had arthritis of the shoulder or wrist.

A contrary view, however, was taken by Hunter et al.[7] who found a low frequency of elbow osteoarthritis in heavy manual workers using the same type of equipment. They reported seven cases amongst 78 riveters, eight of 38 caulkers, three of 108 felters and six of 37 holders-up. They stated that there was no convincing evidence that elbow osteoarthritis was caused by using pneumatic tools.

In 1955 Lawrence[8] reporting on occupational factors predisposing to rheumatism in coal miners also examined the relationship between the use of pneumatic drills and the development of osteoarthritis of the elbow. He found that in miners who had not drilled, 16% developed elbow osteoarthritis compared with 31% who had used pneumatic drills for more than 1 year. Although this appears to be a marked difference, the numbers in each group were small and did reach statistical significance. More recent work has also failed to show a definite link between the use of pneumatic drills and the development of degenerative change within the elbow.[9]

Of greater significance in Lawrence's study, however, was the observation that after degenerative changes within the spine and knee, the elbow was the next most frequently affected joint. He concluded that the development of the elbow osteoarthritis was a feature of all types of heavy manual work that he had investigated.[8]

The development of elbow osteoarthritis has been reported in foundry workers by Mintz and Fraga.[10] In this study it was suggested that the use of tongs significantly increased the leverage of the elbow, since the resistance point (the tip of the tongs instead of the hand) was further from the elbow. Thus more force was required to do the same work resulting in an increase of shearing type friction at the articular surface of the elbow. This was advanced as the cause of the premature onset of osteoarthritis in this group of workers.

Stanley[11] in a study of 1000 consecutive fracture clinic patients (2000 elbows) also found an association between heavy manual work and the development of elbow osteoarthritis. A statistically significant difference was noted between men undertaking manual work compared with those doing non-manual tasks (p = 0.016). In addition in this study the prevalence of elbow osteoarthritis in the community was noted to be 2%. This compares favourably with the 1.3% figure quoted by Collins[12] and the 7% prevalence noted by Doherty and Preston for a typical rheumatological practice.[13]

Doherty and Preston[13] also studied the relationship between elbow osteoarthritis and osteoarthritis at other sites in the body. They found that osteoarthritis of the elbow particularly affected middle aged men and was commonly associated with metacarpophalangeal joint osteoarthritis – the so called Missouri metacarpal syndrome (Fig. 28.1).

Intra-articular changes in ageing and osteoarthritis

NORMAL AGEING

The intra-articular changes that occur within the elbow during ageing have been investigated by Goodfellow and Bullough.[14] In a study of 28 autopsy specimens retrieved from subjects aged 18–88 years, they showed that the radiocapitellar joint almost inevitably degenerated with increasing age. Of particular note was the consistent finding of a posteromedial radial head ulcer (Fig. 28.2) which matched a linear ulcer on the posterior part of the crest, separating the trochlea from the capitellum. In contrast the cartilage of the humeroulnar articu-

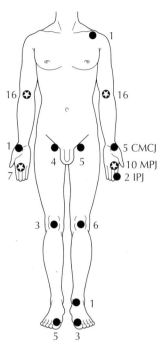

Fig. 28.1 Occurrence of symptomatic and radiographic osteoarthritis at the elbow and at other sites. The association between elbow and metacarpophalangeal joint (MPJ) osteoarthritis (Missouri-metacarpal syndrome) is highlighted. CMCJ: Carpometacarpal joint; IPJ: interphalangeal joint. Redrawn after Ref. 13.

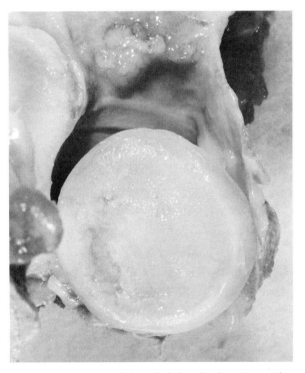

Fig. 28.2 Posteriomedial radial head ulceration. This figure is reproduced in colour in the colour plate section.

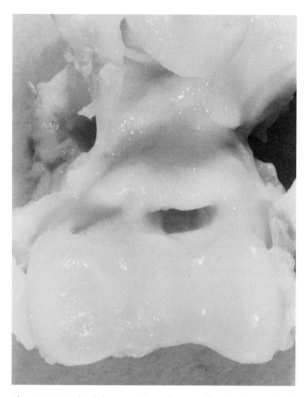

Fig. 28.3 Marked degeneration change affecting the capitellum with preservation of the cartilage over the trochlea. This figure is reproduced in colour in the colour plate section.

lation showed no such pattern of degeneration. In older subjects, however, it was noted that the humeroulnar cartilage was often scored in the line of movement, but the grooves never exposed the underlying bone. It was suggested that these differences were related to the fact that the radiocapitellar joint has a combination of rotation and hinge movements, whilst the humeroulnar joint has only hinge movements.

Murato *et al.*[15] also investigated the articular changes that occur within the elbow during ageing. They found that the degenerative changes in the radiocapitellar joint were always more advanced than those of the humeroulnar joint (Fig. 28.3). They noted that the degenerative changes initially occurred at the capitellum, the crest between the capitellum and trochlea and the ulnar side of the radial head. This observation led them to propose a progression of change from normal ageing to the development of elbow osteoarthritis. It was suggested that excess stress concentration occurred in the central area of the elbow joint, destroying the articular cartilage at the ulnar edge of the radial head and also on the crest. This area of degeneration then increases in size as the radiocapitellar joint passes through a full range of pronation and supination in all positions of flexion and extension. Thus the entire radiocapitellar joint degenerates and becomes osteoarthritic.

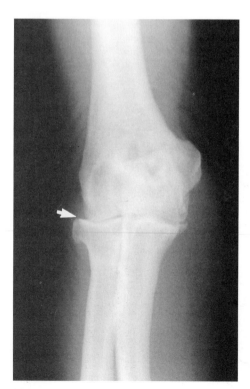

(a)

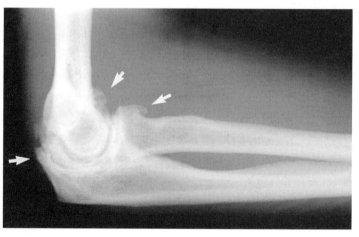

(b)

Fig. 28.4 (a) Anteroposterior radiograph of an osteoarthritic elbow. Joint space narrowing is most marked on the lateral aspect of the joint (arrowed). (b) Lateral radiograph of an osteoarthritic elbow. Osteophytes are seen at the tip of the olecranon, around the radial head and at the coronoid fossa (arrowed).

OSTEOARTHRITIS

The intra-articular changes of osteoarthritis of the elbow are similar to those occurring in other joints namely: joint space narrowing, osteophyte formation, and sclerosis (Fig. 28.4). In addition, thickening of the membrane between the olecranon and coronoid fossae together with loose body formation are important features.

According to Kashiwagi[16] and Tsuge and Mizuseki[17] the radial head cartilage is often eroded at an early stage and with this there is reciprocal loss of cartilage over the capitellum together with sclerosis and eburnation. Degenerative changes affecting the articular surfaces of the humeroulnar joint, however, often remain minor until the condition is well advanced.

Although osteophytes develop around the radial head, they are a more significant feature of the changes that affect the ulna and distal humerus. The coronoid process and tip of the olecranon become osteophytic early and in addition a semi-circle of osteophytes may also be found around the superior border of the olecranon and trochlea fossae (Fig. 28.4). Osteophytes involving the medial aspect of the joint may produce ulnar nerve symptoms.

Thickening of the membrane between the olecranon and coronoid fossae originally described by Kashiwagi can often be marked. This together with the osteophytes on the coronoid process and tip of the olecranon contribute to the reduction in elbow extension and to a lesser extent elbow flexion that is a feature of this condition.

Loose body formation has been reported by Bell[18] to be characteristic of elbow osteoarthritis. Morrey states that loose bodies occur in approximately 50% of patients.[19] The loose bodies may be single, but are more commonly multiple (Fig. 28.5). When present they may further limit elbow motion and can also cause acute locking of the joint.

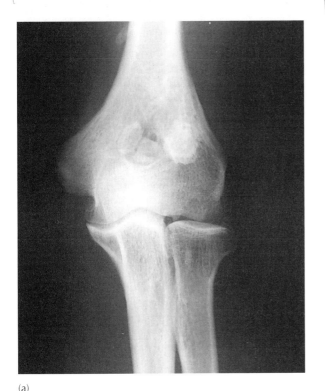

(a)

Fig. 28.5 (a) Anteroposterior radiograph showing loose bodies in the olecranon fossa and between the radiocapitellar joint. (b) Multiple loose bodies removed from an osteoarthritic elbow.

(b)

cm 1   2   3   4   5   6   7   8   9   10   11

Clinical presentation

Although osteoarthritis of the elbow does occur in both sexes, it predominantly affects men.[11,13,16,19] It usually presents after the fourth decade of life, although younger patients have been noted. Most commonly the dominant extremity is involved but either or both elbows may be affected. Clinical presentations can be divided into four main types.

TYPE 1: ACHING DISCOMFORT WITH REDUCED ELBOW MOVEMENT

This is the most common presentation. The symptoms within the elbow are usually described as an aching discomfort rather than pain. Some loss of elbow movement, particularly extension is usually noted by the patient although occasionally this is not appreciated particularly if the shoulder, wrist and hand are normal. At times the abnormality only becomes apparent after a minor injury. Frequently the symptoms are slowly progressive. On clinical examination a functional range of movement is commonly present with a varying but usually greater loss of extension than flexion.

TYPE 2: ACUTE PAIN AND LOCKING

Patients who present with acute pain in the elbow usually link this to episodes of elbow locking. 'Unlocking' of the elbow may occur spontaneously, but there is often a history that the elbow has to be 'shaken free'. This type of presentation occurs most frequently in patients with multiple loose bodies within the joint and it is these that become trapped producing the acute symptoms. In between the acute episodes aching discomfort is experienced and on clinical examination there is terminal restriction of extension and often also flexion.

TYPE 3: ULNAR NERVE ENTRAPMENT

Symptoms of ulnar nerve entrapment may occasionally be the sole reason for specialist orthopaedic referral. Most commonly, however, it is an additional component of a type 1 or type 2 presentation. Kashiwagi reported an incidence of 40.3% ulnar nerve paralysis in his patients with elbow osteoarthritis (75 of 186 patients).[16]

TYPE 4: INCIDENTAL OR INACCURATE DIAGNOSIS

Osteoarthritis of the elbow may at times be identified when the upper limb is being assessed for another orthopaedic problem. The patient usually has minor symptoms and signs at the elbow and radiographs reveal early degenerative change.

The most common elbow condition misdiagnosed and resulting in specialist referral is tennis elbow. Some patients referred with this condition, will following careful assessment be found to be suffering with elbow osteoarthritis.

Investigations

Most cases of elbow osteoarthritis can be diagnosed from anteroposterior and lateral radiographs. These views will show osteophytes on the tip of the olecranon and coronoid processes together with joint space narrowing and the presence of loose bodies (Fig. 28.4). In addition the anteroposterior view will also often show loss of definition of the outline of the olecranon fossa due to thickening of the interfossa membrane. In order to improve visualisation of the olecranon fossa, Kashiwagi advocated a special radiographic view.[16] This involves placing the film cassette behind the distal part of the upper arm and with the elbow flexed to 60 degrees the anteroposterior projection is taken (Fig. 28.6).

When there is doubt as to the presence of intra-articular loose bodies or osteophytes, lateral tomography is the most useful additional investigation (Fig. 28.7).

Computerised tomography and magnetic resonance imaging, also enable visualisation of the bony anatomy and articular surfaces (Fig. 28.8) and can be valuable in patients whose symptoms appear out of proportion to the plain radiographic findings.

Patients presenting with ulnar nerve symptoms should undergo electromyographic evaluation in order to assess the degree of ulnar nerve compromise.

Treatment

CONSERVATIVE

All patients should be advised as to the cause of their symptoms. Those with minor complaints may benefit from taking simple analgesics or non-steroidal anti-inflammatory drugs. In addition physiotherapy and intra-articular steroid injections have been shown to be helpful.[13]

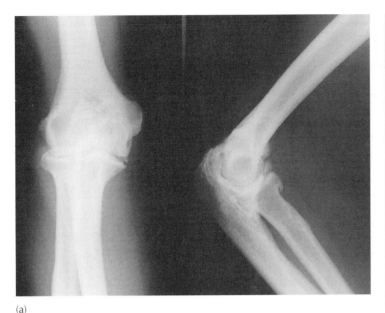

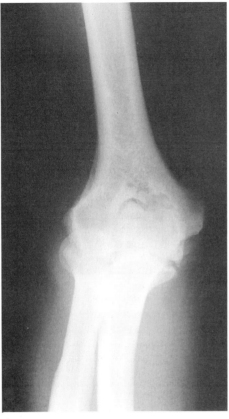

(a)

Fig. 28.6 (a) Anteroposterior and lateral radiographs of an osteo-arthritic elbow. The view of the olecranon fossa is poor on the antero-posterior view due to either osteophytes or loose bodies. (b) The Kashiwagi view improves visualisation of the olecranon fossa and indicates that the abnormality seen in (a) is due predominantly to loose body formation rather than osteophytes. The Kashiwagi view is obtained by placing the film cassette behind the distal part of the upper arm with the elbow flexed to 60 degrees.

(b)

SURGICAL

Surgical treatment of osteoarthritis of the elbow depends on the severity of the disease. The techniques that have been advocated are arthroscopy, debridement procedures, total elbow arthroplasty and ulnar nerve surgery if there is neurological compromise

ARTHROSCOPY

The primary use of arthroscopy is in the removal of intra-articular loose bodies.[20] In addition, in the same way that arthroscopic lavage has been found to be effective in osteoarthritis of the knee[21] it may also be beneficial for the elbow.

Arthroscopy can also be used to perform a variation of the Outerbridge–Kashiwagi debridement procedure. This involves inserting the arthroscope into the anterior compartment of the elbow and then via a small posterior incision and with a drill sleeve to protect the soft tissues, the olecranon fossa is fenestrated using a 1 cm diameter drill. The

passage of the drill into the anterior compartment of the elbow is undertaken with direct visualisation via the arthroscope. This technique described by Redden and Stanley[22] does not allow the posterior compartment of the elbow to be as radically debrided as can be achieved by the open Outerbridge–Kashiwagi operation.

DEBRIDEMENT PROCEDURES

Outerbridge–Kashiwagi procedure

Kashiwagi[23] first reported a debridement procedure for elbow osteoarthritis which he attributed to Outerbridge and described as the Outerbridge–Kashiwagi or OK method. The operation was stated to relieve pain, improve flexion and allow the removal of loose bodies. It did not, however, usually improve extension since this deformity was felt to result from a long-standing contracture of the anterior soft tissues. Since the initial description of this technique, satisfactory results have also been reported by Minami and Ishii[24] and Stanley and

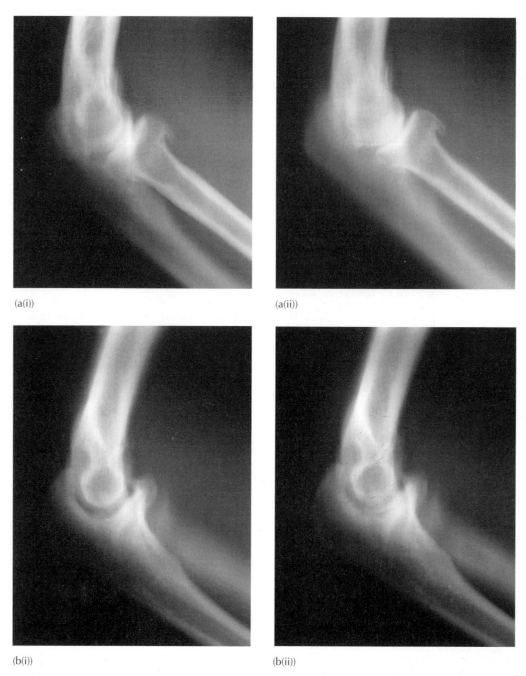

(a(i))   (a(ii))

(b(i))   (b(ii))

Fig. 28.7 (a) Lateral tomography showing joint space narrowing between the radial head and capitellum. (b) Osteophytic changes on the tip of the coronoid process are clearly seen.

Winson.[25] Morrey[19] in his modification of the technique, also obtained good results.

The operation is performed either with the patient supine with a sandbag under the scapula and the patient's arm across their chest or, as is my preference, with the patient in the lateral position. In the lateral position the elbow is supported by a bolster such that the upper arm is horizontal and the forearm hangs vertically. Under tourniquet control, a mid-line incision is made extending proximally for 8 cm from the tip of the olecranon (Fig. 28.9). The incision is deepened, splitting triceps in the line of its fibres and exposing the posterior capsule of the joint. This is opened and any loose bodies in this

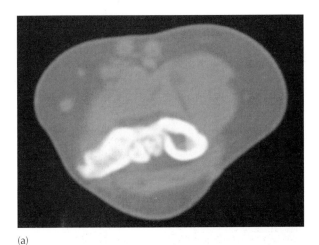

(a)

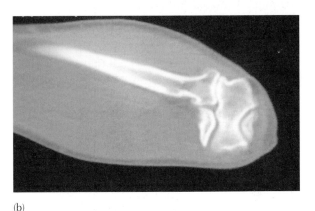

(b)

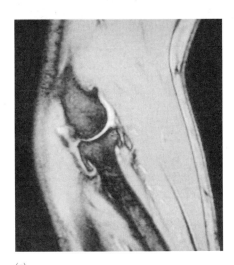

(c)

Fig. 28.8 (a) CT scan showing two loose bodies in the olecranon fossa. (b) CT scan showing preservation of the ulna–trochlea articulation but with marked narrowing of the radiocapitellar joint. (c) Magnetic resonance imaging scan of the radiocapitellar joint. Osteophytes are seen around the radial head with irregularity of the posterior articular surface of the capitellum.

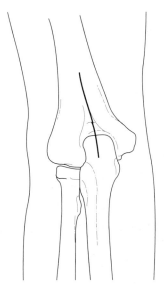

Fig. 28.9 The skin incision for the Outerbridge–Kashiwagi (OK method) debridement procedure.

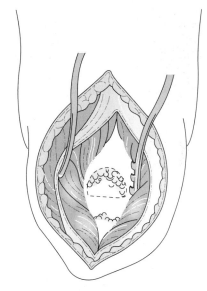

Fig. 28.10 The triceps is split and the posterior elbow compartment entered. Osteophytes around the olecranon fossa and tip of the olecranon can be excised.

compartment are removed. In addition osteophytes around the olecranon fossa and at the tip of the olecranon are excised (Fig. 28.10). The floor of the olecranon fossa is then fenestrated using a bone trephine of approximately 1 cm diameter (Fig. 28.11). Morrey[19] advises this technique for producing the opening into the anterior compartment of the elbow since it causes less bone debris than a drill and provides a more predictable, cleaner resection.

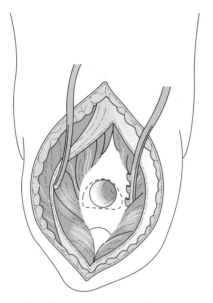

Fig. 28.11 The olecranon fossa is fenestrated using a bone trephine of approximately 1 cm diameter. This allows access to the anterior compartment of the elbow.

Having produced a window into the anterior compartment of the elbow, anterior loose bodies can be removed. Flexion and extension of the elbow displaces loose bodies into the window from where they can be removed with forceps. In addition by operating through the window, osteophytes on the coronoid process can be excised using a fine osteotome (Fig. 28.12).

The elbow is then washed out with warm saline to remove remaining debris and closed over a suction drain. A dressing of orthopaedic gauze, wool and crepe is applied and a broad arm sling used to support the arm. The drain is removed at 28 hours, the dressing reduced and gentle mobilisation of the elbow commenced (Fig. 28.13).

Morrey[19] uses a more aggressive postoperative regime. For the first 3 days after surgery analgesia is provided by a continuous brachial plexus block. In addition continuous passive motion is employed for 6 days and active movement allowed as tolerated. Flexion and extension splintage is also use in order to maximise the operative gain in movement.[26]

Morrey[19] reviewed 15 patients treated using this technique with a mean postoperative follow-up of 33 months. Elbow extension was found to be improved by an average of 11 degrees and elbow flexion by 10 degrees. Twelve patients had good or excellent results and 13 (87%) felt that surgery had been beneficial.

Tsuge debridement procedure

An alternative debridement procedure advocated by Tsuge[27] involves a more extensive surgical approach (Fig. 28.14). Via a posterior incision the ulnar nerve is found and protected and the extensor mechanism reflected medially. The radial collateral ligament together with the posterior portion of the ulnar collateral ligament are divided and the joint dislocated. Loose bodies in

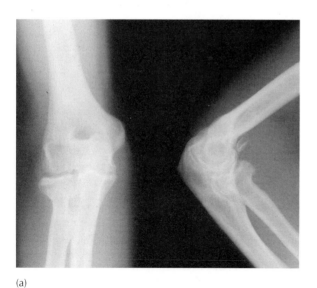

(a)

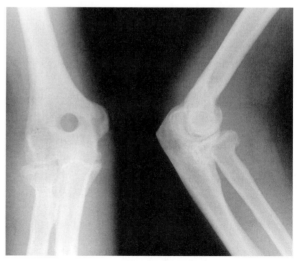

(b)

Fig. 28.12 (a) Preoperative anteroposterior and lateral radiographs of an osteoarthritic elbow. (b) Postoperative anteroposterior and lateral radiographs of the elbow shown in (a). The olecranon fossa fenestration is clearly visible.

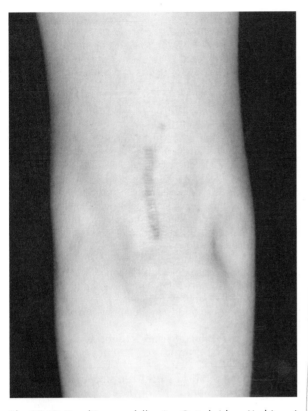

Fig. 28.13 Resulting scar following Outerbridge–Kashiwagi debridement procedure.

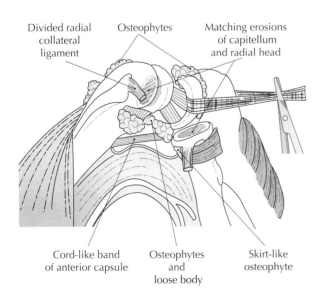

Divided radial collateral ligament | Osteophytes | Matching erosions of capitellum and radial head

Cord-like band of anterior capsule | Osteophytes and loose body | Skirt-like osteophyte

Fig. 28.14 Debridement arthroplasty for advanced primary osteoarthritis of the elbow. Redrawn after Ref. 17.

the posterior compartment are removed and osteophytes around the olecranon fossa and at the tip of the olecranon are excised. The shallow olecranon fossa is deepened using a burr. Anteriorly the coronoid process is trimmed and the coronoid and radial fossae deepened. The anterior joint capsule is released allowing full extension of the elbow. In severe disease with restricted forearm rotation, the radial head is trimmed and reshaped in order to improve pronation and supination. Continuous passive motion is used postoperatively for 7 days. Treating 29 elbows by this technique Tsuge and Mizuseki[17] reported an average gain in range of motion of 34 degrees. Grip strength and pain relief were also improved in most patients.

TOTAL JOINT ARTHROPLASTY

Although total joint arthroplasty is an effective treatment for patients with rheumatoid arthritis, its value in osteoarthritis is limited.[28] Joint replacement is contraindicated in young patients with isolated elbow disease and particularly in those who undertake heavy manual work. However, in retired patients with severe pain and restricted elbow movement elbow replacement may be beneficial.

ULNAR NERVE SURGERY

Impairment of ulnar nerve function is not uncommon in elbow osteoarthritis and may result from medial joint osteophytes or thickening of the fascia overlying the cubital tunnel. The clinical diagnosis should be confirmed electromyographically following which surgical decompression should be performed (Chapter 21).

AUTHOR'S PREFERRED MANAGEMENT

Patients with aching discomfort in the elbow and radiographic signs of early osteoarthritis should be treated conservatively with simple analgesics and non-steroidal anti-inflammatory drugs.

Those presenting with acute pain and locking and in whom radiographs reveal loose bodies should undergo arthroscopy. This will enable removal of the loose bodies from both the anterior and posterior compartments of the elbow joint.

More advanced disease should be treated by the open Outerbridge–Kashiwagi operation. This allows removal of osteophytes from around the olecranon fossa and tip of the olecranon, fenestration of the olecranon fossa with removal of the thickened membrane between the olecranon and coronoid fossae, removal of loose bodies and removal of osteophytes at the tip of the coronoid process.

Older patients who are no longer undertaking heavy manual work and in whom the major symptom is pain should be assessed with a view to total elbow arthroscopy (Chapter 26).

References

1. Sokloff L *The biology of degenerative joint disease.* Chicago, London: The University of Chicago Press, 1969.
2. Harrison MHM, Schajowicz F, Trueta J Osteoarthritis of the hip: A study of the nature and evolution of the disease. *J Bone Joint Surg* 1953; **35B:** 598–626.
3. Muir H Biomechanical basis for cartilage degeneration, destruction and loss of function in osteoarthritis. In: *Mechanism of articular cartilage damage and repair in osteoarthritis.* Muir H, Hirohata K, Shichikawa K (eds) Toronto: Hogrefe and Huber Publishers, 1989: 31–42.
4. Mow VC, Proctor CS, Kelley MA Biomechanics of articular cartilage. In: *Basic biomechanics of the musculoskeletal system* (2nd edn). Nordin M, Frankel VH (eds) Philadelphia: Lea and Febiger, 1989: 31–58.
5. Holtzmann F Erkrankingen Durch Arbeiten Mit Pressluftwerkzeugen. *Zentralb Gewerbehygiene Unfallverhutung* 1929; **50:** 1002–3.
6. Rostock P Gelenkschaden Durch Arbeiten Mit Presluftwerkzeugen und Andere Schwere. *Rorperliche Arbeit Medizinische Klink* 1936; **11:** 341–3.
7. Hunter D, McLaughlin AIG, Perry KMA Clinical effects of the use of pneumatic tools. *Brit J Indust Med* 1945; **2:** 10–16.
8. Lawrence JS Rheumatism in coal miners. *Brit J Indust Med* 1955; **12:** 249–61.
9. Burke MJ, Fear EC, Wright V Bone and joint changes in pneumatic drillers. *Ann Rheum Dis* 1977; **36:** 276–9.
10. Mintz G, Fraga A Severe osteoarthritis of the elbow in foundry workers. *Arch Environ Hlth* 1973; **27:** 78–80.
11. Stanley D Prevalence and aetiology of symptomatic elbow osteoarthritis. *J Shoulder Elbow Surg* 1994; **3:** 386–9.
12. Collins DH *Incidence of cartilage changes and osteoarthritis in joints at different ages in the pathology of articular and spinal diseases.* London: Edward Arnold; 1949.
13. Doherty M, Preston B Primary osteoarthritis of the elbow. *Ann Rheum Dis* 1989; **48:** 743–7.
14. Goodfellow JW, Bullough PG The pattern of ageing of the articular cartilage of the elbow joint. *J Bone Joint Surg* 1967; **49B:** 175–81.
15. Murato H, Ikuta Y, Murakami T Anatomic investigation of the elbow joint with special reference to aging of the aticular cartilage. *J Shoulder Elbow Surg* 1993; **2:** 175–81.
16. Kashiwagi D Osteoarthritis of the elbow joint – intraarticular changes and the special operative procedure, Outerbridge–Kashiwagi method (O>K> method). In: *Elbow joint.* Kashiwagi D (ed) Amsterdam: Elsevier Science Publishers BV (Biomedical Division), 1985: 177–88.
17. Tsuge K, Mizuseki T Debridgement arthroplasty for advanced primary osteoarthritis of the elbow. *J Bone Joint Surg* 1994; **76B:** 641–6.
18. Bell MS Loose bodies in the elbow. *Brit J Surg* 1975; **62:** 921–4.
19. Morrey BF Primary arthritis of the elbow treated by ulno humeral arthroplasty. *J Bone Joint Surg* 1992; **74B:** 409–13.
20. O'Driscoll S, Morrey BF Arthroscopy of the elbow. *J Bone Joint Surg* 1992; **74A:** 84.
21. Livesey PJ, Doherty M, Needoff M, Moulton A Arthroscopic lavage of osteoarthritic knees. *J Bone Joint Surg* 1991; **73B:** 922–6.
22. Redden JF, Stanley D Arthroscopic fenestration of the olecranon fossa in the treatment of osteoarthritis of the elbow. *Arthroscopy* 1993; **9:** 14–16.
23. Kashiwagi D Intra-articular changes of the osteoarthritic elbow, especially about the fossa olecrani. *J Jap Orthop Assoc* 1978; **52:** 1367–82.
24. Minami M, Ishii S Outerbridge–Kashiwagi arthroplasty for osteoarthritis of the elbow joint. In: *Elbow joint.* Kashiwagi D (ed) Amsterdam: Elsevier Science Publishers BV (Biomedical Division), 1985: 189–96.
25. Stanley D, Winson IG A surgical approach to the elbow. *J Bone Joint Surg* 1990; **72B:** 728–9.
26. Morrey BF Post-traumatic contracture of the elbow: Operative treatment including distraction arthroplasty. *J Bone Joint Surg* 1990; **72A:** 601–18.
27. Tsuge K, Mrakami T, Yasunaga Y, Kanaujia RR Arthroscopy of the elbow: Twenty years experience of a new approach. *J Bone Joint Surg* 1987; **69B:** 116–20.
28. Kraay MJ, Figgie MP, Inglis AE *et al.* Primary semiconstrained total elbow arthroplasty. *J Bone Joint Surg* 1994; **76B:** 636–40.

CHAPTER 29

Infections of the elbow

AMIT R TOLAT

Introduction

Primary infections of the elbow are a concern particularly in developing countries with ankylosis and deformity often being the end-point of the disease process, However, with the advent of increased awareness of infection and effective chemotherapy the incidence of both septic and tuberculous elbow infections are on the decline. Early diagnosis and prompt aggressive treatment remains the cornerstone for achieving a good result. Infants, the elderly and immunosuppressed patients often carry a higher risk with a relatively poor prognosis.[1]

Classification of elbow infections

Olecranon bursitis
    Traumatic
    Septic
    Inflammatory
Infections of the elbow joint
    Septic
        primary
        post-surgical
        gonococcal
        in association with sickle cell disease
        in association with rheumatoid arthritis
    Tuberculous
    Miscellaneous
        fungal
        viral

Olecranon bursitis

There are two olecranon bursae of clinical significance – one that separates the tendon of the triceps muscle from the posterior capsule of the elbow joint (deep olecranon bursa) and the other which lies between the attachment of the triceps tendon to the olecranon and the skin (superficial olecranon bursa).

The deep olecranon bursa facilitates the movement of the triceps over the bone. It is usually so small that its presence is not often evident. It is infrequently inflamed but, under the stimulus of repetitive trauma, it may become distended and appear as a rounded swelling.[2]

The superficial olecranon bursa is large and important. It is often the site of infection, which may be of three types:

1.   Traumatic
2.   Septic
3.   Inflammatory (non-septic)

TRAUMATIC

Often termed miner's or student's elbow. It presents as a fluctuant and transilluminant swelling approximately 4 × 3 cm in size over the olecranon. Typically it is painful at the outset, and minimally tender. There is usually no interference with elbow motion. Septic affection of this bursitis is thought to commonly supervene.[2]

SEPTIC

Septic bursitis results in severe pain with increased local warmth and tenderness. A secondary cellulitis may occur with possible superficial bone necrosis. The joint, however, usually remains unaffected.

INFLAMMATORY (NON-SEPTIC)

This is often associated with a systemic inflammatory process such as rheumatoid arthritis, gout and chondrocalcinosis.[3] Communication with the joint may be present in rheumatoid arthritis in which case the bursitis is generally considered a secondary process.

TREATMENT FOR OLECRANON BURSITIS

Traumatic

The primary attack usually responds to aspiration followed by a firm compression bandage or strapping. Recurrent attacks often do not respond to aspiration alone and need surgical excision. Excision of the bursa requires careful and complete dissection of the entire sac. The incision is usually taken away from the mid-line and the dead space must be obliterated by suturing the subcutaneous tissues to the periosteum.[4] A drain is usually retained for 24–48 hours with the elbow splinted in acute flexion for approximately 10 days.

Septic

Acute infection requires urgent incision and drainage. The elbow should then be splinted in 90 degrees of flexion and the patient treated with appropriate antibiotics until the wound has healed. A chronically infected bursa may require surgical excision.

Inflammatory (non-septic)

Treatment of the underlying condition is essential. To this end aspiration of the bursa may assist in the diagnosis. In rheumatoid disease, it is important to exclude joint communication. If this does exist excision of the bursa may result in recurrent swelling or lead to the formation of a continuously discharging sinus.

Infections of the elbow joint

PATHOPHYSIOLOGY AND ROUTES OF INFECTION

Infections of synovial joints require early detection and prompt treatment if a good functional result is to be obtained. Damage to articular cartilage is repaired only by fibrocartilage or fibrous tissue.[5]

Articular cartilage is avascular and aneural and metabolic materials pass to and fro across the cartilage by a diffusion process.[6,7] Synovial fluid is the primary source of nutrition and the synovial membrane is especially adapted for its production. The fluid is a dialysate of plasma with the addition of hyaluronic acid.[8,9] Excessive synovial fluid within a closed space causes increased intra-articular pressure and pain. Thus a person so affected will hold the elbow in the position of minimum pressure and maximum comfort. This is between 30 degrees and 70 degrees of elbow flexion.[10]

As is common for most synovial joints, bacteria gain entrance to the elbow by one of three routes: haematogenous, direct inoculation and by extension from an adjacent focus of infection.[11–13] Haematogenous septic, or tuberculous arthritis is the most common infection of adult elbow joints. Extension from an adjacent focus of sepsis is common only in the infant or child. Direct bacterial inoculation is an infrequent route but may result from penetrating needles used for diagnostic or therapeutic purposes or by drug abusers. It may also follow compound elbow fractures, or occur postoperatively. In tuberculous infections, the primary focus usually lies in the thoracic cavity. Occasionally tuberculous joint disease may be due to direct extension from a lesion in one of the adjacent bones.[14]

CLINICAL PRESENTATIONS

The chief complaints of a patient with a developing septic arthritis are pain, swelling and limitation of joint motion. If the symptoms are of short duration, erythema and swelling may not be marked but the pain on attempted motion will often be severe. In those with immunodeficiency, the general systemic response to sepsis (pyrexia, malaise) may not be apparent.

Physical examination usually reveals the elbow held in 30–70 degrees of flexion. The elbow is guarded by the patient who refuses to allow examination of the joint. An effusion is noted at the 'soft spot' with elimination of the bony prominences. Erythema with warmth are an important clinical sign. There is moderate to severe tenderness of the joint line with limitation of active and passive movements. In the young child spasm is often diagnostic.

ASSESSMENT AND INVESTIGATIONS

Joint aspiration

Although blood investigations may show a leucocytosis and a raised sedimentation, the key to diagnosis is joint aspiration. The distended joint is easy to enter through the 'anconeus triangle' sited laterally (needle A, Fig. 29.1). The triangle is formed by the tip of the lateral epicondyle, the radial head and the tip of the olecranon. It represents a safe and easy route as the needle passes merely through skin, subcutaneous tissue and anconeus to enter the joint. An alternative route is through the posterior olecranon fossa (needle B, Fig. 29.1).

Joint aspiration must be performed under sterile conditions, since inoculation of a sterile joint is possible.[15] Septic joint fluid is usually yellowish–white

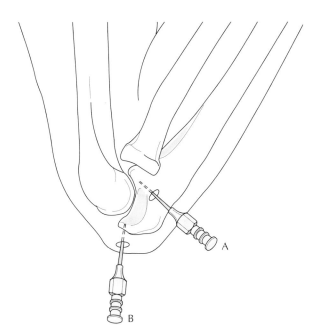

Fig. 29.1 Aspiration routes for the elbow, Needle A and Needle B. Redrawn after Ref. 1 with permission from Churchill Livingstone, New York.

grey, extremely turbid in appearance and often shows pus flakes. It has a very low viscosity and poor mucin clot formation. Microscopically, the features which differentiate it from a non-infected inflammatory exudate include an extremely high leucocyte count (>50 000), a low ratio to plasma glucose (<0.5), a high titre for proteins (up to 8 g/100 ml) and a positive smear for bacteria, which can be isolated on culture. The most common organism in the adult is *Straphylococcus aureus* (70%). In the child up to 3 years old *Haemophilus influenzae* may be more frequently seen.[16] However, in the neonate, coliform and Gram-positive organisms are not uncommon.[17] Above the age of 3 years *Staph. aureus* is again the predominant organism.[16]

Blood culture

Blood cultures are seen to be positive in up to 70% of patients.[15,16] To be useful, blood cultures must be done prior to the initiation of antibiotic treatment.

Radiology

The soft tissues have to be carefully evaluated to see the earliest x-ray changes. A positive fat pad sign related to the visualisation of the dorsal or olecranon fat pad is possible in moderate effusions, at an early stage.[18] The earliest bony change is an osteoporosis of the distal humerus and proximal radius and ulna, due to hyperaemia. Subtle bony erosions at the synovial attachments then occur, progressing to uniform articular cartilage thinning. Finally, more extensive erosions with subchondral disruptions occur, reflected by the radiographic picture 'fuzziness', irregularity and obvious joint space narrowing. In untreated septic joints fibrous or bony ankylosis finally supervenes.

TREATMENT

The principles of treatment are:

1. rest for the joint
2. joint decompression by adequate surgical drainage of the purulent exudate
3. commencement of parenteral antibiotic therapy
4. joint rehabilitation.

1. *Initial rest for the elbow* is essential. This can be achieved with either a removable plastazoate moulded splint or a posterior plaster slab set at approximately a right angle.
2. *Joint decompression* to remove cellular debris, detritus and pus is a vital part of the treatment.

Cartilage is very easily destroyed by the lysosomal enzymes released from neutrophils, synovium and bacteria.[19] Adequate surgical drainage is achieved by arthroscopy or a formal arthrotomy. Repeated aspirations have been advocated in the past but have now been superseded by arthroscopic drainage with lavage.[1] Arthroscopy of the elbow allows inspection, clearance of loculations and adhesions, thorough irrigation, and synovial tissue culture as well as insertion of drainage catheters. For infections which are subacute, postoperative or due to direct inoculation, open surgical drainage via an arthrotomy may be necessary. Posterior drainage by medial and lateral incisions (Fig. 29.2) may be used. These incisions are through the medial and lateral borders of the triceps aponeurosis into the joint. Care must be taken not to injure the ulnar nerve as it crosses the cubital tunnel medially. Alternatively, a single lateral incision centred on the lateral humeral epicondyle may be used.

3. *Initial parenteral antibiotic therapy* is based on age and presentation. This should include a cephalosporin in combination with amikacin or clindamycin (Gram-negative coverage) in the adult patient, and *H. influenzae* cover (intravenous

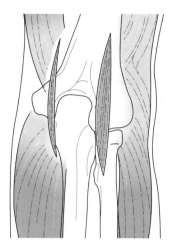

Fig. 29.2 Posteromedial and posterolateral incisions for elbow drainage. Redrawn after Ref. 1 with permission from Churchill Livingstone, New York.

ampicillin 150–200 mg/kg/day) in the child under 3 years of age. Further antibiotic changes are made on the basis of the blood culture and/or fluid aspirate and smear results (Table 29.1).

Table 29.1 Antibiotic therapy for septic arthrtis

Organism	Antibiotic	Dose	Alternative drug
Staphylococcus aureus (penicillin sensitive)	Penicillin G	100–200 mg (160 000– 320 000)/kg body wt/day as six equal intravenous doses	Cefazolin Clindamycin
Staphylococcus aureus (penicillinase producing)	Nafcillin, oxacillin or dicloxacillin	150–200 mg/kg/day as six equal intravenous doses	Cefazolin Clindamycin
Streptococcus pneumoniae Streptococcus pyogenes, Neisseria gonorrheae Neisseria meningitides	Penicillin G	5–6 mg/kg/day as three equal intravenous doses	Cefazolin
Pseudomonas aeruginosa	Gentamicin or tobramycin	5–6 mg/kg/day as three equal intravenous doses	
Proteus sp.	Carbenicillin	300–500 mg/kg/day as six equal intravenous doses	
Serratia sp. *Enterobacter* sp. *Klebsiella* sp.	Gentamicin or tobramicin	5–6 mg/kg/day as three equal intravenous doses	
E. coli Proteus mirabilis	Ampicillin	150–200 mg/kg/day as six equal intravenous doses	Cefazolin Gentamicin
Haemophilus influenzae	Ampicillin	150–200 mg/kg/day as six equal intravenous doses	Chloramphenicol
Brucella sp.	Tetracycline	30–50 mg/kg/day as four equal oral doses	Trimethoprim, Streptomycin

After Ref. 1 with permission from Churchill Livingstone, New York.

Parenteral antibiotic treatment should not be delayed until the blood culture/aspirate smear results are obtained. The duration of intravenous therapy should be dictated by the clinical setting. Generally, however, intravenous therapy is continued for approximately 1 week after serum bactericidal levels have been obtained.[20] Thereafter oral antibiotics need to be continued for a further 4–6 weeks with serial monitoring of the serum antibiotic levels.

4. *Irrespective of the surgical method employed early motion should be undertaken postoperatively.* The basis of the beneficial effects of early motion were studied by Salter *et al.*[21] who concluded that this method prevents adhesion formation, improves the nutrition of articular cartilage and enhances the clearance of the exudate. As the rehabilitation phase progresses, the patient may enhance isotonic or isokinetic muscle strengthening.[1]

AUTHOR'S PREFERRED MANAGEMENT

Following the diagnosis of a septic elbow, the patient is admitted to hospital and appropriate blood investigations (white cell count, erythrocyte sedimentation rate (ESR) and blood cultures) are performed. The joint is placed in a right-angled plaster back slab and a combination of cefazolin (15–20 mg/kg body weight/day) and Amikacin (10–15 mg/kg body weight/day) are initiated. Response to parenteral antibiotic treatment is awaited over a 24-hour period. A failure to respond or an equivocal response requires joint aspiration under a general anaesthetic. If the aspirate appears infective, surgical drainage by arthroscopy is the preferred method. Joint lavage must be thorough and a suction drain is left *in situ* for 3–4 days. Joint motion is initiated after drain removal, and consists initially of active assisted motion, followed by independent active motion at 12–14 days after the wound has healed. Adequate serum antibiotic levels should be maintained by parenteral drug administration for 1 week after which oral antibiotics should be continued for a further 6 weeks or until the ESR approaches normality.

Results

A delay in the diagnosis as well as in the initiation of treatment appears to be the most important factor in the prognosis.[16,22] Degeneration of articular cartilage with fibrous adhesions is likely to be the end-point of a joint for which treatment is delayed for more than a week after the onset of symptoms.[23] Other factors which influence the prognosis include the age of the patient, virulence

and nature of the organism. The younger the patient, the better the host resistance and the better the outcome with early treatment. Virulence of the organism is an important variable. Complete recovery occurs in less than one-third of patients infected with Gram-negative bacteria. Gram-negative infection has a poor prognosis and is often associated with a diminished host resistance. On the other hand, *Staph aureus* infection is associated with approximately a 60% chance of full recovery and *Streptococcus* infection is associated with a 90% chance of full recovery. Loss of function of the joint, as opposed to recurrence is the most common sequela of septic elbows[15] but, the ultimate functional outcome is directly linked to the condition of the joint prior to the infectious process.

Post-surgical

This is often a 'mixed-bag' of organisms, although here too *Staph. aureus* is the most common pathogen involved. Post-surgical sepsis requires prompt detection and early open surgical drainage, followed by catheter drainage for at least 3–4 days. Postoperative immobilisation as opposed to motion may be of value depending on the type of elbow surgery originally performed.

Gonococcal

Gonococcal arthritis affects the elbow in 10% of cases.[24] The causative organism is *Neisseria gonorrhoeae*, which has a known affinity for the synovium.[25] As part of a polyarthritis, it is associated with fever and pustular skin lesions. Synovial fluid aspirate reveals a very high white cell count of several thousand to 100 000 cells, with a positive culture.[1] Treatment of *N. gonorrhoeae* infections gives reasonably good results.

Non-gonococcal *Neisseria* infections have also been reported to involve the elbow, often in association with crystal-induced arthritis.[20] Occasionally, elbow synovitis is seen with a gonococcal or non-gonococcal urinary tract infection. This is usually of a reactive nature, with no true infection.

Septic elbow in association with sickle-cell disease

Such patients may present with a warm, swollen and acutely painful joint during a sickling crisis. Elbow affection is seen second only to the knee and shoulder. Sickle-cell sufferers have a predilection for *Salmonella* or *staphylococcal* sepsis. Treatment should include rehydration along with appropriate antibiotic treatment.[26,27]

Septic elbow in association with rheumatoid disease

Patients with rheumatoid arthritis have been noted to occasionally present with septic elbow joints.[28] Kellgren *et al.*[22] reported that septic joints in four of 12 rheumatoid arthritis patients (33%) involved the elbow. They also noted the high incidence of *Staph. aureus* organisms (83%) and multiple sites of involvement in all 12.

Owing to pre-existing joint disease and immune abnormalities, the diagnosis is often made late.[29] Any sudden or rapid increase in joint inflammation in rheumatoid patients should raise the suspicion of a possible infection.

TUBERCULOSIS OF THE ELBOW

Skeletal tuberculosis remains a major cause of concern in the developing world, including the Asian subcontinent. With the spread of AIDS (Acquired immunodeficiency syndrome) to all countries of the globe there is every likelihood that this infection will recur in the developed world. Overall, the incidence of elbow tuberculosis is between 2 and 5% of all skeletal tuberculosis.[30] In comparison with the shoulder and the wrist, the elbow is more often affected. It is seen, in my experience, as frequently in children as in adults.

Pathology

Mycobacterium tuberculosis is the causative organism, which reaches the joint by a haematogenous route. Less commonly, it may occur following the extension of a focus in the adjacent bone.[14] The pathological process is marked by its chronicity with synovial thickening and tubercles (caseating or non-caseating granulomas) studding the synovium. There is, usually further progression to the formation of tuberculous granulation tissue – pannus – which is seen initially at the margins of the articular cartilage and then progresses centrally, causing cartilage destruction and subchondral erosions. Flakes or loose sheets of necrosed articular cartilage and accumulations of fibrinous material in the synovial fluid may produce 'rice bodies'.[30] Complete joint destruction usually produces a fibrous ankylosis with very little motion. Damage to the physis in childhood may result in shortening or angulation of the extremity.

In the elbow the disease often starts with a bony lesion in the olecranon (Fig. 29.3) or the distal humerus. On other occasions, the onset is from a lesion in the radial head. In up to 50% of cases the onset is synovial. In the developing world the

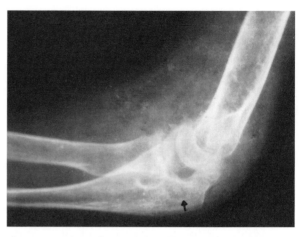

Fig. 29.3 Tuberculosis of the elbow with an olecranon lesion.

patient often seeks medical attention at a much later stage, such that accurate localisation of the disease onset is not possible.

Clinical features

The onset is generally insidious, with constitutional symptoms such as evening rise of temperature, malaise, loss of appetite and weight. Pain on attempted motion of the joint is usually the earliest clinical sign. Soon to follow are muscle spasm, swelling, local warmth and tenderness with restriction of joint motion (Fig. 29.4). Swelling is maximally appreciated over the posterior aspect of the elbow joint, on either side of the olecranon and triceps insertion area. As the synovitis progresses, the bony prominences are obliterated and the synovium may be palpable as a 'doughy' feel.

Muscle spasm is also an early sign, with consequent limitation of motion. Initially there is a restriction of the terminal 5–10 degrees of flexion and extension. Subsequently, if untreated, the articular cartilage undergoes irreversible damage with the range of motion substantially reduced, ultimately leaving the elbow with a mere jog of motion (10–15 degrees) or a complete short fibrous ankylosis with no perceivable movement.

In the active stages local warmth is invariably increased in comparison with the opposite normal side. If an abscess forms, it is more pronounced and may be seen to point lateral to the olecranon. Muscle wasting is a feature typically noted at approximately 4–6 weeks after the onset of the disease. Supratrochlear or axillary lymph nodes are enlarged in nearly one-third of patients.[31] Unless immunodeficient, constitutional symptoms that accompany tuberculosis are usually present.

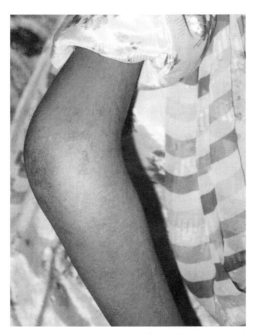

Fig. 29.4 Tuberculosis of the elbow. Clinical features of swelling, secondary proximal muscle wasting.

Radiology

The earliest radiological sign is a localised osteoporosis of the joint, sometimes accompanied by a soft tissue swelling. Over the ensuing weeks the articular margin and bony cortical outline becomes hazy. This early articular cartilage damage is reflected by an irregularity and 'fuzziness' over the joint space. Additionally, areas of tuberculous destruction with an osteolytic focus in the olecranon or the lateral condyle of the humerus usually appear. The radiological stage then progresses to bone resorption with cystic subchondral changes, reflecting the bony destruction and reduction in joint space. The x-ray changes do not necessarily correlate with the loss of motion seen clinically. Rarely, due to marked destruction of the bone and the supporting ligaments, the elbow may develop a pathological posterior dislocation.[30]

Investigations

Blood

A relative lymphocytosis, associated with an anaemia and raised ESR are usually noted in the active stages of the disease.

Mantoux or tuberculin test

This is usually irrelevant in a tuberculosis endemic area, as all adults have had subclinical exposure to tuberculosis. It is useful, however, in the developed world, where the incidence of tuberculosis is low. In this situation it is a useful screening test. It is universally useful in children, when a highly positive test (20 mm reaction with induration at 72 hours) is usually indicative of tuberculous infection. The test may also be helpful if it is negative as this excludes any exposure to tuberculosis. On rare occasions a negative test may occur in patients with low tuberculosis immunity who have miliary tuberculosis and AIDS associated tuberculosis.

Joint aspiration

Aspiration assists the diagnosis in up to 25% of cases though isolation of the organism is rare. The features suggestive of an exudate include a leucocytosis (10 000–20 000 white cell count/ml), markedly reduced glucose, significantly increased protein and poor mucin clot formation.

Immunological tests

Stroebel *et al.*[32] reported that an ELISA (enzyme linked immunosorbent assay) for antibody to mycobacterium antigen-6, when demonstrated at a cut-off of 1:32, revealed a sensitivity of 94% and specificity of 100% in the serological diagnosis of skeletal tuberculosis. The consistency of these observations in the diagnosis of tuberculosis are, however, uncertain.[30]

Chest x-ray

This is seen to be positive for pulmonary tuberculosis in approximately 50% of cases.[33]

Biopsy of the synovium

This may greatly assist in diagnosis. The only method of definitive diagnosis is the actual isolation of tuberculous bacilli, which is not easy, even from tissue specimens. Hence, in most of the developing world the diagnosis is often based on a high index of clinicoradiologic suspicion coupled with positive ancillary investigations. Treatment is then initiated as soon as possible.

Conservative treatment

The aim of conservative treatment is a pain-free, useful range of elbow motion. This is often achievable in those who present early. It involves:

Rest for the elbow

The joint is placed at rest in the position that will be most useful should ankylosis occur. This is at or just above the right angle (100 degrees). It is usually immobilised in a cast or brace for approximately 6 weeks, while the chemotherapeutic response is awaited.

Chemotherapy (anti-tuberculous medication)

The drugs in common usage are:

isoniazid (INH): 5–7 mg/kg/day
rifampicin (RIFA): 10–15 mg/kg/day
pyrazinamide (PZA): 20–30 mg/kg/day
ethambutol (ETB): 15–20 mg/kg/day

Additionally pyridoxine (Vitamin B6) is given at a dose of 50–100 mg/day to counter the side-effect of neuritis associated with isoniazid therapy.

In the past, para-aminosalicylic acid (PAS) and streptomycin (SM) were considered ideal companions to isoniazid for primary therapy. However, these have been associated with numerous side-effects which include drug toxicity and early drug resistance. Hence, over the last decade, ethambutol and rifampicin have successfully taken their place.[34]

The current chemotherapeutic regimen employed at our institution utilises a primary four-drug (INH + RIFA + PZA + ETB) regimen for all tuberculous elbow patients. Pyrazinamide is usually discontinued at 2 months and ethambutol at 3 months. Isoniazid and rifampicin are then continued for a further 6 months (a total of 9 months treatment). In children, ethambutol is used with care owing to the known occular side-effect of retrobulbar neuritis.[34] Hence, in children it is advocated that not more than 15 mg/kg/day dose be given for more than 6 weeks. With the current concern for drug-resistant tuberculosis in association with immunocompromised patients,[35] testing of all adult tuberculosis patients for human immunodeficiency virus (HIV) is necessary. If a patient tests HIV-positive, a minimum of 11 months of anti-tuberculous therapy is necessary (PZA + ETB discontinued at 2 months, and INH + RIFA for 9 months thereafter). Careful monitoring of all HIV-positive patients with tuberculosis is essential, especially to diagnose non-compliance and drug resistance.[35] Those with proven drug resistance need up to 2 years of therapy. As soon as pain in the elbow permits, active assisted flexion/extension and pronation/supination exercises are initiated. The splint is worn for 6–9 months on an intermittent basis and at night. After splint removal the joint should be protected against overuse for another 9–12 months.

In a study of 29 tuberculous elbows treated with chemotherapy alone, 28 achieved a satisfactory joint with a useful arc of painfree motion (30–100 degrees).[36] In another study by Srivastava,[31] similar findings were reported for conservatively treated elbow tuberculosis. Overall the results of chemotherapy alone are best in patients who have only synovial disease, unicompartmental disease or early arthritis.

In advanced tuberculous arthritis with involvement of all the elbow compartments, the result is usually a stiff, ankylosed elbow.

Surgical treatment

The indications for surgical intervention are:

1. Persistent tuberculous elbow synovitis with a poor response to 6 weeks of conservative treatment.
2. Tuberculous arthritis with a significant functional deficit.
3. Large cold abscess.
4. Cubital tunnel syndrome with tuberculous synovitis.

The surgical procedures available include:

Elbow synovectomy with debridement

This procedure is suitable for relatively early disease with no major cartilage damage, but associated with persistent synovitis. It may also involve the curettage of any bone lesions. Usually, a modified Kocher 'J' approach is used with the proximal part of the incision extending slightly posteriorly. As soon as the deep fascia is incised, the synovium is seen to bulge through the thin capsule. A synovectomy is performed with excision of all loose tissue and debris. Tuberculous pannus is often distinct and can gradually be peeled off the articular surface. Excision of the radial head enables a more extensive synovectomy to be undertaken. The postoperative care involves rest for 3 weeks in a plaster back-slab followed by guarded mobilisation.

Excisional arthroplasty

This is usually indicated in adults in whom the disease is extensive and more conservative measures have failed. It usually results in less disability than an arthrodesis.

Excision of the elbow is prone to the development of instability. This may be avoided to some extent by performing what is termed a 'V' notch

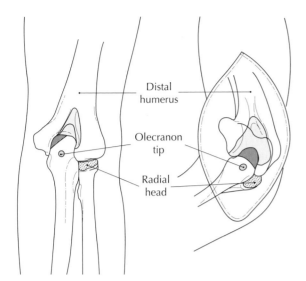

Fig. 29.5 'V' Notch plasty of the elbow. Resection of distal humerus and olecranon tip. The radial head is routinely excised (as shown in hatched areas).

plasty of the elbow.[30] This procedure has been in use at our institution since 1980 with good results. It involves a bony excision in the manner shown (Fig. 29.5a,b), and maximises the preservation of the collateral ligaments. The approach used for surgery is an extended Kocher 'J' incision through the posterolateral aspect. The lateral collateral ligament is divided and in order to open the joint fully, the deep part of the medial collateral ligament, is released from its ulnar attachment. After performing a synovectomy and radial head excision, a 'V'

notch plasty is carried out. The dished-out proximal ulna moves in an inverted 'V' notch created in the distal humerus. The ulnar nerve is not transposed as a routine. However, in those patients who do have symptoms referable to ulnar nerve compression preoperatively, it is advisable to release and transpose the nerve anteriorly through a separate medial incision.

Postoperatively, the joint is rested for a week in a plaster slab set at approximately a right angle. Following this, gentle active and active assisted motion is initiated. A hinged elbow brace is optional, and may be essential if stability is poor. The therapy is often painful at the outset, but as the pseudo joint forms the pain eases and the motion steadily improves. Usually, a gratifying painfree arc of about 80–100 degrees, with good stability is achieved at approximately 8–12 weeks postoperatively (Fig. 29.6a,b).

Late excision arthroplasty (>1 year) usually requires a more extensile posterolateral approach. The triceps insertion may need lengthening and arthrolysis of the elbow together with excision arthroplasty are necessary in order to obtain a satisfactory result. The tendency to re-ankylose is high (50–60%) and careful preoperative planning is necessary. Froimson[37] describes good results using a fascial interposition arthroplasty. This involves the use of a resurfacing dermocutaneous free graft over the refashioned lower end of the humerus.

Arthrodesis of the elbow

This procedure is rarely undertaken today. The acceptance rate even in developing countries like

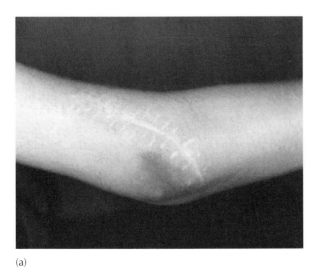

(a)

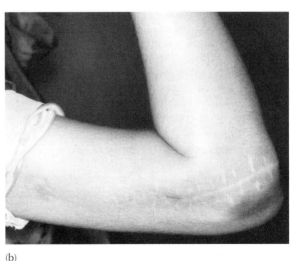

(b)

Fig. 29.6 (a,b) Postoperative follow-up of range of motion at 6 months following 'V' notch plasty for tuberculosis, flexion 110 degrees, extension 15 degrees short of full.

India is extremely low. It has traditionally been indicated for the dominant elbow of a manual labourer with fixation being achieved by means of a compression screw technique. The optimal joint position for fusion is approximately 90 degrees. Immobilisation in an above elbow cast is necessary for 3 months.[2]

Author's preferred management

Elbow tuberculosis which has not responded to a 6-week course of four-drug chemotherapy requires a careful re-evaluation. If the patient has been taking medication regularly, the persistent synovitis needs surgical decompression along with synovectomy and debridement. I prefer to do this through a modified Kocher lateral approach which is extended posterosuperiorly. A completely destroyed joint with painful limitation of motion and a significant functional deficit requires an elbow excisional arthroplasty of the 'V' notch type. Elbow arthrodesis is not recommended since the results of excision arthroplasty are superior.

MISCELLANEOUS

Fungal

This is an extremely rare cause of elbow infection. However, coccidioidomycosis has been reported in up to 12% of elbow joint infections, due to *Coccidioides immitis*.[38] The recommended treatment here is synovectomy with intravenous amphotericin-B for the disseminated disease.

Viral

True viral infections of joints are extremely rare as far as the elbow is concerned. Of historical interest is variola (smallpox arthritis) which has been eradicated from the Asian subcontinent since 1975. Occasionally, an older patient can present with a residue of this condition, in whom despite complete destruction with bony resorption, there is a near full range of motion.

References

1. Petty W In: *Infection of synovial joints.* Evarts McCollister CC, Nelson C (eds) New York: Churchill Livingstone, 1984: 75–100.
2. Duthie RB, Bentley G Infections of the musculoskeletal system. In: *Mercer's orthopaedic surgery* (8th edn). London: Edward Arnold, 1983: 526.
3. Gerster JC, Lagler R, Bolvin G Olecranon bursitis related to calcium phyrophosphate dihydrate crystal deposition disease. *Arth Rheum* 1982; **25:** 989–96.
4. Justis EJ Jr Affections of muscles, tendons and associated structures. In: *Campbell's operative orthopaedics* Vol. 2 (6th edn). Edmonson AS, Crenshaw AH (eds) St Louis: CV Mosby, 1980: 1412.
5. Gardner E The structure and functions of joints. In: *Arthritis and allied conditions* (8th edn). Hollander JHL (ed). Philadelphia: Lea and Febiger, 1972: 32.
6. Gardner E Physiological mechanisms in moveable joints. *Am Acad Orth Surg Instructional Course Lectures* 1953; **10:** 251–61.
7. Hamerman D, Rosenberg LC, Schubert M Diarthrodial joints revisited. *J Bone Joint Surg* 1970; **52A:** 725–74.
8. Davies DV The lymphatics of the synovial membrane. *J Anat* 1946; **80:** 21–3.
9. Jessar R The synovial fluid. In: *Arthritis and allied conditions* (8th edn). Hollander JHL (ed) Philadelphia: Lea and Febiger, 1972: 67.
10. Eyring EJ, Murray WR Effect of joint position on the pressure of intra-articular effusion. *J Bone Joint Surg* 1964; **46A:** 1235–41.
11. Johnson AH, Campbell WG, Callahan B Infection of rabbit knee joint after intra-articular injection of *Staphylococcus aureus. Am J Path* 1970; **60:** 165–202.
12. Jones WC, Miller WE Skeletal tuberculosis. *South Med J* 1964; **57:** 964–71.
13. Schurman DJ, Johnson BL, Amstutz HC Knee joint infections with *Staphylococcus aureus* and micrococcus species. *J Bone Joint Surg* 1975; **57A:** 40–9.
14. Davidson PT, Horowitz I Skeletal tuberculosis. *Am J Med* 1970; **48:** 77–84.
15. Argen RJ, Wilson CH, Wood P Suppurative arthritis. *Arch Intern Med* 1966; **117:** 61–6.
16. Morrey BF, Peterson HA Haematogenous pyogenic osteomyelitis in children. *Orthop Clin North Am* 1975; **6:** 935–51.
17. Nelson JD The bacterial aetiology and antibiotic managament of septic arthritis in infants and children. *Paediatrics* 1972; **50:** 437–40.
18. Norell HG Roentgenologic visualisation of extracapsular fat; its importance in the diagnosis of traumatic injuries to the elbow. *Acta Radiol* 1954; **42:** 205–10.
19. Degan TJ, Rand JA, Morrey BF Musculoskeletal infection with nongonococcal *Neisseria* species not associated with meningitis. *Clin Orthop* 1983; **176:** 206–9.
20. Kolyvas E, Kolyvas E Ahronheim G *et al.* Oral antibiotic therapy of skeletal infections in children. 1980; **65:** 867–71.
21. Salter RB, Bell RS, Keeley FW The protective effect of continous passive motion on living articular cartilage in acute septic arthritis. *Clin Orthop* 1981; **159:** 223–47.
22. Kellgren JH, Ball J, Fairbrother RW, Barnes KL Suppurative arthritis complicating rheumatoid arthritis. *Brit Med J* 1958; **1:** 1193–200.
23. Peterson S, Knudsen FU, Andersen EA, Egebald M Acute haematogenous osteomyelitis and septic arthritis in children. *Acta Orthop Scand* 1980; **51:** 451–7.

24. Masi AT, Eisenstein BI Disseminated gonococcal infection and gonococcal arthritis. *Sem Arth Rheum* 1981; **10**: 173–97.
25. Sharp JT Gonococcal arthritis. In: *Arthritis and allied conditions.* McCarty DJ (ed) Philadelphia: Lea and Febiger, 1979.
26. Vartiainen J, Hurri L Arthritis due to *Salmonella typhimurium. Acta Med Scand* 1964; **175**: 771–6.
27. Barrett-Connor E Bacterial infection and sickle-cell anaemia. *Medicine* 1971; **50**: 97–112.
28. MacGregor RR, Spagnuolo PJ, Lentnek AL Inhibition of granulocyte adherence by ethanol, prednisone and aspirin, measured with an assay system. *New Engl J Med* 1974; **291**: 642–6.
29. Dale DC, Fauci AS, Wolff SM Alternate-day prednisone. *New Engl J Med* 1974; **291**: 1154–8.
30. Tuli SM Tuberculosis of the elbow joint. In: *Tuberculosis of the skeletal system* (1st edn). Tuli SM (ed) Delhi: Jaypee Brothers, 1991: 105.
31. Srivastava T Tuberculosis of the elbow joint. Proceedings of the combined congress of the international bone and joint tuberculosis club and Indian Orthopaedic Association, Madras, India. *Indian Orthop* 1983; **12**: 26–9.
32. Stroebel AB, Daniel TM, Lau JHK Serologic diagnosis of bone and joint tuberculosis by an enzyme-linked immunosorbent assay. *J Infect Dis* 1982; **146**: 280–3.
33. Wolfgang GL Tuberculous joint infection. *Clin Orthop* 1978; **136**: 257–63.
34. Lawrence RM Extra-pulmonary tuberculosis. In: *Infectious diseases.* Hoeprich PD (ed) Hagerstown Md: Harper and Row, 1977.
35. Iseman MD Treatment of multidrug resistant tuberculosis. *New Engl J Med* 1994; **329**: 784–91.
36. Martini M, Gottesmann H Results of conservative treatment in tuberculosis of the elbow. *Int Orthop* 1980; **4**: 83–6.
37. Froimson AI Fascial interposition arthroplasty of the elbow. In: *The elbow: Master techniques in orthopaedic surgery.* Morrey BF (ed) New York: Raven Press, 1994: 329–42.
38. Winter WG, Larson RK, Honeggar MM *et al.* Coggidioidal arthritis and its treatment. *J Bone Joint Surg* 1975; **57A:** 1152–7.

CHAPTER 30

Primary bone tumours around the elbow

SR CANNON

Introduction

The elbow appears to be an area which is rarely afflicted by primary bone tumours. Although it is difficult to give a true incidence of the conditions, a review of 1900 cases referred to the London Bone Tumour Service reveals only 32 cases involving the elbow joint. The pathological diagnoses of these cases is shown in Table 30.1. Although this table may represent the true incidence of primary malignant lesions in the southern half of the United Kingdom, it does not reflect the true incidence of benign lesions, many of which will be treated without referral to a supra-specialist centre.

The most common benign lesion of bone is undoubtedly the solitary osteocartilaginous exostosis (osteochondroma). This condition was first described by Sir Astley Cooper in 1818.[1] A review of 323 solitary lesions revealed only five around the distal humerus.[2] In multiple exostoses (diaphyseal

Table 30.1 Pathological diagnosis of 32 cases involving the elbow joint referred to the London Bone Tumour Service

Malignant	
Osteosarcoma/periosteal osteosarcoma	4
Chondrosarcoma	4
Malignant fibrous histiocytoma	4
Ewing's sarcoma	3
Metastasis	3
Synovial sarcoma	2
Lymphoma	1

Benign	
Giant cell tumour	2
Benign fibrous histiocytoma/fibrous dysplasia	2
Aneurysmal bone cyst	2
Osteoid osteoma/Osteoblastoma	2
Myositis ossificans	1
Chondroblastoma	1
Osteomyelitis	1

aclasis) the distal humerus, in common with other long tubular bones, may be affected and unequal growth of the bones about the elbow may cause radiohumeral subluxation.[3] Diaphyseal aclasis must be distinguished from Ollier's disease or multiple enchondromatosis. This is a cartilage dysplasia which rarely affects the elbow region but involvement of a bone close to an epiphysis may lead to forearm distortion.[4] The association of soft tissue haemangiomas with enchondromatosis is known as Maffucci's syndrome.[5,6] Any bone or area may be affected and the rate of malignant transformation of the enchondritic element is said to be greater than in Ollier's disease.

Sir Astley Cooper is also credited with the first description of a gaint cell tumour and emphasised its benign nature, but the French surgeon, Nelaton, was the first to give a good account of the varied clinical course and histological features.[7] A review of 265 cases of giant cell tumour finds only three occurring around the distal humerus.

None of the four common primary bone malignancies – osteosarcoma, chondrosarcoma, Ewing's sarcoma and malignant fibrous histiocytoma – are commonly found around the elbow joint. Sir James Paget first described osteosarcoma in 1854.[8] Treatment until the mid-1970s has always been by ablation, but with modern chemotherapy, limb-sparing surgical techniques may be attempted. Ewing first described his eponymous disease in 1921[9] and further classified telangiectatic osteosarcoma in 1922.[10] The disease which bears his name is now thought to have been originally recognised by Lucke in 1866.[11] It is considered to be one of a spectrum of small round cell tumours to afflict bone. Considerable skill and immunocytochemistry may be required for a histopathologist to differentiate Ewing's sarcoma from neuroblastoma, primitive neuroectodermal tumour of bone, small cell osteosarcoma, embryonal rhabdomyosarcoma and lymphoma of bone.

Classification of common primary bone tumours

Bone forming tumours
Benign
  osteoma
  osteoid osteoma
  osteoblastoma
Malignant
  osteosarcoma
  parosteal osteosarcoma
  periosteal osteosarcoma

Cartilage forming tumours
Benign
  solitary/multiple osteochondroma
  chondroblastoma
  chondromyxoid fibroma
Malignant
  chondrosarcoma
  dedifferentiated chondrosarcoma
  mesenchymal chondrosarcoma
  clear cell chondrosarcoma
Tumours of histiocytic or fibrohistiocytic origin
Benign
  giant cell tumour
  non-ossifying fibroma
  benign fibrous histiocytoma/fibrous dysplasia
Malignant
  malignant fibrous histiocytoma
  Ewing's sarcoma
Simple bone cyst
Aneurysmal bone cyst
Miscellaneous tumours of soft tissue
  myositis ossificans

Bone-forming tumours

BENIGN

Osteoma

These usually present as small, painless, slowly-enlarging lumps. Although most commonly occurring around the skull, any bone may be affected. Radiological appearance is of a dense well-circumscribed lesion.

Treatment is by surgical excision if the patient is symptomatic.

Osteoid osteoma

This condition usually presents as vague pain, often nocturnal in timing, and relieved characteristically by aspirin and other non-steroidal anti-inflammatory agents.[12] The pain may be associated with tenderness and vasomotor disturbance. Classically, the osteoblastic nidus arises within the cortex or spongiosa of long bones. The nidus is less than 1 cm in diameter and induces intense surrounding reactive change. If the nidus is in a sub-articular location diagnosis can be difficult as the reactive changes may not occur (Fig. 30.1). Intra-capsular osteoid osteomas around the elbow have been mistaken for tuberculous synovitis[13] and rheumatoid arthritis.[14] It is also well recognised that long-standing disease can induce degenerative change.[15]

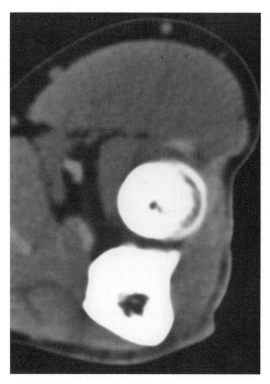

Fig. 30.1 Computed tomography scan of osteoid osteoma of the proximal radius

The radiological investigation consists initially of a plain x-ray. This may or may not reveal the characteristic nidus. When marked reactive bone is seen, the differential diagnosis is between bone abscess, sclerosing osteomyelitis of Garré, osteochondritis and stress fracture.[16] Bone scintigraphy will usually help localise a nidus but is relatively non-specific. Computerised tomography (CT), if applied in close 2 mm sections, will be successful in giving accurate locations of the nidus prior to surgical resection.[17]

The treatment of osteoid osteoma requires excision or ablation of the nidus. As the nidus is surrounded by dense reactive bone this can be difficult to achieve. The traditional approach requires wide exposure with radiological verification of the site. More recently the use of intra-operative scintigraphy has been described although this is rarely required.[18] Excisional biopsy of the nidus under CT control is now performed with success[19] whilst electrothermal coagulation has also been explored and reported as successful.[20]

Osteoblastoma

This is a similar lesion histologically to osteoid osteoma, but larger and not inducing so much reactive surrounding change. It is an extremely rare lesion affecting mainly the axial skeleton, although any bone may be affected. Patients are predominantly male in their second or third decades.[21]

The clinical presentation is of vague pain, less marked than osteoid osteoma, and not particularly relieved by salicylates. Occasionally there may be both swelling and joint dysfunction.

The radiological features classically show an expansile lesion, radiolucent with a thin shell of peripheral new bone.

Treatment consists of either curettage with or without bone grafting or local excision. Local excision gives good local control but reconstruction may be required. Recurrence rate may be as high as 20% following curettage, but the use of radiotherapy in extra-spinal cases is rarely required.[22]

MALIGNANT

Osteosarcoma

Osteosarcoma is the most common primary bone tumour and can occur at any age, although most cases occur in the first two decades of life.[23] Although commonly affecting the metaphyses around the knee, the humerus is the third most frequently affected bone, with tumours often arising at an earlier age than in the lower limb.[24]

Osteosarcomas are usually subtyped on the basis of their histological patterns into fibroblastic, chondroblastic, osteoblastic, telangiectatic or mixed.[25] Although the subtype was originally thought to have a bearing on prognosis, in carefully controlled studies now available this is not the case. Histological grading as a prognostic indication is also unreliable.[26]

Patients present usually with a short history of pain followed by swelling, joint dysfunction and occasionally pathological fracture. The many radiological advances which have occurred in the last decade have allowed very accurate staging of the disease. Plain x-rays remain the initial diagnostic tool but tend to underestimate the local extent of the tumour (Fig. 30.2a); CT scanning will give accurate visualisation of cortical destruction and soft tissue spread but may miss skip lesions in the same bone. It is a useful technique in planning biopsy and local excisions.[27] Now, the accepted staging investigation to assess the potential presence of pulmonary metastases is CT of the chest. Local staging of disease depends heavily on magnetic resonance imaging (MRI) scanning. This, particularly in T2 mode, will delineate accurately the intramedullary extent and soft tissue extent of the lesion. It will outline the relationship to the adjacent joints and to the blood vessels (Fig. 30.2b).

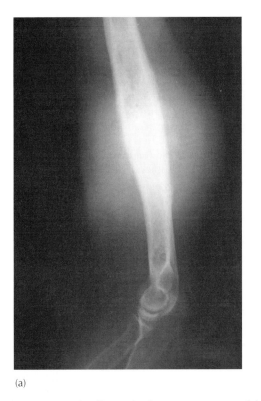
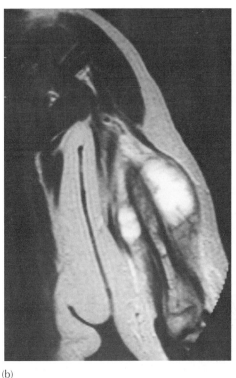

(a)   (b)

Fig. 30.2 (a) Lateral radiograph of an osteosarcoma of the humeral diaphysis. (b) Magnetic resonance imaging scan showing a large osteosarcoma of the humeral diaphysis with large soft tissue extension.

Preoperative scanning using technetium isotopes is useful in identifying skip lesions and metachronous lesions in other bones. The radioisotope scan may also on occasions demonstrate pulmonary metastases.[28]

Having performed the radiological staging procedures, it is necessary to establish the pathological diagnosis. At this stage a biopsy is performed. Many argue that an open biopsy is required, however, Stoker *et al.*[29] have shown the accuracy of Jamshidi needle biopsy cores obtained in a referral centre under local anaesthesia and image intensification.

Historically, the treatment of osteosarcoma has always been surgical ablation. In the upper limb this has led to either disarticulation of the shoulder for lesions in the distal humerus or forequarter amputation for more proximal growths. Survival, however, has been poor with 5-year survival rates varying between 11 and 25%.[30] Cade[31] reported an alternative method of preoperative radiation followed by surgical ablation only in those cases not developing pulmonary metastases. Fewer amputations were performed but the survival rate was unaltered. This has subsequently been confirmed by other series.[32]

By the early 1970s, it became evident that this appalling survival rate might be improved by the use of adjuvant chemotherapy. Many different protocols were produced, some claiming very high survival rates,[33] but controlled trials of therapies were not performed. In the UK, the Medical Research Council combined with the European Organisation for Research into Cancer Treatment (EORTC) to set up controlled trials of adjuvant chemotherapy. These have advanced to neoadjuvant chemotherapy which allows treatment of undetected micrometatases and causes necrosis of the tumour and may allow some shrinkage of the primary tumour. This latter effect may allow easier local resection and reconstruction of the limb. The initial trials compared the effect of adriamycin and cisplatin with or without high-dose methotrexate. The two-drug combination performed better, giving a survival of 65% at 5 years. This combination has also been compared with a Rosen T10 regime. The trial has assessed 400 cases but analysis is awaited. The present trial into which all osteosarcoma cases without metastases should be entered is an attempt at dose intensification using the rescue factor granulocyte cell stimulating factor. It aims to allow three courses of chemotherapy to be given in 6 rather than 9 weeks. The trial design is outlined in Table 30.2.

Surgery is now performed at the 6th week following commencement of chemotherapy which

Table 30.2 Biopsy proven osteosarcoma of long bones of an extremely untreated non-metastatic disease

age < 40 years
<4 weeks since biopsy

↓

Randomise

⤢

Regimen 1	**Regimen 2**
(chemotherapy **without** C-CSF)	(chemotherapy **with** G-CSF)
↓	↓
CDDP + DOX	**CDDP + DOX + G-CSF**
two cycles at 3-weekly intervals	three cycles at 2-weekly intervals
↓	↓
Surgery	Surgery
↓	↓
CDDP + DOX	**CDDP + DOX + G-CSF**
four cycles at 3-weekly intervals	three cycles at 2-weekly intervals

CDDP: cisplatin
DOX: doxorubicin
G-CSF: granulocyte colony stimulating factor

then continues in the postoperative period. In most cases, a 'wide excision' of the tumour is performed outside the tumour pseudocapsule with preservation of the neurovascular bundles, although often in tumours arising in the distal humerus the radial nerve may have to be sacrificed to allow adequate clearance. Following wide excisions, reconstruction is only possible using either customised endoprostheses or allografts.

Parosteal osteosarcoma

This is a low-grade malignant tumour developing on the external surface of large bones. The disease was first reported by Geschickter and Copeland in 1951.[34] It has a long natural history and tends to affect patients in the second and third decades of life. Most patients present with a long-standing swelling associated with dull ache. The elbow is only rarely affected.

Treatment consists of wide local resection of the tumour with appropriate reconstruction. It is generally accepted that in most cases chemotherapy is not indicated. Review of the tumour may show high-grade changes in the fibrous elements. These tumours have a poorer prognosis,[35] and chemotherapy may be indicated. Occasionally the low-grade component may transform or dedifferentiate to a

high-grade osteosarcoma.[36] Treatment is then as for an osteosarcoma.

Periosteal osteosarcoma

This is a very rare tumour, many still doubting its existence,[37] although it probably is a variant of parosteal osteosarcoma with a prominent cartilaginous component.[38] These are usually small unicortical lesions (Fig. 30.3). Treatment is by wide resection and appropriate reconstruction. Whether chemotherapy is required in their management is still unclear.

Cartilage-forming tumours

BENIGN

Osteochondroma

These cartilage-capped bony protrusions may develop in any bone derived from cartilage. They are usually discovered in childhood and many are found only as incidental findings on radiography.

They are usually painless but pain can be invoked by mechanical irritation or nerve compression.

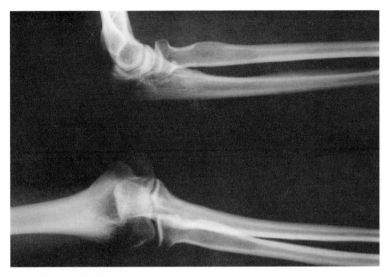

Fig. 30.3 Anteroposterior and lateral radiographs of periosteal osteosarcoma of the proximal ulna.

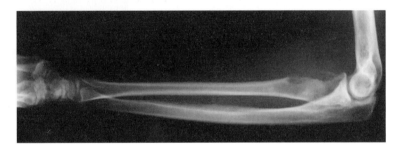

Fig. 30.4 Lateral radiograph of the proximal radius showing a chondroblastoma

Pseudoaneurysm has also been reported specifically in the popliteal region.[39]

If symptomatic, straightforward excision at the base is curative. If asymptomatic, they can be safely left. Growth will continue until skeletal maturity. If growth appears to occur after skeletal maturity then malignant transformation must be considered even if the radiographic appearances do not alter.

In diaphyseal aclasis the patient may also present with growth abnormality and subluxation at the radiohumeral joints. In this condition, removal of the lesions is rarely enough and the patients often require major reconstructions to correct the deformities.[40] The patient should be warned specifically of the possibility of malignant change associated with growth after maturity. Known lesions which cannot be palpated should be monitored by radiography. Unfortunately, bone isotope scanning cannot reliably differentiate benign from malignant cartilage lesions.[41]

Chondroblastoma

This is a rare bone tumour usually located in the epiphyseal plate. It is essentially benign. Jaffe and Lichtenstein[42] consider that it is a tumour developed from cartilaginous germ cells, although Higaki *et al.* considers the cell of origin to be histiocytic.[43] Typically, the patient is in the second decade and is more likely to be male. A long prodromal history is typical and there may be muscle wastage and joint restriction.[44] The most common site of affliction is the upper humeral epiphyseal plate, although they can be associated with any primary or secondary site of ossification.

Typically, the lesion is radiolucent crossing the growth plate – and intralesional calcification can be seen particularly with tomography[45] (Fig. 30.4). Computerised tomography may better illustrate the local invasive properties of the tumour. It is well-recognised that chondroblastoma may exhibit metastatic implantation in the pulmonary tissues. These 'areas' if resected have a 'benign' histological appearance and therefore represent implantation of vascularly transported tumour tissue rather than true metastases.

Treatment of the local lesion is by a combination of curettage and excision of any adjacent soft tissue extension. The recurrence rate is approximately 20% but this may be further reduced by use of cryotherapy.[46] The application of autologous bone graft will lessen the recurrence rate but conversely makes local recurrence more difficult to detect by radiography.

Chondromyxoid fibroma

This is a tumour which arises commonly in the upper tibia. It is most common in the second decade of life but may occur in any decade. There is often a long prodromal history, which may be as long as 2 years.[47] With the exception of the clavicle, any bone may be involved, but it is much more common in the lower limb.

The radiological features are of an eccentric lesion in the metaphyseal area of a long bone. It is well-defined but surrounding subperiosteal reaction may be slight.[48]

As with chondroblastoma, treatment consists of an initial curettage. The recurrence rate can be reduced if the operation is supplemented with autograft.[49]

MALIGNANT

Chondrosarcoma

Chondrosarcoma is divided into two basic subgroups: primary chondrosarcoma which arises in normal bone and secondary chondrosarcoma which arises in a pre-existing benign cartilage tumour, usually an enchondroma or cartilage cap of an exostosis. Primary lesions are twice as common.

Although chondrosarcomas may occur in the young, they predominate after the third decade of life. Both sexes are equally afflicted. Most patients complain of pain but it is well recognised that a presenting mass may be painless.[50] The anatomical distribution favours the axial skeleton, but 10% of tumours occur in the humerus.

Classically the radiological appearance is of a thick-walled radiolucency with irregularly blotchy areas of calcification. On the medullary surfaces the cortex is scalloped and cortical penetration occurs late in the disease. It is frequently difficult to discern radiographically the presence of a pre-existing benign tumour (Fig. 30.5).

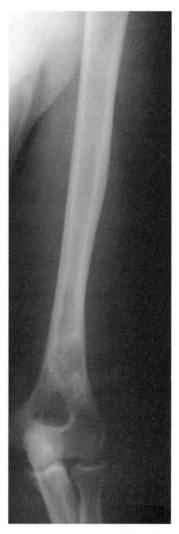

Fig. 30.5 Anteroposterior radiograph of chondrosarcoma of the distal humerus.

The only treatment effective in chondrosarcoma is surgery, the adequacy of which is important in determining the outcome.[51] The survival outcome is also influenced by the degree of malignancy and site. Patients with pelvic lesions do far worse than those with upper limb tumours.[50] Although most lesions require excision, preferably of a wide or radical nature, small corticated low-grade lesions in the elderly may be best served by curettage and adjuvant therapy consisting of cryosurgery, phenolization or 'cement' application.

Dedifferentiated chondrosarcoma

This rare tumour was first described by Dahlin and Beabout in 1971.[52] Additional mesenchymal elements are present as well as the chondrosarcoma. The humerus is the second commonest site. The radiological appearance may give a clue to the probability of this lesion, which may be represented by a purely lytic expansile area in an otherwise typical chondrosarcoma. The overall poor prognosis of patients with this tumour has led to attempts with the use of chemotherapy as a neo-adjuvant therapy in addition to surgery.

Mesenchymal chondrosarcoma

This is a further subtype of chondrosarcoma which rarely affects the upper limb. It is characterised by a highly cellular primitive spindle cell stroma with focal chondroid differentiation.[53] The tumour occurs most frequently in the second decade of life.

In terms of radiography, it is extremely difficult to differentiate the lesion, which may resemble an osteosarcoma, soft tissue extension being heavily calcified.

Treatment is as for dedifferentiated chondrosarcoma, consisting of chemotherapy and surgical resection. In Britain, the chemotherapy consists of the agents cisplatin, ifosfamide and adriamycin.

Clear cell chondrosarcoma

This is an extremely rare tumour which is rather slow-growing, patients often having symptoms for up to 3 years. The most common site is the upper femur but the upper limb may be affected.[54] The tumour appears as an osteolytic expansile lesion, usually at the proximal end of long bones. Treatment consists of complete surgical excision with reconstruction.

Tumours of histiocytic or fibrohistiocytic origin

BENIGN

Giant cell tumour

This is a locally aggressive but essentially benign bone tumour. It accounts for 5% of all primary bone tumours and afflicts the mature skeleton. There is a slight female predominance.[55] Although commonly affecting the knee, distal radius and proximal humerus, the elbow region may be affected (Fig. 30.6) and indeed patients with multiple sites have been recorded.[56] All patients suspected of presenting with a giant cell tumour should have hyperparathyroidism excluded by biochemical testing.

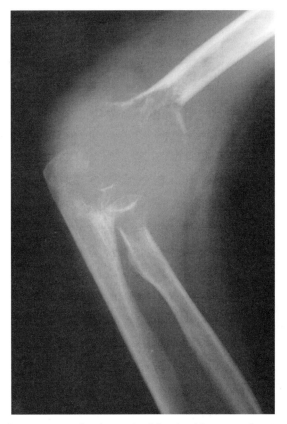

Fig. 30.6 Lateral radiograph of the distal humerus showing a giant cell tumour.

Early lesions present radiographically as expanding lytic lesions, eccentric to the long axis, often with fine trabeculae present. Most people consider that the tumour arises in the epiphysis (subarticular region) and extends to involve the metaphysis. Large lesions progress to cortical destruction and joint dysfunction.

On the basis of the radiological appearance, four subtypes have been proposed which redefine the previously proposed terms of latent, active and aggressive.[57] Unfortunately, grade 1 probably often represents benign fibrous histiocytoma and the other grades do not necessarily predict their clinical behaviour. The picture is further complicated by the histological pattern of the tumour. The osteoclasts which are present are now considered markers of the true tumour which is represented by the stromal background. This background can vary from being inconspicuous to frankly malignant[58] and thus can profoundly affect treatment intentions.

Another poorly understood phenomenon in these tumours is the likelihood of malignant transformation of a benign tumour either following multiple local recurrences or irradiation treatment.[59] It is important to establish whether there has been true malignant transformation of the giant cell tumour or sarcomatous induction by the radiotherapy when this modality of treatment has been used.

Primary *de novo* malignant giant cell tumour is a rare but well-recognised entity. Care is required, however, particularly in its differentiation from an osteoclast-rich osteosarcoma.[60] When diagnosed, their treatment is as for a malignant fibrous tumour.

Given the multiplicity of combinations of local extent and histological appearance, it is difficult to be adamant regarding therapy. It is well-recognised that curettage alone has a 20% or greater local recurrence rate.[61] Recent work by the European Musculoskeletal Oncology Society in a multicentre study suggests that this might be halved if adjuvant therapy (phenolization, cryotherapy or polymethylmethacrylate) is used in combination with intralesional techniques.

Curettage remains the mainstay of treatment; occasionally multiple attempts may be required. Reconstruction may not always be required after curettage and a number of patients have been treated by simple casting or cast-bracing until infilling of the cavity.[62] If articular failure has occurred by fracture or tumour invasion, then reconstruction with a prosthesis or allograft will be required.

Non-ossifying fibroma/benign fibrous histiocytoma

Non-ossifying fibroma is generally the term given to a lesion which is larger than a fibrous cortical defect. The term metaphyseal fibrous defect may be used for both. The lesions are extremely common between the ages of 4 and 8 years and can affect any metaphysis.[63] They are rarely seen in adults, which probably reflects the natural history of the condition. Large lesions may be associated with pathological fractures.[64]

The radiological features are characteristic consisting of an eccentric lesion which may involve the cortex situated at the end of the diaphysis. A sclerotic rim is usually seen on the medullary border. Although the lesion does not usually require biopsy, unusual clinical or radiological features may justify the need for needle biopsy.

Treatment in the majority of cases is only observation. Enlargement or pathological fracture will demand curettage or block excision with or without bone grafting. Fractures occasionally lead to obliteration of the lesion.[65]

Benign fibrous histiocytoma may have a similar histological picture to a non-ossifying fibroma. However, they tend to occur in older patients and are situated away from the metaphysis. Treatment requires either curettage or block excision.

MALIGNANT

Malignant fibrous histiocytoma

This is a rare tumour which tends to affect the diaphysis of the appendicular skeleton. It is a tumour which must be differentiated from the dedifferentiated chondrosarcoma, fibroblastic osteosarcoma and fibrosarcoma. In all, 70% of tumours arise *de novo*, the remaining 30% arising in bones afflicted by infarction, irradiation, Paget's disease and fibrous dysplasia.[66]

The tumour tends to occur in middle age but has a wide age distribution. Men are more commonly afflicted than women. Secondary tumours occur later in life then *de novo* tumours. The clinical findings are similar to other malignant bone tumours, but unlike osteosarcoma it does not particularly afflict the knee region.

The radiological features are usually an area of poorly delineated osteolysis without other features of characterisation (Fig. 30.7). Pathological fracture is a common occurrence. Where the lesion arises secondarily to a pre-existing condition then the pre-existing pathology may be visible. Endosteal scalloping, periosteal reaction or a soft tissue mass are indicative of malignant transformation.[67]

Treatment of malignant fibrous histiocytoma is now very much along the lines as that for osteosarcoma. The fact that this lesion will respond to chemotherapy has been noted for some time,[68] although since the patients are older, (the mean age being around 40 years) this mode of therapy is less well-tolerated. Following neoadjuvant chemotherapy, surgical treatment is by wide excision which around the elbow consists of prosthetic replacement of the distal humerus and proximal ulna.

The overall survival of patients with the disease is approximately 65% at 5 years. Many, particularly the lower grade lesions, may have a significantly better prognosis.

EWING'S SARCOMA

Ewing's sarcoma is the eponym given to a malignant round cell tumour which arises in bone. It is now considered that this tumour represents one end of a spectrum which includes primitive neuroectodermal tumours (PNET), Askin's tumour and neuroblastoma. The tumour is typified by glycogen staining of cytoplasmic granules. It does not usually show any neural markers but may exhibit a t11–22 translocation on chromosomal analysis.

In the UK the incidence is around one case per million per year. It is reported to be rare in both Negroes and the Chinese. Patients may be any age

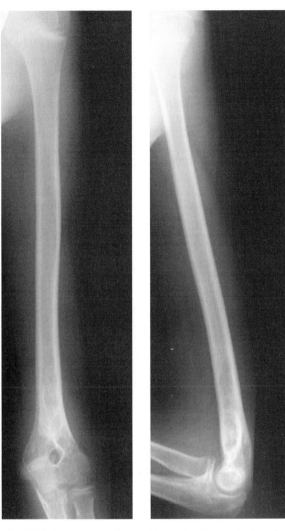

Fig. 30.7 Anteroposterior and lateral radiograph of malignant fibrous histiocytoma of the distal humerus.

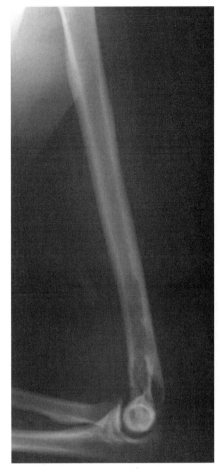

Fig. 30.8 Ewing's sarcoma of the distal humerus (lateral view).

but 80% of cases occur before the age of 20. They present with pain and swelling of any bone which may be accompanied by mild pyrexia and malaise. About 8% of cases arise primarily in the humerus. It is predominantly a diaphyseal or diametaphyseal lesion.

The classical description of the radiological appearance is a moth-eaten medullary bone with periosteal lamination of new bone. Repeated events of lamination will lead to the classical so-called onion skin appearance. This appearance is rare and is not pathognomic.[69] More frequently, a patchy lysis and sclerosis is noted (Fig. 30.8). Staging investigations are particularly important in this condition as with their increasing use and sophistication a greater percentage of patients are

found to have either multifocal bone disease of pulmonary metastases. These findings have a negative effect upon overall survival.

Biopsy material requires extremely careful evaluation and scrutiny. Immunohistochemical techniques will be required to differentiate the lesion from PNET, neuroblastoma, small-cell osteosarcoma, lymphoma of bone and embryonal rhabdomyosarcoma. Having established a diagnosis, the optimal mode of treatment is still unclear. Chemotherapy certainly has a role to play and its usage has increased with overall 5-year survival varying from 20% to 50%.[70] The difficulty remains in that there are a number of variables which are recognised to affect survival rates. Among these are age and sex of the patient, site of the lesion and its measurable volume.[71] Advances in treatment will continue to evolve by use of carefully designed and evaluated controlled trials.

Although the overall role of chemotherapy is not in doubt, the management of the local primary lesion is still in dispute. The traditional local therapy is radiation but the local recurrence rate with this mode of treatment is probably around 30%. Surgery can do better but the results are liable to bias with this method being chosen in smaller more distally-situated lesions. Previous irradiation may also lead to the induction of postirradiation sarcomata.

Simple bone cyst (unicameral bone cyst)

These fluid-filled cysts often arise in the metaphyseal region of long bones juxtaposed to the epiphyseal plate. They are usually brought to the patient's attention either by an incidental x-ray or following a pathological fracture. Fracture may lead to resolution of the cyst, but it is also well-recognised that a traumatic episode may turn a cystic lesion into an aneurysmal bone cyst.[72]

Cysts are commonly found in the proximal humerus and femur but may also occur in both the radius and ulna. They are commonly seen in childhood and adolescence, 90% of cases being younger than 20 years old. When they do occur in the adult, they tend to occur in either the ilium or os calcis.

Plain x-rays usually show a lesion which has a central medullary location. Its length is usually greater than its width. The transverse diameter of the cyst closest to the epiphysis is recognised as being as wide as the epiphysis. With age, the cyst grows towards the diaphysis. This appearance is contrary to an aneurysmal bone cyst, which shows a centrifugal growth pattern. Where the cyst reacts with cancellous bone there is a bony reaction but periosteal reaction is extremely rare. There is no soft tissue component. Further radiological investigation is rarely performed, although it is possible to recognise fluid levels on CT scanning. Treatment can be difficult. Small cysts which are asymptomatic do not require any therapy. However, large cysts may require curettage, bone grafting, en bloc resection or even nailing. It is now fairly universally accepted that these cysts will respond to an injection of methylprednisolone.[73] If surgery is contemplated, incomplete removal of the cyst lining usually leads to local recurrence. The recurrence rate is much higher in children.[74]

Aneurysmal bone cyst

These blood-filled expansile lesions present with pain and swelling and may follow a fracture. It is well recognised that during pregnancy aneurysmal bone cysts may rapidly enlarge.

This is predominantly a disease of the first three decades of life and occurs equally in both sexes. It can affect any bone and 8% are recorded as occurring in the upper limb.

The radiological features are of a purely lytic expansile lesion which usually arises in the metaphysis. Extension may occur into the epiphysis when the growth plate has closed.[75] They may grow alarmingly and may mimic malignant tumours (Fig. 30.9). If further radiological investigation is required, the

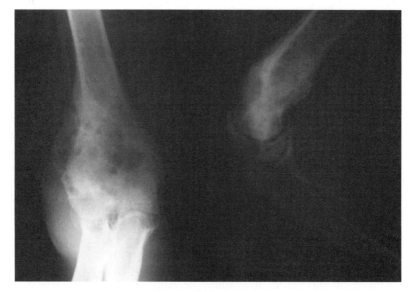

Fig. 30.9 Aneurysmal bone cyst of the distal humerus (anteroposterior view).

multiple fluid levels seen on CT are practically diagnostic of an aneurysmal bone cyst.

The mainstay of treatment is a combination of curettage and bone grafting. Where the tumour arises in inaccessible sites or where excessive blood loss is feared, arterial embolisation may be a helpful adjunct to treatment. In tumours that recur or remain inaccessible, small doses of radiation can be given.[76]

Miscellaneous tumours of soft tissue

MYOSITIS OSSIFICANS

This condition is particularly troublesome when it occurs around the elbow joint. Although it can occur following a single injury, it more usually follows chronic repetitive trauma. The most usual presentation is of a painless mass although some patients may have considerable soft tissue inflammation and pain. The period of symptoms is usually short.

The radiographic features show no abnormality in the first 2–3 weeks and then speckled calcification becomes evident. A fully mature lesion can usually be seen at around 14 weeks. In general, the diagnosis should be made on clinical and radiological grounds as great care is required in the examination of a biopsy. Unfortunately, myositis ossificans can be easily mistaken for osteogenic sarcoma.[77]

Treatment is usually by surgical excision, but this should not be performed until the lesions have matured. Surgical intervention prior to maturity leads to a high rate of local recurrence.

Surgical options

Patients presenting with localised high-grade malignancy around the elbow joint are fortunately very rare. However, in many presenting late with widespread soft tissue spread, the only oncologically correct procedure is disarticulation at the shoulder or forequarter amputation.

Where the disease is contained within the bone (Enneking stage 11A)[78] or is contained beneath the expanded periosteum (stage 11B) and gives clinical and radiographic indication of responding to chemotherapy, then a wide local excision of the lesion may be justified. Where the lesion is of low-grade malignancy (stage 1A or 1B) this type of conservative approach will lead to good local control.[79]

In benign disease such a radical approach is rarely justified unless other methods aimed at maintaining joint integrity have failed.

Following wide excision of the elbow joint, reconstruction can be achieved by a number of different approaches. None is ideal and some are inapplicable if an extra-articular resection of the joint has been performed. Enneking[80] has reported a method of arthodesis which may be difficult to achieve. In smaller resections hemiarthroplasty of the distal humeral or proximal ulna may be appropriate.[81–85] In the USA, Mankin has popularised the use of cadaveric allografts and although function in the upper limb is better than in the lower limb, there are still problems of sizing, stability, fracture, rejection and degeneration.[86,87]

In Europe, America and Japan, prosthetic reconstructions replacing the total elbow have been developed.[88,89] The results in 26 patients have been reported.[79] This shows a local recurrence rate and a loosening rate of 11.5% but no prosthetic failures.

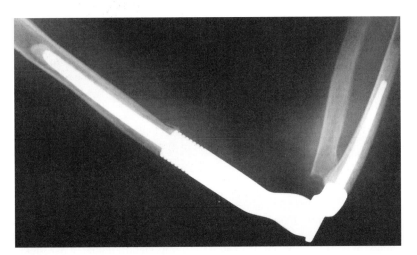

Fig. 30.10 Current design of flexi-elbow prosthesis of the distal humerus and elbow joint.

Since the publication of this paper two important developments have led to a reduction in this complication rate. Firstly, better staging procedures, particularly MRI, have led to more accurate visualisation of the tumours and, therefore, better selection for limb salvage surgery. Secondly, the rate of aseptic loosening has been reduced by the development of a 'flexi-elbow' design instead of the earlier constrained axled type (Fig. 30.10).

The results of customised elbow replacements in malignant disease has recently been reviewed by Lambert *et al.*[90] When assessed by a Mankin functional grading system, 80% of patients were good or excellent. Only one patient reviewed had instability of his prosthetic hinged mechanism. If a second score – the Mayo elbow performance index – is used, the average gain in function is 16.25 points, which is largely due to pain relief achieved by the operation. Radiological evaluation remains good.

References

1. Cooper A Exostosis. In: *Surgical essays* (3rd edn). Cooper A, Travers B (eds) London: Cox & Son, 1818: 169–226.
2. Huvos AG (ed) *Bone tumours* (2nd edn). Philadelphia: WB Saunders Co, 1991: 255.
3. Solomon L Bone growth in diaphyseal aclasis. *J Bone Joint Surg* 1961; **43B:** 700–16.
4. Ollier M Dyschondroplasie. *Lyon Med* 1900; **93:** 23–25.
5. Maffuci A Di un caso di enchondroma ed angiome multiplo. *Mov Med Chir* 1881; **13:** 399–412.
6. Elmore SM, Cantrell WC Maffucci's syndrome – case report with a normal karyotype. *J Bone Joint Surg* 1966; **48A:** 1607–13.
7. Nelaton E D'une nouvelle espèce de tumeurs benignes des os, ou tumeurs a myeloplaxes. Paris: Adrien Delahayle, 1860.
8. Paget J *Lectures in surgical pathology.* Philadelphia: Lindsay & Blackiston, 1854.
9. Ewing J Diffuse endothelioma of bone. *Proc NY Path Soc* 1921; **21:** 17–24.
10. Ewing J A review and classification of bone sarcomas. *Arch Surg* 1922; **4:** 483–533.
11. Lucke A *Beitrage zur Geschwulstlehre Virehars Arch (Patholog Anat)* 1866; **35:** 524–39.
12. Saville PD A medical option for the treatment of osteoid osteoma. *Arthritis Rheum* 1980; **23:** 1409–11.
13. Leonessa C, Savoni E Osteoma osteoide para articulare del gomito. *Chir Organic Mov* 1971; **59:** 487–92.
14. Marcove RC, Freiberger RH Osteoid osteoma of the elbow – a diagnostic problem. *J Bone Joint Surg* 1966; **48A:** 1185–90.
15. Shifrin LZ, Reynolds WA Intra-articular osteoid osteoma of the elbow. *Clin Orthop* 1971; **81:** 126–9.
16. Sim FH, Dahlin DC, Beabout JW Osteoid osteoma – diagnostic problems. *J Bone Joint Surg* 1975; **57A:** 154–9.
17. Gamba JL, Martinez S, Apple J *et al.* Computed tomography of axial skeletal osteoid osteomas. *Am J Roentgenol* 1984; **142:** 769–72.
18. Szypryt EP, Hardy JG, Colton CL An improved technique of intra-operative bone scanning. *J Bone Joint Surg* 1986; **68B:** 643–6.
19. Johnson S, Cannon SR Excision biopsy of osteoid osteoma under CT control. (in preparation).
20. Taminiau A, Berg JC de, Oberman WR Percutaneous computer tomography-guided thermocoagulation for osteoid osteomas. *Trans Int Soc Limb Salvage* 1977: 159.
21. Lepage J, Rigault P, Nezelof C *et al.* Benign osteoblastoma in children. *Rev Clin Orthop* 1984; **70:** 117–27.
22. Camepa G, Defabiani F Osteoblastoma Del radio. *Minerva Ortop* 1965; **16:** 645–8.
23. Williams G, Barrett G, Pratt C Osteosarcoma in two very young children. *Clin Paediat* 1977; **16:** 548–51.
24. Price CHG Primary bone-forming tumours and their relationship to skeletal growth. *J Bone Joint Surg* 1958; **40B:** 574–93.
25. Simmons CC Bone sarcoma: Factors influencing prognosis. *Surg Gynecol Obstet* 1939; **68:** 67–75.
26. Mankin HJ, Connor JF, Schiller AC *et al.* Grading of bone tumours by analysis of nucleus DNA content using flow cytometry. *J Bone Joint Surg* 1985; **67A:** 404–13.
27. Coffre E, Vanel D, Contesso G *et al.* Problems and pitfalls in the use of computed tomography for the local evaluation of long bone osteosarcoma. *Skeletal Radiol* 1985; **13:** 147–153.
28. Flowers JM Jr 99m Tc-polyphosphate up-take within pulmonary and soft tissue metastases from osteosarcoma. *Radiology* 1974; **112:** 377–8.
29. Stoker DJ, Cobb JP, Pringle JAS Needle biopsy of musculoskeletal lesions. *J Bone Joint Surg* 1991; **73B:** 498–500.
30. Sweetnam DR, Knowelden J, Seddon H Bone sarcoma – treatment by irradiation, amputation and a combination of the two. *Brit Med J* 1971; **2:** 363–7.
31. Cade S Sarcoma of bone. *Ann Roy Col Surg Eng* 1951; **9:** 211–23.
32. Beck JC, Wara WM, Bovill EG Jr, Philips TL The role of radiation therapy in the treatment of osteosarcoma. *Radiology* 1976; **120:** 163–5.
33. Rosen G, Tan C, Exelby P Vincristine, high-dose methotrexate with citrovarum factor rescue, cyclophosphamide and adriamycin cyclic therapy following surgery in childhood osteogenic sarcoma. *Proc Am Assoc Cancer Res* 1974; **15:** 172.
34. Geschickter CF, Copeland MM Parosteal osteosarcoma of bone: A new entity. *Ann Surg* 1951; **133:** 790–807.
35. Campanacci M, Picci P, Gherlinzoni F *et al.* Parosteal osteosarcoma. *J Bone Joint Surg* 1984; **66B:** 313–21.
36. Wold LE, Unni KK, Beabout JW, Sim FM, Dahlin DC Dedifferentiated parosteal osteosarcoma. *J Bone Joint Surg* 1984; **66A:** 53–9.

37. Hall FM Periosteal sarcoma. *Radiology* 1978; **129:** 835–6.
38. Campanacci M, Giunti A Periosteal osteosarcoma – review of 41 cases. *Ital J Orthop Trauma* 1976; **2:** 23–35.
39. Tomsu M, Procek J, Wagner K *et al.* Vascular complications in osteochondromatosis. *Rozhl Chir* 1977; **56:** 696–9.
40. Fogel G, McElfresh EC, Peterson HA, Wicklund PT Management of deformities of the forearm in multiple heredity osteochondromas. *J Bone Joint Surg* 1984; **66A:** 670–80.
41. Hudson TM, Chew FS, Manaster BJ Scintigraphy of benign exostoses and exostotic chondrosarcomas. *Am J Rad* 1983; **140:** 581–6.
42. Jaffe HL, Lichtenstein C Benign chondroblastoma of bone. *Am J Path* 1942; **18:** 969–83.
43. Higaki S, Takeyama S, Tateishi A Clinicol pathological study of twenty-two cases of benign chondroblastoma. *Nippon Seikeigeha Gahhai Zasshi* 1981; **55:** 647–64.
44. Bloem JL, Mulder JD Chondroblastoma: A clinical and radiological study of 104 cases. *Am J Surg Path* 1984; **8:** 223–30.
45. Hudson TM, Hawkins IF Jr Radiological evaluation of chondroblastoma. *Radiology* 1981; **139:** 1–10.
46. Huvos AG, Marcove RC Chondroblastoma of bone – a critical review. *Clin Orthop* 1973; **95:** 300–12.
47. Rahimi A, Beabout JW, Ivins JC, Dahlini DC Chondromyxoid fibroma – a clinical pathological study of 76 cases. *Cancer* 1972; **30:** 726–36.
48. Schajowicz F Chondromyxoid fibroma – a report of three cases with predominant cortical involvement. *Radiology* 1987; **164:** 783–6.
49. Gerlinzoni F, Rock M, Picci P Chondromyxoid fibroma. *J Bone Joint Surg* 1983; **65A:** 198–204.
50. Marcove RC, Mike V, Hutter RVP *et al.* Chondrosarcoma of the pelvis and upper end of the femur. *J Bone Joint Surg* 1972; **54A:** 561–72.
51. Kaufman JH, Douglass HO Jr, Blake W *et al.* The importance of initial presentation and treatment upon the survival of patients with chondrosarcoma. *Surg Gynaecol Obstet* 1977; **145:** 357–63.
52. Dahlin DC, Beabout JW Dedifferentation of low-grade chondrosarcoma. *Cancer* 1971; **28:** 461–6.
53. Lichtenstein L, Bernstein D Unusual benign and malignant chondroid tumours of bone. *Cancer* 1959; **12:** 1142–57.
54. Bjornsson J, Unni KK, Dahlin DC *et al.* Clear cell chondrosarcoma of bone – observations in 47 cases. *Am J Surg Path* 1984; **8:** 223–30.
55. Hutter RVP, Worcester JN Jr, Francis KC *et al.* Benign and malignant giant cell tumours of bone. *Cancer* 1962; **15:** 653–90.
56. Singson R, Feldman F Case report 229: Diagnosis of multiple (multicentric) giant cell tumours of bone. *Skeletal Radiol* 1983; **9:** 276–81.
57. Campanacci M, Baldini N, Boriani S, Sudanese A Giant cell tumour of bone. *J Bone Joint Surg* 1987; **69A:** 106–14.
58. Hadders H.N Some remarks on the histology of bone tumours. *Year Book Cancer Res Amsterdam* 1973; **22:** 7–10.
59. Tudway RC Giant cell tumour of bone. *Brit J Radiol* 1959; **32:** 315–21.
60. Nascimento AG, Huvos AG, Marcove RC Primary malignant giant cell tumour of bone. *Cancer* 1979; **44:** 1393–402.
61. Johnson EW Jr Adjacent and distal spread of giant cell tumours. *Am J Surg* 1965; **109:** 163–6.
62. Kemp HBS, Cannon SR, Briggs TWR *et al.* Shark-bite: A conservative method for the treatment of cysts, bengin tumours, and selected malignant tumours of bone. *J Bone Joint Surg* 1996; **78B:**(Supp 1): 58.
63. Caffey J On fibrous defects in cortical walls of frowing tubular bones. *Adv Pediatr* 1955; **7:** 13–51.
64. Arata MA, Peterson HA, Dahlin DC Pathological fractures through non-ossifying fibromas. *J Bone Joint Surg* 1981; **63A:** 980–8.
65. Cunningham JB, Ackerman LV Metaphyseal fibrous defects. *J Bone Joint Surg* 1956; **38A:** 797–808.
66. Huvos AG, Heilwell M, Bretsky SS The pathology of malignant fibrous histiocytoma of bone. *Am J Path* 1985; **9:** 853–71.
67. Taconis WK, Mulder JD Fibrosarcoma and malignant fibrous histiocytoma of long bones: Radiographic features and grading. *Skeletal Radiol* 1984; **11:** 237–45.
68. Bacci G, Springfield D, Capanna P *et al.* Adjuvant chemotherapy for malignant fibrous histiocytoma of the femur and tibia. *J Bone Joint Surg* 1985; **67A:** 620–5.
69. Feldman F Round cell lesions of bone. In: *Diagnostic radiology.* St Louis: CV Mosby, 1977: 437–54.
70. Rosen G The current management of malignant bone tumours. *Med J Austral* 1988; **148:** 373–8.
71. Gobel V, Jurghens H, Etspuler G *et al.* Prognostic significance of tumour volume in localised Ewing's sarcoma of bone in children and adolescents. *J Cancer Res Clin Oncol* 1987; **113:** 187–91.
72. Johnston CE, Fletcher RR Traumatic transformation of unicameral bone cyst into aneurysmal bone cyst. *Orthopedics* 1986; **9:** 1441–77.
73. Campanacci M, Capanna R, Picci P Unicameral and aneurysmal bone cysts. *Clin Orthop* 1986; **204:** 35–6.
74. Norman A, Schiffman M Simple bone cysts: Factors of age dependency. *Radiology* 1977; **124:** 779–82.
75. Dyer R, Stelling CB, Fechner RE Epiphyseal extension of an aneurysmal bone cyst. *Am J Rad* 1981; **137:** 153–68.
76. Biesecker JL, Marcove RC, Huvos AG, Mike V Aneurysmal bone cysts. A clinicopathologic study of 66 cases. *Cancer* 1970; **26:** 615–25.
77. Ackerman L, Ramamurthy S, Jablokow V *et al.* Case report 488: Post-traumatic myositis ossificans mimicking a soft tissue neoplasm. *Skeletal Radiol* 1988; **17:** 310–4.
78. Enneking WF, Spanier SS, Goodman MA A system for the surgical staging of musculoskeletal sarcoma. *Clin Orthop* 1980; **153:** 106–20.
79. Ross AC, Sneath RS, Scales JT Endoprosthetic replacement of the humerus and elbow joint. *J Bone Joint Surg* 1987; **69B:** 652–5.
80. Enneking WF *Musculoskeletal tumour surgery.* New York: Churchill Livingstone, 1983.

81. Mellen RH, Phalen GS Arthroplasty of the elbow by replacement of the distal portion of the humerus with an acrylic prosthesis. *J Bone Joint Surg* 1947; **29:** 348–53.

82. Barr JS, Eaton RG Elbow reconstruction with a new prosthesis to replace the distal end of the humerus: A case report. *J Bone Joint Surg* 1965; **47A:** 1408–13.

83. Kestler OC Replacement of the distal humerus for reconstruction of the elbow joint: Report of two cases with long follow-up. *Bull Hosp Joint Dis* 1970; **31:**85–90.

84. Dunn AW A distal humeral prosthesis. *Clin Orthop* 1971; **77:** 199–202.

85. Johnson EW Jr, Schlein AP Vitallium prosthesis for the olecranon and proximal part of the ulna: Case report with thirteen year follow-up. *J Bone Joint Surg* 1970; **52A:** 721–4.

86. Mankin HJ, Dopperts S, Tomford W Clinical experience with allograft implantation: The first ten years. *Clin Orthop* 1983; **174:** 69–86.

87. Urbaniak JR, Black KE Jr Cadaveric elbow allografts: A six year experience. *Clin Orthop* 1985; **197:** 131–40.

88. Scales JlT, Lettin AWF, Bayley I The evolution of the Stanmore hinged total elbow replacement 1967–1976. In: *Joint replacement in the upper limb*. Conference held by the Institution of Mechanical Engineers and the BOA. London: Mechanical Engineers Publications Ltd for the Institution of Mechanical Engineers: 1977: 53–62.

89. Yoshimoto S, Kaneso H, Tatematsu M Total prosthetic replacement of the humerus for chronic osteomyelitis with a pathological fracture: Report of case. *J Bone Joint Surg* 1977; **59B:** 360–2.

90. Lambert S, Davis J, Cannon S Endoprosthetic reconstruction for tumours of the elbow region. *Trans Int Soc Limb Salvage* 1995: 96.

Index